Medical Terminology

An Illustrated Guide

THIRD EDITION

Barbara Janson Cohen, MS

Assistant Professor
Delaware County Community College
Media, Pennsylvania

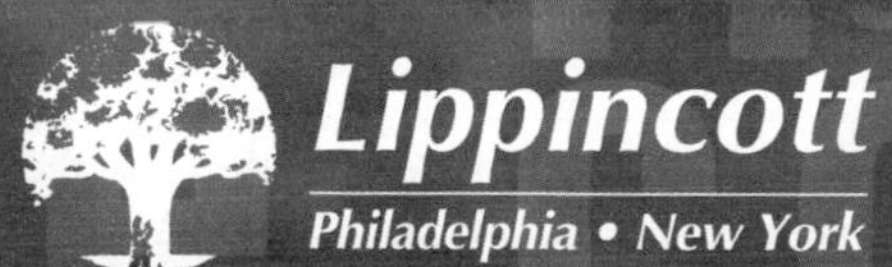

Executive Editor: Margaret Biblis
Assistant Editor: Patricia Moore
Associate Managing Editor: Barbara Ryalls
Senior Production Manager: Helen Ewan
Production Coordinator: Sharon McCarthy
Designer: Doug Smock
Cover Designer: Matt Suhanec
Indexer: Alexandra Nickerson

Edition 3

9 8 7 6 5 4 3 2 1

Library of Congress Cataloging in Publications Data

Cohen, Barbara J.
Medical terminology : an illustrated guide / Barbara Janson Cohen. — 3rd ed.
p. cm.
Includes bibliographical references and index.
ISBN (invalid) 0-07-817144-7 (alk. paper)
1. Medicine—Terminology. I. Title.
[DNLM: 1. Nomenclature. W 15 C678m 1998]
R123.C56 1998
610′.1′4—dc21
DNLM/DLC
for Library of Congress 97-4344
CIP

Care has been taken to confirm the accuracy of the information presented and to describe generally accepted practices. However, the authors, editors, and publisher are not responsible for errors or omissions or for any consequences from application of the information in this book and make no warranty, express or implied, with respect to the contents of the publication.

The authors, editors and publisher have exerted every effort to ensure that drug selection and dosage set forth in this text are in accordance with current recommendations and practice at the time of publication. However, in view of ongoing research, changes in government regulations, and the constant flow of information relating to drug therapy and drug reactions, the reader is urged to check the package insert for each drug for any change in indications and dosage and for added warnings and precautions. This is particularly important when the recommended agent is a new or infrequently employed drug.

Some drugs and medical devices presented in this publication have Food and Drug Administration (FDA) clearance for limited use in restricted research settings. It is the responsibility of the health care provider to ascertain the FDA status of each drug or device planned for use in their clinical practice.

Preface

Medical Terminology: An Illustrated Guide is an introduction to the study of medical language. It can be used as part of classroom instruction, for independent study, or for distance learning. Through word analysis and labeling exercises the student learns the anatomic and clinical terms pertaining to each body system. At all times the student participates in the learning experience, answering questions on new material, checking responses with nearby answer keys, and verifying progress with chapter reviews.

Many learning aids are provided. Each chapter opens with a chapter outline and a set of student objectives to guide and measure learning. Word parts used in medical terms are introduced early in each chapter. Overviews summarize both normal and clinical subjects. All key terms are clearly defined, and roots have been included with these definitions when possible. Crossword puzzles now appear with each chapter on the body systems. Flashcards are also provided.

The glossary has complementary lists of word parts and their meanings to help with exercises. Each of these is referenced to the page on which the word part first appears. There is also a comprehensive list of abbreviations with chapter references.

This book places great emphasis on pronunciation. It is important for the students to practice saying the terms that are learned and to be able to recognize them when heard. Therefore, every opportunity is taken to include phonetic pronunciations in the text. Audio tapes to aid in pronunciation are also available to instructors and may be copied for students. In addition to a brief overview and definitions, they give practice with pronunciation for Chapters 4 to 21.

New for instructors with this edition is a set of color transparencies of both normal and clinical illustrations taken from the text. Also availabe now is a test bank in both computerized and printed form. This includes a variety of questions that can be sorted according to chapter, question style, subject (normal or clinical), chapter objective, and page. The Instructor's Manual has also been revised and expanded.

Acknowledgments

In addition to everyone who helped with the first two editions of *Medical Terminology: An Illustrated Guide*, I wish to thank the following people, who assisted with this third edition.

At Lippincott-Raven Publishers: Andrew Allen helped in planning major revisions of the text. Patty Moore assisted in every part of manuscript preparation, including artwork and case studies. Doris Wray coordinated production of all ancillary materials. Many others on the staff contributed their expertise as well.

Several reviewers were kind enough to evaluate portions of the manuscript. Linda Fulton, Marie Janes, and Mary Ann Woods reviewed the second edition text. Marie Janes, Sara Wellman, and Mary Ann Woods reviewed sample revised manuscript chapters. Elizabeth Christoff, Sue Hunt and Nancy Thomas reviewed Chapters 1 through 8 of the final manuscript. Beverly Baker, Toni Cade, Betty Jones, and Midge Ray reviewed Chapters 9 through 15 of the final manuscript. Rebecca Hageman, Diane Herschfelt, and Sandra Liming reviewed Chapters 16 through 21 of the final manuscript.

To the many friends, relatives, and relative strangers who contributed their personal case studies, I wish to express my gratitude. All of these appear anonymously to illustrate subjects in the text. Thanks also to the Hoffman family and the LaVan family, friends and advisors whenever I need to call on them.

Finally, and at last, I dedicate this book with unending thanks to Matthew, who shares in every aspect of my life.

Contents

Expanded Contents

Part 1

Introduction to Medical Terminology

Chapters 1 to 8 present the basics of medical terminology. Work through these chapters in order before proceeding to chapters on the body systems in Part II.

1 Concepts of Medical Terminology

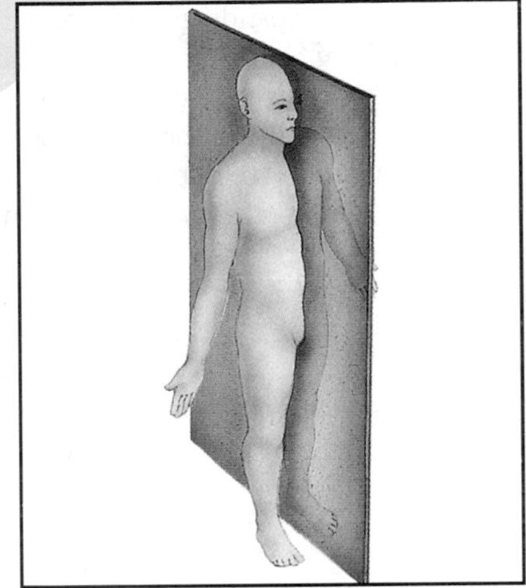

Chapter Contents

Word Parts
Combining Vowels
Word Derivations
Study Aids
Pronunciation
Abbreviations
Words Ending in *x*
Suffixes Beginning With *rh*
Medical Terminology: An Illustrated Guide

Objectives

After study to this chapter you should be able to:

1. Explain the purpose of medical terminology
2. Define the terms *root, suffix,* and *prefix*
3. Explain how combining vowels are used in forming medical words
4. Name the languages from which most medical word parts are derived
5. Pronounce words according to the pronunciation guide used in this text

Medical terminology is a special vocabulary used by health care professionals. It is needed, not to bewilder the uninformed, but to aid in communication. Think how difficult it is to get by in a foreign country when you don't know the language or to use an unfamiliar computer program. Because it is based mainly on Greek and Latin words, medical terminology is consistent and uniform throughout the world. It is also efficient; although some of the terms are long, they often reduce an entire phrase to a single word. The one word *acrodermatitis*, for example, conveys "inflammation of the skin of the hands and feet."

Undeniably, the medical vocabulary is vast. Moreover, like the jargon in all forward-moving fields, it is ever expanding. Think of the words that have been added to our vocabulary with the development of computers—software, hard drives, megabyte, and internet, for example. There are methods, however, that can aid in learning and remembering words and even help in making informed guesses as to the meaning of unfamiliar words. Most medical terms can be divided into component parts—roots, prefixes, and suffixes—that maintain the same meaning whenever they appear. By learning these meanings, you can analyze and remember many words.

Word Parts

The fundamental unit of each medical word is the **root**. This establishes the basic meaning of the word and is the part to which modifying prefixes and suffixes are added.

A **suffix** is a short word part or series of parts added at the end of a root to modify its meaning. In this book suffixes are indicated by a dash before the suffix, such as *-sis*.

A **prefix** is a short word part added before a root to modify its meaning. In this book prefixes are indicated by a dash after the prefix, such as *pre-*.

The simple word *write* can be used as a root to illustrate. If we add the suffix *-er* to form *writer*, we have "one who writes." If we add the prefix *re-* to form *rewrite*, we have "to write again."

Not all roots are complete words. In fact, most medical roots are derived from other languages and are meant to be used in combinations. The Greek word kardia, for example, meaning "heart," gives us the root *cardi*. The Latin word *pulmo*, meaning "lung," gives us the root *pulm*. In a few instances, both the Greek and Latin roots are used. We find both the Greek root *nephr* and the Latin root *ren* used in words pertaining to the kidney.

Conversely, the same root may have different meanings in different fields of study. The root *myel* means "marrow" and may apply to either the bone marrow or the spinal cord. The root *scler* means "hard," but may also apply to the white of the eye. *Cyst* means "a filled sac or pouch," but also refers specifically to the urinary bladder. You will sometimes have to consider the context of a word before assigning its meaning.

Compound words contain more than one root. The words *eyeball, bedpan, frostbite*, or *wheelchair* are examples. Some compound medical words are *cardiovascular* (pertaining to the heart and blood vessels), *gastrointestinal* (pertaining to the stomach and intestines), and *lymphocyte* (a white blood cell found in the lymphatic system).

Combining Vowels

When a suffix beginning with a consonant is added to a root, a vowel (usually an o) is inserted to aid in pronunciation. Thus, when the suffix *-logy* meaning "study of" is added to the root *neur* meaning "nerve or nervous system," a combining vowel is added.

---

neur + o + logy = neurology (study of the nervous system)

In this text, the combining vowel is always included with the root and is separated from it by a slash, as *neur/o*. In this format, the root is often referred to as a **combining form**.

A combining vowel is not used if the ending begins with a vowel. The root *neur* is combined with the suffix *-itis*, meaning "inflammation of" in this way:

neur + itis = neuritis (inflammation of a nerve)

There are some exceptions to this rule, particularly when pronunciation or meaning is affected, but you will observe these as you work.

Word Derivations

As mentioned, most medical word parts come from Greek (G) and Latin (L). The original words and their meanings are included in this text only in a few cases. They are interesting, however, and may aid in learning. For example, *muscle* comes from a Latin word that means "mouse" because the movement of a muscle under the skin was thought to resemble the scampering of a mouse. The coccyx, the tail end of the spine, is named for the cuckoo, because it was thought to resemble the cuckoo's bill. If you are interested in the derivations of medical words, a good medical dictionary will provide this information. Several such books are listed in the bibliography at the end of this text.

Study Aids

Chapter Organization

Each chapter opens with a chapter outline and a list of student objectives—goals to be accomplished by the completion of the chapter. In Part II, the chapters begin with an overview of the normal structure and function of the system under study followed by a list of key terms with definitions. The roots for most of the key terms are included with the definitions. Word parts related to each topic are then presented and illustrated along with exercises on the new material. Next, there is an overview of clinical information pertaining to the system, also followed by a list of key terms with definitions. Many chapters contain tables that unify and simplify material on specific topics.

Illustrations

Detailed, 4-color anatomic drawings illustrate the text. More than 50 clinical illustrations also are included.

Exercises

Exercises accompany the introduction of all material, and review exercises conclude each chapter. Most of the illustrations are accompanied by labeling exercises. Each has an alphabetical word list to assist in the labeling. Answers are given at the end of each chapter so that you can check your progress and correct any mistakes as you work.

Case Studies

Case studies are included in Chapters 6 to 21. These illustrate terminology in the context of a medical report. They may include information learned in previous chapters, so they also serve as a review. There are questions pertaining to these studies, but you should look up any unfamiliar words and be sure that you understand the meaning of the report.

Glossary of Word Parts

In working through the exercises, you will need to refer to reciprocal lists at the end of the text. One of these is a list of word parts and their meanings; the other is a list of meanings with corresponding word parts. There is also an index to topics and terms in the text.

Crossword Puzzles

To exercise your newfound knowledge, there is a crossword puzzle in each chapter on body systems. These are based on material from the chapter with some review terms. The answers to these puzzles are at the end of the chapter.

Flashcards

An excellent way to learn this new vocabulary is by means of flashcards. These have proved so successful that a section of flashcards has been included. They are presented in chapter order so that they can be removed in sequence as you progress through the book. Of course, these cards represent only a portion of the necessary vocabulary, and you should add to the collection with cards of your own. Blank cards are included for this purpose. Note also that the flashcards are exactly the size of one half of a 3″ × 5″ index card. You can make additional cards by cutting index cards in half.

You can create a self-test by covering lists of words and testing yourself on the definitions, or by covering definitions and testing yourself on the words. The same can be done with the charts on word parts and their definitions. It is also helpful to keep a personal list of words that you find difficult to spell or pronounce.

Help yourself in your studies by devising mental images or devices to help remember words. For example, to remember the root for the heart, *cardi*, think of a playing card—the ace of hearts. To differentiate the word *supine*, meaning "face up" from the word *prone*, meaning "face down," picture someone carrying hot soup—straight up, of course. Join classmates in spelling bees and quizzes. Try to make associations with words that are already in your vocabulary. You will find that these studies increase your understanding and appreciation of your own language.

Audiotapes

Audiotapes drawn from the text are available. They give a brief overview, exercises, and practice with pronunciation for Chapters 4 to 21.

Pronunciation

Phonetic pronunciations are provided in the text at every opportunity, even in the answer keys. Take advantage of these aids. Repeat the word aloud as you learn to recognize it in print. Be aware that word parts may change in pronunciation when they are combined in different ways.

The following pronunciation guidelines apply throughout the text.

A vowel (a, e, i, o, u) gets a short pronunciation if it has no pronunciation mark over it, such as:

a as in bat
e as in met
i as in sin
o as in pond
u as in run

A short line over the vowel gives it a long pronunciation:

ā as in say
ē as in tea
ī as in tie
ō as in hoe
ū as in sue

The accented syllable in each word is shown with capital letters.

Note that pronunciations may vary from place to place. Only one for each word is given here, but be prepared for differences.

Soft and Hard *c* and *g*

A soft *c*, as in *racer*, will be written as *s* *(RA-ser)*. A hard *c*, as in *candy*, will be written as *k* *(KAN-de)*. A soft g, as in *page*, will be written as *j* *(paj)*. A hard g, as in *grow*, will be written as g *(gro)*.

Silent Letters and Unusual Pronunciations

A silent letter or unusual pronunciation can be a problem especially if it appears at the start of a word that you are trying to look up in the dictionary. Some examples include the following:

Letter(s)	Pronunciation	Example
ch	k	chemical *(KEM-i-kl)*—pertaining to chemistry
dys	dis	dystrophy *(DIS-trō-fē)*—poor nourishment of tissue
eu	u	euphoria *(ū-FOR-ē-a)*—exaggerated feeling of well-being
gn	n	gnathic *(NATH-ik)*—pertaining to the jaw
ph	f	pharmacy *(FAR-ma-sē)*—a drug dispensary
pn	n	pneumonia *(nū-MŌ-nē-a)*—inflammation of the lungs
ps	s	pseudo- *(SŪ-dō)*—false
pt	t	ptosis *(TŌ-sis)*—dropping
rh	r	rheumatic *(rū-MAT-ik)*—pertaining to rheumatism, a disorder of muscles and joints
x	z	xiphoid *(ZIF-oyd)*—pertaining to cartilage attached to the sternum

These combinations may be pronounced differently when they appear within a word, as in apnea *(ap-NĒ-a)*, meaning cessation of breathing; nephroptosis *(nef-rop-TŌ-sis)*, meaning dropping of the kidney; prognosis *(prog-NŌ-sis)*, meaning prediction of the outcome of disease.

Abbreviations

Abbreviations can save time, but they can also cause confusion if they are not universally understood. Usage varies in different institutions, and the same abbreviation may have different meanings in different fields. Only the most commonly used abbreviations are given. These are listed at the end of each chapter, but a complete alphabetical list appears at the end of the book. An abbreviation dictionary also is helpful.

Words Ending in *x*

When a word ending in *x* has a suffix added, the *x* is changed to a g or a *c*. For example, pharynx (throat) becomes pharyngeal *(fa-RIN-jē-al),* to mean "pertaining to the throat"; *coccyx* (terminal portion of the vertebral column) becomes *coccygeal (kok-SIJ-ē-al),* to mean "pertaining to the coccyx"; *thorax* (chest) becomes *thoracotomy (thor-a-KOT-ō-mē)* to mean "an incision into the chest."

---

hem/o (blood) + -rhage (bursting forth) = hemorrhage (a bursting forth of blood)
men/o (menses) + -rhea (flow, discharge) = menorrhea (menstrual flow)

Suffixes Beginning With *rh*

When a suffix beginning with *rh* is added to a root, the *r* is doubled:

Medical Terminology: An Illustrated Guide

This book may be used with an instructor or as an independent study. The overview in each chapter contains the most common terms pertaining to the topic. After introduction of word parts and exercises, terms that do not lend themselves to analysis, such as words derived from proper names, or words that need further explanation are listed in a section titled "Additional Terms."

Chapters 1 to 8 present the basics of medical terminology. These include chapters on word parts, a general orientation to body structure, chapters on disease, diagnosis and treatment, and a chapter on drugs. Work through these chapters in order before proceeding to chapters on the body systems in Part II.

This book will be a good beginning to your studies of medical terminology. You will continue to learn as you work in your chosen field. Ask questions, look up new words, and read the medical literature. New terms arise continually as the fields of medicine evolve.

2 *Suffixes*

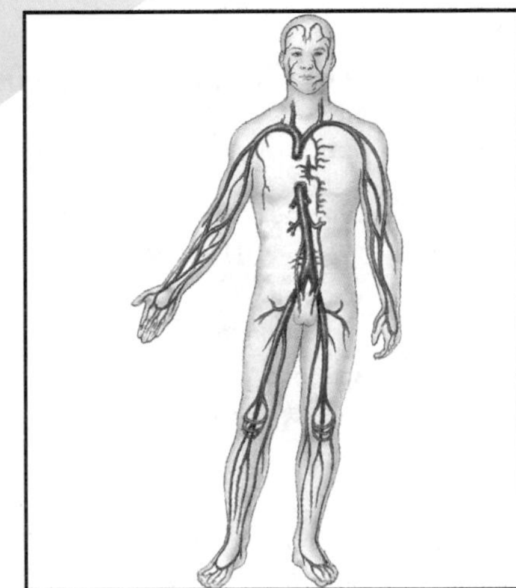

Chapter Contents

Objectives

After study of this chapter you should be able to:

1. Define a suffix
2. Give examples of how suffixes are used
3. Recognize and use some general noun, adjective, and plural suffixes employed in medical terminology

A suffix is a word ending that modifies a root. A suffix may indicate that the word is a noun or an adjective, and often determines how the definition of the word will begin. For example, using the root *myel/o* meaning "bone marrow," the adjective ending *-oid* gives the word *myeloid* which means "like or pertaining to bone marrow." The ending *-oma* gives *myeloma*, a tumor of the bone marrow, and *myelogenous* means "originating in bone marrow."

The suffixes given in this chapter are general ones that are used throughout medical terminology. Some additional suffixes will be presented in later chapters.

Suffixes That Mean "Condition Of"

Suffix	Example	Definition of Example
-ia	anesthesia *an-es-THĒ-zē-a*	loss of sensation
-ism	egotism *Ē-go-tizm*	exaggerated self-importance
-sis*	sclerosis *skle-RŌ-sis*	hardening
-y	atony *AT-ō-nē*	lack of muscle tone

* The ending *-sis* may appear with a combining vowel as *-osis*, *-iasis*, *-esis*, or *-asis*. The first two of these denote an abnormal condition.

Exercise 2-1

Write the suffix that means "condition of" in each of the following words:

	Suffix
1. insomnia (inability to sleep) *in-SOM-nē-a*	-ia
2. stenosis (narrowing of a vessel) *ste-NŌ-sis*	
3. psoriasis (skin disease) *sō-RĪ-a-sis*	
4. alcoholism (chronic dependence on or addiction to alcohol) *AL-ko-hol-izm*	
5. dysentery (intestinal disorder) *DIS-en-ter-ē*	
6. thrombosis (having a blood clot in a vessel) *throm-BŌ-sis*	
7. parasitism (infection with parasites or behaving as a parasite) *PAR-a-sit-izm*	

8. tetany (sustained muscle contraction)
   TET-a-nē ____________________

9. analgesia (absence of pain)
   an-al-JĒ-zē-a ____________________

Adjective Suffixes

The suffixes below are all adjective endings that mean "pertaining to," "characterized by," or "resembling." There are no rules for which ending to use for a given noun. Familiarity comes with practice. When necessary, tips on proper usage are given in the text.

Suffix	Example	Definition of Example
-ac	cardiac *CAR-dē-ak*	pertaining to the heart
-al	skeletal *SKEL-e-tal*	pertaining to the skeleton
-ar	muscular *MUS-kū-lar*	pertaining to muscles
-ary	dietary *DĪ-e-tar-ē*	pertaining to the diet
-ic	pelvic *PEL-vik*	pertaining to the pelvis
-ical (ic + al)	surgical *SUR-ji-kal*	pertaining to surgery
-ile	febrile *FEB-rīl*	pertaining to fever
-ous	venous *VĒ-nus*	pertaining to a vein
-form	epileptiform *ep-i-LEP-ti-form*	like or resembling epilepsy
-oid	ovoid *OV-oyd*	resembling an egg

For words ending with the suffix *-sis*, the ending is changed to *-tic* to form the adjective, as in *neurotic*, pertaining to neurosis, or *diuretic*, pertaining to diuresis (increased urination).

Exercise 2-2

Identify the suffix meaning "pertaining to" or "resembling" in each of the following words:

Suffix

1. salivary
   (*SAL-i-var-ē*) -ary

2. metric
   (*ME-trik*) ____________________

3. fibrous
 (FĪ-brus) ____________________

4. muciform
 (MŪ-si-form) ____________________

5. toxoid
 (TOK-soyd) ____________________

6. topical
 (TOP-i-kal) ____________________

7. virile
 (VIR-il) ____________________

8. vocal
 (VŌ-kal) ____________________

9. anatomical
 (an-a-TOM-i-kal) ____________________

10. circular
 (SIR-kū-lar) ____________________

11. urinary
 (Ū-ri-nar-ē) ____________________

Suffixes for Medical Specialties

Suffix	Meaning	Example	Definition of Example
-logy	study of	physiology *fiz-ē-OL-ō-jē*	study of function in a living organism
-ist	specialist in a field of study	dentist *DEN-tist*	specialist in study and treatment of the teeth and mouth
-ian	specialist in a field of study	physician *fi-ZISH-un*	practitioner of medicine (from root meaning "nature," "medicine")
-iatrics, -iatry	medical specialty	psychiatry *sī-KĪ-a-trē*	study and treatment of mental illness

Exercise 2-3

Write a word for a specialist in each of the following fields:

1. anatomy
 (a-NAT-ō-mē) anatomist

2. pediatrics
 (pē-dē-AT-riks) ____________________

3. radiology
 (rā-dē-OL-ō-jē) ____________________

4. obstetrics
   (ob-STET-riks) ____________________

5. allergy
   (AL-er-jē) ____________________

6. technology
   (tek-NOL-ō-jē) ____________________

7. psychiatry
   (sī-KĪ-a-trē) ____________________

Plural Endings

Many medical words have special plural forms based on the ending of the word. The following chart gives some general rules for the formation of plurals along with examples. The plural endings listed in column 2 are substituted for the word endings in column 1.

Word Ending	Plural Ending	Example	
		Singular	**Plural**
a	ae	patella (kneecap)	patellae *pa-TEL-ē*
en	ina	foramen (opening)	foramina *fō-RAM-i-na*
ex, ix	ices	index (indicator)	indices *IN-di-sēz*
is	es	diagnosis (identification of disease)	diagnoses *dī-ag-NŌ-sēz*
nx (anx, inx, ynx)	nges	phalanx (bone of finger or toe)	phalanges *fa-LAN-jēz*
on	a	ganglion (mass of nerve tissue)	ganglia *GANG-lē-a*
um	a	ovum (egg)	ova *Ō-va*
us	i	focus (center)	foci *FŌ-sī*

Exercise 2-4

Write the plural form of each of the following words. The word ending is underlined in each.

1. gingiva (gum) *(JIN-ji-va)* gingivae

2. protozoon (microscopic animal)
   (prō-tō-ZŌ-an) ____________________

3. omentum (abdominal membrane)
   (ō-MEN-tum) ____________________

4. lum*en* (central opening)
 (LŪ-min) ________________

5. test*is* (male gonad)
 (TES-tis) ________________

6. ap*ex* (top, peak)
 (Ā-peks) ________________

7. ser*um* (liquid)
 (SĒ-rum) ________________

8. men*inx* (membrane around the brain and spinal cord)
 (ME-ninks) ________________

9. embol*us* (a blockage in the circulation)
 (EM-bō-lus) ________________

10. pelv*is* (bony hip girdle)
 (PEL-vis) ________________

CHAPTER REVIEW 2

Identify the suffix that means "condition of" in each of the following words.

	Suffix
1. stenosis *(ste-NŌ-sis)*	
2. dystrophy *(DIS-trō-fē)*	
3. embolism *(EM-bō-lizm)*	
4. acidosis *(as-i-DŌ-sis)*	
5. phobia *(FŌ-bē-a)*	

Identify the adjective suffix in each of the following words that means "pertaining to" or "resembling."

	Suffix
6. biologic	
7. oral	
8. basic	
9. cutaneous	
10. lymphoid	
11. cellular	
12. virile	

13. salivary ______

14. nuclear ______

15. rheumatoid ______

Give the name of the specialist in each of the following fields.

16. pharmacy *(FAR-ma-sē)* ______

17. dermatology *(der-ma-TOL-ō-jē)* ______

18. obstetrics *(ob-STET-riks)* ______

19. gynecology *(gī-ne-KOL-ō-jē)* ______

20. podiatry *(pō-DĪ-a-trē)* ______

Write the plural for each of the following words. The word ending is underlined.

21. vertebra (bone of the spine) *(VER-te-bra)* ______

22. prognosis (prediction of disease outcome) *(prog-NŌ-sis)* ______

23. bacterium *(bak-TĒ-rē-um)* ______

24. nucleus *(NŪ-klē-us)* ______

25. spermatozoon *(sper-ma-tō-ZŌ-an)* ______

26. larynx (voice box) *(LAR-inks)* ______

Write the singular for each of the following words. The word ending is underlined.

27. lumina *(LŪ-min-a)* ______

28. fungi *(FUN-jī)* ______

29. ganglia *(GANG-lē-a)* ______

30. patellae *(pa-TEL-ē)* ______

31. appendices *(a-PEN-di-sēz)* ______

Chapter 2
Answer Section

Answers to Chapter Exercises

Exercise 2-1

1. -ia
2. -sis, -osis
3. -sis, -iasis
4. -ism
5. -y
6. -sis, -osis
7. -ism
8. -y
9. -ia

Exercise 2-2

1. -ary
2. -ic
3. -ous
4. -form
5. -oid
6. -al
7. -ile
8. -al
9. -ical
10. -ar
11. -ary

Exercise 2-3

1. anatomist
2. pediatrician
3. radiologist
4. obstetrician
5. allergist
6. technologist, technician
7. psychiatrist

Exercise 2-4

1. gingivae *(JIN-ji-vē)*
2. protozoa *(prō-tō-ZŌ-a)*
3. omenta *(ō-MEN-ta)*
4. lumina *(LŪ-min-a)*
5. testes *(TES-tēz)*
6. apices *(Ā-pi-sēz)*
7. sera *(SĒ-ra)*
8. meninges *(me-NIN-jēz)*
9. emboli *(EM-bō-lī)*
10. pelves *(PEL-vēz)*

Answers to Chapter Review 2

1. -sis, -osis
2. -y
3. -ism
4. -sis, -osis
5. -ia
6. -ic
7. -al
8. -ic
9. -ous
10. -oid
11. -ar
12. -ile
13. -ary
14. -ar

15. -oid
16. pharmacist
17. dermatologist
18. obstetrician
19. gynecologist
20. podiatrist
21. vertebrae
22. prognoses
23. bacteria
24. nuclei
25. spermatozoa
26. larynges
27. lumen
28. fungus
29. ganglion
30. patella
31. appendix

3 Prefixes

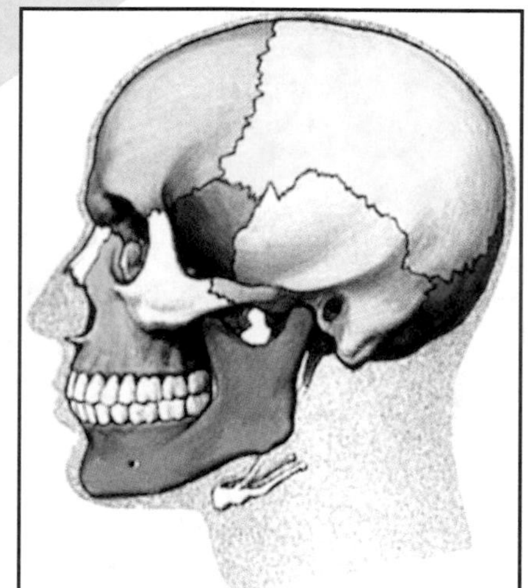

Chapter Contents

Objectives

After study of this chapter you should be able to:

1. Identify, define, and use the main prefixes employed in medical terminology

This chapter introduces most of the prefixes used in medical terminology. Although the list is long, almost all of the prefixes you will need to work through this book are presented here. There is just one short additional chart of prefixes related to position in Chapter 5 on body structure.

The meaning of many of these prefixes will be familiar to you from words that are already in your vocabulary. The words in the charts are given as examples of usage. Almost all of them will reappear in later chapters. If you forget a prefix as you work, you can refer to this chapter or to the alphabetical lists of word parts and meanings in the glossary.

Common Prefixes

*Prefixes for Numbers**

Prefix	Meaning	Example	Definition of Example
prim/i-	first	primary *PRĪ-mar-ē*	first, principal
mon/o-	one	monoclonal *mon-ō-KLŌN-al*	pertaining to a cell colony (clone) arising from a single cell
uni-	one	unify *Ū-ni-fi*	to make two or more parts into one
bi-	two, twice	bipolar *bī-PŌL-ar*	having two poles or processes
di-	two, twice	dichotomy *dī-KOT-ō-mē*	division into two parts
dipl/o-	double	diploid *DIP-loyd*	having two sets of chromosomes
hemi-	half, one side	hemithorax *hem-ē-THŌ-raks*	one side of the chest
semi-	half,partial	semisolid *sem-ē-SOL-id*	partially solid
tri-	three	triad *TRĪ-ad*	a group of three
quadr/i-	four	quadrant *KWOD-rant*	one-fourth of an area
tetra-	four	tetrad *TET-rad*	a group of four similar components
multi-	many	multicellular *mul-ti-SEL-ū-lar*	consisting of many cells
poly-	many, much	polymorphic *pol-ē-MOR-fik*	having many shapes (morph/o)

*Prefixes pertaining to the metric system are in the appendix.

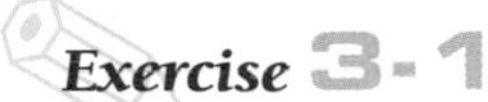

Exercise 3-1

Fill in the blanks:

1. Monarthritis *(mon-ar-THRĪ-tis)* is arthritis affecting ______________________ joint(s).
2. The quadriceps *(KWAD-ri-seps)* muscle has ______________________ parts.

3. The term semilunar (*sem-ē-LŪ-nar*) means ______________ moon.
4. Unipolar (*ū-ni-PŌ-lar*) means having ______________ pole(s).
5. A tetralogy (*te-TRAL-ō-jē*) is composed of ______________ elements or factors.
6. A triplet (*TRIP-let*) is one of ______________ offspring produced in a single birth.
7. A bicuspid (*bī-KUS-pid*) tooth has ______________ points, or cusps.

Give a prefix similar in meaning to each of the following:

8. di- ______________
9. poly- ______________
10. hemi- ______________

Prefixes for Colors

Prefix	Meaning	Example	Definition of Example
cyan/o-	blue	cyanosis *sī-a-NŌ-sis*	bluish discoloration of the skin due to lack of oxygen
erythr/o-	red	erythrocyte *e-RITH-rō-sīt*	a red blood cell
leuk/o-	white, colorless	leukoplakia *lū-kō-PLĀ-kē-a*	white patches in the mouth
melan/o-	black, dark	melanin *MEL-a-nin*	the dark pigment that colors the hair and skin
xanth/o-	yellow	xanthoma *zan-THŌ-ma*	a yellow raised area on the skin

Exercise 3-2

Match the following terms and write the appropriate letter to the left of each number:

______ 1. melanoma (*mel-a-NŌ-ma*)	a. pertaining to bluish discoloration
______ 2. xanthoderma (*zan-thō-DER-ma*)	b. redness of the skin
______ 3. cyanotic (*sī-a-NOT-ik*)	c. yellow coloration of the skin
______ 4. erythroderma (*e-rith-rō-DER-ma*)	d. a dark growth on the skin
______ 5. leukocyte (*LŪ-kō-sīt*)	e. white blood cell

Negative Prefixes

Prefix	Meaning	Example	Definition of Example
a-, an-	not, without	aseptic *ā-SEP-tik*	free of infectious organisms
anti-	against	antidote *AN-ti-dōt*	means for counteracting a poison
contra-	against	contraception *kon-tra-SEP-shun*	prevention of conception
de-	down, without	depilatory *dē-PIL-a-tor-ē*	agent used to remove hair (pil/o)
dis-	absence, removal, separation	dissect *di-SEKT*	to separate tissues for anatomical study
in-*, im- (before b,m,p)	not	incontinent *in-KON-ti-nent*	having no control over excretion
un-	not	unconscious *un-KON-shus*	not responsive

*May also mean "in" or "into" as in *inject, inhale.*

Exercise 3-3

Identify and define the prefix in each of the following words:

	Prefix	Meaning of Prefix
1. amorphous (without form; root morph/o) (*a-MOR-fus*)	a-	not, without, lack of, absence
2. antibody		
3. amnesia		
4. disintegrate		
5. contralateral		
6. inadequate		
7. decongestant		

Write the negative of each of the following words:

8. responsive ______unresponsive______
9. sufficient ____________
10. infect ____________
11. permeable (capable of being penetrated) ____________

12. humidify ______________________

13. compatible ______________________

Prefixes for Direction

Prefix	Meaning	Example	Definition of Example
ab-	away from	abduct *ab-DUKT*	to move away from the midline
ad-	toward, near	adhere *ad-HĒR*	to attach or stick together
dia-	through	dialysis *dī-AL-i-sis*	separation (-lysis) by passage through a membrane
per-	through	percutaneous *per-kū-TĀ-nē-us*	through the skin
trans-	through	transfusion *trans-FŪ-zhun*	introduction of blood or blood components into the bloodstream

Exercise 3-4

Identify and define the prefix in each of the following words:

	Prefix	Meaning of Prefix
1. transfer		
2. diarrhea		
3. adjacent		
4. abnormal		
5. perforate		

Prefixes for Degree

Prefix	Meaning	Example	Definition of Example
hyper-	over, excess, abnormally high, increased	hypertension *hī-per-TEN-shun*	high blood pressure
hypo-*	under, below	hypoxia *hi-POK-sē-a*	decreased oxygen in the tissues
olig/o-	few, scanty	oligomenorrhea *ol-i-gō-men-ō-RĒ-a*	scanty menstrual flow
pan-	all	panplegia *pan-PLĒ-jē-a*	total paralysis (-plegia)
super-*	above, excess	supernumerary *sū-per-NŪ-mer-ar-ē*	in excess number

*Also show position, as in *hypodermic, superficial.*

Exercise 3-5

Match the following terms and write the appropriate letter to the left of each number:

_____ 1. pandemic *(pan-DEM-ik)*	a. excess movement
_____ 2. hyperventilation *(hī-per-ven-ti-LĀ-shun)*	b. less than the normal number of teeth
_____ 3. hypotension *(hī-pō-TEN-shun)*	c. increased breathing
_____ 4. oligodontia *(ol-i-gō-DON-shē-a)*	d. disease affecting an entire population
_____ 5. supermotility *(sū-per-mō-TIL-i-tē)*	e. low blood pressure

Prefixes for Size and Comparison

Prefix	Meaning	Example	Definition of Example
eu-	true, good, easy, normal	euthanasia *ū-tha-NĀ-zhē-a*	easy or painless death (thanat/o)
hetero-	other, different, unequal	heterosexual *het-er-ō-SEX-ū-al*	pertaining to the opposite sex
homo-, homeo-	same, unchanging	homothermic *hō-mō-THER-mik*	maintaining a constant body temperature (therm/o); warm blooded
iso-	equal, same	isograft *Ī-sō-graft*	graft between two genetically identical individuals
macro-	large, abnormally large	macroscopic *mak rō SKOP-ik*	visible with the naked eye (without a microscope)
mega-,* megalo-	large, abnormally large	megacolon *meg-a-KŌ-lon*	enlargement of the colon
micro-†	small	microsurgery *MĪ-krō-sur-jer-ē*	surgery of extremely small structures under the microscope
neo-	new	neonate *NĒ-ō-nāt*	a newborn infant
normo-	normal	normovolemia *nor-mō-vol-Ē-mē-a*	normal blood volume
ortho-	straight, correct, upright	orthosis *or-THŌ-sis*	an appliance used to correct or prevent deformities
poikilo-	varied, irregular	poikiloderma *poy-ki-lō-DER-ma*	mottled condition of the skin
pseudo-	false	pseudoreaction *sū-dō-rē-AK-shun*	false reaction
re-	again, back	reflux *RĒ-fluks*	backward or return flow

**Mega-* also means "one million" as in *megahertz*.
†*Micro-* also means "one millionth" as in *microsecond*.

Exercise 3-6

Match the following terms and write the appropriate letter (a–e) to the left of each number:

_____ 1. regurgitation *(rē-gur-ji-TĀ-shun)*	a. an irregularly shaped cell
_____ 2. orthodontic *(or-thō-DON-tik)*	b. pertaining to normal body temperature
_____ 3. pseudoplegia *(sū-dō-PLĒ-jē-a)*	c. backward flow, as of blood or stomach contents
_____ 4. poikilocyte *(POY-kil-ō-sīt)*	d. false paralysis
_____ 5. normothermic *(nor-mō-THER-mik)*	e. pertaining to straight teeth

Identify and define the prefix in each of the following words:

	Prefix	Meaning of Prefix
6. orthopedics	_____	_____
7. recuperate	_____	_____
8. euthyroidism	_____	_____
9. neocortex	_____	_____
10. megabladder	_____	_____
11. isometric	_____	_____

Write the opposite of each of the following words:

12. heterogeneous (composed of different materials) _____

13. microscopic (visible only with a microscope) _____

Prefixes for Time and/or Position

Prefix	Meaning	Example	Definition of Example
ante-	before	antenatal *an-tē-NĀ-tal*	before birth
pre-	before, in front of	predisposing *prē-dis-POZ-ing*	leading toward a condition, such as disease
pro-	before, in front of	prodrome *PRŌ-drōm*	symptom that precedes a disease
post-	after, behind	post-traumatic *pōst-traw-MAT-ik*	after injury or traumatic event

An exercise on this chart is included in Exercise 3-7.

Prefixes for Position

Prefix	Meaning	Example	Definition of Example
dextr/o-	right	dextrocardia *deks-trō-KAR-dē-a*	location of the heart (cardi/o) in the right side of the chest
sinistr/o-	left	sinistrad *sin-IS-trad*	toward the left
ec-, ecto-	out, outside	ectoderm *EK-tō-derm*	outermost layer of the developing embryo
ex/o-	away from, outside	excise *ek-SĪZ*	to cut out
end/o-	in, within	endoscope *EN-dō-skōp*	device for viewing the inside of a cavity or organ
mes/o-	middle	mesencephalon *mes-en-SEF-a-lon*	midbrain
syn-, sym- (before b,m,p,)	together	synapse *SIN-aps*	a junction between two nerve cells
tel/e-, tel/o-	end	telangion *tel-AN-jē-on*	a terminal vessel (angi/o)

Exercise 3-7

Match the following terms and write the appropriate letter (a–e) to the left of each number:

_____ 1. endonasal *(en dō-NĀ-zal)*	a. displacement of the heart from its normal position
_____ 2. syndrome *(SIN-drōm)*	b. middle layer of the developing embryo
_____ 3. mesoderm *(MES-ō-derm)*	c. behind the nose
_____ 4. ectocardia *(ek-tō-KAR-dē-a)*	d. within the nose
_____ 5. postnasal *(post-NĀ-zal)*	e. group of symptoms occurring together

Identify and define the prefix in each of the following words:

	Prefix	Meaning of Prefix
6. synthesis	________	________
7. extract	________	________
8. antecedent *(an-tē-SĒ-dent)*	________	________
9. symbiosis *(sim-bī-Ō-sis)*	________	________
10. protrude	________	________

Write the opposite of each of the following words:

11. antepartum (before childbirth) ______postpartum______
12. exogenous (outside the organism) (*eks-OJ-e-nus*) ____________
13. premenopausal ____________
14. postadolescent ____________
15. sinistromanual (left handed) ____________
16. ectoderm ____________

CHAPTER REVIEW 3

Multiple choice. Match the terms in each of the sets below with their definitions and write the appropriate letter (a–e) to the left of each number:

_____ 1. primigravida	a. paralysis on both sides of the body
_____ 2. trisect	b. compound made of many subunits
_____ 3. unilateral	c. to cut into three parts
_____ 4. polymer	d. pertaining to one side of the body
_____ 5. diplegia	e. woman pregnant for the first time

_____ 6. neonatal	a. cell with yellow color
_____ 7. melanocyte	b. through the skin
_____ 8. xanthocyte	c. dark-colored cell
_____ 9. percutaneous	d. pertaining to a newborn
_____ 10. leukoderma	e. loss of color in the skin

_____ 11. adhesion	a. endbrain
_____ 12. mesencephalon	b. attachment of parts
_____ 13. oligomenorrhea	c. scanty menstrual flow
_____ 14. telencephalon	d. location or movement toward the right
_____ 15. dextroversion	e. midbrain

Match each of the following prefixes with its meaning:

_____ 16. pan-	a. equal, same
_____ 17. pseudo-	b. straight
_____ 18. eu-	c. all
_____ 19. iso-	d. good, true, easy
_____ 20. ortho-	e. false

Fill in the blanks:

21. A binocular microscope has ______________________ eyepiece(s).
22. Trifocal glasses have ______________________ lens(es).
23. A quadrant is one of ______________________ parts.
24. Sinistrad means toward the ______________________.
25. A unicellular organism is composed of ______________________ cell(s).
26. A tetratomic molecule has ______________________ atoms.

Identify and define the prefix in each of the following words:

	Prefix	**Meaning of Prefix**
27. transmit	________	________
28. react	________	________
29. exhale	________	________
30. contraindication	________	________
31. detoxify	________	________
32. perforate	________	________
33. dialyze *(DĪ-a-līz)*	________	________
34. antiserum	________	________
35. disease	________	________
36. ectopic *(ek-TOP-ik)*	________	________
37. symbiotic	________	________
38. prognosis	________	________

Opposites. Write a word that means the opposite of each of the following:

39. coordinated ______________________
40. mature ______________________
41. active ______________________
42. adduct ______________________
43. ectoparasite ______________________
44. macroscopic ______________________
45. homosexual ______________________
46. hypersensitivity ______________________
47. postoperative ______________________

Synonyms. Write a word that means the same as each of the following:

48. supersecretion ______________________
49. megalocyte (extremely large red blood cell) ______________________
50. antenatal ______________________

Chapter 3 Answer Section

Answers to Chapter Exercises

Exercise 3-1

1. one
2. four
3. half
4. one
5. four
6. three
7. two
8. bi-
9. multi-
10. semi-

Exercise 3-2

1. d
2. c
3. a
4. b
5. e

Exercise 3-3

1. a-; not, without, lack of, absence
2. anti-; against
3. a-; not, without (root *mnem/o* means "memory")
4. dis-; absence, removal, separation
5. contra-; against
6. in-; not
7. de-; down, without, removal, loss
8. unresponsive
9. insufficient
10. disinfect
11. impermeable
12. dehumidify
13. incompatible

Exercise 3-4

1. trans-; through, across, beyond
2. dia-; through
3. ad-; toward, near
4. ab-; away from
5. per-; through

Exercise 3-5

1. d
2. c
3. e
4. b
5. a

Exercise 3-6

1. c
2. e
3. d
4. a
5. b
6. ortho-; straight, correct, upright

7. re-; again, back
8. eu-; true, good, easy, normal
9. neo-; new
10. mega-; large, abnormally large
11. iso-; equal, same
12. homogeneous *(hō-mō-JĒ-nē-us)*
13. macroscopic

Exercise 3-7

1. d
2. e
3. b
4. a
5. c
6. syn-; together
7. ex/o; away from, outside
8. ante-; before
9. sym-; together
10. pro-; before, in front of
11. postpartum
12. endogenous *(en-DOJ-e-nus)*
13. postmenopausal
14. preadolescent
15. dextromanual
16. endoderm

Answers to Chapter Review 3

1. e
2. c
3. d
4. b
5. a
6. d
7. c
8. a
9. b
10. e
11. b
12. e
13. c
14. a
15. d
16. c
17. e
18. d
19. a
20. b
21. two
22. three
23. four
24. left
25. one
26. four
27. trans-; through, across, beyond
28. re-; again, back
29. ex/o-; away from, outside
30. contra-; against
31. de-; down, without, removal, loss
32. per-; through
33. dia-; through
34. anti-; against
35. dis-; absence, removal, separation
36. ec-; out, outside
37. sym-; together
38. pro-; before, in front of
39. uncoordinated
40. immature
41. inactive
42. abduct
43. endoparasite
44. microscopic
45. heterosexual
46. hyposensitivity
47. preoperative
48. hypersecretion
49. macrocyte
50. prenatal

4 Cells, Tissues, and Organs

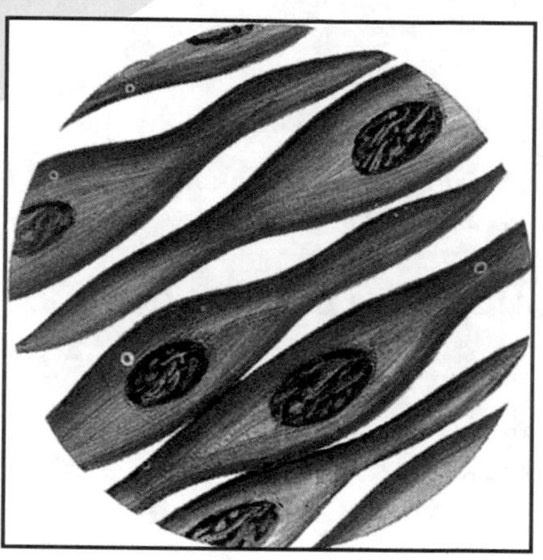

Chapter Contents

Objectives

After study of this chapter you should be able to:

1. Describe the main parts of a cell
2. Label a diagram of a typical cell
3. Name and give the functions of the four basic types of tissues in the body
4. Define basic terms pertaining to the structure and function of body tissues.
5. Recognize and use roots and suffixes pertaining to cells, tissues, and organs

The Cell

The body can be studied from its simplest to its most complex level, beginning with the **cell**, the basic unit of living organisms (Fig. 4-1). All body functions derive from the activities of billions of specialized cells.

Within the **cytoplasm** that fills the cell are subunits, organelles, each with a specific function. The main cell structures are named and described in Table 4-1.

The **nucleus** is the control region of the cell. It contains the **chromosomes** which carry genetic information. Each human cell, aside from the sex cells, contains 46 chromosomes. The chromosomes are composed of a complex organic substance, **DNA**, which is organized into separate units called **genes**. When a body cell divides, by the process of **mitosis**, the chromosomes are doubled and then equally distributed to the two daughter cells. Sex cells (egg and sperm) divide by another process (meiosis) that halves the chromosomes in preparation for fertilization.

Tissues

Cells are organized into **tissues** which perform specific functions. The four basic tissue types are:

1. epithelial *(ep-i-THĒ-lē-al)* tissue—covers and protects body structures and lines organs, vessels, and cavities.

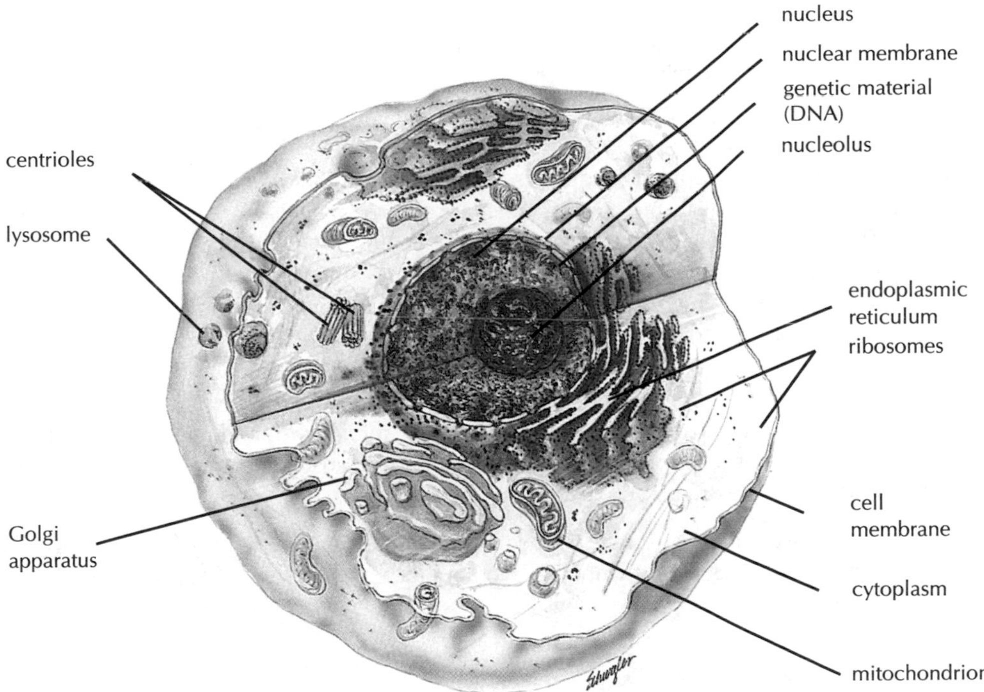

FIGURE 4-1. Diagram of a typical animal cell showing the main organelles.

TABLE 4-1 Cell Structures

Name	Description	Function
Cell membrane	Outer layer of the cell; composed mainly of lipids and proteins	Limits the cell; regulates what enters and leaves the cell
Cytoplasm	Colloidal suspension that fills cell	Holds cell contents
Nucleus	Large, dark-staining body near the center of the cell; composed of DNA and proteins	Contains the chromosomes with the genes (the hereditary material that directs all cell activities)
Nucleolus	Small body in the nucleus; composed of RNA, DNA, and protein	Needed for protein manufacture
Endoplasmic reticulum (ER)	Network of membranes in the cytoplasm	Used for storage and transport; holds ribosomes
Ribosomes	Small bodies attached to the ER; composed of RNA and protein	Manufacture proteins
Mitochondria	Large organelles with folded membranes inside	Convert energy from nutrients into ATP
Golgi apparatus	Layers of membranes	Put together special substances such as mucus
Lysosomes	Small sacs of digestive enzymes	Digest substances within the cell
Centrioles	Rod-shaped bodies (usually 2) near the nucleus	Help separate the chromosomes in cell division
Cilia	Short, hairlike projections from the cell	Create movement around the cell
Flagellum	Long, whiplike extension from the cell	Moves the cell

2. connective tissue—supports and binds body structures. It contains fibers and other nonliving material between the cells. Included are adipose (fat) tissue, cartilage, bone (Chapter 19), and blood (Chapter 10).
3. muscle tissue (root *my/o*)—contracts to produce movement. The three types are: skeletal or voluntary muscle that moves the skeleton; the cardiac muscle of the heart; smooth or visceral muscle that forms the walls of the abdominal organs. Cardiac and smooth muscle can function without conscious control and are thus described as involuntary. Skeletal muscle is studied in greater detail in Chapter 20.
4. nervous tissue (root *neur/o*)—makes up the brain, spinal cord, and nerves. It coordinates and controls body responses by the transmission of electrical impulses. The nervous system and senses are discussed in Chapters 17 and 18.

The simplest tissues are membranes. Mucous membranes secrete a thick fluid (mucus) that protects underlying tissue. Serous membranes secrete a thin, watery fluid. They line body cavities and cover organs.

Organs and Organ Systems

Tissues are arranged into organs which serve specific functions. The organs, in turn, are grouped into systems. Each of the body systems is discussed in turn in Part II. Bear in mind, however, that the body functions as a whole—no system is independent of the others. They work together to maintain the body's state of internal stability termed **homeostasis**.

KEY TERMS

ATP — The energy compound of the cell; stores energy needed for cell activities. ATP stands for adenosine triphosphate *(a-DEN-ō-sēn trī-FOS-fāt).*

cell — The basic structural and functional unit of the living organism; a microscopic unit that combines with other cells to form tissues (root *cyt/o*)

chromosome *(KRŌ-mō-sōm)* — A threadlike body in the nucleus of a cell that contains genetic information

cytoplasm *(SĪ-tō-plazm)* — The fluid that fills a cell and holds the organelles

DNA — The genetic compound of the cell; makes up the genes. DNA stands for deoxyribonucleic *(dē-ok-sē-rī-bō-nū-KLĒ-ik)* acid.

enzyme *(EN-zīm)* — An organic substance that speeds the rate of metabolic reactions

gene *(jēn)* — A hereditary unit composed of DNA and combined with other genes to form the chromosomes

glucose *(GLŪ-kōs)* — A simple sugar that circulates in the blood; the main energy source for metabolism (roots *gluc/o, glyc/o*)

homeostasis *(hō-mē-ō-STĀ-sis)* — A steady state; a condition of internal stability and constancy

lipid *(LIP-id)* — A category of organic compounds which includes fats (root *lip/o*)

metabolism *(me-TA-bō-lizm)* — The sum of all the physical and chemical changes that occur within an organism

mitosis *(mī-TŌ-sis)* — Cell division

mucus *(MŪ-kus)* — A thick fluid secreted by cells in membranes and glands that lubricates and protects tissues (roots *muc/o, myx/o*); the adjective is *mucous*

nucleus *(NŪ-klē-us)* — The control center of the cell; directs all cell activities based on the information contained in its chromosomes (roots *nucle/o, kary/o*)

RNA — An organic compound involved in the manufacture of proteins within cells. RNA stands for ribonucleic *(rī-bō-nū-KLĒ-ik)* acid.

tissue — A group of cells that acts together for a specific purpose (root *hist/o, histi/o*)

Word Parts Pertaining to Cells, Tissues, and Organs

Roots for Cells and Tissues

Root	Meaning	Example	Definition of Example
morph/o	form	polymorphic *pol-ē-MOR-fik*	having many forms
cyt/o	cell	cytogenesis *sī-tō-JEN-e-sis*	the formation (-genesis) of cells
nucle/o	nucleus	nuclear *NŪ-klē-ar*	pertaining to a nucleus
kary/o	nucleus	karyomegaly *kar-ē-ō-MEG-a-lē*	enlargement (-megaly) of the nucleus of a cell
hist/o, histi/o	tissue	histologist *his-TOL-ō-jist*	specialist in the study of tissue
fibr/o	fiber	fibrosis *fī-BRŌ-sis*	abnormal formation of fibrous tissue
reticul/o	network	reticulum *re-TIK-ū-lum*	a network
aden/o	gland	adenitis *ad-e-NĪ-tis*	tumor (-oma) of a gland
papill/o	nipple	papilla *pa-PIL-a*	nipplelike projection
myx/o	mucus	myxadenitis *miks-ad-e-NĪ-tis*	inflammation of gland that secretes mucus
muc/o	mucus, mucous membrane	mucorrhea *mū-kō-RĒ-a*	increased flow (-rhea) of mucus
somat/o	body	somatic *sō-MAT-ik*	pertaining to the body (as compared to the germ cells or to the mind)

Exercise 4-1

Fill in the blanks:

1. Morphology *(mor-FOL-ō-jē)* is the study of ____________________.
2. A megakaryocyte *(meg-a-KAR-ē-ō-sīt)* is a cell with a very large ____________________.
3. The term *adenoid (AD-e-noyd)* means resembling or pertaining to a(n) ____________________.
4. The adjective *papilliform (pa-PIL-i-form)* means resembling a(n) ____________________.
5. A fibril *(FĪ-bril)* is a small ____________________.
6. Histogenesis is the formation (-genesis) of ____________________.
7. A myxoma *(mik-SŌ-ma)* is a tumor of tissue that secretes ____________________.

8. The term *reticular (re-TIK-ū-lar)* means resembling or pertaining to a(n) ______________________.

9. The term *mucosa (mu-KŌ-sa)* is used to describe a membrane that secretes ______________________.

10. Nucleoplasm *(NŪ-klē-ō-plazm)* is the material that fills the ______________________.

11. Somatotropin *(sō-ma-tō-TRŌ-pin)*, also called growth hormone, has a general stimulating effect on the ______________________.

Use the suffix *-logy* to build a word with each of the following meanings:

12. The study of cells ______________________

13. The study of tissues ______________________

Roots for Cell Activity

Root	Meaning	Example	Definition of Example
blast/o	immature cell, productive cell, embryonic cell	erythroblast *e-RITH-rō-blast*	an immature red blood cell
gen	origin, formation	genesis JEN-e-sis	the origin of something
phag/o	eat, ingest	phagocyte *FAG-ō-sīt*	cell that ingests waste and foreign matter
phil	attract, absorb	chromophilic *krō-mō-FIL-ik*	attracting color (stain)
trop	act on, affect	inotropic *in-ō-TROP-ik*	affecting contraction of muscle fibers (-ino)
troph/o	feeding, growth, nourishment	atrophy *AT-rō-fē*	wasting away (lack of nourishment)
plas	formation, molding, development	hypoplasia *hī-pō-PLĀ-zha*	underdevelopment of an organ or tissue
some	small body	ribosome *RĪ-bō-sōm*	small body in the cytoplasm that contains RNA

The above roots are often combined with a simple noun suffix (*-in*, *-y*, or *-ia*) or an adjective suffix (*-ic*) and used as word endings. Such combined forms that routinely appear as word endings will simply be described and used as suffixes in this book. Examples from the above list are *-trophy*, *-plasia*, *-tropin*, *-philic*.

Exercise 4-2

Multiple choice. Match the terms in the sets below with their definitions and write the appropriate letter (a–e) to the left of each number:

_____ 1. leukoblast (*LŪ-kō-blast*) a. small body containing digestive enzymes
_____ 2. hypertrophy (*hī-PER-trō-fē*) b. attracting water
_____ 3. phagocytosis (*fag-ō-sī-TŌ-sis*) c. increased growth of tissue
_____ 4. hydrophilic (*hī-drō-FIL-ik*) d. ingestion of waste by a cell
_____ 5. lysosome (*LĪ-sō-sōm*) e. immature white blood cell

_____ 6. myotropic (*mī-ō-TROP-ik*) a. formation of a nucleus
_____ 7. neoplasia (*nē-ō-PLĀ-zha*) b. substance that acts on the sex glands
_____ 8. karyogenesis (*kar-ē-ō-JEN-e-sis*) c. acting on muscle tissue
_____ 9. aplasia (*a-PLĀ-zha*) d. new formation of tissue
_____ 10. gonadotropin (*gon-a-dō-TRŌ-pin*) e. lack of development

Identify and define the root in each of the following words:

	Root	Meaning of Root
11. esophagus (*e-SOF-a-gus*)	_____	_____
12. genetics (*je-NET-iks*)	_____	_____
13. normoblast (*NOR-mō-blast*)	_____	_____
14. dystrophy (*DIS-trō-fē*)	_____	_____
15. aplastic (*a-PLAS-tik*)	_____	_____

Word Parts for Body Chemistry

Part	Meaning	Example	Definition of Example
Suffixes			
-ase	enzyme	carbohydrase *kar-bō-HĪ-drās*	enzyme that digests carbohydrates
-ose	sugar	fructose *FRUK-tōs*	fruit sugar
Roots			
hydr/o	water, fluid	hydrated *HĪ-drāt-ed*	combined with water

(continued)

Word Parts for Body Chemistry (Continued)

Part	Meaning	Example	Definition of Example
lip/o	lipid, fat	lipoma *lī-PŌ-ma*	tumor containing fat
adip/o	fat	adipoid *AD-i-poyd*	like or resembling fat
steat/o	fatty	steatorrhea *stē-a-tō-RĒ-a*	discharge (-rhea) of fatty stools
gluc/o	glucose	glucosuria *glu-kō-SŪ-rē-a*	presence of glucose in the urine (-ur/o)
glyc/o	sugar, glucose	hyperglycemia *hī-per-glī-SĒ-mē-a*	high blood sugar
amyl/o	starch	amylase *AM-i-lās*	enzyme that digests starch
prote/o	protein	proteolysis *prō-tē-OL-i-sis*	dissolving (-lysis) of proteins

Exercise 4-3

Fill in the blanks:

1. The term *amyloid (AM-i-loyd)* means resembling ____________________.
2. The ending *-ose* indicates that maltose is a(n) ____________________.
3. Glucogenesis *(glū-kō-JEN-e-sis)* is the formation of ____________________.
4. Hydrotherapy is treatment using ____________________.
5. Liposuction is the surgical removal of ____________________.
6. Adiposuria *(ad-i-pō-SŪ-rē-a)* is the presence of ____________________ in the urine.

Identify and define the root in each of the following words:

	Root	Meaning of Root
7. protease *(PRŌ-tē-ās)*	________	________
8. glucolytic *(glū-kō-LIT-ik)*	________	________
9. asteatosis *(as-tē-a-TŌ-sis)*	________	________
10. normoglycemia *(nor-mō-glī-SĒ-mē-a)*	________	________

ADDITIONAL TERMS

amino acids *(a-mē-nō)*	The nitrogen-containing compounds that make up proteins
anabolism *(a-NAB-ō-lizm)*	The type of metabolism in which body substances are made; the building phase of metabolism
catabolism *(ka-TAB-ō-lizm)*	The type of metabolism in which substances are broken down for energy and simple compounds
collagen *(KOL-a-jen)*	A fibrous protein found in connective tissue
cortex *(KOR-tex)*	The outer region of an organ
glycogen *(GLĪ-kō-jen)*	A complex sugar compound stored in liver and muscles; broken down into glucose when needed for energy
interstitial *(in-ter-STISH-al)*	Between parts, such as the spaces between cells in a tissue
medulla *(me-DUL-la)*	The inner region of an organ; marrow (root *medull/o*)
parenchyma *(par-EN-ki-ma)*	The functional tissue of an organ
parietal *(pa-RĪ-e-tal)*	Pertaining to a wall; describes a membrane that lines a body cavity
soma *(SŌ-ma)*	The body
visceral *(VIS-er-al)*	Pertaining to the internal organs; describes a membrane on the surface of an organ

Chapter 4
Labeling Exercise

Write the name of each numbered part on the corresponding line of the answer sheet.

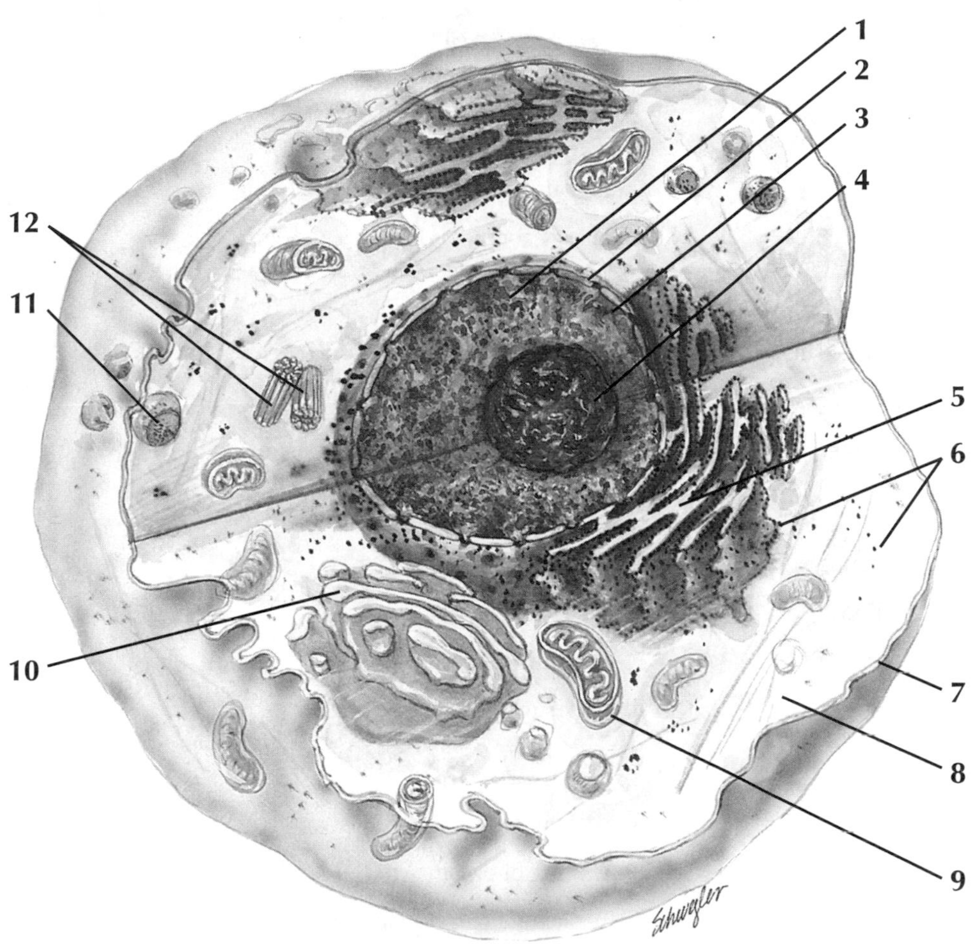

Diagram of a typical animal cell

cell membrane	genetic material (DNA)	nuclear membrane
centrioles	Golgi apparatus	nucleolus
cytoplasm	lysosome	nucleus
endoplasmic reticulum	mitochondrion	ribosomes

1. ____________________ 7. ____________________

2. ____________________ 8. ____________________

3. ____________________ 9. ____________________

4. ____________________ 10. ____________________

5. ____________________ 11. ____________________

6. ____________________ 12. ____________________

CHAPTER REVIEW 4

Matching. Match the terms in the sets below with their definitions and write the appropriate letter (a–e) to the left of each number:

_____ 1. ribosomes	a. genetic material
_____ 2. ATP	b. state of internal stability
_____ 3. homeostasis	c. organelles that contain RNA
_____ 4. DNA	d. fibrous protein in connective tissue
_____ 5. collagen	e. energy compound of the cells
_____ 6. cytoplasm	a. organelles that produce ATP
_____ 7. anabolism	b. cell that contains a network
_____ 8. mitochondria	c. material that fills the cell
_____ 9. reticulocyte	d. breakdown phase of metabolism
_____ 10. catabolism	e. building phase of metabolism
_____ 11. adenitis	a. enzyme that digests fats
_____ 12. adipose	b. inflammation of a gland
_____ 13. fibroma	c. pertaining to fat
_____ 14. lactose	d. milk sugar
_____ 15. lipase	e. fibrous tumor
_____ 16. fibroplasia	a. without form
_____ 17. amorphous	b. wasting of tissue
_____ 18. papillary	c. attracting neutral stain
_____ 19. atrophy	d. formation of fibrous tissue
_____ 20. neutrophilic	e. like or resembling a nipple
_____ 21. hyperplasia	a. resembling mucus
_____ 22. hypoglycemia	b. low blood sugar
_____ 23. amylase	c. immature red blood cell
_____ 24. mucoid	d. overdevelopment of an organ or tissue
_____ 25. erythroblast	e. enzyme that digests starch
_____ 26. adipocyte	a. pertaining to the body and the mind
_____ 27. nucleosome	b. destroying or dissolving protein
_____ 28. somatotropic	c. cell that contains fat

_____ 29. proteolytic d. small body in the nucleus

_____ 30. somatopsychic e. acting on the body

Fill in the blanks:

31. The four basic tissue types are ______________________________.

32. The simple sugar that is the main energy source for metabolism is ______________.

33. The control center of the cell is the ______________.

34. The number of chromosomes in each human cell aside from the sex cells is ______________.

35. An organic compound that speeds the rate of metabolic reactions is a(n) ______________.

36. A karyotype *(KAR-ē-ō-tīp)* is a study of the chromosomes found in the ______________ of a cell.

37. A cytotoxic substance is damaging or poisonous to ______________.

38. The term *hydration* refers to the amount of ______________ in a substance.

39. A myxocyte is found in tissue that secretes ______________.

Word building. Write a word for each of the following definitions.

40. The study of form and structure ______________

41. The study of tissues ______________

42. The formation of cells (use *-genesis*) as an ending ______________

Chapter 4
Answer Section

Answers to Chapter Exercises

Exercise 4-1

1. form, structure
2. nucleus
3. gland
4. nipple
5. fiber
6. tissue
7. mucus
8. network
9. mucus
10. nucleus
11. body
12. cytology (sī-*TOL-ō-jē*)
13. histology (his-*TOL-ō-jē*)

Exercise 4-2

1. e
2. c
3. d
4. b
5. a
6. c
7. d
8. a
9. e
10. b
11. phag/o; eat, ingest
12. gen; origin, formation
13. blast/o; immature cell, productive cell
14. troph; feeding, growth, nourishment
15. plas; formation, molding, development

Exercise 4-3

1. starch
2. sugar
3. glucose
4. water
5. fat
6. fat
7. prote/o; protein
8. glyc/o; sugar, glucose
9. steat/o; fatty
10. glyc/o; sugar, glucose

Labeling Exercise

Diagram of a Typical Animal Cell

1. nucleus
2. nuclear membrane
3. genetic material (DNA)
4. nucleolus
5. endoplasmic reticulum (ER)
6. ribosomes
7. cell membrane
8. cytoplasm
9. mitochondrion
10. Golgi apparatus
11. lysosome
12. centrioles

Answers to Chapter Review 4

1. c
2. e
3. b
4. a
5. d
6. c
7. e
8. a
9. b
10. d
11. b
12. c
13. e
14. d
15. a
16. d
17. a
18. e
19. b
20. c
21. d
22. b
23. e
24. a
25. c
26. c
27. d
28. e
29. b
30. a
31. epithelial, connective, muscle, nervous
32. glucose
33. nucleus
34. 46
35. enzyme
36. nucleus
37. cells
38. water
39. mucus
40. morphology
41. histology
42. cytogenesis

5 *Body Structure*

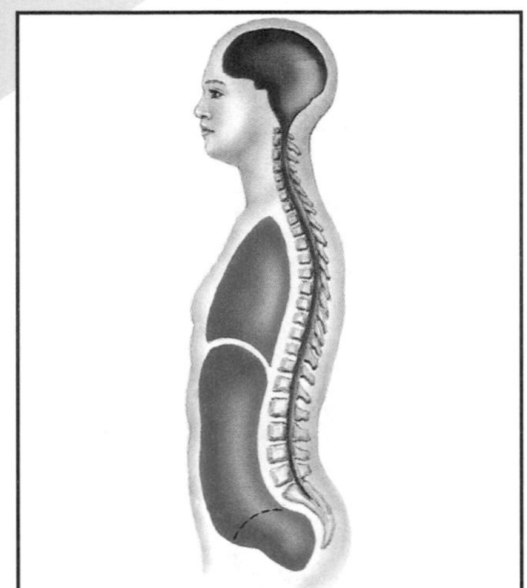

Chapter Contents

Objectives

After study of this chapter you should be able to:

1. Define the main directional terms used in anatomy
2. Describe division of the body along three different planes
3. Locate the dorsal and ventral body cavities
4. Locate the nine divisions of the abdomen
5. Describe the main body positions used in medical practice
6. Define basic terms describing body structure
7. Recognize and use roots pertaining to body regions
8. Recognize and use prefixes pertaining to position and direction

Directional Terms

In describing the location or direction of a given point in the body, it is always assumed that the subject is in the **anatomic position**, that is, upright, with face front, arms at the sides with palms forward, and feet parallel. In this stance, the terms illustrated in Figure 5-1 and listed in Table 5-1 are used to designate relative position.

Figure 5-2 illustrates planes of section, that is, directions in which the body can be cut. A **frontal plane**, also called a coronal plane, is made at right angles to the midline and divides the body into anterior and posterior parts. A **sagittal** *(SAJ-i-tal)* **plane** passes from front to back and

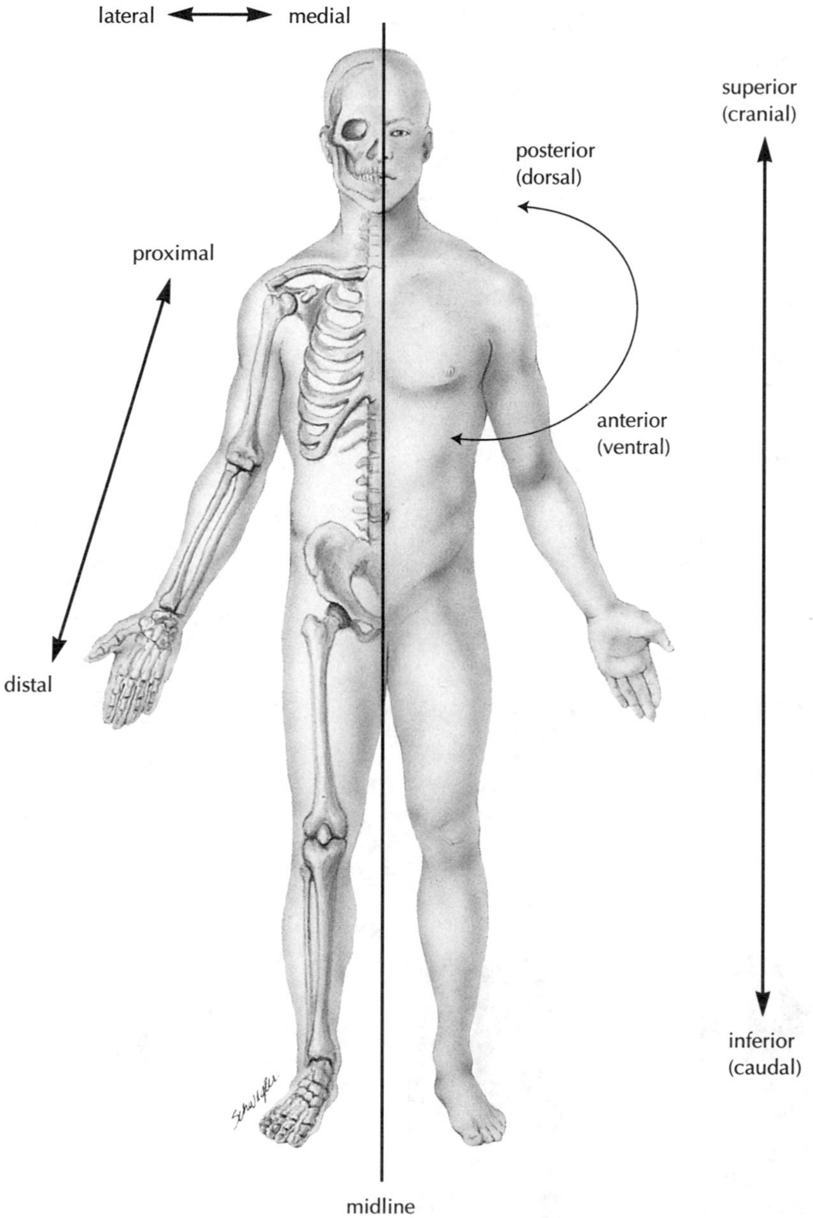

FIGURE 5-1. Directional terms.

TABLE 5-1 Anatomic Directions

Term	Definition
anterior (ventral)	toward the front (belly) of the body
posterior (dorsal)	toward the back of the body
medial	toward the midline of the body
lateral	toward the side of the body
proximal	nearer to the point of attachment or to a given reference point
distal	farther from the point of attachment or from a given reference point
superior	above
inferior	below
cranial (cephalic)	toward the head
caudal	toward the lower end of the spine (L. *cauda* means "tail")
superficial (external)	close to the surface of the body
deep (internal)	close to the center of the body

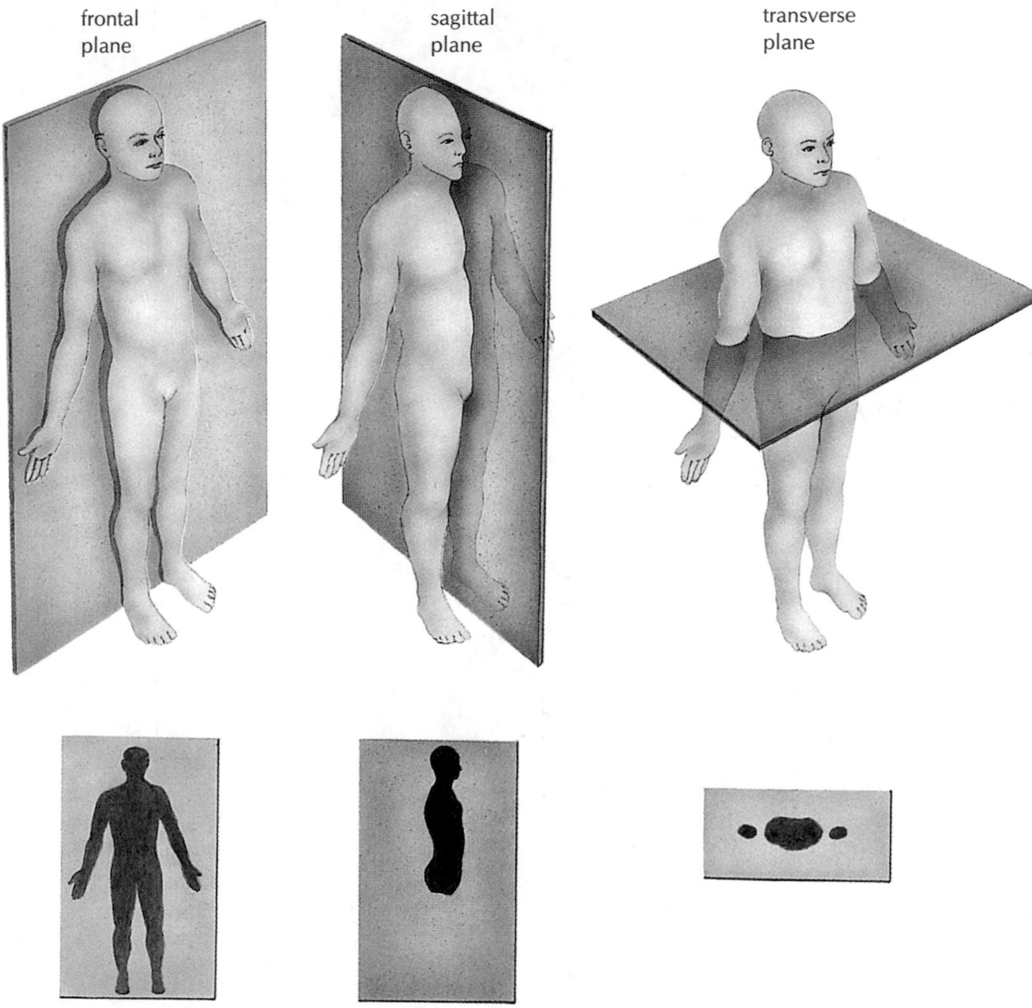

FIGURE 5-2. Planes of division.

divides the body into right and left portions. If the plane passes through the midline, it is a midsagittal or medial plane. A **transverse plane** passes horizontally dividing the body into superior and inferior parts.

Body Cavities

Internal organs are located within dorsal and ventral cavities (Fig. 5-3). The dorsal cavity contains the brain and the spinal cord. The uppermost ventral space, the **thoracic cavity**, is separated from the **abdominal cavity** by the **diaphragm**. There is no anatomic separation between the abdominal cavity and the **pelvic cavity**, which together make up the **abdominopelvic cavity**. The large membrane that lines the abdominopelvic cavity and covers the organs within it is the **peritoneum** *(per-i-tō-NĒ-um)*.

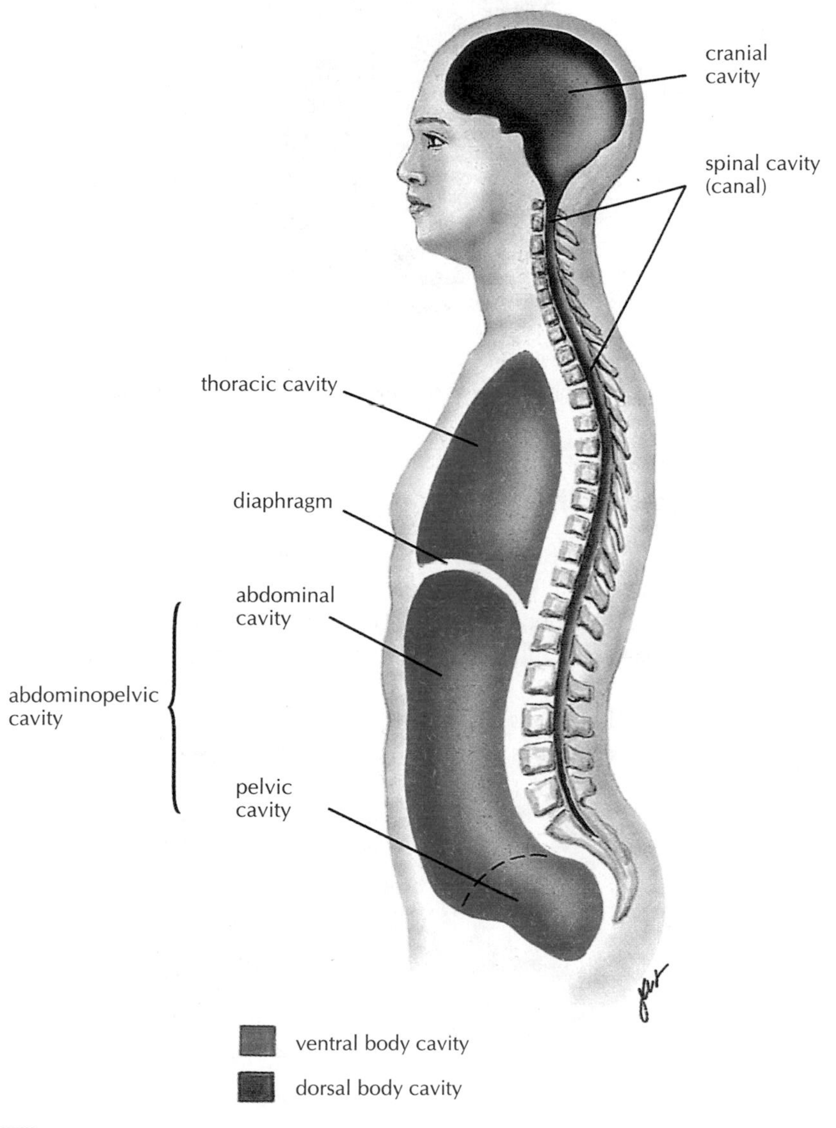

FIGURE 5-3. Side view of the body cavities.

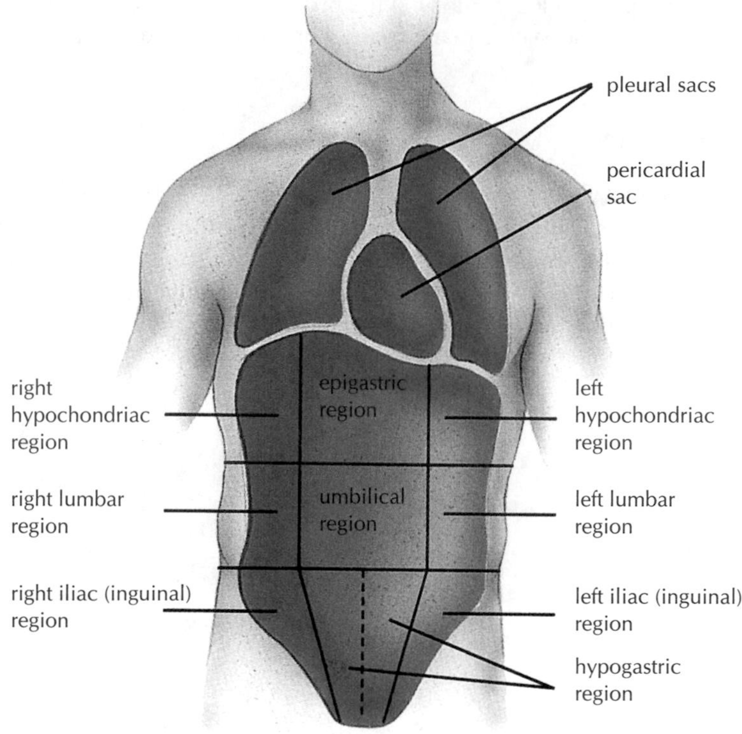

FIGURE 5-4. Front view of the thoracic cavity and the nine regions of the abdomen.

✳ Body Regions

For orientation the abdomen can be divided by imaginary lines into nine regions. These are named as shown in Figure 5-4. More simply, but less specifically, the abdomen can be divided by a single vertical line and a single horizontal line into 4 sections (Fig. 5-5), designated the right upper quadrant (RUQ), left upper quadrant (LUQ), right lower quadrant (RLQ), and left lower quadrant (LLQ).

Additional terms for body regions are shown in Figures 5-6 and 5-7. You may need to refer to these illustrations as you work through the book.

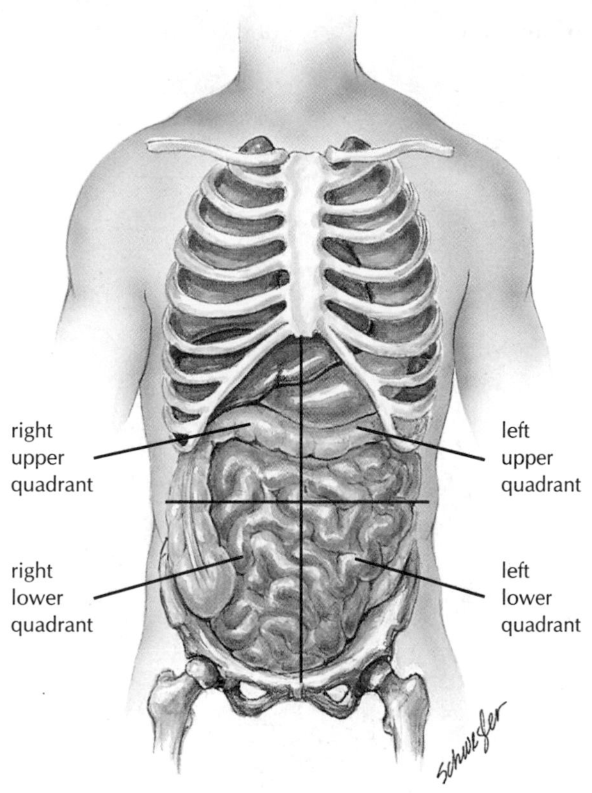

FIGURE 5-5. Quadrants of the abdomen showing the organs within each quadrant.

Word Parts Pertaining to Body Structure

Roots for Regions of the Head and Trunk

Root	Meaning	Example	Definition of Example
cephal/o	head	macrocephaly *mak-rō-SEF-a-lē*	abnormal largeness of the head
cervic/o	neck	cervicofacial *ser-vi-kō-FĀ-shal*	pertaining to the neck and face
thorac/o	chest, thorax	intrathoracic *in-tra-thō-RAS-ik*	within the thorax
abdomin/o	abdomen	subabdominal *sub-ab-DOM-i-nal*	below the abdomen
celi/o	abdomen	celiac *SĒ-lē-ac*	pertaining to the abdomen
lapar/o	abdominal wall	laparotomy *lap-a-ROT-ō-mē*	incision (-tomy) through the abdominal wall
lumb/o	lumbar region, lower back	thoracolumbar *thō-rak-ō-LUM-bar*	pertaining to the chest and lumbar region
periton, peritone/o	peritoneum	peritoneal *per-i-tō-NĒ-al*	pertaining to the peritoneum

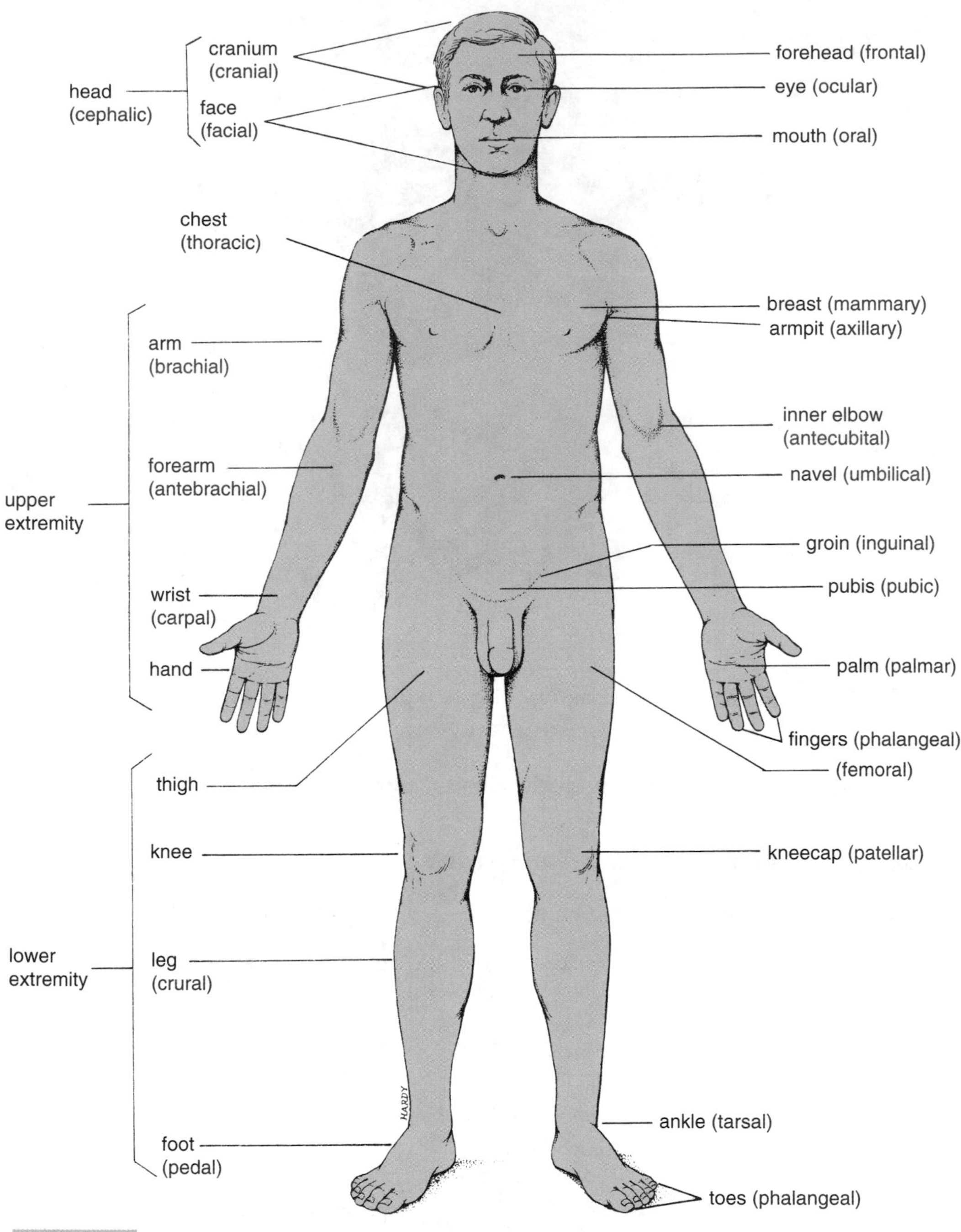

FIGURE 5-6. Common terms for body regions; anterior view. Anatomic terms for regions are in parentheses.

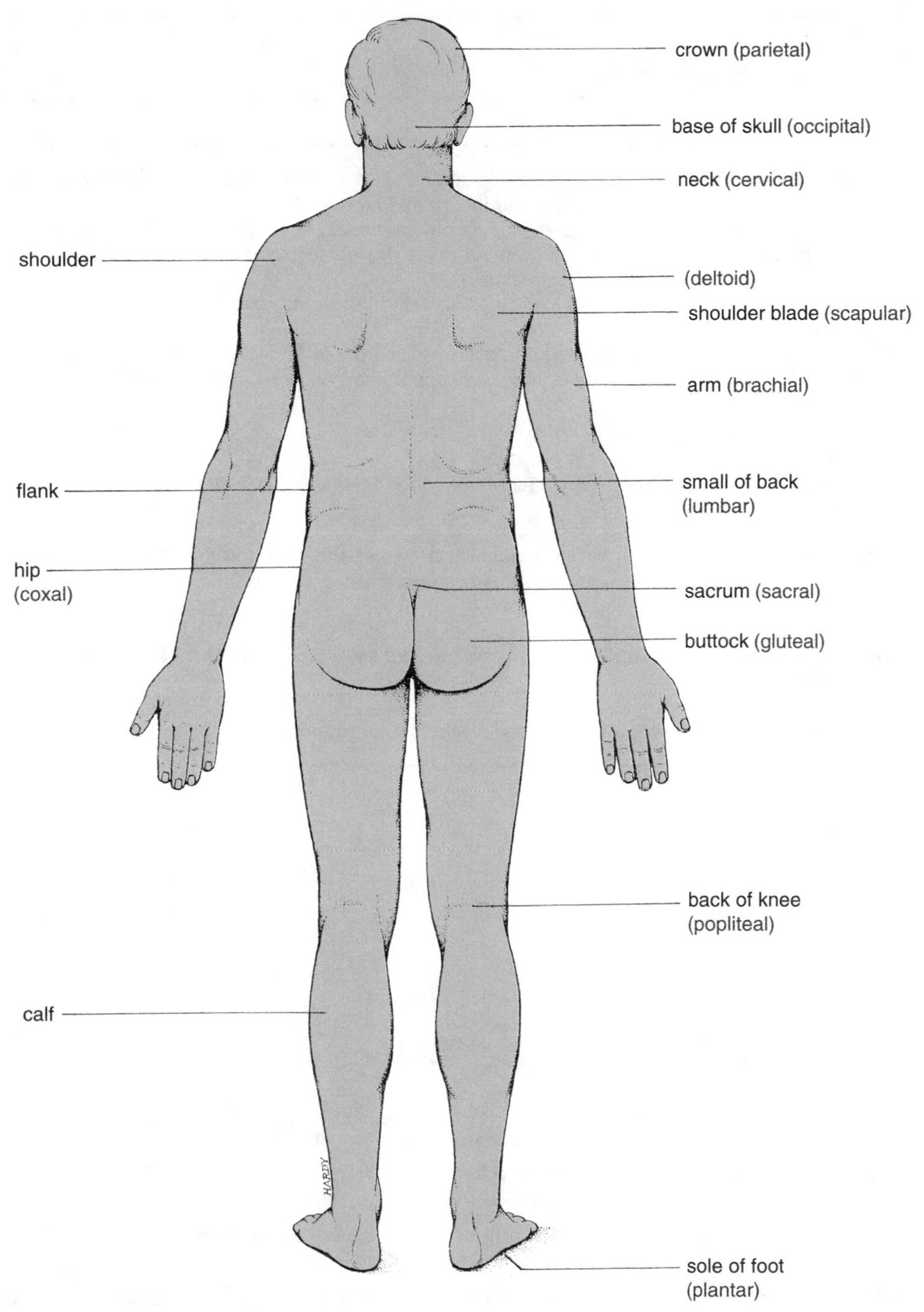

FIGURE 5-7. Common terms for body regions; posterior view.

TABLE 5-2 Body Positions

Position	Description
anatomic position	standing erect, facing forward, arms at sides, palms forward, legs parallel, and toes pointed forward
decubitus position *dē-KŪ-bi-tus*	lying down, specifically according to the part of the body resting on a flat surface, as in left or right lateral decubitus, or dorsal or ventral decubitus
dorsal recumbent position	on back, with legs bent and separated, feet flat
Fowler position	on back, head of bed raised about 18 inches and knees elevated
knee–chest position	on knees, head and upper chest on table, arms crossed above head
left lateral recumbent position	on left side, right leg drawn up
lithotomy position *li-THOT-ō-mē*	on back, legs flexed on abdomen, thighs apart
prone	lying face down
Sims position	on left side, right leg drawn up high and forward, left arm along back, and chest forward resting on bed
supine* *SU-pin*	lying face up
Trendelenburg position *tren-DEL-en-berg*	on back with head lowered by tilting bed back at 45° angle

*To remember the difference between prone and supine, look for the word *up* in supine.

Positions

In addition to the anatomic position, there are other standard positions in which the body is placed for examination or medical procedures. The most common of these are described in Table 5-2.

Roots for the Extremities

Root	Meaning	Example	Definition of Example
acro	extremity, end	acrocyanosis *ak-rō-si-a-NŌ-sis*	bluish discoloration (cyanosis) of the extremities
brachi/o	arm	antebrachium *an-tē-BRĀ-kē-um*	forearm
cheir/o, chir/o	hand	cheirospasm *KĪ-rō-spazm*	spasm of the hand muscles; writer's cramp
ped/o	foot	dextropedal *deks-TROP-e-dal*	using the right foot in preference to the left
pod/o	foot	podiatry *pō-DĪ-a-trē*	study and treatment of the foot
dactyl/o	finger, toe	polydactyly *pol-ē-DAK-tile-ē*	having more than the normal number of fingers or toes

Exercise 5-1

Write the adjective that fits each of the following definitions. The correct suffix is given in parentheses.

1. Pertaining to (-ic) the head ________________
2. Pertaining to (-ic) the chest ________________
3. Pertaining to (-al) the neck ________________
4. Pertaining to (-ar) the lower back ________________
5. Pertaining to (-al) the abdomen ________________

Fill in the blanks:

6. Peritonitis *(per-i-tō-NĪ-tis)* is inflammation (-itis) of the ________________.
7. Celiocentesis *(sē-lē-ō-sen-TĒ-sis)* is surgical puncture (centesis) of the ________________.
8. A laparoscope *(LAP-a-rō-skōp)* is a viewing instrument (-scope) for examining the inside of the body through the ________________.

Exercise 5-2

Fill in the blanks:

1. Acrodermatitis *(ak-rō-der-ma-TĪ-tis)* is inflammation of the skin of the ________________.
2. Macrobrachia *(mak-rō-BRĀ-ke-a)* refers to excessive size of the ________________.
3. A chiropractor is one who treats disorders by use of his or her ________________.
4. Adactyly *(a-DAK-til-ē)* is an absence of the ________________.

Define the following terms:

5. brachiocephalic *(brā-kē-ō-se-FAL-ik)* ________________.
6. podiatrist *(pō-DĪ-a-trist)* ________________.
7. pedal *(PED-al)* ________________.

Prefixes for Position and Direction

Prefix	Meaning	Example	Definition of Example
circum-	around	circumocular *ser-kum-OK-ū-lar*	around the eye
peri-	around	perioral *per-ē-Ō-ral*	around the mouth
intra-	in, within	intrauterine *in-tra-Ū-ter-in*	within the uterus
epi-	upon, over	epidermis *ep-i-DER-mis*	outer layer of the skin (above the dermis)
extra-	outside	extravascular *eks-tra-VAS-kū-lar*	outside the vessels (vascul/o)
infra-*	below	infrascapular *in-fra-SKAP-ū-lar*	below the shoulder blade (scapula)
sub-*	below, under	sublingual *sub-LING-gwal*	under the tongue (lingu/o)
inter-	between	intercostal *in-ter-KOS-tal*	between the ribs (cost/o)
juxta-	near, beside	juxtaposition *juks-ta-pō-zi-shun*	a position near or beside
para-	near, beside	parasagittal *par-a-SAJ-i-tal*	near or beside a sagittal plane
retro-	behind, backward	retroperitoneal *re-trō-per-i-tō-NĒ-al*	behind the peritoneum
supra-	above	suprarenal *su-pra-RĒ-nal*	above the kidney (ren/o)

*Also indicates degree.

Exercise 5-3

Synonyms. Write a word that has the same meaning as each of the words below:

1. perioral ______circumoral______
2. subscapular ____________
3. circumvascular ____________

Define each of the following terms:

4. paranasal
   (par-a-NĀ-zal) ____________

5. retrouterine
   (re-trō-Ū-ter-in) ______________________

6. suprapelvic
   (sū-pra-pel-vik) ______________________

7. intracellular
   (in-tra-SEL-ū-lar) ______________________

Refer to Figures 5-6 and 5-8 to define the following terms:

8. suprapatellar
   (sū-pra-pa-TEL-ar) ______________________

9. extraocular
   (eks-tra-OK-ū-lar) ______________________

10. epicranial
    (ep-i-KRĀ-nē-al) ______________________

11. inframammary
    (in-fra-MAM-a-rē) ______________________

12. intergluteal
    (in-ter-GLŪ-tē-al) ______________________

ADDITIONAL TERMS

digit
(DIJ it)
A finger or toe (adj. digital)

epigastrium
(ep-i-GAS-trē-um)
The epigastric region

fundus
(FUN-dus)
The base or body of a hollow organ; the area of an organ farthest from its opening

hypochondrium
(hī-pō-KON-drē-um)
The hypochondriac region (left or right)

lumen
(LŪ-men)
The central opening within a tube or vessel

meatus
(mē-Ā-tus)
A passage or opening

orifice
(OR-i-fis)
The opening of a cavity

os
Mouth; any body opening

septum
(SEP-tum)
A wall dividing two cavities

sinus
(SĪ-nus)
A cavity, as within a bone

sphincter
(SFINK-ter)
A circular muscle that regulates an opening

ABBREVIATIONS

LLQ Left lower quadrant
LUQ Left upper quadrant
RLQ Right lower quadrant
RUQ Right upper quadrant

Chapter 5
Labeling Exercise

For each of the following illustrations, write the name of each numbered part on the corresponding line of the answer sheet.

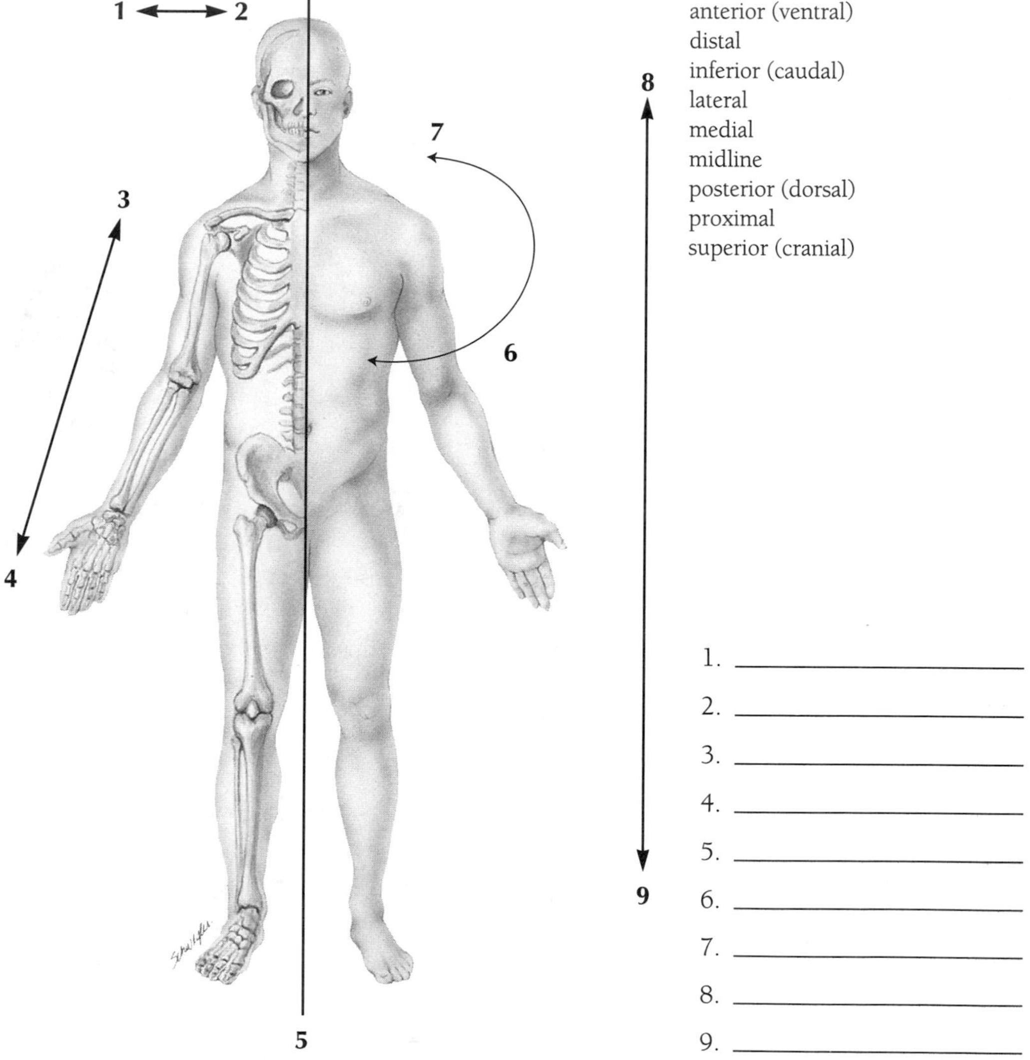

Directional terms

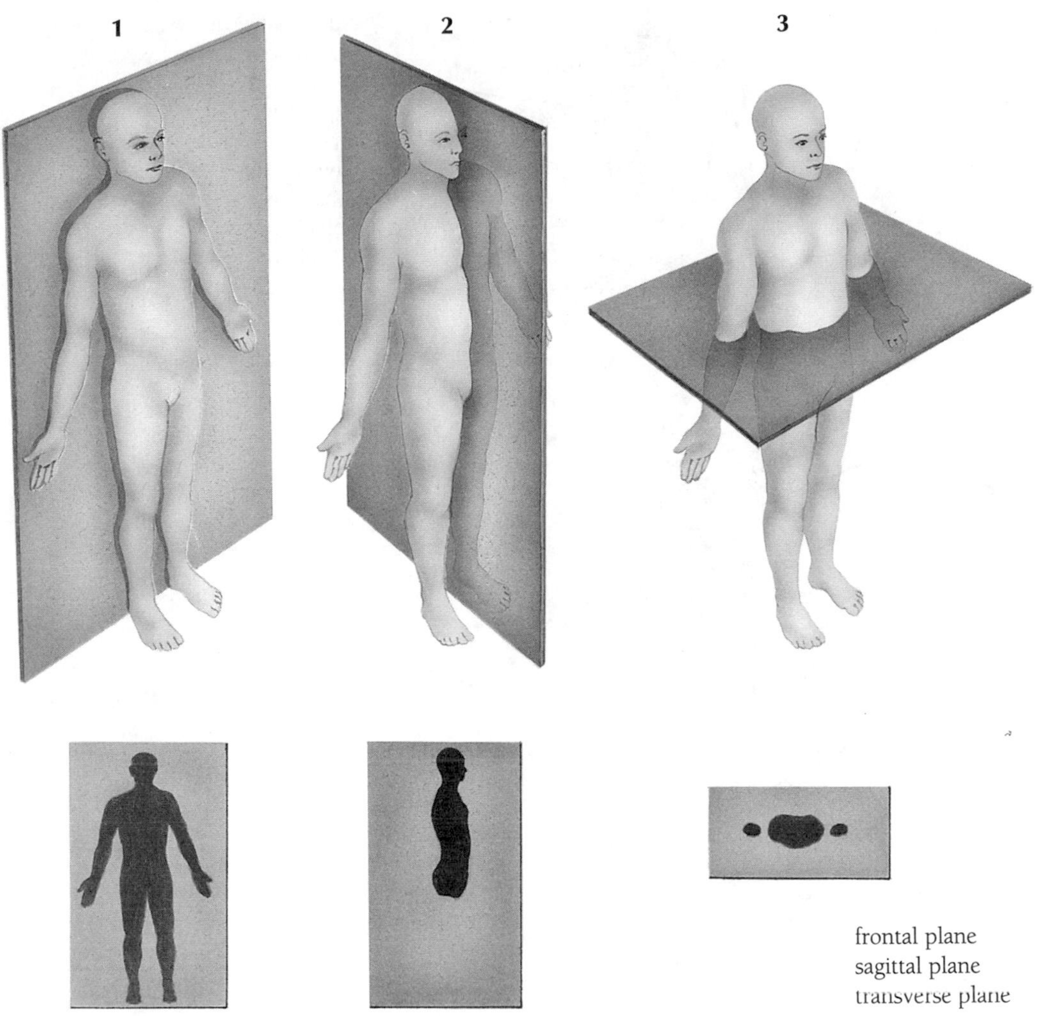

frontal plane
sagittal plane
transverse plane

Planes of division

1. ______________________ 2. ______________________ 3. ______________________

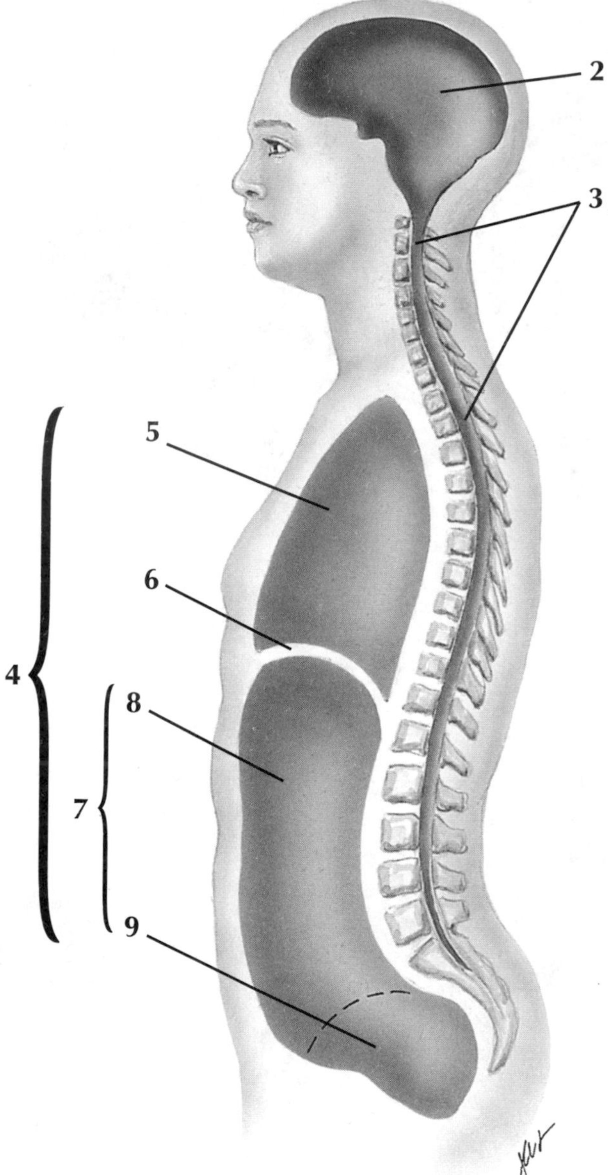

abdominal cavity
abdominopelvic cavity
cranial cavity
diaphragm
dorsal body cavity
pelvic cavity
spinal cavity (canal)
thoracic cavity
ventral body cavity

1. ____________________
2. ____________________
3. ____________________
4. ____________________
5. ____________________
6. ____________________
7. ____________________
8. ____________________
9. ____________________

Side view of body cavities

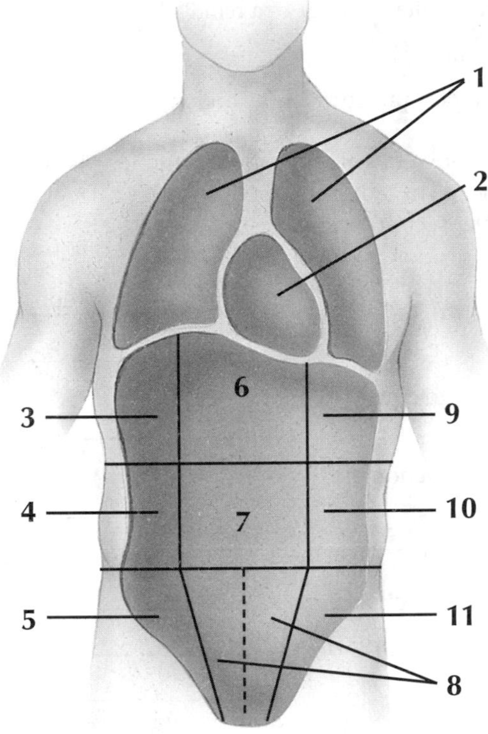

epigastric region
hypogastric region
left hypochondriac region
left iliac (inguinal) region
left lumbar region
pericardial sacs
pleural sacs
right hypochondriac region
right iliac (inguinal) region
right lumbar region
umbilical region

Front view of thoracic cavity and nine regions of the abdomen

1. ____________________
2. ____________________
3. ____________________
4. ____________________
5. ____________________
6. ____________________
7. ____________________
8. ____________________
9. ____________________
10. ____________________
11. ____________________

CHAPTER REVIEW 5

Multiple choice. Match the terms in each of the sets below with their definitions and write the appropriate letter (a–e) to the left of each number:

_____	1. abrachia	a. incision into the chest
_____	2. acrokinesia	b. absence of an arm
_____	3. laparotomy	c. pertaining to the neck and arm
_____	4. cervicobrachial	d. excess motion of the extremities
_____	5. thoracotomy	e. incision through the abdominal wall

_____	6. dactylospasm	a. fusion of the fingers or toes
_____	7. celiocentesis	b. excessive size of the feet

_____ 8. macropodia c. congenital absence of a hand

_____ 9. acheiria d. cramp of a finger or toe

_____ 10. syndactyly e. surgical puncture of the abdomen

True-False. Examine each of the following statements. If the statement is true, write T in the first blank. If the statement is false, write F in the first blank and correct the statement by replacing the underlined word in the second blank.

11. The cranial and spinal cavities are the ventral body cavities. F dorsal
12. The wrist is proximal to the elbow. _____ _____
13. A midsagittal plane divides the body into equal right and left parts. _____ _____
14. A frontal plane divides the body into superior and inferior parts. _____ _____
15. The abdominal cavity is inferior to the thoracic cavity. _____ _____
16. The left hypochondriac region is in the RUQ. _____ _____
17. In the prone position the patient is lying face down. _____ _____
18. Retroversion is a bending backward. _____ _____

Define the following words:

19. intravenous _____
20. retroperitoneal _____
21. subscapular _____
22. sphincter _____
23. lumen _____
24. suprapelvic _____

Synonyms. Write a word that has the same meaning as each of the following words:

25. periocular _____
26. submammary _____
27. dorsal _____
28. anterior _____

Opposites. Write a word that means the opposite of each of the following words:

29. microcephaly _____
30. extracellular _____
31. distal _____
32. inferior _____
33. infrapubic _____
34. superficial _____

Chapter 5
Answer Section

Answers to Chapter Exercises

Exercise 5-1

1. cephalic *(se-FAL-ik)*
2. thoracic *(thō-RAS-ik)*
3. cervical *(SER-vi-kal)*
4. lumbar *(LUM-bar)*
5. abdominal *(ab-DOM-i-nal)*
6. peritoneum
7. abdomen
8. abdominal wall

Exercise 5-2

1. extremities (hands and feet)
2. arms
3. hands
4. fingers or toes
5. pertaining to the arms and head
6. one who studies and treats the foot
7. pertaining to the foot

Exercise 5-3

1. circumoral
2. infrascapular
3. perivascular
4. near the nose
5. behind the uterus
6. above the pelvis
7. within the cell
8. above the kneecap
9. outside the eye
10. upon or over the cranium
11. below the breast
12. between the buttocks

Answers to Labeling Exercises

Directional Terms

1. lateral
2. medial
3. proximal
4. distal
5. midline
6. anterior (ventral)
7. posterior (dorsal)
8. superior (cranial)
9. inferior (caudal)

Planes of Division

1. frontal plane
2. sagittal plane
3. transverse plane

Side View of the Body Cavities

1. dorsal body activity
2. cranial cavity
3. spinal cavity (canal)
4. ventral body cavity
5. thoracic cavity
6. diaphragm
7. abdominopelvic cavity
8. abdominal cavity
9. pelvic cavity

Front View of the Thoracic Cavity and the Nine Regions of the Abdomen

1. pleural sacs
2. pericardial sac
3. right hypochondriac *(hī-pō-KON-drē-ak)* region
4. right lumbar *(LUM-bar)* region
5. right iliac *(IL-ē-ak)* region; also inguinal *(ING-gwi-nal)* region
6. epigastric *(ep-i-GAS-trik)* region
7. umbilical *(um-BIL-i-kal)* region
8. hypogastric *(hī-pō-GAS-trik)* region
9. left hypochondriac region
10. left lumbar region
11. left iliac region; also inguinal *(ING-gwi-nal)* region

Answers to Chapter Review 5

1. b
2. d
3. e
4. c
5. a
6. d
7. e
8. b
9. c
10. a
11. F dorsal
12. F distal
13. T
14. F transverse
15. T
16. F LUQ
17. T
18. T
19. within or into a vein
20. behind the peritoneum
21. below the scapula (shoulder blade)
22. a circular muscle that regulates an opening
23. the central opening within a tube or vessel
24. above the pelvis
25. circumocular
26. inframammary
27. posterior
28. ventral
29. macrocephaly
30. intracellular
31. proximal
32. superior
33. suprapubic
34. deep

6 Disease

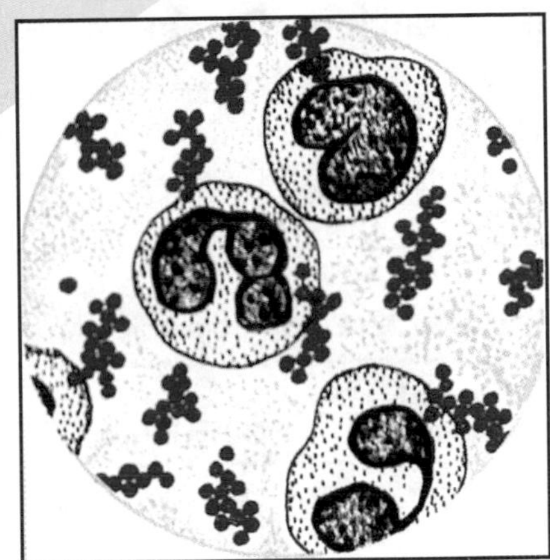

Chapter Contents

Infectious Diseases
Inflammation
Neoplasia
Key Terms
Word Parts Pertaining to Disease
Additional Terms
Abbreviations
Chapter Review
Case Studies
Answers to Exercises

Objectives

After study of this chapter you should be able to:

1. List the major categories of diseases
2. Compare the common types of infectious organisms and list some diseases caused by each
3. Define and give examples of neoplasms
4. Compare the terms *benign* and *malignant*
5. Identify and use the roots, prefixes, and suffixes pertaining to diseases
6. Define the major terms describing types of diseases
7. List and define the major manifestations of diseases

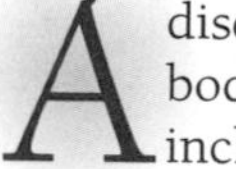
A disease is any alteration from the normal structure or function of any part of the body. Diseases fall into a number of different, but often overlapping, categories. These include:

1. Infectious diseases
2. Degenerative diseases
3. Hormonal and metabolic disorders
4. Immune disorders, including allergies
5. Neoplasia
6. Psychiatric disorders

Infectious Diseases

Infectious diseases are caused by viruses, bacteria, fungi (yeasts and molds), protozoa (single-celled animals), and worms (Table 6-1). Bacteria are either round (cocci), rod-shaped (bacilli), or spiral (spirochetes). They may be named according to their shape and also by the arrangements

TABLE 6-1 Common Infectious Organisms

Type of Organism	Description	Examples of Diseases Caused
Bacteria *bak-TĒ-rē-a*	simple microscopic organisms that are widespread throughout the world, and some of which can produce disease. Sing. bacterium *(bak-TĒ-rē-um)*	
cocci *KOK-sī*	round bacteria. May be in clusters (staphylococci), chains (streptococci), and other formations. Sing. coccus *(KOK-us)*	pneumonia, rheumatic fever, food poisoning, septicemia, urinary tract infections, gonorrhea
bacilli *ba-SIL-ī*	rod-shaped bacteria. Sing. bacillus *(ba-SIL-us)*	typhoid, dysentery, salmonellosis, tuberculosis, botulism, tetanus
spi-rochetes *SPĪ-rō-kētz*	corkscrew-shaped bacteria	Lyme disease, syphilis, Vincent's disease
chlamydia *kla-MID-ē-a*	organisms smaller than bacteria that, like viruses, grow in living cells, but are susceptible to antibiotics	conjunctivitis, trachoma, pelvic inflammatory disease (PID), and other sexually transmitted diseases (STDs)
rickettsia *ri-KET-sē-a*	similar in growth to chlamydia	typhus, Rocky Mountain spotted fever
Viruses *VĪ-rus-es*	submicroscopic infectious agents that can live and reproduce only within living cells	colds, herpes, hepatitis, measles, chickenpox, influenza, AIDS
Fungi *FUN-jī*	simple, nongreen plants, some of which are parasitic; includes yeasts and molds. Sing. fungus *(FUN-gus)*	candidiasis, skin infections (tinea, ringworm), valley fever
Protozoa *prō-tō-ZŌ-a*	single-celled animals. Sing. protozoon *(prō-tō-ZŌ-on)*	dysentery, *Trichomonas* infection, malaria
Helminths *HEL-minths*	worms	trichinosis, infestations with roundworms, pinworms, hookworms

KEY TERMS*

R T E M S

benign (*bē-NĪN*) — Not recurrent or malignant; favorable for recovery; describing tumors which do not spread

carcinoma (*kar-si-NŌ-ma*) — A malignant neoplasm composed of epithelial cells (from G. root *carcin* meaning "crab") (adj. carcinomatous)

cyst (*sist*) — A filled sac or pouch that is usually abnormal; also used as a root meaning a normal bladder or sac, such as the urinary bladder or gallbladder (root cyst/o, cyst/i)

hernia (*HER-nē-a*) — Protrusion of an organ through an abnormal opening; a rupture (Fig. 6-1)

malignant (*ma-LIG-nant*) — Growing worse; harmful; tending to cause death; describing tumors that spread (metastasize)

metastasis (*me-TAS-ta-sis*) — A spreading from one part of the body to another; characteristic of cancer

neoplasm (*NĒ-ō-plazm*) — An abnormal and uncontrolled growth of tissue, namely, a tumor; may be benign or malignant

parasite (*PAR-a-sīt*) — An organism that grows on or in another organism (the host), causing damage to it

pathogen (*PATH-ō-jen*) — An organism capable of causing disease (root path/o)

*See also Table 6-1 on infectious diseases.

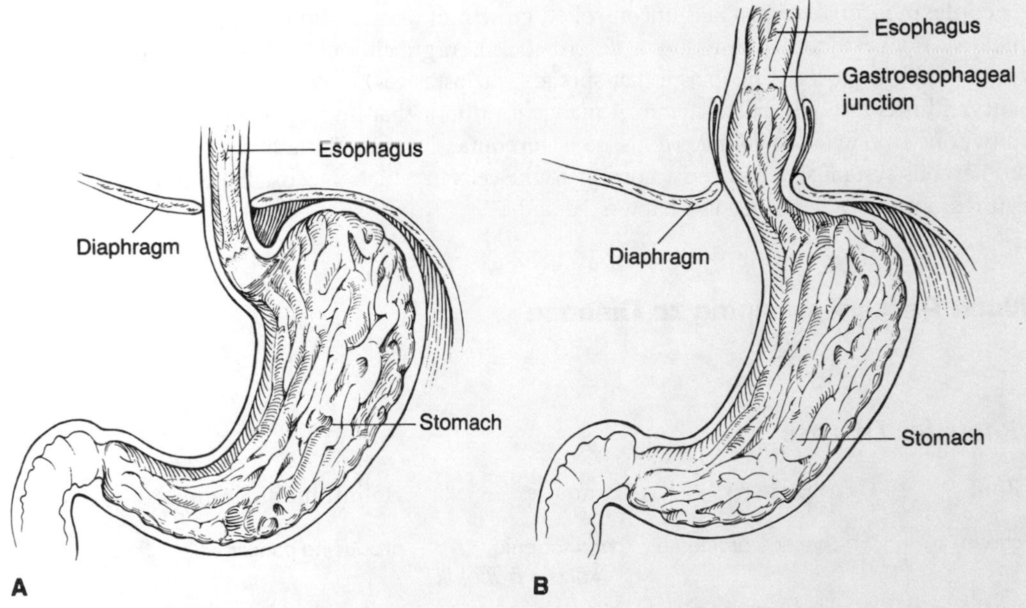

FIGURE 6-1. **(A)** Normal. **(B)** Hiatal hernia. The stomach protrudes through the diaphragm into the thoracic cavity, raising the level of the junction between the esophagus and the stomach.

(continued)

prolapse *(PRŌ-laps)*	A dropping of an organ or part; ptosis
pus	A product of inflammation consisting of fluid and white blood cells (root py/o)
sarcoma *(sar-KŌ-ma)*	A malignant neoplasm arising from connective tissue (from G. root *sarco* meaning "flesh") (adj. sarcomatous)
toxin *(TOKS-in)*	A poison (adj. toxic); (roots tox/o, toxic/o)

they form. They also are described according to the dyes they take up when stained in the laboratory.

Inflammation

A common response to infection, irritation, and other forms of disease is **inflammation**. When cells are injured, blood is quickly delivered to the damaged tissue by the circulation. This inrush of blood results in the four signs of inflammation: heat, pain, redness, and swelling.

Neoplasia

A **neoplasm** is an abnormal and uncontrolled growth of tissue, a tumor or growth. A neoplasm that does not spread to other tissues is described as **benign**, although it may cause damage at the site in which it grows. A neoplasm that spreads (metastasizes) to other tissues is termed **malignant**, and is commonly called *cancer*. A malignant tumor that involves epithelial tissue is **carcinoma**; one that involves connective tissue is **sarcoma**. Cancers of the blood, lymphatic system, and nervous system are classified according to the cells in which they originate and other clinical features. These are described in Chapters 10 and 17.

Word Parts Pertaining to Disease

Roots for Disease

Root	Meaning	Example	Definition of Example
carcin/o	cancer, carcinoma	carcinogenic *kar-sin-ō-JEN-ik*	producing cancer
cyst/o, cyst/i	filled sac or pouch, cyst, bladder	cystic *SIS-tik*	pertaining to or having cysts
lith	calculus, stone	lithiasis *lith-Ī-a-sis*	stone formation

(continued)

Roots for Disease (Continued)

Root	Meaning	Example	Definition of Example
onc/o	tumor	oncology *on-KOL-ō-jē*	study and treatment of tumors
path/o	disease	pathogen *PATH-ō-jen*	organism that produces disease
py/o	pus	pyorrhea *pī-ō-RĒ-a*	a discharge (-rhea) of pus
pyr/o, pyret/o	fever, fire	pyretic *pī-RET-ik*	pertaining to fever
scler/o	hard	sclerosis *skle-RŌ-sis*	hardening of tissue
tox/o, toxic/o	poison	endotoxin *en-dō-TOK-sin*	toxin present within bacterial cells

Exercise 6-1

Identify and define the root in each of the following words:

	Root	Meaning of Root
1. pyrexia *(pī-REK-sē-a)*	______	______
2. intoxicate *(in-TOK-si-kāt)*	______	______
3. empyema *(em-pī-Ē-ma)*	______	______

Fill in the blanks:

4. Carcinolysis *(kar-sin-OL-i-sis)* is the destruction (-lysis) of a(n) ______.
5. A urolith *(Ū-rō-lith)* is a(n) ______ in the urinary tract (ur/o).
6. An oncogene *(ON-kō-jēn)* is a gene that causes a(n) ______.
7. Pathology *(pa-THOL-ō-jē)* is the study of ______.
8. A pyocyst *(PĪ-ō-sist)* is a sac or cyst containing ______.
9. Arteriosclerosis *(ar-tē-rē-ō-skle-RŌ-sis)* is a(n) ______ of the arteries.
10. The term *toxoid (TOK-soyd)* means like a(n) ______.

Prefixes for Disease

Prefix	Meaning	Example	Definition of Example
brady-	slow	bradycardia *brad-ē-KAR-dē-a*	slow heart (cardi/o) rate

(continued)

Prefixes for Disease (Continued)

Prefix	Meaning	Example	Definition of Example
dys-	abnormal, painful, difficult	dysplasia *dis-PLĀ-zha*	abnormal development of tissue
mal-	bad, poor	malabsorption *mal-ab-SORP-shun*	poor absorption of food from the digestive tract
pachy-	thick	pachyemia *pak-ē-Ē-mē-a*	thickness of the blood (-emia)
tachy-	rapid	tachypnea *tak-ip-NĒ-a*	rapid breathing (-pnea)
xero-	dry	xerosis *zē-RŌ-sis*	dryness of the skin or membranes

Exercise 6-2

Match each of the five terms below with its definition and write the appropriate letter (a–e) to the left of each number:

_____ 1. dystrophy *(DIS-trō-fē)*
_____ 2. tachycardia *(tak-i-KAR-dē-a)*
_____ 3. bradypnea *(brad-ip-NĒ-a)*
_____ 4. xeroderma *(zē-rō-DER-ma)*
_____ 5. dysphagia *(dis-FĀ-jē-a)*

a. dryness of the skin
b. rapid heart rate
c. difficulty in eating
d. slow breathing rate
e. poor nourishment of tissue

Identify and define the prefix in each of the following words:

	Prefix	Meaning of Prefix
6. malnutrition *(mal-nu-TRISH-un)*	_____	_____
7. dysentery *(DIS-en-ter-ē)*	_____	_____
8. pachyderma *(pak-ē-DER-ma)*	_____	_____

Suffixes for Disease

Suffix	Meaning	Example	Definition of Example
-algia, -algesia	pain	gastralgia *gas-TRAL-jē-a*	pain in the stomach (gastr/o)
-cele	hernia, localized dilation	hydrocele *HĪ-drō-sēl*	localized dilation containing fluid

(continued)

Suffixes for Disease (Continued)

Suffix	Meaning	Example	Definition of Example
-clasis, -clasia	breaking	osteoclasis *os-tē-OK-la-sis*	breaking of a bone (oste/o)
-itis	inflammation	encephalitis *en-sef-a-LĪ-tis*	inflammation of the brain (encephal/o)
-megaly	enlargement	splenomegaly *splē-nō-MEG-a-lē*	enlargement of the spleen (splen/o)
-odynia	pain	urodynia *ū-rō-DIN-ē-a*	pain on urination (ur/o)
-oma*	tumor	lipoma *lip-Ō-ma*	a fatty tumor
-pathy	any disease of	myopathy *mi-OP-a-thē*	any disease of muscle (my/o)
-rhage†, -rhagia†	bursting forth, profuse flow, hemorrhage	hemorrhage *HEM-or-ij*	profuse flow of blood
-rhea†	flow, discharge	diarrhea *dī-a-RĒ-a*	frequent passage of watery stool
-rhexis†	rupture	amniorrhexis *am-nē-ō-REK-sis*	rupture of the amniotic sac (bag of waters)
-schisis	fissure, splitting	retinoschisis *ret-i-NOS-ki-sis*	splitting of the retina of the eye

*Plural: -omas, -omata

†Remember to double the *r* when adding this suffix to a root.

Exercise 6-3

Matching. Match the terms in each of the sets below with their definitions and write the appropriate letter (a–e) to the left of each number:

_____	1. thoracoschisis *(thō-ra-KOS-ki-sis)*	a. breaking of a nucleus
_____	2. adipocele *(AD-i-pō-sēl)*	b. congenital fissure of the chest
_____	3. karyoclasis *(kar-ē-OK-la-sis)*	c. any disease of a gland
_____	4. blastoma *(blas-TŌ ma)*	d. hernia containing fat
_____	5. adenopathy *(ad-e-NOP-a-thē)*	e. tumor of immature cells

_____	6. hemorrhagic *(hem-or-AJ-ik)*	a. rupture of the liver
_____	7. hepatorrhexis *(hep-a-tō-REK-sis)*	b. discharge of mucus
_____	8. analgesia *(an-al-JĒ-zē-a)*	c. absence of pain
_____	9. mucorrhea *(mū-kō-RĒ-a)*	d. pain in a gland
_____	10. adenodynia *(ad-e-nō-DIN-ē-a)*	e. pertaining to a profuse flow of blood

The root *gastr/o* means "stomach". Define the following terms:

11. gastromegaly (*gas-trō-MEG-a-lē*) enlargement of the stomach
12. gastritis (*gas-TRĪ-tis*) ____________
13. gastropathy (*gas-TROP-a-thē*) ____________
14. gastrocele (*GAS-trō-sēl*) ____________

Some words pertaining to disease are used as suffixes in compound words. As previously noted, the term *suffix* is used in this book to mean any word part that consistently appears at the end of words. This may be a simple suffix (such as -y, -ia, -ic), a word, or a root–suffix combination (such as -megaly, -rhagia, -pathy).

Words for Disease Used as Suffixes

Word	Meaning	Example	Definition of Example
dilation*, dilatation*	expansion, widening	vasodilation *vas-ō-dī-LĀ-shun*	widening of blood vessels (vas/o)
ectasia, ectasis	dilation	bronchiectasis *brong-kē-EK-ta-sis*	chronic dilation of a bronchus (bronchi/o)
edema	accumulation of fluid, swelling	lymphedema *lim-fe-DĒ-ma*	swelling of tissues as a result of lymphatic blockage
lysis*	separation, loosening, dissolving, destruction	dialysis *dī-AL-i-sis*	separation of substances by passage through a membrane
malacia	softening	hepatomalacia *hep-at-ō-ma-LĀ-shē-a*	softening of the liver (hepat/o)
necrosis	death of	osteonecrosis *os-tē-ō-ne-KRŌ-sis*	death of bone tissue (oste/o)
ptosis	dropping, downward displacement, prolapse	blepharoptosis *blef-e-rop-TŌ-sis*	drooping of the eyelid (blephar/o) (Fig. 6-2)
spasm	sudden contraction, cramp	bronchospasm *BRONG-kō-spazm*	spasm of a bronchus (bronch/o)
stasis*	suppression, stoppage	menostasis *men-OS-ta-sis*	suppression of menstrual (men/o) flow
stenosis	narrowing, constriction	tracheostenosis *trā-kē-ō-ste-NŌ-sis*	narrowing of the trachea

*May also refer to treatment.

The words toxic, toxin, and sclerosis are also used as suffixes in compound words. The words carcinoma and sarcoma are used as suffixes to indicate malignant tumors, as in adenocarcinoma, fibrosarcoma.

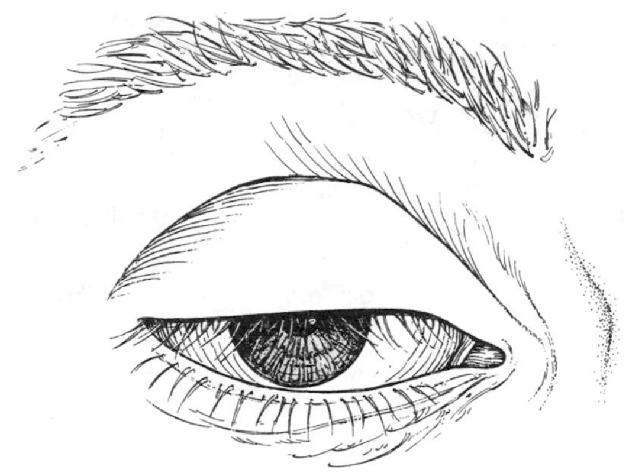

FIGURE 6-2. Blepharoptosis. Drooping of the eyelid.

Exercise 6-4

Match each of the five terms below with its definition and write the appropriate letter (a–e) to the left of each number:

_____ 1. hemolysis *(hē-MOL-i-sis)* a. death of bone tissue

_____ 2. gastrectasia *(gas-trek-TĀ-sē-a)* b. dilatation of the stomach

_____ 3. hemostasis *(hē mō-STĀ-sis)* c. softening of the skull

_____ 4. osteonecrosis *(os-tē-ō-ne-KRŌ-sis)* d. destruction of red blood cells

_____ 5. craniomalacia *(krā-nē-ō-ma-LĀ-shē-a)* e. stoppage of blood flow

The root *bronch/o* means "bronchus," an air passageway in the lungs. Define the following words:

6. bronchodilation *(brong-kō-dī-LĀ-shun)* widening of a bronchus
7. bronchoedema *(brong-kō-e-DĒ-ma)* _____________
8. bronchospasm *(BRONG-kō-spazm)* _____________
9. bronchostenosis *(brong-kō-ste-NO-sis)* _____________

Word Parts for Infectious Diseases

Word Part	Meaning	Example	Definition of Example
Prefixes			
staphyl/o	grapelike cluster	staphylococcus *staf-i-lō-KOK-us*	a round bacterium that forms clusters
strept/o	twisted chain	streptobacillus *strep-tō-ba-SIL-us*	a rod-shaped bacterium that forms chains

(continued)

Word Parts for Infectious Diseases (Continued)

Word Part	Meaning	Example	Definition of Example
Roots			
bacill/i, bacill/o	bacillus	bacilluria *bas-i-LŪ-rē-a*	bacilli in the urine (-uria)
bacteri/o	bacterium	bactericide *bak-TER-i-sīd*	agent that kills (-cide) bacteria
myc/o	fungus, mold	mycosis *mī-KŌ-sis*	any disease condition caused by a fungus
vir/o	virus	viremia *vī-RĒ-mē-a*	presence of viruses in the blood (-emia)

Exercise 6-5

Fill in the blanks:

1. The term *bacillary* (*BAS-il-a-rē*) means pertaining to ____________
2. The prefix *staphylo-* means ____________
3. The prefix *strepto-* means ____________

Use the suffix *-logy* to write a word that means each of the following:

4. Study of viruses ____________
5. Study of fungi ____________
6. Study of bacteria ____________

ADDITIONAL TERMS

General Terms Pertaining to Disease

acid-fast stain
A laboratory staining procedure used mainly to identify the tuberculosis organism

acute (*a-KŪT*)
Sudden, severe; having a short course

chronic (*KRON-ik*)
Of long duration; progressing slowly

etiology (*ē-tē-OL-ō-jē*)
The cause of a disease

exacerbation (*eks-zas-er-BĀ-shun*)
Worsening of disease; increase in severity of a disease or its symptoms

(continued)

Gram stain — A laboratory staining procedure that divides bacteria into two groups: Gram positive, which stain blue, and Gram negative, which stain red

iatrogenic *(ī-at-rō-JEN-ik)* — Caused by the effects of treatment (from G. root *iatro-* meaning "physician")

idiopathic *(id-ē-ō-PATH-ik)* — Having no known cause

in situ *(in SĪ-tū)* — Localized, noninvasive (literally "in position"); said of tumors that do not spread, such as carcinoma *in situ* (CIS)

nosocomial *(nos-ō-KŌ-mē-al)* — Describing an infection acquired in a hospital (root *nos/o* means "disease," and *comial* refers to a hospital)

opportunistic *(op-por-tū-NIS-tik)* — Describing an infection that occurs because of a poor or altered condition of the host

remission *(rē-MISH-un)* — A lessening of disease symptoms; the period during which such lessening occurs

sepsis *(SEP-sis)* — The presence of harmful microorganisms or their toxins in the blood or other tissues (adj. septic)

septicemia *(sep-ti-SĒ-mē-a)* — Presence of pathogenic bacteria in the blood; blood poisoning

systemic *(sis-TEM-ik)* — Pertaining to the whole body

trauma *(TRAW-ma)* — A physical or psychological wound or injury (adj. traumatic)

Manifestations of Disease

abscess *(AB-ses)* — A localized collection of pus

adhesion *(ad-HĒ-zhun)* — A uniting of two surfaces or parts that may normally be separated

anaplasia *(a-na-PLĀ-zha)* — Lack of normal differentiation shown by cancer cells

ascites *(a-SĪ-tēz)* — Accumulation of fluid in the peritoneal cavity

cellulitis *(sel-ū-LĪ-tis)* — A spreading inflammation of tissue

effusion *(e-FŪ-zhun)* — Escape of fluid into a cavity or other body part

exudate *(EKS-ū-dāt)* — Material that escapes from blood vessels as a result of injury to tissues

fissure *(FISH-ur)* — A groove or split

fistula *(FIS-tū-la)* — An abnormal passage between two organs or from an organ to the surface of the body

gangrene *(GANG-grēn)* — Death of tissue, usually caused by lack of blood supply. May be associated with bacterial infection and decomposition.

hyperplasia *(hī-per-PLĀ-zha)*	Excessive growth of normal cells in normal arrangement
hypertrophy *(hī-PER-trō-fē)*	An increase in size of an organ without increase in the number of cells; may result from an increase in activity, as in muscles
induration *(in-dū-RĀ-shun)*	Hardening; an abnormally hard spot or place
lesion *(LĒ-zhun)*	A distinct area of damaged tissue; an injury or wound
metaplasia *(met-a-PLĀ-zha)*	Conversion of cells to a form that is not normal for that tissue (prefix *meta* means "change")
polyp *(POL-ip)*	A tumor attached by a thin stalk
prolapse *(prō-LAPS)*	A dropping of an organ or part; ptosis
purulent *(PUR-ū-lent)*	Forming or containing pus
suppuration *(sup-ū-RĀ-shun)*	Pus formation

ABBREVIATIONS

CA cancer

CIS carcinoma *in situ*

FUO fever of unknown origin

staph staphylococcus

strep streptococcus

CHAPTER REVIEW 6

Multiple choice. Match the terms in each of the sets below with their definitions and write the appropriate letter (a–e) to the left of each number:

_____ 1. apyrexia	a. incision to remove a stone
_____ 2. detoxification	b. hardened
_____ 3. sclerotic	c. absence of a fever
_____ 4. oncolysis	d. destruction of a tumor
_____ 5. lithotomy	e. removal of poisons

_____ 6. xerotic	a. dry
_____ 7. dyskinesia	b. thickness of the blood
_____ 8. pachyemia	c. swelling of the fingers or toes

_____ 9. pyorrhea d. abnormal movement

_____ 10. dactyledema e. discharge of pus

_____ 11. lesion a. self destruction

_____ 12. nephroptosis b. local wound or injury

_____ 13. hemostasis c. dilatation

_____ 14. ectasia d. stoppage of blood flow

_____ 15. autolysis e. dropping of the kidney

_____ 16. cardiorrhexis a. inflammation of a gland

_____ 17. stenosis b. rupture of the heart

_____ 18. cephaledema c. narrowing

_____ 19. adenitis d. presence of pathogens in the blood

_____ 20. septicemia e. accumulation of fluid in the head

_____ 21. bacilli a. round bacteria in clusters

_____ 22. helminths b. round bacteria in chains

_____ 23. streptococci c. fungal infection

_____ 24. mycosis d. rod-shaped bacteria

_____ 25. staphylococci e. worms

Fill in the blanks:

26. Any abnormal and uncontrolled growth of tissue, whether benign or malignant, is called a(n) _____________________.
27. Heat, pain, redness, and swelling are the four major signs of _____________________.
28. The spreading of cancer to other parts of the body is called _____________________.
29. A malignant tumor of connective tissue is called _____________________.
30. Another name for a poison is _____________________.
31. Death of tissue is called _____________________.
32. A sudden contraction or cramp is called a(n) _____________________.
33. Protrusion of an organ through an abnormal opening is a(n) _____________________.

Word building. Use *-genesis* as a suffix to write words with the following meanings:

34. Formation of cancer carcinogenesis
35. Origin of any disease _____________________
36. Formation of a tumor _____________________
37. Formation of pus _____________________

The root *neur/o* pertains to the nervous system or a nerve. Add a suffix to this root to form words with the following meanings:

38. Any disease of the nervous system ____________________
39. Inflammation of a nerve ____________________
40. Pain in a nerve ____________________
41. Tumor of the nervous system ____________________

Use the root *oste/o*, meaning "bone," to form words with the following meanings:

42. Softening of a bone ____________________
43. Tumor of a bone ____________________
44. Destruction of bone tissue ____________________
45. Breaking of a bone ____________________

Chapter 6

Case Studies

1. Esophageal Spasm

This patient is a 53-year-old female who has consulted for occasional episodes of dysphagia with moderate to severe tight, gripping pain in the mid-thorax. The onset is sudden following ingestion of food or beverage. The pain is retrosternal at first and then radiates to the cervical and dorsal regions. It is not improved by assuming a supine position. There is no vomiting or dyspnea. In the absence of other symptoms, esophageal spasm is suspected. If difficulties persist, fluoroscopy with a barium swallow will be done to rule out paraesophageal hiatal hernia.

2. HIV Infection and Tuberculosis

This patient is a 48-year-old male who for 4 weeks has experienced fever, night sweats, coughing, malaise, and a 10-pound loss of weight. He admits to intravenous drug use and ingests approximately 12 oz of alcohol daily. Physical examination shows bilateral anterior cervical and axillary adenopathy and pyrexia of 38.9°C. Chest x-ray shows paratracheal adenopathy and bilateral interstitial infiltrates. Laboratory tests are positive for HIV and show a low lymphocyte count. Sputum and bronchoscopic lavage (wash) fluid is positive for an acid-fast organism. A PPD test is scheduled for TB, to be done with a control for immunologic deficiency. Results of a chest radiograph will be evaluated before determining therapy.

3. Laparoscopy and Laparotomy

The patient was taken to the operating room under general anesthetic. A pneumoperitoneum was performed for usual laparoscopy procedure per an infra-umbilical incision. Visualization of the abdominal viscera was complicated by multiple small bowel adhesions. The laparoscopy instruments were therefore withdrawn. Interrupted 3-0 Vicryl sutures were placed periumbilically. An exploratory laparotomy was then performed by means of a midline incision. Intestinal adhesions were lysed. The remainder of the abdomen appeared normal, but a small nodule was removed from the posterior pelvis. Copious irrigation was performed followed by closure of the peritoneal cavity. The skin was approximated with staples. Blood loss was less than 100 mL. The patient tolerated the procedure well and was taken to the recovery room in satisfactory condition.

Chapter 6
Case Study Questions

Multiple choice. Select the best answer and write the letter of your choice in the blank to the left of each number:

_____ 1. The term *supine* means
a. lying face down
b. standing in the anatomic position
c. sitting
d. lying face up
e. lying on one's side

_____ 2. The cervical region is the region of the
a. heart
b. arm
c. neck
d. head
e. leg

_____ 3. A word that means the same as *dorsal* is
a. anterior
b. inferior
c. posterior
d. superior
e. caudal

_____ 4. In referring to tissues, the term *interstitial* means
a. around cells
b. within cells
c. through cells
d. between cells
e. under cells

_____ 5. The term *axillary* refers to the region of the
a. bladder
b. armpit
c. abdomen
d. leg
e. wrist

_____ 6. The term *pyrexia* refers to a
a. fever
b. spasm
c. stone
d. poison
e. tumor

_____ 7. The phrase "adhesions were lysed" means that
a. parts were joined together
b. joined parts were separated
c. parts were removed
d. specimens were taken
e. parts were measured

_____ 8. The term *pneumoperitoneum* refers to inflation (pneum/o) of the:
a. thoracic cavity
b. abdominal cavity
c. dorsal cavity
d. pleural cavity
e. cranial cavity

_____ 9. The main disease organism identified by the acid-fast stain is
a. the common cold virus
b. staphylococcus
c. a protozoon
d. the diphtheria bacillus
e. the tuberculosis bacillus

Identify and define the prefix in each of the following words:

	Prefix	Meaning of Prefix
10. retrosternal	______	______
11. paraesophageal	______	______
12. dyspnea	______	______
13. Infra-umbilical	______	______

Fill in the blanks:

14. The word in the case studies that means "pain or difficulty in swallowing" is ____________________

15. The word that means "protrusion of an organ through an abnormal body opening" is ____________________

16. Adenopathy is any disease of a(n) ____________________

17. The word that means "on both sides" is ____________________

18. The root *lapar/o* in laparotomy and laparoscopy means ____________________

Chapter 6
Answer Section

Answers to Chapter Exercises

Exercise 6-1

1. pyr/o; fever
2. toxic/o; poison
3. py/o; pus
4. cancer, carcinoma
5. calculus, stone
6. tumor
7. disease
8. pus
9. hardening
10. poison, toxin

Exercise 6-2

1. e
2. b
3. d
4. a
5. c
6. mal; bad, poor
7. dys; abnormal, painful, difficult
8. pachy; thick

Exercise 6-3

1. b
2. d
3. a
4. e
5. c
6. e
7. a
8. c
9. b
10. d
11. enlargement of the stomach
12. inflammation of the stomach
13. any disease of the stomach
14. hernia of the stomach

Exercise 6-4

1. d
2. b
3. e
4. a
5. c
6. widening of a bronchus
7. accumulation of fluid in or swelling of a bronchus
8. sudden contraction (spasm) of a bronchus
9. narrowing of a bronchus

Exercise 6-5

1. bacilli or a bacillus
2. grapelike cluster
3. twisted chains
4. virology *(vī-ROL-ō-jē)*
5. mycology *(mī-KOL-ō-jē)*
6. bacteriology *(bak-tēr-ē-OL-ō-jē)*

Answers to Chapter Review 6

1. c
2. e
3. b
4. d
5. a
6. a
7. d
8. b
9. e
10. c
11. b
12. e
13. d
14. c
15. a
16. b
17. c
18. e
19. a
20. d
21. d
22. e
23. b
24. c
25. a
26. neoplasm
27. inflammation
28. metastasis
29. sarcoma
30. toxin
31. necrosis
32. spasm
33. hernia
34. carcinogenesis
35. pathogenesis
36. oncogenesis
37. pyogenesis
38. neuropathy *(nū-ROP-a-thē)*
39. neuritis *(nū-RĪ-tis)*
40. neuralgia *(nū-RAL-jē-a)*
41. neuroma *(nū-RŌ-ma)*
42. osteomalacia *(os-tē-ō-ma-LĀ-shē-a)*
43. osteoma *(os-tē-Ō-ma)*
44. osteolysis *(os-tē-OL-i-sis)*
45. osteoclasis *(os-tē-OK-la-sis)*

Answers to Case Study Questions

1. d
2. c
3. c
4. d
5. b
6. a
7. b
8. b
9. e
10. retro-; behind
11. para-; near, beside
12. dys-; abnormal, painful, difficult
13. infra-; below
14. dysphagia
15. hernia
16. gland
17. bilateral
18. abdominal wall

7 Diagnosis and Treatment; Surgery

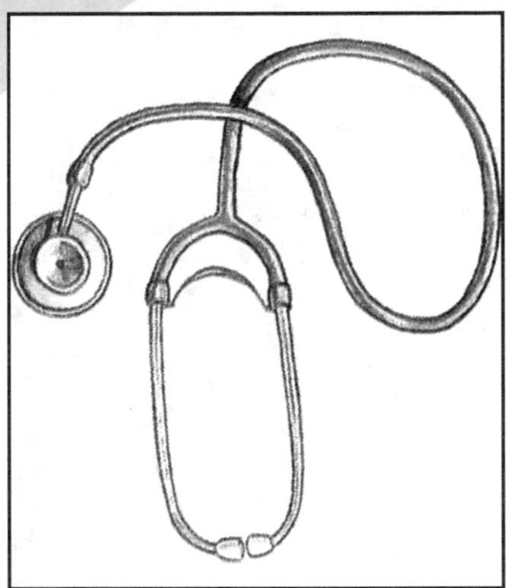

Chapter Contents

Diagnosis
Imaging Techniques
Treatment
Cancer
Key Terms
Word Parts Pertaining to Diagnosis and Treatment
Additional Terms
Abbreviations
Chapter Review
Case Studies
Answers to Exercises

Objectives

After study of this chapter you should be able to:

1. Describe the main methods used in examination of a patient
2. List the main components of a medical history
3. Name seven forms of treatment
4. Describe how staging is used in treatment of cancer
5. Name and describe nine imaging techniques
6. Define basic terms pertaining to medical examination, diagnosis, and treatment
7. Identify and use the roots and suffixes pertaining to diagnosis and surgery
8. Interpret abbreviations used in diagnosis and treatment

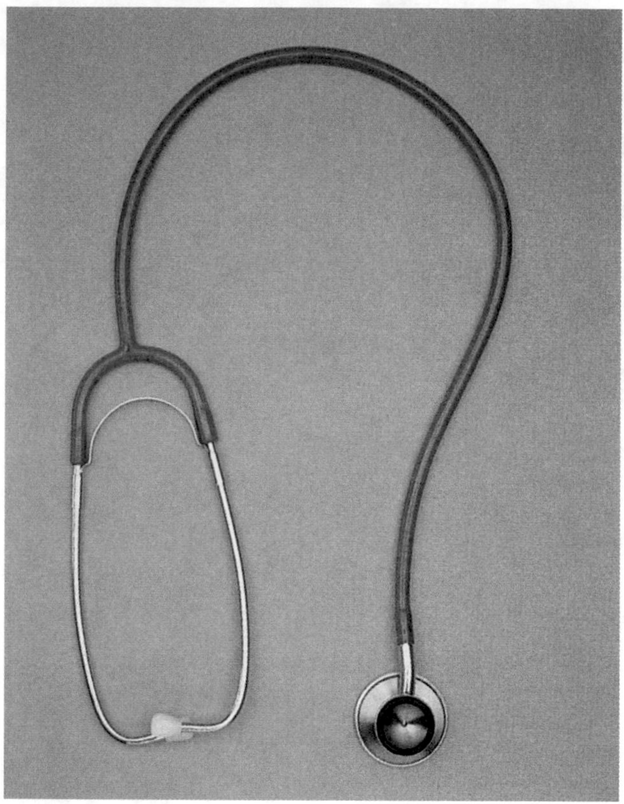

FIGURE 7-1. Stethoscope. (Photograph © Ken Kasper. From Taylor C, Lillis CA, LeMone P: Fundamentals of Nursing, 2nd ed, p 413. Philadelphia: JB Lippincott, 1993.)

Diagnosis

Medical diagnosis begins with a patient history. This includes a history of the present illness with a description of **symptoms**, a past medical history, a family and a social history.

A physical examination, which includes a review of all systems, follows the history taking. Practitioners use techniques of **inspection**, **palpation**, **percussion**, and **auscultation** (see Key Terms) to perform physicals. Tools such as the **stethoscope** (Fig. 7-1), for listening to body sounds; **ophthalmoscope** (Fig. 7-2A), for examination of the eyes; **otoscope** (Fig. 7-2B), for examination of the ears; and blood pressure apparatus also are employed.

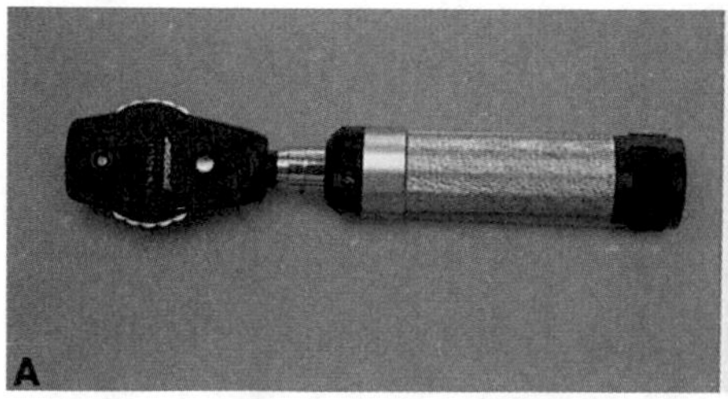

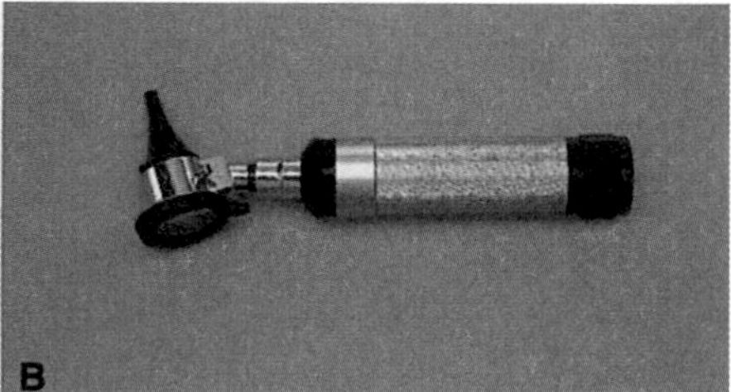

FIGURE 7-2. (A) Ophthalmoscope. (B) Otoscope. (Photographs © Ken Kasper. From Taylor C, Lillis CA, LeMone P: Fundamentals of Nursing, 2nd ed, p 426. Philadelphia: JB Lippincott, 1993.)

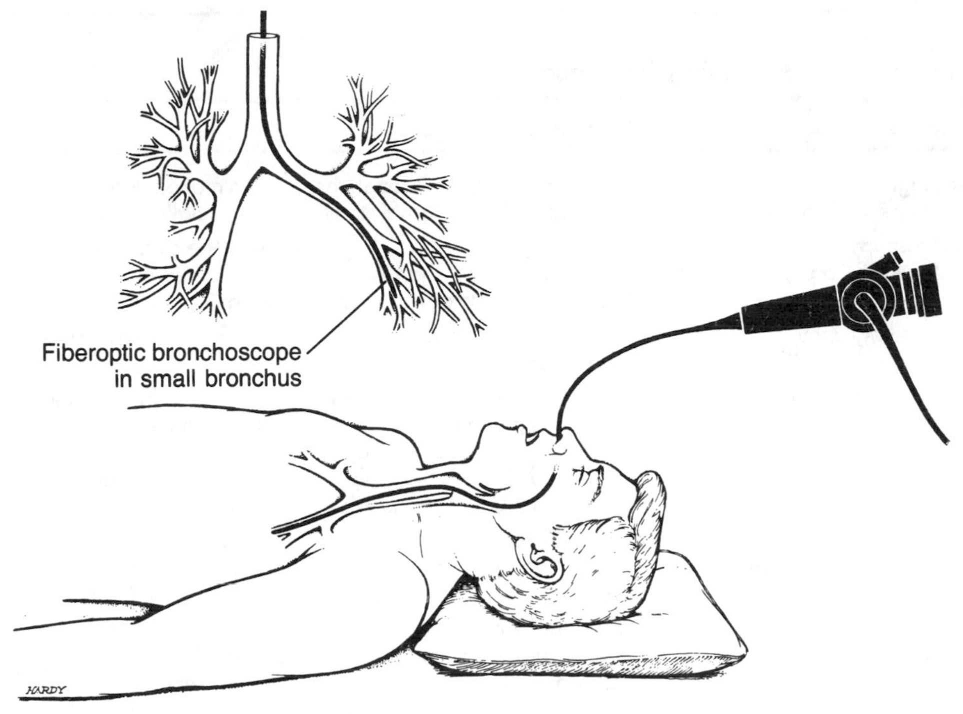

FIGURE 7-3. A fiberoptic bronchoscope, a type of endoscope. The flexible scope can be used to examine the airways and to take biopsy specimens. (Smeltzer SC, Bare BG: Brunner and Suddarth's Textbook of Medical-Surgical Nursing, 7th ed, p 516. Philadelphia: JB Lippincott, 1992.)

Diagnosis is further aided by laboratory tests. These may include tests on blood, urine, and other body fluids, study of specimens taken by **biopsy**, and the identification of infectious organisms. Additional tests may include study of the electrical activity of tissues such as the brain and heart, examination of body cavities by means of an **endoscope** (Fig. 7-3), and imaging techniques.

The skin, hair, and nails provide indications of a person's state of health. Such features of the skin as color, texture, thickness, and presence of lesions (local injuries) are noted throughout the course of the physical examination. Chapter 21 contains a discussion of the skin and skin diseases.

Imaging Techniques

Imaging techniques are methods used to visualize body structure or function. The most fundamental imaging method is radiography, which uses x-rays to produce a picture on sensitized film. The value of this method may be increased with a contrast medium, such as a barium mixture, to outline soft tissue. See Table 7-1 for a description of imaging methods currently in use.

Treatment

If diagnosis so indicates, treatment is begun. This may consist of counseling, drugs, surgery, radiation, physical therapy, occupational therapy, psychiatric treatment, or a combination of these. See Chapter 8 for a discussion of drugs and their actions.

TABLE 7-1 Imaging Techniques

Method	Description
radiography *(rā-dē-OG-ra-fē)*	Use of x-rays passed through the body to make a visual record (radiograph) of internal structures on specially sensitized film
fluoroscopy *(flū-ROS-kō-pē)*	Use of x-rays to examine deep structures. The shadows cast by x-rays passed through the body are observed on a fluorescent screen. The device used is called a fluoroscope.
cineradiography *(sin-e-rā-dē-OG-ra-fē)*	Making of a motion picture of successive images appearing on a fluoroscopic screen
computed tomography (CT, CT scan) *(tō-MOG-ra-fē)*	Use of a computer to generate an image from a large number of x-rays passed at different angles through the body. A 3-dimensional picture of a cross-section of the body is obtained. Reveals more about soft tissues than simple x-rays; also called CAT (computerized axial tomography)
ultrasonography *(ul-tra-son-OG-ra-fē)*	Generation of a visual image from the echoes of high frequency sound waves traveling back from different tissues; also called sonography *(so-NOG-ra-fē)* and echography *(ek-OG-ra-fē)*
scintigraphy *(sin-TIG-ra-fē)*	Production of an image of the distribution of radioactivity in tissues after internal administration of a radioactive substance (radionuclide). The images are obtained with a scintillation camera. The record produced is a scintiscan *(SIN-ti-skan)* and usually specifies the part examined or the isotope used for the test, as in bone scan, gallium scan.
magnetic resonance imaging (MRI)	Production of images through the use of a magnetic field and radiowaves. The characteristics of soft tissue are revealed by differences in molecular properties; eliminates the need for x-rays and contrast media.
positron emission tomography (PET)	Production of sectional body images by administration of a natural substance, such as glucose, labeled with a positron-emitting isotope. The rays subsequently emitted are interpreted by computer to show the internal distribution of the substance administered. PET has been used to follow blood flow through an organ and to measure metabolic activity within an organ, such as the brain, under different conditions.
single photon emission computed tomography (SPECT)	Scintigraphic technique which permits visualization of the cross-sectional distribution of a radioisotope

Cancer

Methods used in the diagnosis of cancer include physical examination, biopsy, imaging techniques, and laboratory tests for abnormalities, or "markers," associated with specific types of malignancies. Some cancer markers are byproducts, such as enzymes, hormones, and cellular proteins, that are abnormal or are produced in abnormal amounts. Researchers are also linking specific genetic mutations to certain forms of cancer.

Staging is a procedure for establishing the extent of tumor spread, both at the original site and in other parts of the body (metastases). Staging is important for selecting and evaluating therapy, and for estimating the outcome of the disease. The TNM system is commonly used. These letters stand for primary tumor (T), regional lymph nodes (N), and distant metastases (M). Eval-

KEY TERMS

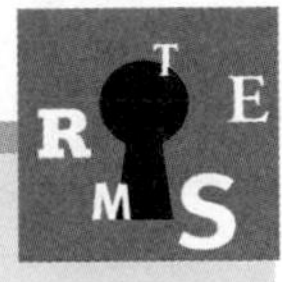

Term	Definition
auscultation *(aws-kul-TĀ-shun)*	Listening for sounds within the body, usually within the chest or abdomen
biopsy *(BĪ-op-sē)*	Removal of a small amount of tissue for microscopic examination
chemotherapy *(kē-mō-THER-a-pē)*	The use of chemicals to treat disease
diagnosis *(dī-ag-NŌ-sis)*	The process of determining the cause and nature of an illness
endoscope *(EN-dō-skōp)*	An instrument for examining the inside of an organ or cavity through a body opening or small incision. Most endoscopes use fiberoptics for viewing (see Figure 7-3).
excision *(ek-SIZH-un)*	Removal by cutting
incision *(in-SIZH-un)*	A cut, as for surgery; also the act of cutting
inspection *(in-SPEK-shun)*	Visual examination of the body
ophthalmoscope *(of-THAL-mō-skōp)*	An instrument for examining the interior of the eye (see Figure 7-2A)
palpation *(pal-PĀ-shun)*	Examining by placing the hands or fingers on the surface of the body
percussion *(per-KUSH-un)*	Tapping the body lightly but sharply in order to assess the condition of the underlying part by the sounds obtained
prognosis *(prog-NŌ-sis)*	Prediction of the course and outcome of a disease
radionuclide *(rā-dē-ō-NŪ-klīd)*	A substance that gives off radiation; used for diagnosis and treatment; also called radioisotope or radiopharmaceutical
sign	An objective evidence of disease that can be observed or tested. Examples are fever, rash, high blood pressure, blood or urine abnormalities; an objective symptom
staging	The process of classifying malignant tumors for diagnosis, treatment, and prognosis
stethoscope *(STETH-ō-skōp)*	An instrument used for listening to sounds produced within the body (from G. root *steth/o* meaning "chest") (see Figure 7-1)
suture *(SŪ-chur)*	To unite parts by stitching them together; also the thread or other material used in that process or the seam formed by surgical stitching
symptom *(SIM-tum)*	Any evidence of disease; sometimes limited to subjective evidence of disease, as experienced by the individual, such as pain, dizziness, weakness
syndrome *(SIN-drōm)*	A group of signs and symptoms that together characterize a disease condition
therapy *(THER-a-pē)*	Treatment; intervention

uation in these categories varies for each type of tumor. Based on TNM results, a stage ranging in Roman numerals from I–IV in severity is assigned. Cancers of the blood, lymphatic system, and nervous system are evaluated by different standards.

The most widely used methods for treatment of cancer are surgery, radiation therapy, and **chemotherapy** (treatment with chemicals).

Word Parts Pertaining to Diagnosis and Treatment

Roots for Physical Forces

Root	Meaning	Example	Definition of Example
aer/o	air, gas	aerobic *er-Ō-bik*	requiring air (oxygen)
bar/o	pressure	hypobaric *hī-pō-BAR-ik*	pertaining to decreased atmospheric pressure
chrom/o, chromat/o	color, stain	chromophilic *krō-mō-FIL-ik*	staining easily
chron/o	time	chronic *KRON-ik*	occurring over a long period of time
cry/o	cold	cryalgesia *krī-al-JĒ-zē-a*	pain caused by cold
electro/o	electricity	electrolysis *ē-lek-TROL-i-sis*	destruction (-lysis) by means of electric current
erg/o	work	synergistic *sin-er-JIS-tik*	working together with increased effect, like drugs in combination
phon/o	sound, voice	phonostethograph *fō-nō-STETH-ō-graf*	instrument used to record chest sounds
phot/o	light	photosensitive *fō-tō-SEN-si-tiv*	abnormally sensitive to (sun)light
radi/o	radiation, x-ray	radiotherapy *rā-dē-ō-THER-a-pē*	treatment with radiation
son/o	sound	ultrasonic *ul-tra-SON-ik*	pertaining to high-frequency sound waves (beyond human hearing)
therm/o	heat, temperature	hyperthermia *hī-pō-THER-mē-a*	abnormally high body temperature

Exercise 7-1

Match each of the following words with its meaning and write the appropriate letter (a–e) to the left of each number:

_____ 1 photoreaction *(fō-tō-rē-AK-shun)* — a. maintaining a constant body temperature

_____ 2 barotrauma *(bar-ō-TRAW-ma)* — b. giving off radiation

_____ 3 achromatous *(a-KRŌ-ma-tus)* — c. injury caused by pressure

_____ 4 homeothermic *(hō-mē-ō-THER-mik)* — d. response to light

_____ 5 radioactive *(rā-dē-ō-AK-tiv)* — e. colorless

Identify and define the root in each of the following words:

	Root	Meaning of Root
6. thermal	therm/o	heat
7. anaerobic	________	________
8. exergonic	________	________
9. synchronize	________	________

Fill in the blanks:

10. A cryoprobe *(KRĪ-ō-prōb)* is an instrument used to apply extreme ________________.

11. A phonogram *(FŌ-nō-gram)* is a record of ________________.

12. The term *electroconvulsive (ē-lek-trō-con-VUL-siv)* means causing convulsions by means of ________________.

13. Ultrasonography *(ul-tra-son-OG-ra-fē)* is a method for diagnosis that uses ________________.

Suffixes for Diagnosis

Suffix	Meaning	Example	Definition of Example
-graph	instrument for recording data	polygraph *POL-ē-graf*	instrument used to record many physiologic responses simultaneously; lie detector
-graphy	act of recording data*	radiography *rā-dē-OG-ra-fē*	obtaining pictures with x-rays
-gram†	a record of data	echogram *EK-ō-gram*	record obtained by ultrasonography; sonogram
-meter	instrument for measuring	calorimeter *kal-ō-RIM-e-ter*	instrument for measuring heat in calories
metry	measurement of	audiometry *aw-dē-OM-e-trē*	measurement of hearing (audi/o)
-scope	instrument for viewing or examining	laryngoscope *lar-RING-gō-skōp*	endoscope used to examine the larynx (laryng/o)
-scopy	examination of	laparoscopy *lap-a-ROS-kō-pē*	examination of the abdomen through the abdominal wall (lapar/o)

*This ending is often used to mean not only the recording of data but also the evaluation and interpretation of the data.

†A simple x-ray picture is called a radio*graph*. When special techniques are used to x-ray an organ or region, the ending *-gram* is used with the root for that area, as in urogram (urinary tract), angiogram (blood vessels), mammogram (breast).

Exercise 7-2

Matching. Match the terms in each of these sets with their definitions and write the appropriate letter (a–e) to the left of each number:

_____	1. ergometry *(er-GOM-e-trē)*	a. instrument for recording time
_____	2. microscope *(MĪ-krō-skōp)*	b. instrument for measuring temperature
_____	3. chronograph *(KRON-ō-graf)*	c. measurement of work done
_____	4. photography *(fō-TOG-ra-fē)*	d. instrument for examining very small objects
_____	5. thermometer	e. use of light to record data
_____	6. barometer *(ba-ROM-e-ter)*	a. instrument for examining the abdominal cavity
_____	7. cardiogram *(KAR-dē-ō-gram)*	b. echogram
_____	8. bronchoscopy *(brong-KOS-kō-pē)*	c. instrument for measuring pressure
_____	9. celioscope *(SĒ-lē-ō-skōp)*	d. endoscopic examination of breathing passages
_____	10. sonogram *(SON-ō-gram)*	e. record of the heart's electrical activity

Suffixes for Surgery

Suffix	Meaning	Example	Definition of Example
-centesis	puncture, tap	thoracentesis *thor-a-sen-TĒ-sis*	puncture of the chest
-desis	binding, fusion	pleurodesis *plū-ROD-e-sis*	binding of the pleural membranes (around the lungs)
-ectomy	excision, surgical removal	hysterectomy *his-te-REK-tō-mē*	excision of the uterus (hyster/o)
-pexy	surgical fixation	gastropexy *GAS-trō-pek-sē*	surgical fixation of the stomach (gastr/o)
-plasty	plastic repair, plastic surgery, reconstruction	arthroplasty *AR-thrō-plas-tē*	plastic repair of a joint (arthr/o)
-rhaphy	surgical repair, suture	herniorrhaphy *her-nē-OR-a-fē*	surgical repair of a hernia (herni/o)
-stomy	surgical creation of an opening	tracheostomy *trā-kē-OS-tō-mē*	creation of an opening into the trachea (trache/o)
-tome	instrument for incising (cutting)	microtome *MĪ-krō-tōm*	instrument for cutting thin sections of tissue for microscopic study
-tomy	incision, cutting	laparotomy *lap-a-ROT-ō-mē*	surgical incision of the abdomen
-tripsy	crushing	lithotripsy *LITH-ō-trip-sē*	crushing of a stone

Exercise 7-3

Matching. Match the words in the list with their meanings and write the appropriate letter (a–e) to the left of each number:

_____ 1. gastrorrhaphy *(gas-TROR-a-fē)*	a. plastic surgery of the breast
_____ 2. neurotripsy *(NŪ-rō-trip-sē)*	b. excision of a gland
_____ 3. mammoplasty *(MAM-ō-plas-tē)*	c. suture of the stomach
_____ 4. celiocentesis *(sē-lē-ō-sen-TĒ-sis)*	d. crushing of a nerve
_____ 5. adenectomy *(ad-e-NEK-tō-mē)*	e. puncture of the abdomen

The root *arthr/o* means "joint." Use this root to write a word that means each of the following:

6. Fusion of a joint ______arthrodesis______
7. Incision of a joint ____________
8. Surgical puncture of a joint ____________
9. Plastic repair of a joint ____________

The root *hepat/o* means "liver." Use this root to write a word that means each of the following:

10. Surgical repair of the liver ____________
11. Incision into the liver ____________
12. Excision of liver tissue ____________
13. Surgical fixation of the liver ____________

Build a word for each of the following definitions using the roots given:

14. Creation of an opening in the colon (root *col/o*) ____________
15. Incision into the stomach (root gastr/o) ____________
16. An instrument for cutting skin (derm/o) ____________

ADDITIONAL TERMS

Symptoms

clubbing *(KLUB-ing)*	Enlargement of the ends of the fingers and toes due to growth of the soft tissue around the nails. Seen in a variety of diseases, especially lung and heart diseases (Fig. 7-4)

(continued)

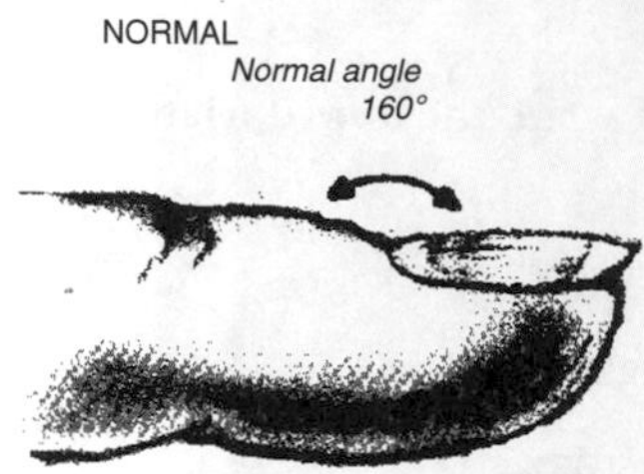

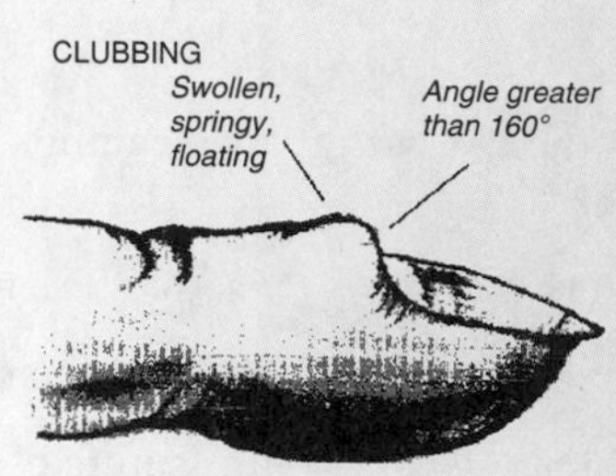

FIGURE 7-4. Clubbing. (Adapted from Bates B, Bickley LS, Hoekelman RA: A Guide to Physical Examination, 5th ed, p 149, Philadelphia: JB Lippincott, 1991.)

colic *(KOL-ik)* — Acute abdominal pain associated with smooth muscle spasms

cyanosis *(sī-a-NŌ-sis)* — Bluish discoloration of the skin due to lack of oxygen

diaphoresis *(dī-a-fō-RĒ-sis)* — Profuse sweating

malaise *(ma-LĀZ)* — A feeling of discomfort or uneasiness, often indicative of infection

nocturnal *(nok-TUR-nal)* — Pertaining to or occurring at night (roots *noct/i* and *nyct/o* mean "night")

pallor *(PAL-or)* — Paleness; lack of color

prodrome *(PRŌ-drōm)* — A symptom indicating an approaching disease

sequela *(sē-KWĒ-la)* — A lasting effect of a disease (pl. sequelaē)

syncope *(SIN-kō-pē)* — A temporary loss of consciousness due to inadequate blood flow to the brain; fainting

Diagnosis

alpha-fetoprotein (AFP) *(al-fa fē-to-prō-tēn)* — A fetal protein that appears in the blood of adults with certain types of cancer.

bruit *(brwē)* — A sound, usually abnormal, heard in auscultation

facies *(FĀ-shē-ēz)* — The expression or appearance of the face

febrile *(FEB-ril)* — Pertaining to fever

nuclear medicine — The branch of medicine concerned with the use of radioactive substances (radionuclides) for diagnosis, therapy, and research

radiology *(rā-dē-OL-ō-jē)* — The branch of medicine that uses radiation, such as x-rays, in the diagnosis and treatment of disease. A specialist in this field is a radiologist.

speculum *(SPEK-ū-lum)* — An instrument for examining a canal (Fig. 7-5)

(continued)

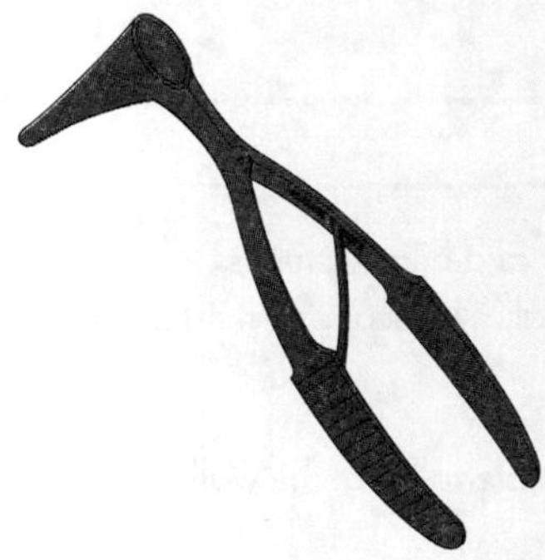

FIGURE 7-5. Nasal speculum. (Taylor C, Lillis CA, LeMone P: Fundamentals of Nursing, 2nd ed, p 426. Philadelphia: JB Lippincott, 1993.)

Treatment

catheter
(KATH-e-ter)
A thin tube that can be passed into the body; used to remove fluids from or introduce fluids into a body cavity

clysis
(KLĪ-sis)
The introduction of fluid into the body, other than orally, as into the rectum or abdominal cavity; also refers to the solution thus used

lavage
(la-VAZH)
The washing out of a cavity; irrigation

paracentesis
(par-a-sen-TĒ-sis)
Puncture of a cavity for removal of fluid

palliative treatment
(PAL-ē-at-iv)
Treatment that is designed to relieve pain and distress but does not attempt a cure

prophylaxis
(prō-fi-LAK-sis)
Prevention of disease

Surgery*

cautery
(KAW-ter-ē)
Destruction of tissue by means of a caustic substance, heat, electricity, or other agent

drain
Device for allowing matter to escape from a wound or cavity. Common types include Penrose (cigarette), T-tube, Jackson-Pratt (J-P), and Hemovac

laser
(LĀ-zer)
A device that transforms light into a beam of intense heat and power; used for surgery and diagnosis

ligature
(LIG-a-chur)
A tie or bandage; the process of binding or tying (also called ligation)

resection
(rē-SEK-shun)
Partial excision of a structure

stapling
(STĀ-pling)
In surgery, the joining of tissue by using wire staples that are pushed through the tissue and then bent

*See Table 7-2 for a description of surgical instruments and Figure 7-6 for pictures of surgical instruments.

TABLE 7-2 Surgical Instruments

Instrument	Description
bougie *(BOO-zhē)*	slender, flexible instrument for exploring and dilating tubes
cannula *(KAN-ū-la)*	tube enclosing a trocar (see below) that allows escape of fluid or air after removal of the trocar
clamp	instrument used to compress tissue
curet (curette) *(KŪ-ret)*	spoon-shaped instrument for removing material from the wall of a cavity or other surface (see Fig. 7-6)
elevator *(EL-e-vā-tor)*	instrument for lifting tissue or bone
forceps *(FOR-seps)*	instrument for holding or extracting (see Fig. 7-6)
Gigli's saw *(JĒL-yēz)*	flexible wire saw
hemostat *(HĒ-mō-stat)*	small clamp for stopping blood flow from a vessel (see Fig. 7-6)
rasp	surgical file
retractor *(rē-TRAK-tor)*	instrument used to maintain exposure by separating a wound and holding back organs or tissues (see Fig. 7-6)
rongeur *(ron-ZHUR)*	gouge forceps
scalpel *(SKAL-pel)*	surgical knife with a sharp blade (see Fig. 7-6)
sound *(sownd)*	instrument for exploring a cavity or canal (see Fig. 7-6).
trocar *(TRŌ-kar)*	sharp pointed instrument contained in a cannula used to puncture a cavity

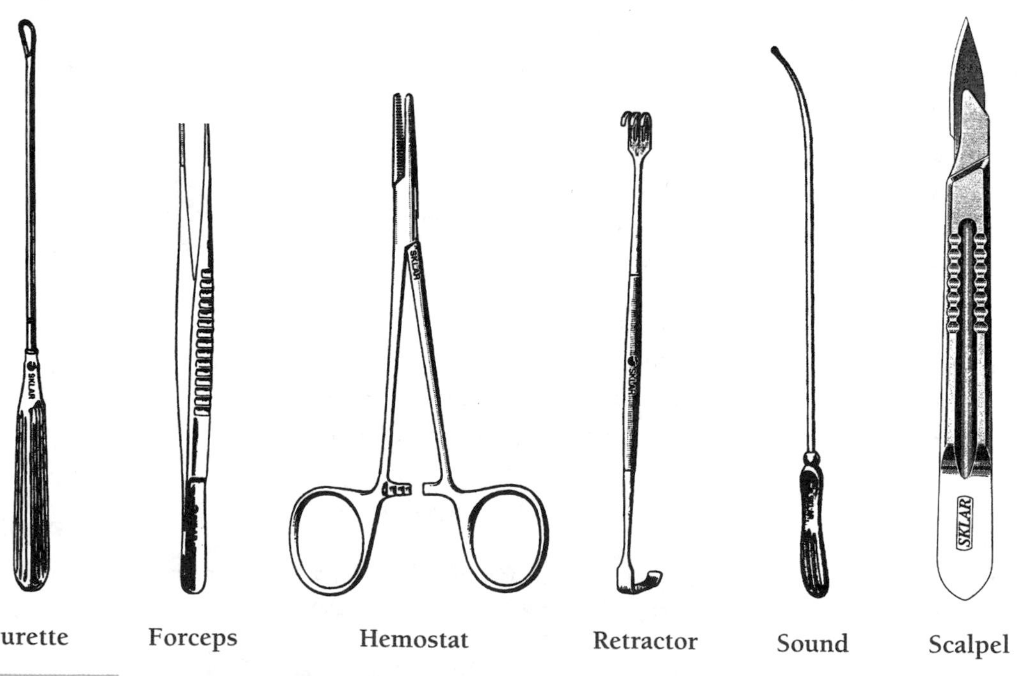

FIGURE 7-6. Surgical instruments.

ABBREVIATIONS

History and Physical Examination

BP blood pressure

C Celsius (centrigrade)

CC chief complaint

c/o complains of

EOMI extraocular muscles intact

F Fahrenheit

HEENT head, eyes, ears, nose, and throat

h/o history of

H & P history and physical

HPI history of present illness

HR heart rate

Hx history

I & O intake and output

IPPA inspection, palpation, percussion, auscultation

NAD no apparent distress

P pulse

PE physical examination

PE(R)RLA pupils equal (regular) react to light and accommodation

PMH past medical history

pt patient

R respiration

R/O rule out

ROS review of systems

T temperature

TPR temperature, pulse, respiration

VS vital signs

WD well developed

WNL within normal limits

Diagnosis and Treatment

ABC aspiration biopsy cytology

AFP alpha-fetoprotein

bx biopsy

Ci Curie (unit of radioactivity)

C&S culture and (drug) sensitivity (of bacteria)

CT computed tomography

Dx diagnosis

ICU intensive care unit

I&D incision and drainage

MET metastasis

MRI magnetic resonance imaging

PCA patient controlled analgesia

PET positron emission tomography

postop postoperative

preop preoperative

RATx radiation therapy

Rx drug, prescription, therapy

SPECT single photon emission computed tomography

TNM (primary) tumor, (regional lymph) nodes, (distant) metastases

UV ultraviolet

Views for X-ray

AP anteroposterior

LL left lateral

PA posteroanterior

RL right lateral

Orders

AMA against medical advice

AMB ambulatory

BRP bathroom privileges

CBR complete bed rest

KVO keep vein open

NPO nothing my mouth (L. *non per os*)

OOB out of bed

QNS quantity not sufficient

QS quantity sufficient

STAT immediately

TKO to keep open

Drug abbreviations are in Chapter 8.

CHAPTER REVIEW 7

Matching. Match the terms in each of the sets below with their definitions and write the appropriate letter (a–e) to the left of each number:

_____ 1. biopsy	a. classification of malignant tumors
_____ 2. prognosis	b. prediction of the outcome of disease
_____ 3. staging	c. to unite parts by stitching them together
_____ 4. palpation	d. removal of tissue for microscopic examination
_____ 5. suture	e. examination by touch
_____ 6. chromogenesis	a. listening for body sounds
_____ 7. scintiscan	b. destruction of tissue with chemicals
_____ 8. cryotherapy	c. formation of color
_____ 9. auscultation	d. image obtained with a radionuclide
_____ 10. chemocautery	e. treatment by use of cold
_____ 11. radiograph	a. instrument for cutting bone
_____ 12. opthalmoscope	b. x-ray picture
_____ 13. osteotome	c. device for examining the inside of a joint
_____ 14. catheter	d. thin tube
_____ 15. arthroscope	e. instrument used to examine the eye
_____ 16. malaise	a. partial excision
_____ 17. paracentesis	b. feeling of discomfort
_____ 18. resection	c. crushing of a stone
_____ 19. lithotripsy	d. plastic repair of the hand
_____ 20. chiroplasty	e. puncture of a cavity for removal of fluid
_____ 21. febrile	a. occurring at night
_____ 22. nocturnal	b. symptom of an approaching disease
_____ 23. clubbing	c. a group of symptoms that characterizes a disease
_____ 24. prodrome	d. enlargement of the ends of the fingers and toes
_____ 25. syndrome	e. pertaining to fever
_____ 26. bruit	a. profuse sweating
_____ 27. prophylaxis	b. washing out of a cavity
_____ 28. diaphoresis	c. prevention of disease
_____ 29. colic	d. sound heard on auscultation
_____ 30. lavage	e. acute abdominal pain

Identify and define the root in each of the following words:

	Root	Meaning of Root
31. allergy	__________	__________
32. radiology	__________	__________
33. synchronous	__________	__________
34. hyperbaric	__________	__________
35. aerobic	__________	__________

Word building. Use the root *-cyst/o* meaning "urinary bladder" to write a word with each of the following meanings:

36. Suture of the bladder ____________________
37. Plastic repair of the bladder ____________________
38. Incision of the bladder ____________________
39. Surgical fixation of the bladder ____________________
40. Surgical creation of an opening in the bladder ____________________

Eliminations. Underline the word in each of the sets below that does not fit in with the rest and explain the reasons for your choice.

41. otoscope stethoscope speculum syncope endoscope

____

42. trocar scalpel sequela hemostat forceps

____

Word analysis. Define each of the following words and give the meaning of the word parts in each. Use a dictionary if necessary.

43. anergic (an-ER-jik) ____________________
    a. an- ____________________
    b. erg/o ____________________
    c. -ic ____________________
44. hypothermia *(hī-pō-THER-mē-a)* ____________________
    a. hypo- ____________________
    b. therm/o ____________________
    c. -ia ____________________
45. phonocardiography *(fō-nō-kar-dē-OG-ra-fē)* ____________________
    a. phon/o ____________________
    b. cardi/o ____________________
    c. -graphy ____________________

Chapter 7

Case Studies

1. Physical Examination

Female 5′2″ tall, weight 114 pounds. T-98; P-80; R-17; BP 110/60.
HEENT: fundi benign; PERRLA. Mouth clear. Neck supple without thyromegaly or cervical adenopathy.
LUNGS: Clear to auscultation
HEART: Rate regular without murmurs, gallops, or rubs
BREASTS: Without masses or discharges
ABDOMEN: No hepatosplenomegaly. No suprapubic tenderness. Bowel sounds are normal
EXTREMITIES: Without acrocyanosis or edema
Neurological: Grossly intact

2. Sarcoma of the Left Lung

History and physical findings: Patient is a 65-year-old male with a history of primary giant cell carcinoma in the left lung. The left lung was resected 10 weeks prior to admission. He was readmitted with increasing pain, dyspnea, and diaphoresis. Medical Hx is remarkable for renal artery stenosis of the right kidney causing hypertension. Social Hx was negative for alcohol use. He had smoked 1 pack a day for 35 years but had stopped smoking 5 years prior to surgery.

Physical examination revealed an elderly cooperative male. T- 98; HR- 72; R- 22; BP 175/95. Thoracotomy scar in the left chest. There were decreased breath sounds and dullness to percussion of the left base. Abdomen was soft, mild tenderness in the LLQ. The examination was otherwise unremarkable.

3. Biliary Colic

Chief complaint: The patient is a 28-year-old female who was 3 weeks status post cholecystectomy (removal of the gallbladder). She did well at home for 2 weeks but presented with the sudden onset of retrosternal, upper abdominal, and back pain, identical to the pain which led to the diagnosis of her gallstones. There was some nausea and vomiting. Zantac and Reglan in large doses for several days were not helpful. The patient was afebrile. Vital signs were normal. Chest was clear. Heart sounds were normal. There was diffuse abdominal tenderness but no guarding or rebound. Bowel sounds, although quiet, were present.

The clinical impression was clearly that of biliary colic with retained stone. A radiographic study of the biliary and pancreatic ducts was performed. Although no stones were seen on the preliminary film of her biliary tree, the presentation was so classic for biliary obstruction that it was felt reasonable to undergo sphincterotomy.

Following the procedure, her condition improved and she had no clinical findings to suggest pancreatitis or other complication. She was discharged in improved condition with orders for Zantac 300 mg once daily for several weeks and a follow-up liver profile in 2–3 weeks.

Chapter 7

Case Study Questions

Write the meaning of the following abbreviations:

1. T ____________________
2. P ____________________

3. R ______________________________
4. BP ______________________________
5. HEENT ______________________________
6. PERRLA ______________________________
7. LLQ ______________________________
8. Hx ______________________________
9. HR ______________________________

Multiple choice. Select the best answer and write the letter of your choice to the left of each number:

_____ 10. In referring to the eyes, the fundi are the
- a. eyelids
- b. eyelashes
- c. areas around the eyes
- d. back regions of the eyes
- e. fronts of the eyes

_____ 11. The suffix in the terms *thyromegaly* and *hepatosplenomegaly* means
- a. shrinking
- b. enlargement
- c. disease
- d. washing
- e. pain

_____ 12. The term *dyspnea* means
- a. difficulty in breathing
- b. vomiting
- c. loss of consciousness
- d. paleness
- e. facial expression

_____ 13. When the left lung was resected it was
- a. irradiated
- b. washed
- c. sutured
- d. partially removed
- e. examined with an endoscope

_____ 14. A sphincterotomy is
- a. cutting of a circular muscle
- b. endoscopic examination of an organ
- c. surgical repair of a muscle
- d. crushing of a stone
- e. removal of muscle tissue for examination

Find the word in the case studies that means:

15. Profuse sweating ______________________________
16. Narrowing of a part ______________________________
17. High blood pressure ______________________________
18. Tapping the body and listening for sounds ______________________________
19. Acute abdominal pain ______________________________
20. Pertaining to an x-ray study ______________________________

Define the following terms:

21. edema ______________________________
22. carcinoma ______________________________
23. afebrile ______________________________
24. restrosternal ______________________________

Chapter 7
Answer Section

Answers to Chapter Exercises

Exercise 7-1

1. d
2. c
3. e
4. a
5. b
6. therm/o; heat
7. aer/o; air (oxygen)
8. erg/o; work
9. chron/o; time
10. cold
11. sound
12. electricity
13. sound, ultrasound

Exercise 7-2

1. c
2. d
3. a
4. e
5. b
6. c
7. e
8. d
9. a
10. b

Exercise 7-3

1. c
2. d
3. a
4. e
5. b
6. arthrodesis *(ar-thrō-DĒ-sis)*
7. arthrotomy *(ar-THROT-ō-mē)*
8. arthrocentesis *(ar-thrō-sen-TĒ-sis)*
9. arthroplasty *(AR-thrō-plas-tē)*
10. hepatorrhaphy *(hep-a-TOR-a-fē)*
11. hepatotomy *(hep-a-TOT-ō-mē)*
12. hepatectomy *(hep-a-TEK-tō-mē)*
13. hepatopexy *(HEP-a tō-pek-sē)*
14. colostomy *(kō-LOS-tō-mē)*
15. gastrotomy *(gas-TROT-ō-mē)*
16. dermatome *(DER-ma-tōm)*

Chapter Review 7

1. d
2. b
3. a
4. e
5. c
6. c
7. d
8. e
9. a
10. b
11. b
12. e
13. a
14. d
15. c
16. b
17. d
18. a
19. c
20. d

21. e
22. a
23. d
24. b
25. c
26. d
27. c
28. a
29. e
30. b
31. erg/o; work
32. radi/o; radiation, x-ray
33. chron/o; time
34. bar/o; pressure
35. aer/o; air
36. cystorrhaphy *(sis-TOR-a-fē)*
37. cystoplasty *(SIS-tō-plas-tē)*
38. cystotomy *(sis-TOT-ō-mē)*
39. cystopexy *(SIS-tō-pek-sē)*
40. cystostomy *(sis-TOS-tō-mē)*
41. syncope. The others are examining instruments; syncope is loss of consciousness, fainting
42. sequela. The others are surgical instruments; sequela is a lasting effect of disease
43. Lacking energy; inactive; listless
    a. not, without, lack of
    b. work
    c. pertaining to
44. Excessively low body temperature
    a. under, below, abnormally low, decreased
    b. heat
    c. condition of
45. The act of recording heart sounds
    a. sound
    b. heart
    c. the act of recording data

Answers to Case Study Questions

1. temperature
2. pulse
3. respiration
4. blood pressure
5. head, eyes, ears, nose, and throat
6. pupils equal, regular, react to light and accommodation
7. left lower quadrant
8. history
9. heart rate
10. d
11. b
12. a
13. d
14. a
15. diaphoresis
16. stenosis
17. hypertension
18. percussion
19. colic
20. radiographic
21. swelling, accumulation of fluid
22. malignant tumor of epithelial tissue
23. without fever
24. behind the sternum

8 Drugs

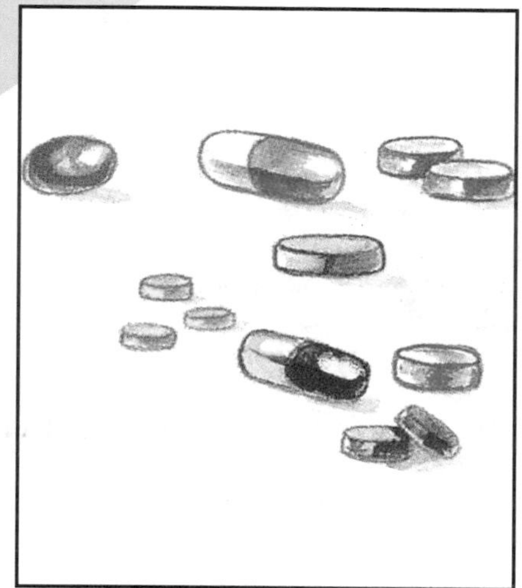

Chapter Contents

Objectives

After study of this chapter you should be able to:

1. Compare over-the-counter and prescription drugs
2. Compare the generic and trade names of drugs
3. List some potential side effects of drugs
4. Explain ways in which drugs can interact
5. List several drug references
6. Identify and use word parts pertaining to drugs
7. Recognize the major categories of drugs and how they act
8. List common routes for drug administration
9. List standard forms in which liquid and solid drugs are prepared
10. Define abbreviations related to drugs and their use

A **drug** is a substance that alters body function. Traditionally, drugs have been derived from natural plant, animal, and mineral sources. Today, most are manufactured synthetically in pharmaceutical companies. A few, such as certain hormones and enzymes, have been produced by genetic engineering.

Many drugs, described as over-the-counter (OTC) drugs, are available without **prescription**. Others require a physician's prescription for use. Responsibility for the safety and **efficacy** of all drugs sold in the United States lies with the Federal Food and Drug Administration (FDA), which must approve all drugs before they are sold.

Most drugs have potential **side effects** or risks that must be evaluated before being prescribed. On an individual basis, there may be **contraindications** to the use of a particular drug. Also, while a patient is under treatment, it is important to watch for signs of adverse effects, such as allergy, digestive upset, or changes in the blood. Because drugs given in combination may interact, the physician must know of any drugs the patient is taking before prescribing another. In some cases, the combination results in **synergy** or **potentiation**; in others one drug may act as an **antagonist** of another.

Drug Names

Drugs may be cited by either their generic or their trade names. The **generic name** is usually a simple version of the chemical name for the drug and is not capitalized. The **trade name** (brand name, proprietary name) is a registered trademark of the manufacturer and is written with a capital. The same drug may be marketed by different companies under different trade names. See Table 8-1 for a summary of the major categories of drugs with examples cited by both generic and trade names. Tables 8-2 to 8-4 define terms pertaining to drug preparation and use.

Drug Information

The official United States listing of drugs is the *United States Pharmacopeia* (USP). There is also the *Hospital Formulary*, published by the American Society of Hospital Pharmacists, and the *Physicians' Desk Reference*, published yearly by Medical Economics Books, with information supplied by the manufacturers. Another excellent source of up-to-date information on drugs is a community or hospital pharmacist.

The remainder of this chapter is an introduction to drugs and their applications. Use it as a reference when working on Part II of this book.

text continues on page 109

TABLE 8-1 Common Drugs and Their Actions

Category	Action; Applications	Example: Generic Name	Example: Trade Name
Adrenergics *(ad-ren-ER-jiks)* (sympathomimetics) *(sim-pa-thō-mi-MET-iks)*	Mimic the action of the sympathetic nervous system, which responds to stress	epinephrine norepinephrine phenylephrine pseudoephedrine	Bronkaid Levo-Phed Neo-Synephrine Sudafed

(continued)

TABLE 8-1 Common Drugs and Their Actions *(Continued)*

Category	Action; Applications	Example: Generic Name	Example: Trade Name
Analgesics *(an-al-JĒ-siks)*	Alleviate pain		
narcotic *(nar-KO-tik)*	Decrease pain sensation in CNS. They are highly addictive.	meperidine morphine propoxyphene	Demerol Duramorph Darvon
nonnarcotic *(non-nar-KO-tik)*	Act peripherally to inhibit prostaglandins (local hormones). They may also be anti-inflammatory and antipyretic (reduce) fever).	aspirin (acetylsalicylic acid; ASA) acetaminophen (APAP) ibuprofen	 Tylenol Motrin
Anesthetics *(an-es-THET-iks)*	Reduce or eliminate sensation	lidocaine (local) procaine (local)	Xylocaine Novocaine
Anticoagulants *(an-ti-kō-AG-ū-lants)*	Prevent coagulation and formation of blood clots	heparin warfarin	 Coumadin
Anticonvulsants *(an-ti-kon-VUL-sants)*	Suppress or reduce the number and/or intensity of seizures	phenobarbital phenytoin carbamazepine valproic acid	 Dilantin Tegretol Depakene
Antiemetics *(an-tē-e-MET-iks)*	Relieve symptoms of nausea and prevent vomiting (emesis)	ondansetron dimenhydrinate prochlorperazine scopolamine	Zofran Dramamine Compazine Transderm-Scop
Antihistamines *(an-ti-HIS-ta-mēnz)*	Prevent responses mediated by histamine: allergic and inflammatory reactions	diphenhydramine brompheniramine promethazine loratadine terfenadine astemizole	Benadryl Dimetane Phenergan Claritin Seldane Hismanal
Antihypertensives *(an-ti-hī-per-TEN-sivs)*	Lower blood pressure by reducing cardiac output, dilating vessels, or promoting excretion of water by the kidneys. See also calcium channel blockers, beta blockers, and diuretics under cardiac drugs.	clonidine prazosin minoxidil captopril (ACE inhibitor; see Chap. 9)	Catapres Minipress Loniten Capoten

(continued)

TABLE 8-1 Common Drugs and Their Actions *(Continued)*

Category	Action; Applications	Example: Generic Name	Example: Trade Name
Anti-inflammatory Drugs *(an-tē-in-FLAM-a-tō-rē)*	Counteract inflammation and swelling		
corticosteroids *kor-ti-kō-STER-oyds*	Hormones from the cortex of the adrenal gland. Used for allergy, respiratory and blood diseases, injury, and malignancy. Suppress the immune system.	dexamethasone cortisone prednisone hydrocortisone	Decadron Cortone Deltasone Hydrocortone, Cortef
nonsteroidal anti-inflammatory drugs (NSAIDs) *(non-ster-OYD-al)*	Reduce inflammation and pain by interfering with synthesis of prostaglandins. Also antipyretic.	aspirin ibuprofen indomethacin naproxen diclofenac	 Motrin Indocin Naprosyn Aleve Voltaren
Anti-infective Agents	Kill or prevent the growth of infectious organisms		
antibacterials *(an-ti-bak-TĒ-rē-als)*	Effective against bacteria; antibiotic (term sometimes used for any antimicrobial agent)	amoxicillin penicillin V cephalexin sulfisoxazole tetracycline methenamine mandelate (urinary tract) isoniazid (INH) (anti-tubercular)	Polymox Pen-Vee K Keflex Gantrisin Achromycin Mandelamine Nydrazid
antifungals *(an-ti-FUNG-gals)*	Effective against fungi	amphotericin B miconazole nystatin fluconazole itraconazole	Fungizone Monistat Nilstat Diflucan Sporanox
antiparasitics *(an-ti-par-a-SIT-iks)*	Effective against parasites: protozoa, worms	iodoquinol (amebae) quinacrine	Yodoxin Atabrine
antivirals *(an-ti-VI-rals)*	Effective against viruses	acyclovir amantadine zidovudine indinavir (anti-HIV protease inhibitor)	Zovirax Symmetrel Retrovir Crixivan
Antineoplastics *(an-ti-nē-ō-PLAS-tiks)*	Destroy cancer cells. They are toxic for all cells but have greater	cyclophosphamide doxorubicin methotrexate	Cytoxan Adriamycin Folex

(continued)

TABLE 8-1 Common Drugs and Their Actions *(Continued)*

Category	Action; Applications	Example	
		Generic Name	Trade Name
	effect on cells that are actively growing and dividing. Hormones and hormone inhibitors are used to slow tumor growth.	vincristine tamoxifen (estrogen inhibitor)	Oncovin Nolvadex
Cardiac drugs *(KAR-dē-ak)*			
antiarrhythmics *(an-tē-a-RITH-miks)*	Correct or prevent abnormalities of heart rhythm	quinidine lidocaine digoxin	Quinidex Xylocaine Lanoxin
beta-adrenergic blockers (beta blockers) *(be-ta-ad-ren-ER-jik)*	Inhibit sympathetic nervous system; reduce rate and force of heart contractions	propranolol metoprolol atenolol	Inderal Lopressor Tenormin
calcium channel blockers *(KAL-sē-um)*	Dilate coronary arteries, slow heart rate, reduce contractions	diltiazem nifedipine verapamil	Cardizem Procardia Calan
nitrates *(NĪ-trātz)*	Dilate coronary arteries and reduce workload of heart by lowering blood pressure and reducing venous return; antianginal	nitroglycerin isosorbide	Nitrostat Isordil
Diuretics *(dī-ū-RET-iks)*	Promote excretion of water, sodium, and other electrolytes by the kidneys; used to reduce edema and blood pressure	bumetanide furosemide mannitol hydrochlorothiazide (HCTZ) triamterine + HCTZ	Bumex Lasix Osmitrol Hydrodiuril Dyazide
Gastrointestinal Drugs *(gas-trō-in-TES-tin-al)*			
antidiarrheals *(an-ti-di-a-RĒ-als)*	Treat or prevent diarrhea by reducing intestinal motility or absorbing irritants and soothing the intestinal lining	diphenoxylate loperamide attapulgite	Lomotil Imodium Kaopectate
histamine H_2 antagonists *(HIS-ta-mēn)*	Decrease secretion of stomach acid by interfering with the action of histamine at H_2 receptors; used to treat ulcers and other GI problems	cimetidine ranitidine	Tagamet Zantac

(continued)

TABLE 8-1 Common Drugs and Their Actions *(Continued)*

Category	Action; Applications	Example: Generic Name	Example: Trade Name
laxatives *(LAK-sa-tivs)*	Promote elimination from the large intestine. Types include:		
	stimulants	bisacodyl	Dulcolax
	hyperosmotics (retain water)	lactulose	Constilac, Chronulac
	stool softeners	docusate	Colase, Surfak
	bulk-forming agents	psyllium	Metamucil
Hypnotics *(hip-NOT-iks)*	Induce sleep or dull the senses. See antianxiety agents.		
Hypolipidemics *(hī-pō-lip-i-DĒ-miks)*	Lower cholesterol in patients with high serum levels that cannot be controlled with diet alone	cholestyramine lovastatin pravastatin	Questran Mevacor Pravachol
Muscle relaxants *(rē-LAK-sants)*	Depress nervous system stimulation of skeletal muscles. Used to control muscle spasms and pain.	baclofen carisoprodol methocarbamol	Lioresal Soma Robaxin
Psychotropics *(sī-kō-TROP-iks)*	Affect the mind, altering mental activity, mental state, or behavior		
antianxiety agents *(an-tē-ang-ZĪ-e-tē)*	Reduce or dispel anxiety; tranquilizers; anxiolytic agents	chlordiazepoxide diazepam hydroxyzine alprazolam buspirone	Librium Valium Atarax Xanax BuSpar
antidepressants *(an-ti-dē-PRES-sants)*	Relieve depression by raising brain levels of neurotransmitters (chemicals active in the nervous system)	amitriptyline imipramine fluoxetine paroxetine sertraline	Elavil Tofranil Prozac Paxil Zoloft
antipsychotics *(an-ti-sī-KOT-iks)*	Act on nervous system to relieve symptoms of psychoses	chlorpromazine haloperidol clozapine risperidone	Thorazine Haldol Clozaril Risperdal
Respiratory Drugs			
antitussives *(an-ti-TUS-sivs)*	Suppress coughing	dextromethorphan	Benylin DM
bronchodilators *(brong-kō-dī-LĀ-tors)*	Prevent or eliminate spasm of the bronchi	albuterol epinephrine	Proventil Sus-Phrine

(continued)

TABLE 8-1 Common Drugs and Their Actions *(Continued)*

Category	Action; Applications	Example: Generic Name	Example: Trade Name
	(breathing tubes) by relaxing bronchial smooth muscle; used to treat asthma and bronchitis	metaproterenol ephedrine	Alupent
expectorants *(ek-SPEK-tō-rants)*	Induce productive coughing to eliminate respiratory secretions	guaifenesin	Robitussin
mucolytics *(mū-kō-LIT-iks)*	Loosen mucus to promote its elimination	acetylcysteine	Mucomyst
sedatives/ hypnotics *(SED-a-tivs)/ (hip-NOT-iks)*	Induce relaxation and sleep. Lower (sedative) doses promote relaxation leading to sleep. Higher (hypnotic) doses induce sleep.	pentobarbital secobarbital phenobarbital	Nembutal Seconal
tranquilizers *(tran-kwi-LĪZ-ers)*	Reduce mental tension and anxiety. See anti-anxiety agents.		

TABLE 8-2 Routes of Drug Administration

Route	Description
instillation *(in-stil-LĀ-shun)*	liquid is dropped or poured slowly into a body cavity or on the surface of the body, such as into the ear or onto the conjunctiva of the eye
intradermal (ID) *(in-tra-DER-mal)*	injected into the skin
intramuscular (IM) *(in-tra-MUS-kū-lar)*	injected into a muscle
intrathecal *(in-tra-THĒ-kal)*	injected into the meninges around the spinal cord
oral *(OR-al)*	given by mouth; per os (po)
parenteral *(pa-REN-ter-al)*	administered by other than oral route, specifically, by injection
rectal *(REK-tal)*	administered by rectal suppository or enema
subcutaneous (SC) *(sub-kū-TĀ-nē-us)*	injected beneath the skin; hypodermic
sublingual (SL) *(sub-LING-gwal)*	administered under the tongue
topical *(TOP-i-kal)*	applied to the surface of the skin
transdermal *(trans-DER-mal)*	absorbed through the skin

TABLE 8-3 Drug Preparations *(Continued)*

Form	Description
Liquid	
aerosol *(AR-o-sol)*	solution dispersed as a mist to be inhaled
aqueous solution *(A-kwē-us)*	substance dissolved in water
elixir (elix) *(ē-LIK-sar)*	a clear, pleasantly flavored and sweetened hydro-alcoholic liquid intended for oral use
emulsion *(ē-MUL-shun)*	a mixture in which one liquid is dispersed but not dissolved in another liquid
liniment *(LIN-i-ment)*	mixture in oil, soap solution, or other liquid intended for external application
lotion *(LŌ-shun)*	solution prepared for topical use
ointment (ung) *(OYNT-ment)*	drug in a base that keeps it in contact with the skin
suspension (susp) *(sus-PEN-shun)*	fine particles dispersed in a liquid; must be shaken before use
tincture (tinct) *(TINK-chur)*	substance dissolved in an alcoholic solution
Solid	
capsule (cap) *(KAP-sūl)*	material in a gelatin container that dissolves easily in the stomach
suppository (supp) *(su-POZ-i-tor-ē)*	substance mixed and molded with a base that melts easily when inserted into a body opening
tablet (tab) *(TAB-let)*	a solid dosage form containing a drug in a pure state or mixed with a non-active ingredient and prepared by compression or molding. Also called a pill.

TABLE 8-4 Terms Pertaining to Injectable Drugs

Term	Meaning
ampule *(AM-pūl)*	A small sealed glass or plastic container used for sterile intravenous solutions
bolus *(BŌ-lus)*	A concentrated amount of a diagnostic or therapeutic substance given rapidly IV
catheter *(KATH-e-ter)*	A thin tube that can be passed into a body cavity, organ, or vessel
syringe *(sir-INJ)*	An instrument for injecting fluid
vial *(VĪ-al)*	A small glass or plastic container

KEY TERMS

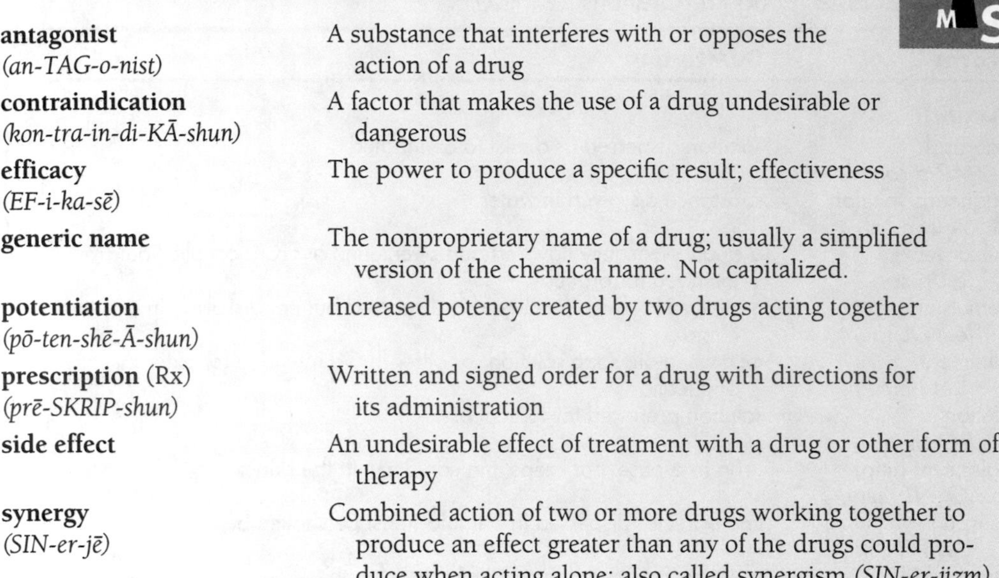

Term	Definition
antagonist *(an-TAG-o-nist)*	A substance that interferes with or opposes the action of a drug
contraindication *(kon-tra-in-di-KĀ-shun)*	A factor that makes the use of a drug undesirable or dangerous
efficacy *(EF-i-ka-sē)*	The power to produce a specific result; effectiveness
generic name	The nonproprietary name of a drug; usually a simplified version of the chemical name. Not capitalized.
potentiation *(pō-ten-shē-Ā-shun)*	Increased potency created by two drugs acting together
prescription (Rx) *(prē-SKRIP-shun)*	Written and signed order for a drug with directions for its administration
side effect	An undesirable effect of treatment with a drug or other form of therapy
synergy *(SIN-er-jē)*	Combined action of two or more drugs working together to produce an effect greater than any of the drugs could produce when acting alone; also called synergism *(SIN-er-jizm)*
trade name	The brand name of a drug, a registered trademark of the manufacturer. Written with a capital letter.

Word Parts for Drugs

Word part	Meaning	Example	Definition of Example
Suffixes			
-lytic	lysing, destroying	thrombolytic *throm-bō-LIT-ik*	dissolving blood clots
-mimetic	mimicking, simulating	sympathomimetic *sim-pa-thō-mi-MET-ik*	mimicking the effects of the sympathetic nervous system
-tropic	acting on	inotropic *in-ō-TROP-ik*	acting on the force of muscle contraction (*in/o* means "fiber")
Prefixes			
anti-	against	antidote *AN-ti-dōt*	substance that counteracts a poison
contra-	against	contraceptive *kon-tra-SEP-tiv*	preventing conception
Roots			
algi/o, algesi/o	pain	algesic *al-JĒ-sik*	painful
chem/o	chemical	chemotherapy *kē-mō-THER-a-pē*	treatment with drugs
hypn/o	sleep	hypnogenic *hip-nō-JEN-ik*	inducing sleep

(continued)

Word Parts for Drugs (Continued)

Word part	Meaning	Example	Definition of Example
narc/o	stupor	narcosis *nar-KŌ-sis*	drug-induced stupor
pharmac/o	drung	pharmacist *FAR-ma-sist*	one who prepares, sells, or dispenses drugs
pyr/o, pyret/o	fever	antipyretic *an-ti-pī-RET-ik*	counteracting fever
tox/o, toxic/o	poison, toxin	toxicolgy *tox-i-KOL-ō-jē*	the study of poisons
vas/o	vessel	vasomotor *vas-ō-MŌ-tor*	pertaining to change in vessel diameter

Exercise 8-1

Identify and define the suffix in each of the following words:

	Suffix	Meaning of Suffix
1. anxiolytic (*ang-zī-ō-LIT-ik*)	______	______
2. parasympathomimetic (*par-a-sim-pa-thō-mi-MET-ik*)	______	______
3. psychotropic (*sī-kō-TROP-ik*)	______	______

Give the opposite of each of the following words:

4. pyretic ______
5. indicated ______
6. inflammatory ______
7. convulsant ______
8. algesic ______

Identify and define the roots in each of the following words:

	Root	Meaning of Root
9. hypnosis	______	______
10. toxicity	______	______
11. chemistry	______	______
12. narcotic	______	______
13. pharmacy	______	______

Define the following words:

14. vasodilation ______________________
15. pharmacology ______________________
16. gonadotropic ______________________
17. toxicology ______________________

ABBREVIATIONS (Use of capitals and periods may vary)

Drugs and Drug Formulations

APAP acetaminophen

ASA acetylsalicylic acid (aspirin)

cap capsule

elix elixir

FDA Food and Drug Administration

INH isoniazid (anti-tubercular drug)

MED(s) medicine(s), medication(s)

NSAID(s) nonsteroidal anti-inflammatory drug(s)

OTC over-the-counter

PDR Physicians' Desk Reference

Rx prescription

supp suppository

susp suspension

tab tablet

tinct tincture

USP United States Pharmacopeia

ung ointment

Dosages and Directions

ā before (L. *ante*)

a̅a̅ of each (G. *ana*)

ac before meals (L. *ante cibum*)

ad lib as desired (L. *ad libitum*)

aq water (L. *aqua*)

bid twice a day (L. *bis in die*)

c̄ with (L. *cum*)

dc discontinue

gt(t) drop(s) (L. *gutta*)

hs at bedtime (L. *hora somni*)

IM intramuscular(ly)

IU international unit

IV intravenous(ly)

IVPB IV piggyback

NS normal saline

p after, post

pc after meals (L. *post cibum*)

po by mouth (L. *per os*)

pp postprandial (following a meal)

prn as needed (L. *pro re nata*)

qd every day (L. *quaque die*)

qh every hour (L. *quaque hora*)

q ___ h every ___ hours

qid four times a day (L. *quater in die*)

qm every morning (L. *quaque matin*)

qn every night (L. *quaque nox*)

qod every other day (L. *quaque* [other] *die*)

s̄ without (L. *sine*)

SC, subcu subcutaneous(ly)

s̄s̄ half (L. *semis*)

tid three times a day (L. *ter in die*)

U unit(s)

x times

CHAPTER REVIEW 8

Matching. Match the terms in each of these sets with their meanings and write the appropriate letter (a–e) to the left of each number:

_____ 1. antineoplastic — a. cough inducer
_____ 2. corticosteroid — b. agent that destroys cancer cells
_____ 3. expectorant — c. cough suppressant
_____ 4. antitussive — d. anti-inflammatory agent
_____ 5. adrenergic — e. sympathomimetic

_____ 6. diuretic — a. prevents blood clotting
_____ 7. sedative — b. suppresses seizures
_____ 8. anticonvulsant — c. promotes excretion of water
_____ 9. anticoagulant — d. induces relaxation
_____ 10. antiemetic — e. relieves nausea

_____ 11. tid — a. as needed
_____ 12. qh — b. by mouth
_____ 13. prn — c. every hour
_____ 14. pc — d. three times a day
_____ 15. po — e. after meals

Multiple choice. Select the best answer and write the letter of your choice in the blank to the left of each number.

_____ 16. Another term for trade name is

a. indicated name
b. generic name
c. prescription name
d. chemical name
e. brand name

_____ 17. An analgesic is used to treat

a. diarrhea
b. arrhythmia
c. psychosis
d. pain
e. thrombosis

_____ 18. Another term for subcutaneous is

a. intrathecal
b. hypodermic
c. sublingual
d. topical
e. instillation

_____ 19. Nitrates, beta blockers, and calcium channel blockers are used to treat disorders of the

a. liver
b. brain
c. spleen
d. heart
e. spinal cord

Fill in the blanks:

20. A thin tube that can be passed into a body cavity, organ, or vessel is a(n) _____________________.

21. A psychotropic drug is one that has an effect on the ____________________.
22. Pharmacokinetics is study of the action and behavior of ____________________.
23. A hypnogenic agent is one that induces ____________________.
24. An intradermal injection is given into the ____________________.

Definitions. Write the meaning of the following terms:

25. Mucolytic ____________________
26. Vasoconstriction ____________________
27. Bronchodilation ____________________
28. Anti-infective ____________________
29. Sublingual ____________________

Word building. Write a word for each of the following definitions:

30. Counteracting fever ____________________
31. Dissolving blood clots (root *thromb/o*) ____________________
32. One who prepares, sells, or dispenses drugs ____________________
33. One who studies poisons ____________________

Write the meaning of the following abbreviations:

34. Rx ____________________
35. IM ____________________
36. U.S.P. ____________________
37. ad lib ____________________
38. ung ____________________
39. NSAIDs ____________________
40. bid ____________________

Word analysis. Define each of the following words and give the meaning of the word parts in each. Use a dictionary if necessary.

41. Chronotropic *(kron-ō-TROP-ik)* ____________________
    a. chron/o ____________________
    b. trop ____________________
    c. -ic ____________________
42. Adrenergic *(ad-ren-ER-jik)* ____________________
    a. adren/o ____________________
    b. erg/o ____________________
    c. -ic ____________________

Chapter 8

Case Studies

1. Pneumonia

This 42-year-old female was in her usual state of health when she developed an acute pyrexia associated with dry cough, nausea, anorexia and pain in the left lower back. These symptoms had persisted for approximately 10 days prior to admission. She was treated as an out-patient with Keflex and antitussive agents.

These MEDs brought only slight relief of symptoms. X-rays done as an outpatient showed pneumonia of the left lower lobe. She was treated at home with bronchodilators Alupent, Ventolin, and Lufyllin 400 mg qid. She began to have productive cough which was blood tinged and then turned into a thick, yellow-brown sputum. Her generalized condition did not improve and hospitalization was recommended.

2. Pericarditis

This patient, on the morning of admission, noted the gradual onset of substernal chest pain which increased with deep inspiration and lying down and decreased with sitting forward. She denied shortness of breath or cough. Several days prior to admission she had begun radiotherapy to the chest for the treatment of non-Hodgkins lymphoma of the mediastinum (area between the lungs).

Echocardiography showed a small pericardial effusion adjacent to the right atrium. She was admitted for parenteral analgesic therapy because of her inability to take oral analgesics. The patient received intermittent doses of IV and IM morphine and, with clinical improvement, Indocin (NSAID) 50 mg tid. Electrocardiogram showed findings consistent with acute pericarditis.

The patient was asymptomatic on the 3rd day and was discharged with follow-up recommended. Discharge medications: Indocin, 50 mg po tid.

3. *E. coli* Sepsis

HPI: This is a 48-year-old male who was admitted from the Dialysis Unit with hypotension, fevers, and myalgia which began 3 days prior to admission. The patient took Demerol and Tylenol #3 without relief of pain. Blood cultures grew out *E. coli*. Physical examination showed that the region of the left olecranon (elbow) was warm and tender. C&S of pus aspirated from the bursa (sac) also showed *E. coli* sensitive to a number of antibiotics. Plans were for 2 weeks of Fortaz 1 gm IV post each hemodialysis. Additional discharge MEDs: calcium carbonate 650 mg 3 tabs po tid with meals, Nephrocaps qd, Tylenol #4 1 po q4h prn for pain, Colase bid.

Chapter 8
Case Study Questions

Matching. Select the best answer and write the letter of your choice to the left of each number:

_____ 1. A drug administered parenterally is given

a. orally
b. topically
c. into the eye
d. by injection
e. sublingually

_____ 2. Effusion is

a. escape of fluid into a cavity
b. dropping of an organ

c. infectious organisms in the blood
d. overgrowth of tissue
e. death of tissue

_____ 3. Myalgia is

a. paleness
b. fusion of muscles
c. pain in a muscle
d. spasm of muscle
e. fainting

Write the meaning of the following abbreviations:

4. HPI _______________
5. MEDs _______________
6. IV _______________
7. tid _______________
8. po _______________
9. C&S _______________
10. q4h _______________
11. qd _______________

Define the following terms:

12. pyrexia _______________
13. antitussive _______________
14. bronchodilator _______________
15. analgesic _______________

Identify and define the suffix in each of the following words:

	Suffix	Meaning of Suffix
16. lymphoma	_______	_______________
17. pericarditis	_______	_______________
18. electrocardiogram	_______	_______________

Chapter 8
Answer Section

Answers to Chapter Exercise

1. -lytic; lysing, destroying
2. -mimetic; mimicking, simulating
3. -tropic; acting on
4. antipyretic
5. contraindicated
6. anti-inflammatory
7. anticonvulsant
8. analgesic
9. hypn/o; sleep
10. tox, toxic/o; poison
11. chem/o; chemical
12. narc/o; stupor
13. pharmac/o; drug
14. widening of a blood vessel
15. the study of drugs
16. acting on the gonads (sex glands)
17. the study of poisons

Answers to Chapter Review 8

1. b
2. d
3. a
4. c
5. e
6. c
7. d
8. b
9. a
10. e
11. d
12. c
13. a
14. e
15. b
16. e
17. d
18. b
19. d
20. catheter
21. mind
22. drugs
23. sleep
24. skin
25. loosening or dissolving mucus
26. narrowing of a blood vessel
27. widening of a bronchus
28. killing or preventing the growth of infectious organisms
29. under the tongue
30. antipyretic
31. thrombolytic
32. pharmacist
33. toxicologist
34. prescription
35. intramuscular(ly)
36. United States Pharmacopeia
37. as desired
38. ointment
39. nonsteroidal anti-inflammatory drugs
40. twice a day
41. acting on the heart rate
    a. time
    b. acting on
    c. pertaining to
42. Activated by or secreting adrenaline (epinephrine)
    a. adrenaline
    b. work
    c. pertaining to

Answers to Case Study Questions

1. d
2. a
3. c
4. history of present illness
5. medication(s)
6. intravenous(ly)
7. three times a day
8. by mouth
9. culture and sensitivity
10. every 4 hours
11. every day
12. fever
13. agent that suppresses coughing
14. agent that relaxes bronchial smooth muscle, widens bronchi
15. agent that alleviates pain
16. -oma; tumor
17. -itis; inflammation
18. -gram; record of data

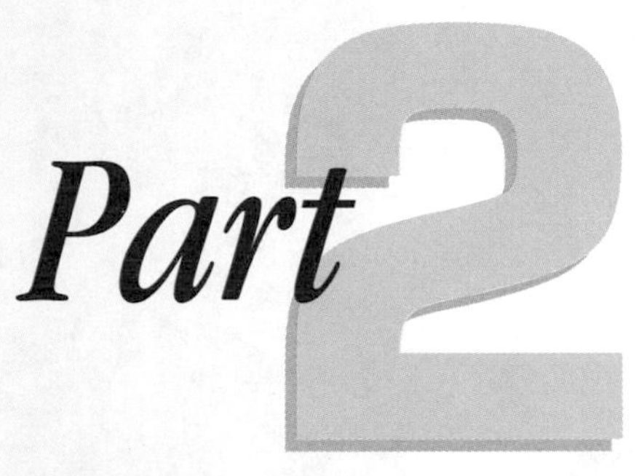

Part 2 Body Systems

In this section, the basics of medical terminology are applied to the body systems. Each chapter begins with a description of normal structure and function, as these form the basis for all medical studies.

The case studies illustrate terminology in the context of a medical report. In most, only significant findings are given. Look up any unfamiliar words and be sure you understand the meaning of the report.

9 Circulation: The Cardiovascular and Lymphatic Systems

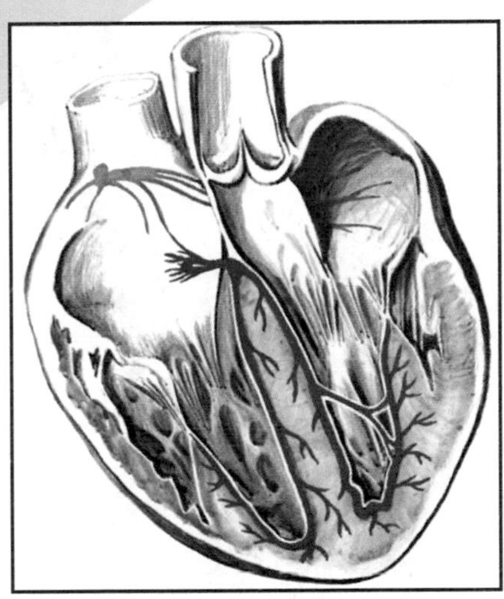

Chapter Contents

Objectives

After study of this chapter you should be able to:

1. Label a diagram of the heart
2. Trace the path of blood flow through the heart
3. Trace the pathway of electrical conduction through the heart
4. Differentiate among arteries, veins, and capillaries
5. Name and locate the main components of the lymphatic system
6. Identify and use the roots pertaining to the cardiovascular and lymphatic systems
7. List and describe the main disorders that affect the heart and the blood vessels
8. Define the main medical terms pertaining to the circulatory system
9. Interpret medical abbreviations referring to the heart and circulation
10. Analyze several case studies concerning the heart and circulation

Blood circulates throughout the body in the **cardiovascular system**, which consists of the heart and the blood vessels (Fig. 9-1). This system forms a continuous circuit that delivers oxygen and nutrients to all cells and carries away waste products. Also functioning in circulation is the **lymphatic system**, which drains fluid and proteins from the tissues and returns them to the bloodstream.

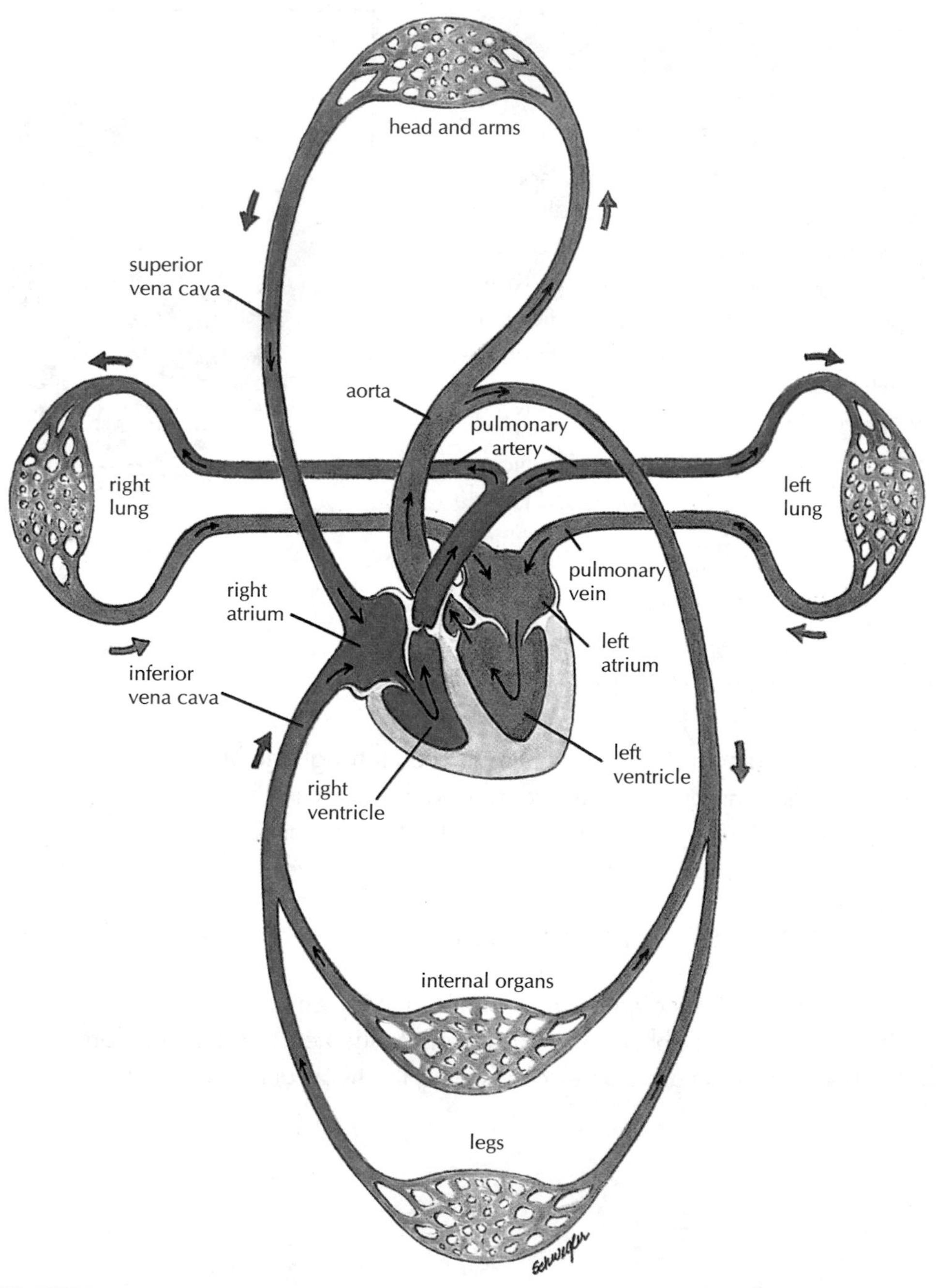

FIGURE 9-1. The cardiovascular system.

The Heart

The **heart** is located between the lungs with its point or **apex** directed toward left (Fig. 9-2). The thick muscle layer of the heart wall is the **myocardium.** This is lined on the inside with a thin **endocardium** and is covered on the outside with a thin **epicardium.** The heart is contained within a fibrous sac, the **pericardium**.

The upper receiving chambers of the heart are the **atria** (sing. atrium). The lower pumping chambers are the ventricles. The chambers are divided by walls, each of which is called a **septum**. The interventricular septum separates the two ventricles; the interatrial septum divides the two atria. There is also a septum between the atrium and ventricle on each side.

The heart pumps blood through two circuits. The right side pumps blood to the lungs to be oxygenated through the **pulmonary circuit**. The left side pumps to the remainder of the body through the **systemic circuit**.

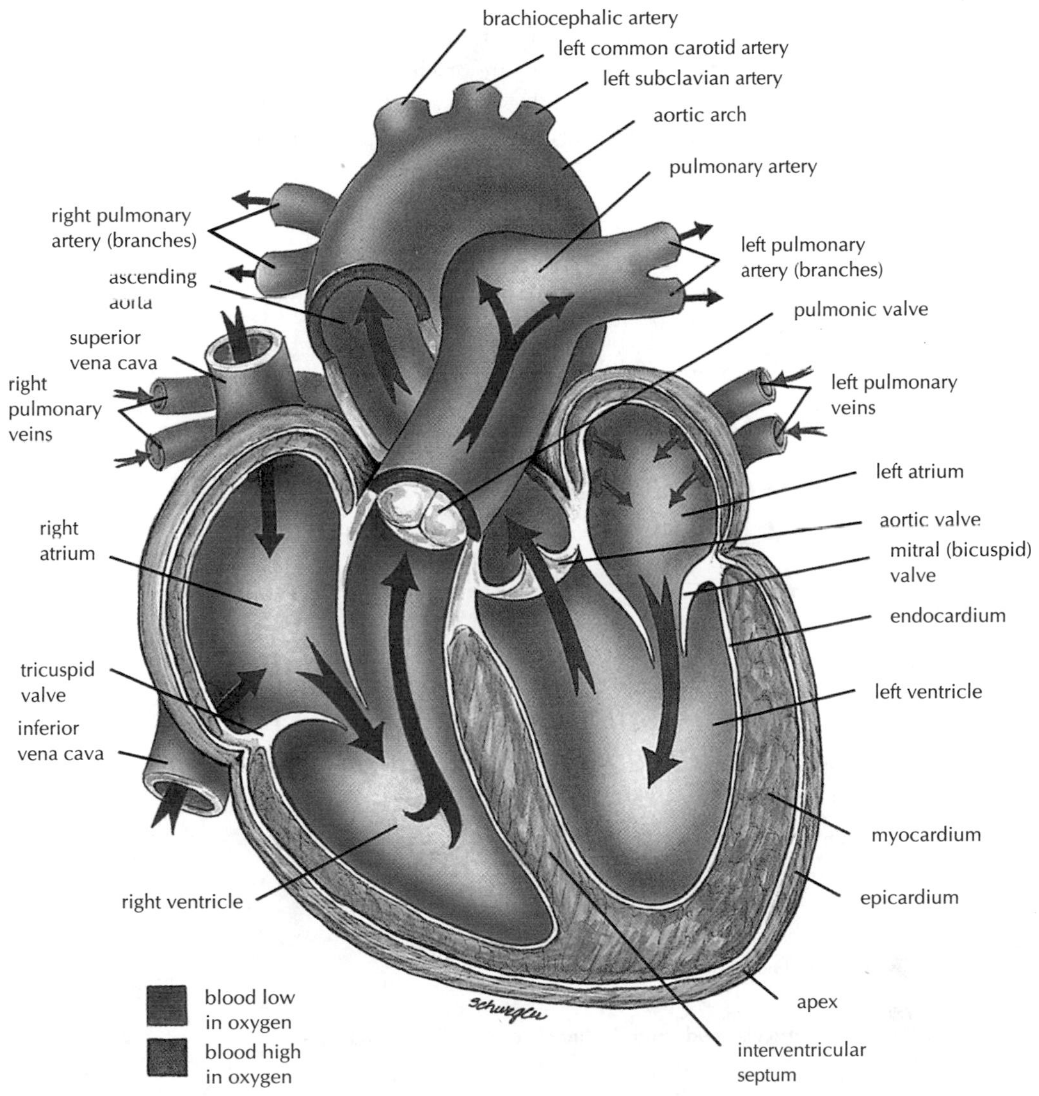

FIGURE 9-2. Heart and great vessels.

Blood Flow Through the Heart

The pathway of blood through the heart is shown by the arrows in Figure 9-2. The right atrium receives blood low in oxygen from all body tissues through the **superior vena cava** and the **inferior vena cava**. The blood then enters the right ventricle and is pumped to the lungs through the **pulmonary artery**. Blood returns from the lungs high in oxygen and enters the left atrium through the **pulmonary veins**. From here it enters the left ventricle and is forcefully pumped into the **aorta** to be distributed to all tissues.

Blood is kept moving in a forward direction by one-way **valves**. The valve in the septum between the right atrium and ventricle is the **tricuspid** (meaning three cusps or flaps); the valve in the septum between the left atrium and ventricle is the bicuspid valve (having two cusps), usually called the **mitral valve** (so named because it resembles a bishop's miter). The valves leading into the pulmonary artery and the aorta have three cusps. Each cusp is shaped like a half-moon, so these valves are described as **semilunar valves**. The valve at the entrance to the pulmonary artery is specifically named the **pulmonic valve**; the valve at the entrance to the aorta is the **aortic valve**.

Heart sounds are produced as the heart functions. The loudest of these, the familiar lubb-dupp that can be heard through the chest wall, are produced by alternate closing of the valves. The first heart sound (S_1) is heard when the valves between the chambers close. The second heart sound (S_2) is produced when the valves leading into the aorta and pulmonary artery close. An abnormal sound is termed a **murmur**.

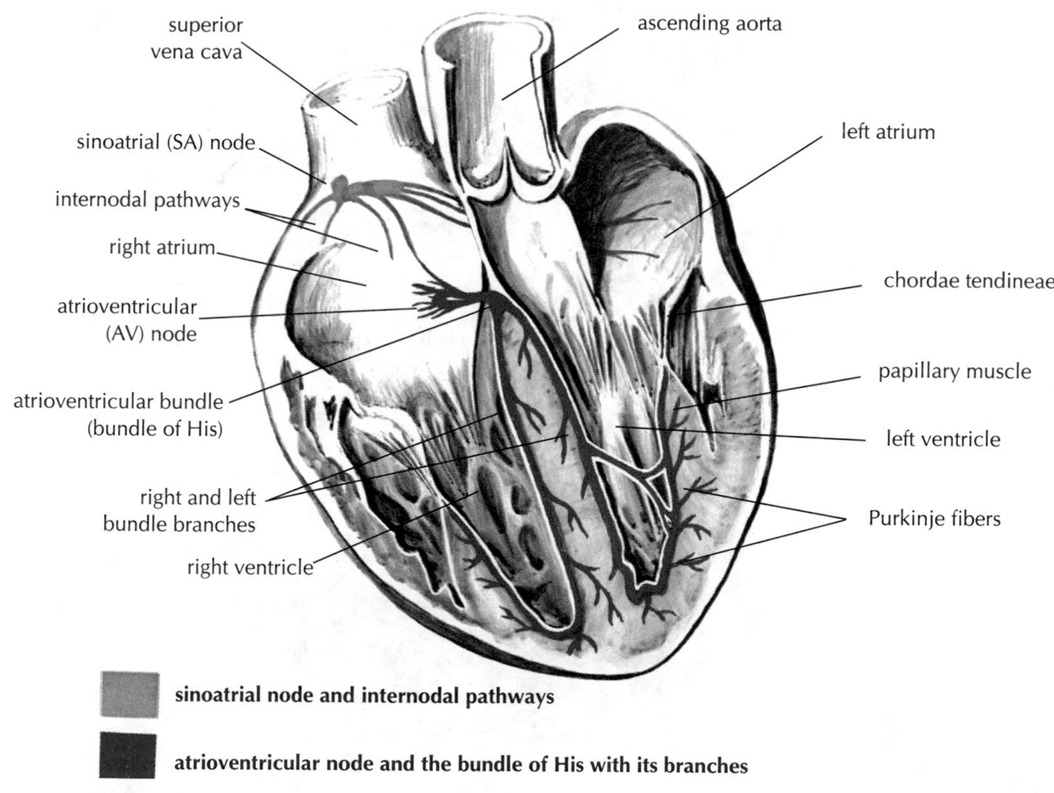

FIGURE 9-3. Conduction system of the heart.

The Heartbeat

Each contraction of the heart, termed **systole** *(SIS-tō-lē)*, is followed by a relaxation phase, during which the chambers fill. The relaxation is termed **diastole** *(dī-AS-tō-lē)*. Each time the heart beats, both atria contract and immediately thereafter both ventricles contract. The wave of increased pressure produced in the vessels each time the ventricles contract is the **pulse.**

The contractions are stimulated by a built-in system that regularly transmits electrical impulses through the heart. The components of this **conduction system** are shown in Figure 9-3. They include the **SA** (sinoatrial) **node**, called the *pacemaker* because it sets the rate of the heartbeat, the **AV** (atrioventricular) **node**, the **AV bundle** (bundle of His), the left and right **bundle branches**, and **Purkinje** *(pur-KIN-jē)* **fibers**.

Although the heart itself generates the heartbeat, factors such as nervous system stimulation, hormones, and drugs can influence the rate and the force of heart contractions.

Blood Pressure

Blood pressure is the force exerted by blood against the wall of a blood vessel. It is commonly measured in a large artery with an inflatable cuff (Fig. 9-4), known as a blood pressure cuff or blood pressure apparatus, but technically called a **sphygmomanometer**. Both systolic and diastolic pressures are measured and reported as systolic then diastolic separated by a slash, such as 120/80. Pressure is expressed as millimeters mercury (mm Hg), that is, the height to which the pressure can push a column of mercury in a tube. Blood pressure is a valuable diagnostic measurement that is easily obtained.

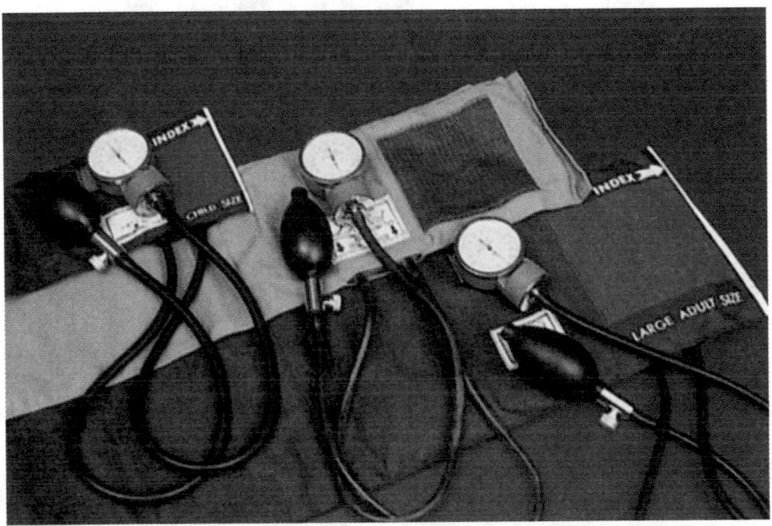

FIGURE 9-4. Blood pressure cuffs in three sizes. Shown are the cuff, the bulb to inflate the cuff, and the manometer to measure pressure. (Photograph © Ken Kasper. From Taylor C, Lillis CA, LeMone P: Fundamentals of Nursing, 2nd ed, p 419. Philadelphia: JB Lippincott, 1993.)

The Vascular System

The vascular system consists of:

1. **Arteries** that carry blood away from the heart (Fig. 9-5). **Arterioles** are small arteries that lead into the capillaries.
2. **Capillaries**, the smallest vessels, through which exchanges take place between the blood and the tissues.

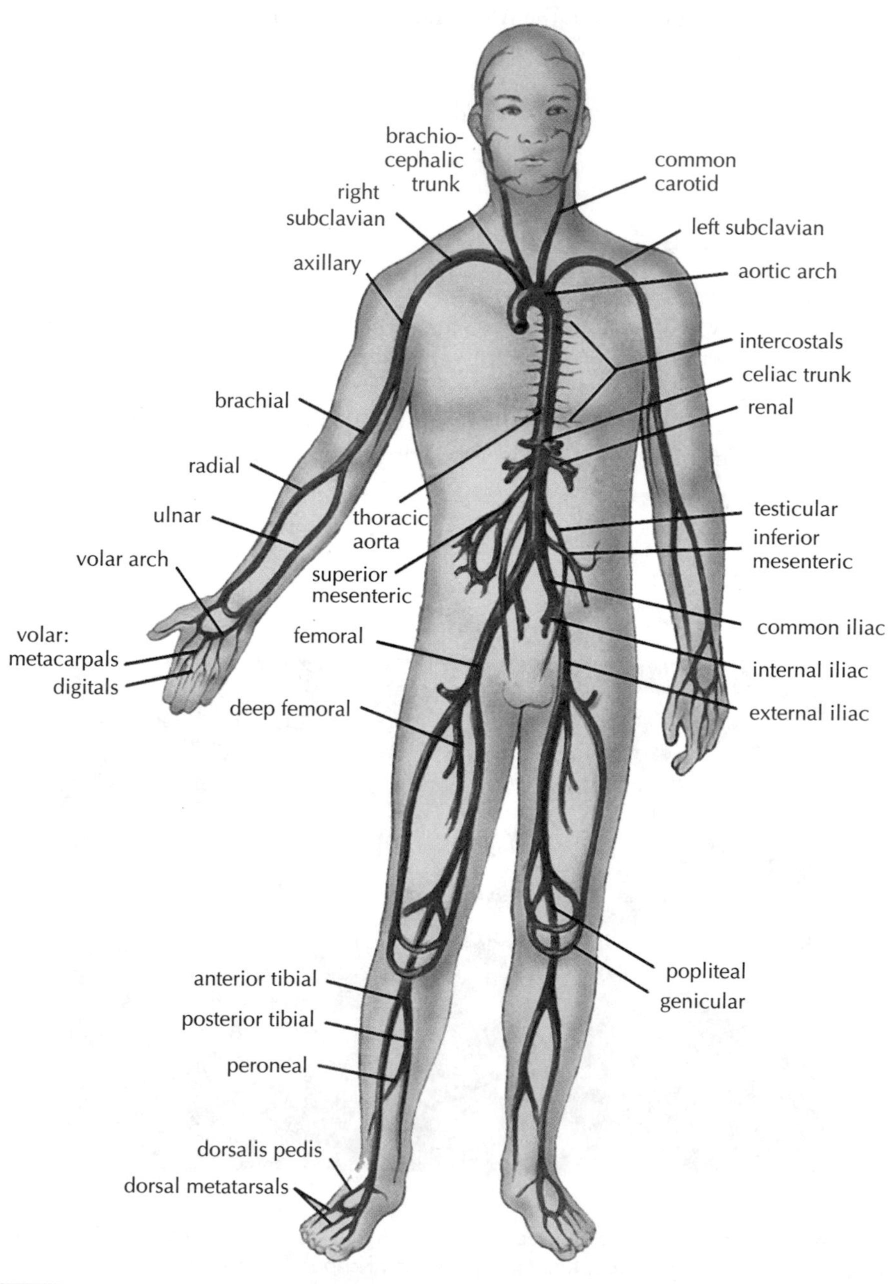

FIGURE 9-5. Principal systemic arteries.

3. **Veins** that carry blood back to the heart (Fig. 9-6). The small veins that receive blood from the capillaries and drain into the veins are **venules**.

All arteries, except the pulmonary artery (and the umbilical artery in the fetus), carry blood high in oxygen. They are thick-walled, elastic vessels that carry blood under high pressure. All veins, except the pulmonary vein (and the umbilical vein in the fetus), carry blood low in oxygen. Veins have thinner, less elastic walls and tend to give way under pressure. Like the heart, veins have one-way valves that keep blood flowing forward.

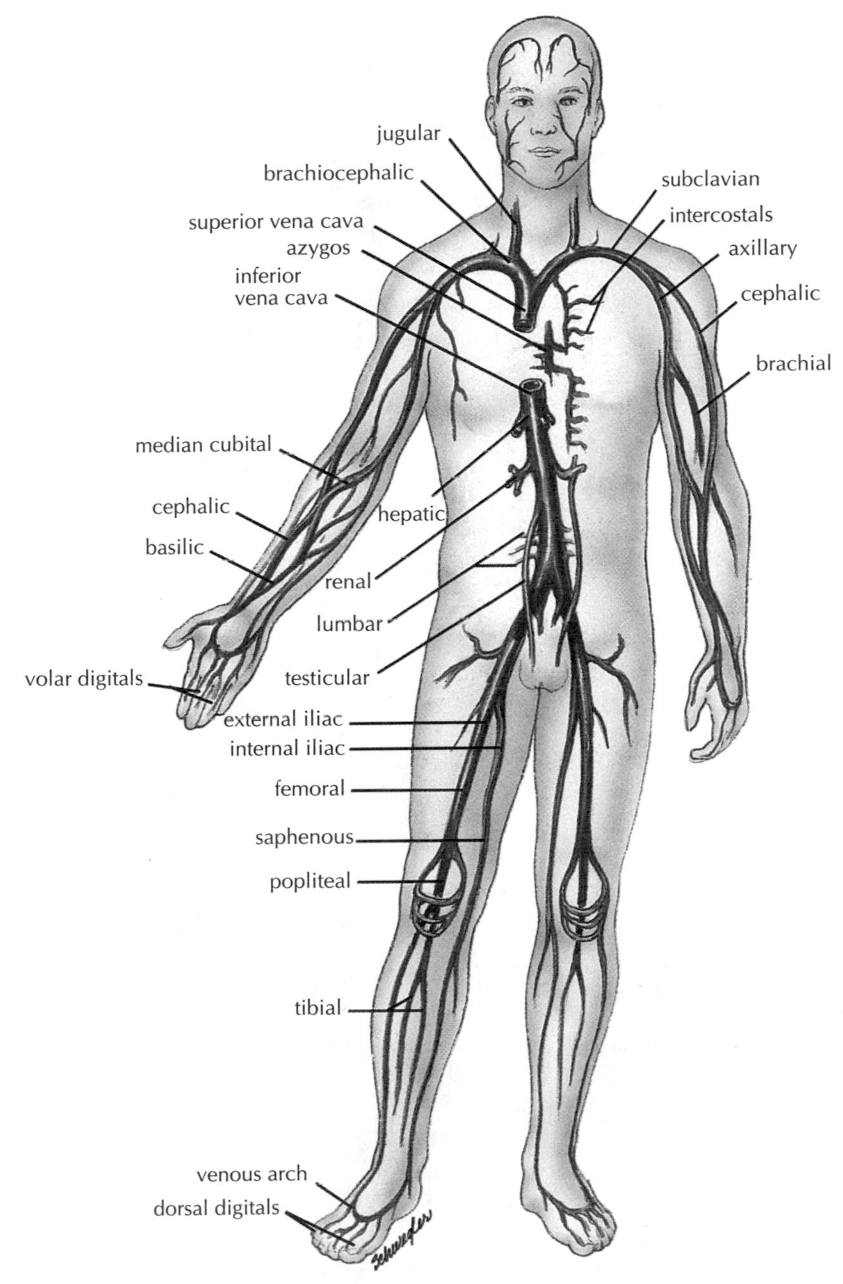

FIGURE 9-6. Principal systemic veins.

Nervous system stimulation can cause the diameter of a vessel to increase (vasodilation) or decrease (vasoconstriction). These changes alter blood flow to the tissues and affect blood pressure.

The Lymphatic System

The lymphatic system is a widely distributed system with multiple functions (Fig. 9-7). Its role in circulation is to return excess fluid and proteins from the tissues to the bloodstream. The fluid

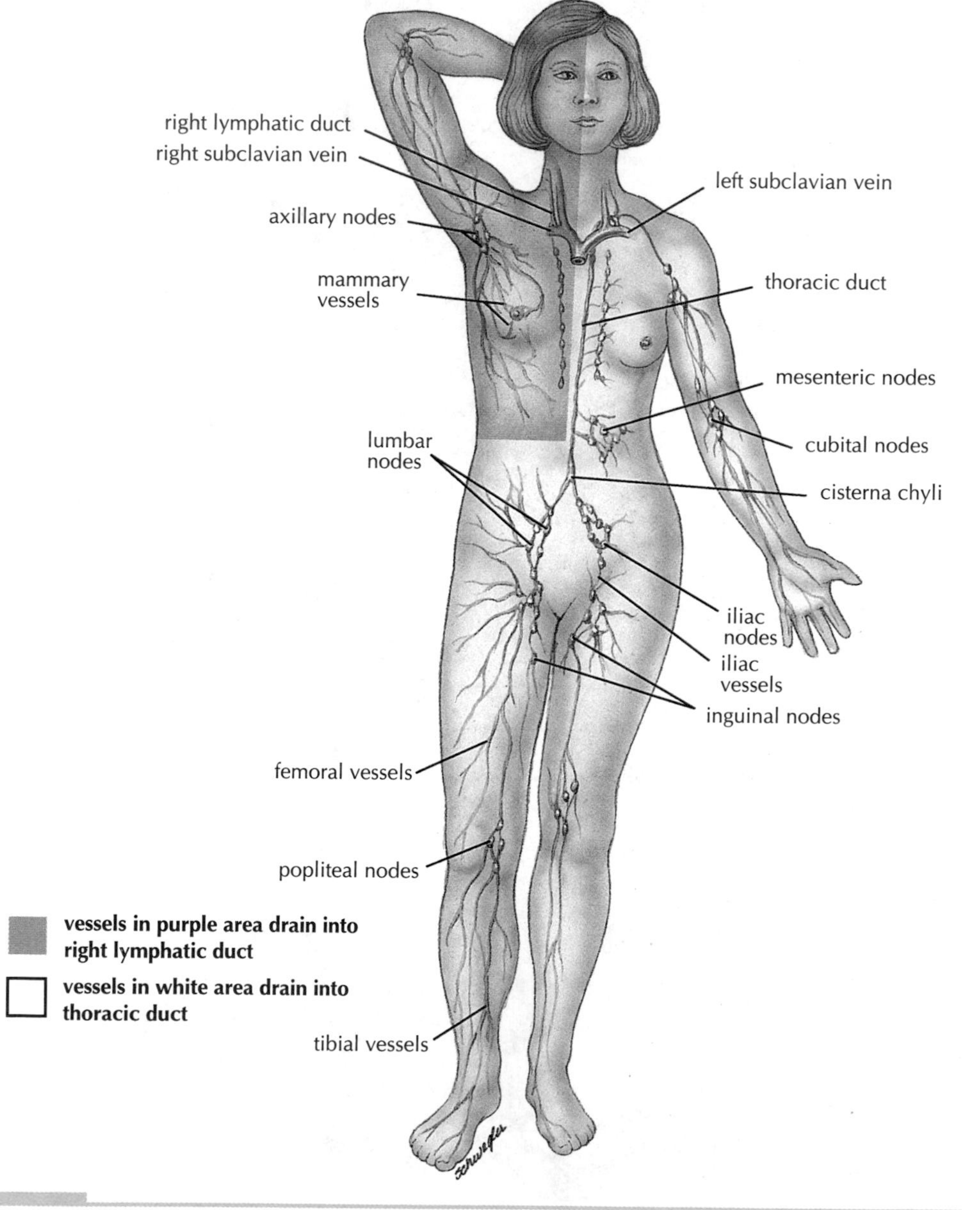

FIGURE 9-7. Lymphatic system.

carried in the lymphatic system is called **lymph**. Lymph drains from the lower part of the body and the upper left side into the **thoracic duct**, which travels upward through the chest and empties into the left subclavian vein near the heart. The **right lymphatic duct** drains the upper right half of the body and empties into the right subclavian vein.

The lymphatic system also absorbs digested fat from the small intestine (see Chapter 12). These fats are then added to the blood near the heart.

Another major function of the lymphatic system is to protect the body from impurities and foreign microorganisms. Along the path of the lymphatic vessels are small masses of lymphoid tissue, the **lymph nodes** (see Figure 9-7). Their function is to filter the lymph as it passes through. They are concentrated in the cervical (neck), axillary (armpit), mediastinal (chest), and inguinal (groin) regions. The lymph nodes and the remainder of the lymphatic system also play a role in immunity (see Chapter 10). Other organs and tissues of the lymphatic system include the **tonsils**, located in the throat (described in Chapter 11), the **thymus gland** in the chest, and the **spleen** in the upper left region of the abdomen (see Figure 12-l).

KEY TERMS

Normal Structure and Function

Cardiovascular System

Term	Definition
aorta *(ā-OR-ta)*	The largest artery. It receives blood from the left ventricle and branches to all parts of the body. (root aort/o)
aortic valve *(ā-OR-tik)*	The semilunar valve at the entrance to the aorta
apex *(Ā-peks)*	The point of a cone-shaped structure (adj. apical). The apex of the heart is formed by the left ventricle. It is inferior and pointed toward the left (see Figure 9-2).
artery *(AR-ter-ē)*	A vessel that carries blood away from the heart. Most arteries carry oxygenated blood. (root arter, arteri/o)
arteriole *(ar-TĒ-rē-ōl)*	A small artery (root arteriol/o)
atrioventricular (AV) node *(ā-trē-ō-ven-TRIK-ū-lar)*	A small mass in the lower septum of the right atrium that passes impulses from the sinoatrial (SA) node toward the ventricles
AV bundle	A band of fibers that transmits impulses from the atrioventricular (AV) node to the top of the interventricular septum. It divides into the right and left bundle branches which descend along the two sides of the septum. Also called bundle of His.
atrium *(Ā-trē-um)*	An entrance chamber. One of the two upper receiving chambers of the heart (root atri/o).
blood pressure	The force exerted by blood against the wall of a vessel
capillary *(KAP-i-lar-ē)*	One of the millions of microscopic blood vessels through which materials are exchanged between the blood and the tissues
diastole *(dī-AS-tō-lē)*	The relaxation phase of the heart cycle

endocardium *(en-dō-KAR-dē-um)*	The thin membrane that lines the chambers of the heart and covers the valves
epicardium *(ep-i-KAR-dē-um)*	The thin outermost layer of the heart wall
heart *(hart)*	The muscular organ with four chambers that contracts rhythmically to propel blood through vessels to all parts of the body (root cardi/o)
heart sounds	Sounds produced as the heart functions. The two loudest sounds are produced by alternate closing of the valves and are desginated S_1 and S_2.
mitral valve *(MĪ-tral)*	The valve between the left atrium and the left ventricle; the bicuspid valve
myocardium *(mī-ō-KAR-dē-um)*	The thick middle layer of the heart wall composed of cardiac muscle
pericardium *(per-i-KAR-dē-um)*	The fibrous sac that surrounds the heart
pulmonary circuit *(PUL-mō-nar-ē)*	The system of vessels that carries blood from the right side of the heart to the lungs to be oxygenated and then back to the left side of the heart
pulmonic valve *(pul-MON-ik)*	The semilunar valve at the entrance to the pulmonary artery
Purkinje fibers *(pur-KIN-jē)*	The terminal fibers of the conducting system of the heart. They carry impulses through the walls of the ventricles.
septum *(SEP-tum)*	A wall dividing two cavities, such as the chambers of the heart
sinoatrial (SA) node *(sī-nō-Ā-trē-al)*	A small mass in the upper part of the right atrium that initiates the impulse for each heartbeat; the pacemaker
sphygmomanometer *(sfig-mō-man-OM-e-ter)*	An instrument for determining arterial blood pressure (root *sphygm/o* means "pulse"); blood pressure apparatus or cuff (see Figure 9-4)
systemic circuit *(sis-TEM-ik)*	The system of vessels that carries oxygenated blood from the left side of the heart to all tissues except the lungs and returns deoxygenated blood to the right side of the heart
systole *(SIS-tō-lē)*	The contraction phase of the heart cycle
tricuspid valve *(trī-KUS-pid)*	The valve between the right atrium and the right ventricle
valve	A structure that keeps fluid flowing in a forward direction (root valv/o, valvul/o)
vein *(vān)*	A vessel that carries blood back to the heart. Most veins carry blood low in oxygen. (root ven, phleb/o)
vena cava *(VĒ-na-KĀ-va)*	One of the two veins (superior and inferior) that carry deoxygenated blood back to the right atrium of the heart (pl. venae cavae)
ventricle *(VEN-trik-l)*	A small cavity. One of the two lower pumping chambers of the heart (root ventricul/o)

venule (*VEN-ūl*) A small vein

vessel (*VES-el*) A tube or duct to transport fluid (root angi/o, vas/o, vascul/o)

Lymphatic System

lymph (*limf*) The thin plasmalike fluid that drains from the tissues and is transported in lymphatic vessels (root lymph/o)

lymph node A small mass of lymphoid tissue along the path of a lymphatic vessel that filters lymph (root lymphaden/o)

spleen A large reddish-brown organ in the upper left region of the abdomen. It filters blood and destroys old red blood cells. (root splen/o)

thymus gland (*THĪ-mus*) A gland in the upper part of the chest beneath the sternum. It functions in immunity. (root thym/o)

tonsil (*TON-sil*) A small mass of lymphoid tissue in the throat that filters impurities (root tonsill/o)

Roots Pertaining to the Cardiovascular and Lymphatic Systems

Roots for the Heart

Root	Meaning	Example	Definition of Example
cardi/o	heart	cardiomyopathy* *kar-dē-ō-mi-OP-a-thē*	any disease of the the heart muscle
atri/o	atrium	atriotomy *ā-trē-OT-ō-mē*	surgical incision of an atrium
ventricul/o	cavity, ventricle	interventricular *in-ter-ven-TRIK-ū-lar*	between the ventricles
valv/o, valvul/o	valve	valvectomy *val-VEK-tō-mē*	surgical removal of a valve

*Preferred over *myocardiopathy*

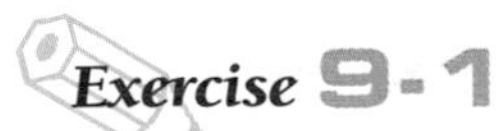

Fill in the blanks:

1. The word *cardiomegaly* (*kar-dē-ō-MEG-a-lē*) means enlargement of the ____________________

2. *Interatrial* (*in-ter-Ā-trē-al*) means between the ____________________

3. The word *ventriculotomy (ven-trik-ū-LOT-ō-mē)* means surgical incision of a(n) ____________________

4. A *valvuloplasty (val-vū-lō-PLAS-tē)* is plastic repair of a(n) ____________________

Write the adjective for each of the following definitions. The proper suffix is given for each.

5. Pertaining to the heart (-ac) *cardiac*
6. Pertaining to the myocardium (-al; ending differs from adjective ending for the heart) __________
7. Pertaining to an atrium (-al) __________
8. Pertaining to the pericardium (-al) __________
9. Pertaining to a ventricle (-ar) __________
10. Pertaining to a valve (-ar) __________

Following the example, write a word for each of the following definitions pertaining to the tissues of the heart:

11. Inflammation of the lining of the heart (usually at a valve) *endocarditis*
12. Inflammation of the heart muscle __________
13. Inflammation of the fibrous sac around the heart __________

Write a word for each of the following definitions:

14. Study (-logy) of the heart __________
15. Downward displacement (-ptosis) of the heart __________
16. Above (supra-) a ventricle __________
17. Pertaining to an atrium and a ventricle __________
18. Surgical incision of a valve __________

Roots for the Blood Vessels

Root	Meaning	Example	Definition of Example
angi/o*	vessel	angiography *an-jē-OG-ra-fē*	radiographic study of blood vessels
vas/o, vascul/o	vessel, duct	vasoconstriction *vas-ō-con-STRIK-shun*	narrowing of a blood vessel
arter/o, arteri/o	artery	endarterial *end-ar-TĒ-rē-al*	within an artery
arteriol/o	arteriole	arteriolitis *ar-tē-rē-ō-LĪ-tis*	inflammation of arterioles

(continued)

Roots for the Blood Vessels (Continued)

Root	Meaning	Example	Definition of Example
aort/o	aorta	aortosclerosis *ā-or-tō-skle-RŌ-sis*	hardening of the aorta
ven/o, ven/i	vein	venous *VĒ-nus*	pertaining to a vein
phleb/o	vein	phlebectasia *fleb-ek-TĀ-zē-a*	dilatation of a vein

*The root *angi/o* usually refers to a blood vessel, but is used for other types of vessels as well. *Hemangi/o* refers specifically to a blood vessel.

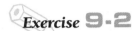

Exercise 9-2

Fill in the blanks:

1. *Vasodilation (vas-ō-dī-LĀ-shun)* means widening of a(n) ____________
2. *Endarterectomy (end-ar-ter-EK-tō-mē)* is removal of the inner lining of a(n) ____________
3. The word *arteriolar (ar-tē-RĒ-ō-lar)* means pertaining to a(n) ____________

Define the following words:

4. angiitis *(an-jē-Ī-tis)* (note spelling); also angitis or vasculitis; ____________
5. cardiovascular *(kar-dē-ō-VAS-kū-lar)* ____________
6. arteriorrhexis *(ar-tē-rē-ō-REK-sis)* ____________
7. aortoptosis *(ā-or-top-TŌ-sis)* ____________
8. phlebitis *(fleb-Ī-tis)* ____________

Use the root *angi/o* to write words with the following meanings:

9. Surgical removal (-ectomy) of a vessel ____________
10. Dilatation (-ectasis) of a vessel ____________
11. Formation (-genesis) of a vessel ____________
12. Plastic repair of a vessel ____________

Use the appropriate root to write a word that means each of the following:

13. Narrowing (-stenosis) of the aorta ____________
14. Inflammation of an artery ____________
15. Within (intra-) a vein ____________
16. Radiographic study (-graphy) of a vein ____________
17. Incision of a vein ____________

Roots for the Lymphatic System

Root	Meaning	Example	Definition of Example
lymph/o	lymph, lymphatic system	lymphoid *LIM-foyd*	resembling lymph or lymphatic tissue
lymphaden/o	lymph node	lymphadenectomy *lim-fad-ē-NEK-tō-mē*	surgical removal of a lymph node
lymphangi/o	lymphatic vessel	lymphangioma *lim-fan-jē-Ō-ma*	tumor of lymphatic vessels
splen/o	spleen	splenomegaly *splē-nō-MEG-a-lē*	enlargement of the spleen
thym/o	thymus gland	athymia *a-THĪ-mē-a*	absence of the thymus gland
tonsill/o	tonsil	tonsillar *TON-sil-ar*	pertaining to a tonsil

Exercise 9-3

Fill in the blanks:

1. Lymphedema *(limf-e-DĒ-ma)* means swelling due to obstruction of the flow of __________
2. Lymphadenitis *(lim-fad-e-NĪ-tis)* is inflammation of a(n) __________
3. A lymphangiogram *(lim-FAN-jē-ō-gram)* is an x-ray of __________
4. The adjective *splenic (SPLEN-ik)* means pertaining to the __________
5. Thymectomy *(thī-MEK-tō-mē)* is surgical removal of the __________
6. Tonsillopathy *(ton-sil-OP-a-thē)* is any disease of the __________

Identify and define the root in each of the following words:

	Root	Meaning of Root
7. lymphangial *(lim-FAN-jē-al)*	*lymphangi/o*	*lymphatic vessel*
8. lymphadenography *(lim-fad-e-NOG-ra-fē)*	________	________
9. perisplenitis *(per-i-sple-NĪ-tis)*	________	________
10. hypothymism *(hī-pō-THĪ-mizm)*	________	________
11. tonsillectomy *(ton-sil-EK-tō-mē)*	________	________

Use the appropriate root to write a word that means:

12. Inflammation of lymphatic vessels __________

13. A tumor (-oma) of lymphatic tissue ____________
14. Any disease (-pathy) of the lymph nodes ____________
15. Pain (-algia) in the spleen ____________
16. Inflammation of a tonsil ____________

Clinical Aspects of the Circulatory System

Atherosclerosis

The accumulation of fatty deposits within the lining of an artery is termed **atherosclerosis** (Fig. 9-8). These areas, called **plaques**, gradually thicken and harden with fibrous material, cells, and other deposits, restricting the lumen (opening) of the vessel and reducing blood flow to the tissues, a condition known as **ischemia**.

Atherosclerosis of the coronary vessels is a primary cause of heart disease. One sign of such coronary artery disease (CAD) is the type of chest pain known as **angina pectoris**. This is a feeling of constriction around the heart or pain that may radiate to the left arm or shoulder, usually brought on by exertion. Often there is anxiety, **diaphoresis** (profuse sweating), and **dyspnea** (difficulty in breathing). Angina pectoris is treated by control of exercise and administration of nitroglycerin to dilate coronary vessels. Other drugs may be used to regulate the heartbeat, strengthen the force of heart contraction, or prevent formation of blood clots. Severe cases may be candidates for **angioplasty**, which is surgical dilatation of the blocked vessel by means of a catheter. Still further, the blocked vessel may be surgically bypassed with a vascular graft.

Atherosclerosis also predisposes to **thrombosis**, the formation of a blood clot or **thrombus** in a vessel. Sudden **occlusion** (obstruction) of a coronary artery by a thrombus causes local necrosis (death) of tissue and formation of an **infarct** (Fig. 9-9). This is the **myocardial infarction** (MI) or "heart attack" that is a leading cause of sudden death. Symptoms include pain over the heart (precordial pain) or upper part of the abdomen (epigastric pain) that may extend to the jaw or arms, pallor (paleness), diaphoresis, nausea, and dyspnea. There may be a burning sensation similar to indigestion or heartburn. Often there is an abnormality of heart rhythm, or **arrhythmia**, usually **fibrillation**, an extremely rapid, ineffective beating of the heart. Outcome is based on the degree of damage and early treatment to dissolve the clot and reestablish normal heart rhythm. **Cardioversion** is the general term for restoration of a normal heart rhythm, either by drugs or application of electric current.

MI can be diagnosed by **electrocardiography** (EKG), study of the electrical impulses given off by the heart as it functions, by measurement of certain enzymes (CPK, LDH, AST) released into the blood from the damaged heart muscle, and by a variety of other methods described later in this chapter.

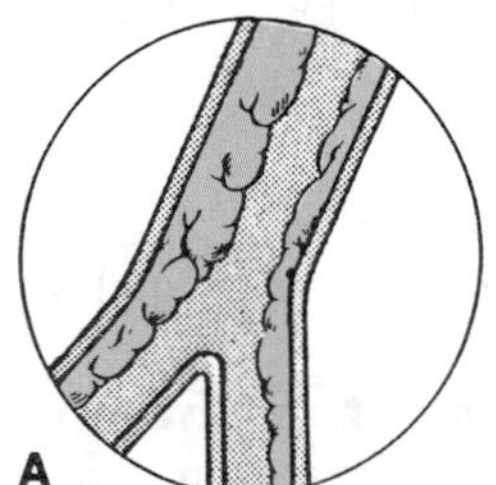

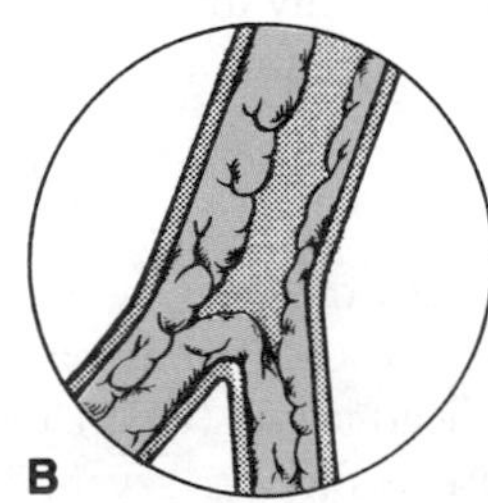

FIGURE 9-8. Atherosclerosis. **(A)** Narrowing of a coronary artery. **(B)** Complete blockage of a coronary artery leading to localized death of heart tissue. (Jones SA, Weigel A, White RD, McSwain NE Jr, Breiter M: Advanced Emergency Care for Paramedic Practice, p 419. Philadelphia: JB Lippincott, 1992).

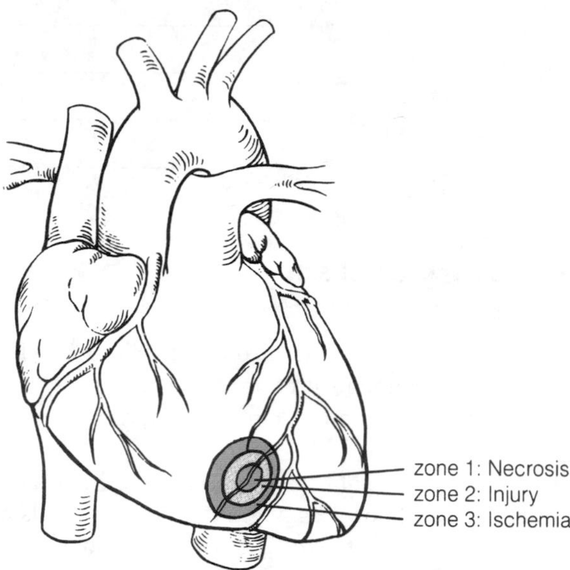

FIGURE 9-9. Myocardial infarction. (Jones SA, Weigel A, White RD, McSwain NE Jr, Breiter M: Advanced Emergency Care for Paramedic Practice, p 420. Philadelphia: JB Lippincott, 1992.)

Atherosclerosis is a major cause of disease in industrialized countries, and the factors that contribute to it are familiar to most people: heredity, high blood pressure, cigarette smoking, a diet high in fat, lack of exercise, and stress. Other vessels commonly affected are the aorta, the carotid arteries leading to the head, the cerebral arteries, and arteries in the leg. Atherosclerosis also contributes to other disorders described below.

Embolism

Occlusion of a vessel by a thrombus or other mass carried in the bloodstream is **embolism**, and the mass itself is called an **embolus**. Usually the mass is a blood clot that breaks loose from the wall of a vessel, but it may also be air (as from injection or trauma), fat (as from marrow released after a bone break), bacteria, or other solid materials. Often a venous thrombus will travel through the heart and then lodge in an artery of the lungs resulting in a life-threatening pulmonary embolism. An embolus from a carotid artery often blocks a cerebral vessel causing a **cerebrovascular accident (CVA)** commonly called **stroke**.

Aneurysm

An arterial wall weakened by atherosclerosis or other cause may balloon out, forming an **aneurysm**. If the aneurysm ruptures, hemorrhage results, causing a stroke, or cerebrovascular accident (CVA) if a cerebral artery is involved. In a **dissecting aneurysm** (Fig. 9-10) blood hemorrhages into the thick middle layer of the artery wall, separating the muscle as it spreads and sometimes rupturing the vessel. The aorta is most commonly involved. It may be possible to repair a dissecting aneurysm surgically with a graft.

Heart Failure

When the heart fails to empty effectively for any reason, the general term **heart failure** is applied. The resulting increased pressure in the venous system leads to **edema**, often in the lungs (pulmonary edema), and justifies the description congestive heart failure (CHF). Other symptoms are **cyanosis**, dyspnea, and **syncope.** Heart failure is one cause of **shock**, a severe disturbance in the circulatory

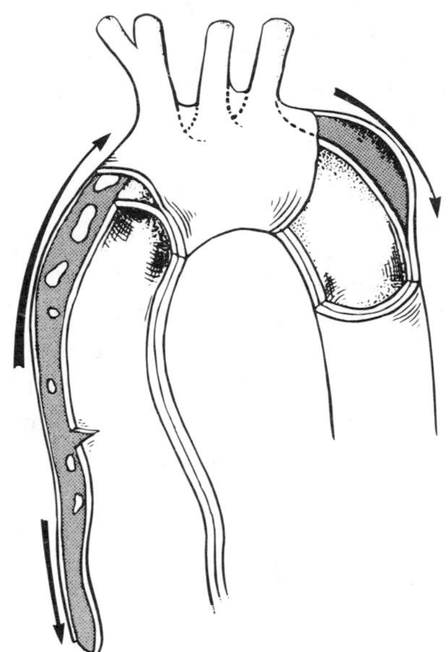

FIGURE 9-10. Dissecting aortic aneurysm. (Jones SA, Weigel A, White RD, McSwain NE Jr, Breiter M: Advanced Emergency Care for Paramedic Practice, p 429. Philadelphia: JB Lippincott, 1992.)

system resulting in inadequate delivery of blood to the tissues. Heart failure is treated with rest, drugs to strengthen heart contractions, diuretics to eliminate fluid, and restriction of salt in the diet.

Hypertension

Hypertension, or high blood pressure, is a contributing factor in all the conditions described above. In simple terms, hypertension is defined as a systolic pressure greater than 140 mm Hg or a diastolic pressure greater than 90 mm Hg. It causes the left ventricle to enlarge (hypertrophy) as a result of increased work. Some cases are secondary to other disorders, such as kidney malfunction or endocrine disturbance, but most cases of hypertension are due to unknown causes and are described as primary or essential hypertension. The condition is controlled with diuretics, vasodilators, and with drugs (ACE inhibitors) that prevent formation of angiotensin, a substance in the blood which acts to raise blood pressure.

Congenital Heart Disease

A congenital defect is any defect that is present at birth. The most common type of congenital heart defect is a hole in the septum (wall) that separates the atria or the ventricles. If not corrected, this may stress the heart and cause it to work harder. Symptoms include cyanosis (leading to the description "blue baby"), syncope, and clubbing of the fingers. Most such congenital defects can be corrected surgically. Another type of congenital defect is malformation of a heart valve.

Rheumatic Heart Disease

In **rheumatic heart disease** infection with a specific type of streptococcus sets up an immune reaction that ultimately damages the heart valves. The infection usually begins as a "strep throat," and most often it is the mitral valve that is involved. Scar tissue fuses the leaflets of the valve causing a narrowing or **stenosis** that interferes with proper function. Persons with rheumatic heart disease are subject to repeated infections of the valves and must take antibiotics prophylactically (preventively) before even minor surgery, such as dental work.

A key sign in cases of valvular defects as well as other heart abnormalities is the presence of a **murmur**, an abnormal sound heard as the heart cycles. Severe cases may require surgical correction or even valve replacement. The incidence of rheumatic heart disease has declined with the use of antibiotics.

Disorders of the Veins

A breakdown in the valves of the veins in combination with a chronic dilatation of these vessels results in **varicose veins**. These appear twisted and swollen under the skin, most commonly in the legs. Contributing factors include heredity, obesity, prolonged standing, and pregnancy, which increases pressure in the pelvic veins. This condition can impede blood flow, and lead to edema, thrombosis, hemorrhage, or ulceration. Treatment includes the wearing of elastic stockings and, in some cases, surgical removal of the varicosities, after which collateral circulation is established. Varicose veins in the rectum and anal canal are referred to as **hemorrhoids**.

Any inflammation of the veins is termed **phlebitis**. This usually involves the deep leg veins and may lead to thrombosis, in which case the condition is termed *thrombophlebitis*.

KEY CLINICAL TERMS

Cardiovascular Disorders

Term	Definition
aneurysm *(AN-ū-rizm)*	A localized abnormal dilation of a blood vessel, usually an artery, caused by weakness of the vessel wall. May eventually burst.
angina pectoris *(an-JĪ-na PEK-tō-ris)*	A feeling of constriction around the heart or pain that may radiate to the left arm or shoulder, usually brought on by exertion; caused by insufficient blood supply to the heart
arrhythmia *(a-RITH-mē-a)*	Any abnormality in the rate or rhythm of the heartbeat (literally "without rhythm." Note doubled *r*.) Also called *dysrhythmia.*
atherosclerosis *(ath-er-ō-skle-RŌ-sis)*	The development of fatty, fibrous patches (plaques) in the lining of arteries causing narrowing of the lumen and hardening of the vessel wall. The most common form of arteriosclerosis. (Root *ather/o* means "porridge" or "gruel").
cerebrovascular accident (CVA) *(ser-e-brō-VAS-kū-lar)*	Sudden damage to the brain resulting from reduction of blood flow. Causes include atherosclerosis, embolism, thrombosis, or hemorrhage from a ruptured aneurysm; commonly called *stroke.*
clubbing *(KLUB-ing)*	Enlargement of the ends of the fingers and toes due to growth of the soft tissue around the nails (see Figure 7-4). Seen in a variety of diseases in which there is poor peripheral circulation.
cyanosis *(sī-a-NŌ-sis)*	Bluish discoloration of the skin due to lack of oxygen

dissecting aneurysm — An aneurysm in which blood enters the arterial wall and separates the layers. Usually involves the aorta (see Figure 9-10).

dyspnea *(DYSP-nē-a)* — Difficult or labored breathing (-pnea)

edema *(e-DĒ-ma)* — Swelling of body tissues due to the presence of excess fluid. Causes include cardiovascular disturbances, kidney failure, inflammation, and malnutrition.

embolism *(EM-bō-lizm)* — Obstruction of a blood vessel by a blood clot or other matter carried in the circulation

embolus *(EM-bō-lus)* — A mass carried in the circulation. Usually a blood clot, but may also be air, fat, bacteria, or other solid matter from within or from outside the body.

fibrillation *(fi-bri-LĀ-shun)* — Spontaneous, quivering, and ineffectual contraction of muscle fibers, as in the atria or the ventricles

heart block — An interference in the conduction system of the heart resulting in arrhythmia (Fig. 9-11). The condition is classified in order of increasing severity as first, second, or third degree heart block. Block in a bundle branch is designated as a left or right bundle branch block (BBB).

heart failure — A condition caused by the inability of the heart to maintain adequate circulation of blood

hypertension *(hī-per-TEN-shun)* — A condition of higher than normal blood pressure. Essential (primary, idiopathic) hypertension has no known cause.

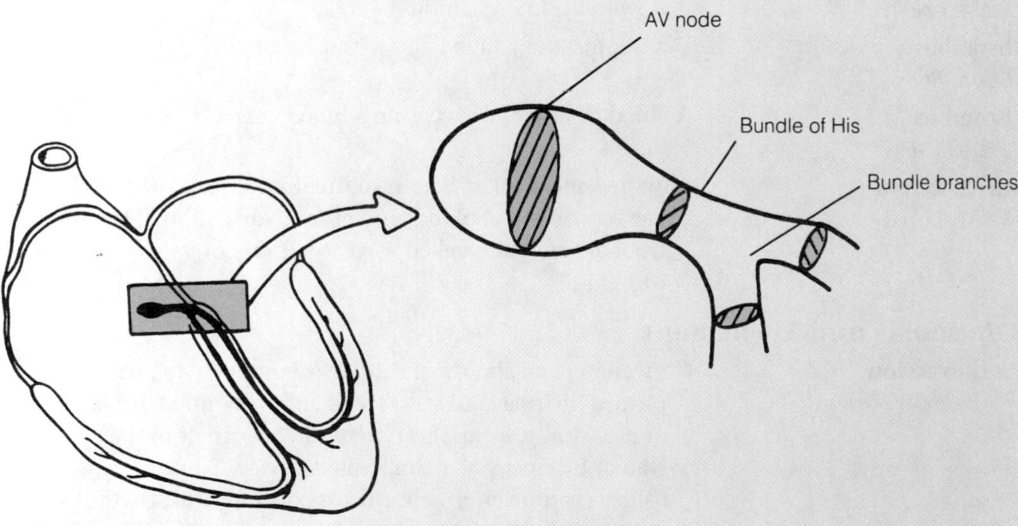

FIGURE 9-11. Potential sites for heart block in the atrioventricular (AV) portion of the heart's conduction system. (Jones SA, Weigel A, White RD, McSwain NE Jr, Breiter M: Advanced Emergency Care for Paramedic Practice, p 484. Philadelphia: JB Lippincott, 1992.)

(continued)

electrocardiography *(ē-lek-trō-kar-dē-OG-ra-fē)* *(EKG, ECG)* — Study of the electrical activity of the heart as detected by electrodes (leads) placed on the surface of the body. The components of the EKG include the P wave, QRS complex, T wave, ST segment, PR (PQ) interval, and the QT interval (Fig. 9-12).

Lymphatic Disorders

Hodgkin's disease — A malignant disease causing progressive enlargement of lymphoid tissue

lymphoma *(lim-FŌ-ma)* — Any neoplastic disease of lymphoid tissue

lymphadenitis *(lim-fad-e-NI-tis)* — Inflammation and enlargement of lymph nodes, usually as a result of infection

lymphadenopathy *(lim-fad-e-NOP-a-thē)* — Any disease of the lymph nodes; often used to mean enlarged lymph nodes

lymphangiitis *(lim-fan-jē-Ī-tis)* — Inflammation of lymphatic vessels as a result of bacterial infection. Appears as painful red streaks under the skin. (Also spelled lymphangitis).

lymphedema *(lim-fe-DĒ-ma)* — Swelling of tissues with lymph due to obstruction or excision of lymphatic vessels

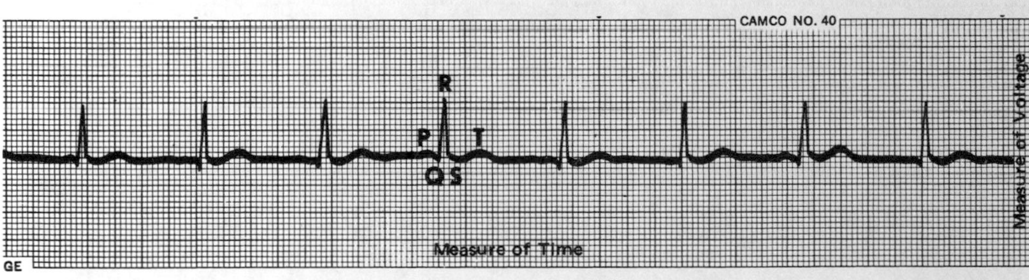

FIGURE 9-12. A normal EKG tracing with main wave components labeled. (Sharp LN, Rubin B: Nursing in the Coronary Care Unit, p. 546. Philadelphia: JB Lippincott, 1970.)

ADDITIONAL TERMS

Normal Structure and Function

apex beat — The pulsing of the heart that can be felt over the apex in the fifth left intercostal space (between the ribs) about 8–9 centimeters from the midline

cardiac output — The amount of blood pumped from the right or left ventricle per minute

ductus arteriosus (*DUK-tus ar-tē-rē-O-sus*) A vessel between the pulmonary artery and the aorta that bypasses the lungs in fetal circulation. Failure to close after birth is called *patent* (PA-tent) *ductus arteriosus*.

foramen ovale (*for-Ā-men ō-VAL-ē*) An opening between the two atria that allows blood to bypass the lungs in fetal circulation. Failure to close after birth results in a septal defect.

Korotkoff's sounds (*ko-rot-KOFS*) Arterial sounds heard with a stethoscope during determination of blood pressure with a cuff

perfusion (*per-FŪ-zhun*) The passage of fluid, such as blood, through an organ or tissue

precordium (*prē-KOR-dē-um*) The anterior region over the heart and the lower part of the thorax; adj. precordial

pulse pressure The difference between systolic and diastolic pressure

sinus rhythm A normal heart rhythm originating from the sinoatrial (SA) node

stroke volume The amount of blood ejected by the left ventricle with each beat

Valsalva's maneuver (*val-SAL-vaz*) Bearing down, as in childbirth or defecation, by attempting to exhale forcefully with the nose and throat closed. This action has an effect on the cardiovascular system.

Symptoms and Conditions

bradycardia (*brad-ē-KAR-de-a*) A slow heart rate of less than 60 beats per minute

bruit (*brwē*) An abnormal sound heard in auscultation

cardiac tamponade (*tam-pon-ĀD*) Pathologic accumulation of fluid in the pericardial sac. May result from pericarditis or injury to the heart or great vessels.

coarctation of the aorta (*kō-ark-TĀ-shun*) Localized narrowing of the aorta

extrasystole (*eks-tra-SIS-tō-lē*) Premature contraction of the heart

flutter Very rapid (200–300 per minute) but regular contractions, as in the atria or the ventricles

hypotension (*hī-po-TEN-shun*) A condition of lower than normal blood pressure.

intermittent claudication (*claw-di-KĀ-shun*) Pain in a muscle during exercise due to inadequate blood supply. The pain disappears with rest.

mitral valve prolapse Movement of the cusps of the mitral valve into the left atrium when the ventricles contract

occlusive vascular disease Arteriosclerotic disease of the vessels, usually peripheral vessels

palpitation (*pal-pi-TĀ-shun*) A sensation of abnormally rapid or irregular heartbeat

pitting edema Edema that retains the impression of a finger pressed firmly into the skin

polyarteritis nodosa (*nō-DŌ-sa*) Potentially fatal collagen disease causing inflammation of small visceral arteries. Symptoms depend on the organ affected.

Raynaud's disease (*rā-NŌZ*) — A disorder characterized by abnormal constriction of peripheral vessels in the arms and legs on exposure to cold

regurgitation (*rē-gur-ji-TĀ-shun*) — A backward flow, such as the backflow of blood through a defective valve

subacute bacterial endocarditis (SBE) — Growth of bacteria in a heart or valves previously damaged by rheumatic fever

tachycardia (*tak-i-KAR-dē-a*) — An abnormally rapid heart rate, usually over 100 beats per minute

tetralogy of Fallot (*fal-Ō*) — A combination of four congenital heart abnormalities: pulmonary artery stenosis, interventricular septal defect, displacement of the aorta to the right, right ventricular hypertrophy

thromboangiitis obliterans — Thrombotic occlusion of leg vessels in young men leading to gangrene of the feet. Patients show a hypersensitivity to tobacco. Also called Buerger's disease.

vegetation — Irregular outgrowths of bacteria on the heart valves; associated with rheumatic fever

Wolff-Parkinson-White syndrome (WPW) — A cardiac arrhythmia consisting of tachycardia and a premature ventricular beat caused by an alternate conduction pathway

Diagnosis

cardiac catheterization — Passage of a catheter into the heart through a vessel to inject a contrast medium for imaging, diagnose abnormalities, obtain samples, or measure pressure

central venous pressure (CVP) — Pressure in the superior vena cava

coronary angiography (*an-jē-OG-ra-fē*) — Radiographic study of the coronary arteries following introduction of an opaque dye by means of a catheter

Doppler ultrasonography — An imaging method used to study the rate and pattern of blood flow

enzyme studies — Measurement of serum levels of enzymes that are released in increased amounts from damaged heart tissue. These include CPK (creatine phosphokinase), LDH (lactic dehydrogenase), AST (aspartate aminotranferase; SGOT), and ALT (alanine aminotransferase; SGPT).

heart scan — Imaging of the heart following injection of a radioactive isotope. The PYP (pyrophosphate) scan using technetium-99m (^{99m}Tc) is used to test for myocardial infarction, as the isotope is taken up by damaged tissue. The MUGA (multigated acquisition) scan gives information on heart function.

Holter monitor — A portable device that can record up to 24 hours of an individual's EKG readings during normal activity

lipoprotein (*lip-ō-PRŌ-tēn*) (L) — A compound of protein with lipid. Lipoproteins are classified according to density as very low density (VLDL), low density (LDL), and high density (HDL). Relatively higher levels of high density lipoproteins have been correlated with health of the cardiovascular system.

(continued)

phonocardiography
(fō-nō-kar-dē-OG-ra-fē)
Electronic recording of heart sounds

pulmonary wedge pressure (PWP)
Pressure measured by a catheter in a branch of the pulmonary artery. It is an indirect measure of pressure in the left atrium.

stress test
Evaluation of physical fitness by continuous EKG monitoring during exercise. In a thallium stress test, a radioactive isotope of thallium is administered to trace blood flow through the heart.

triglycerides
(trī-GLIS-er-īdz)
Fats that appear in the blood in combination with protein as lipoproteins

ventriculography
(ven-trik-ū-LOG-ra-fē)
X-ray study of the ventricles of the heart following introduction of an opaque dye by means of a catheter

Treatment and Surgical Procedures

artificial pacemaker
A device that controls the beating of the heart by emitting a regular electrical discharge, thus substituting for a defective conduction pathway (Fig. 9-13)

atherectomy
(ath-er-EK-tō-mē)
Removal of atheromatous plaque from the lining of a vessel. May be done by open surgery or through the lumen of the vessel.

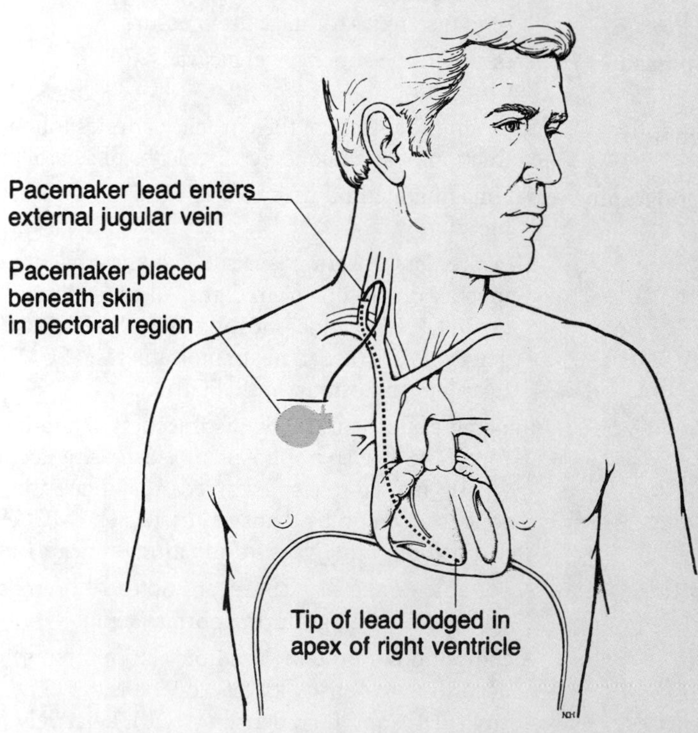

FIGURE 9-13. Placement of a pacemaker. (Rosdahl C: Textbook of Basic Nursing, 5th ed, p 802. Philadelphia: JB Lippincott, 1991.)

commissurotomy *(kom-i-shur-OT-ō-mē)* — Surgical incision of a scarred mitral valve to increase the size of the valve opening

coronary artery bypass graft (CABG) — Surgical creation of a shunt to bypass a blocked coronary artery. The aorta is connected to a point past the obstruction with another vessel or a piece of another vessel, usually the saphenous vein of the leg or the left internal mammary artery (Fig. 9-14).

defibrillation *(dē-fib-ri-LĀ-shun)* — Termination of atrial or ventricular fibrillation, usually by electric shock delivered directly to the chest wall with two paddles; see cardioversion

left ventriciular assist device (LVAD) — A pump that takes over the function of the left ventricle in delivering blood into the systemic circuit. They are used to assist patients awaiting heart transplants or those who are recovering from heart failure.

percutaneous transluminal coronary angioplasty (PTCA) — Dilatation of a sclerotic blood vessel by means of a balloon catheter inserted into the vessel and then inflated to flatten plaque against the artery wall (Fig. 9-15)

stent — A small metal device in the shape of a coil or slotted tube that is placed inside an artery to keep the vessel open following balloon angioplasty

Medications

angiotensin converting enzyme (ACE) inhibitor — A drug that lowers blood pressure by blocking the formation in the blood of angiotensin II, a substance that normally acts to raise blood pressure

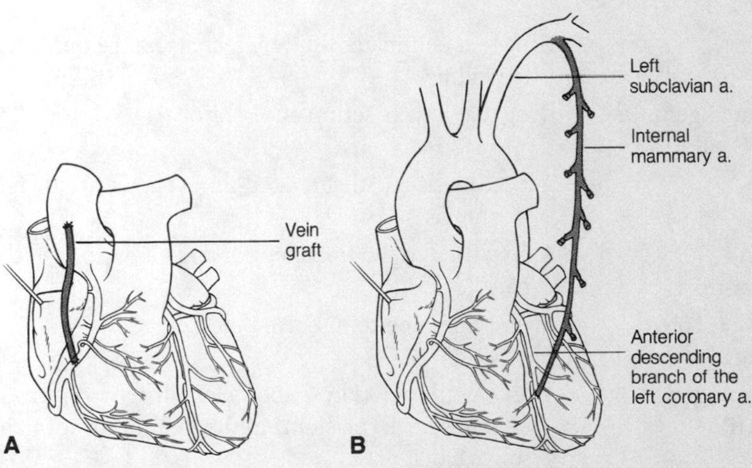

FIGURE 9-14. Coronary artery bypass graft (CABG). **(A)** A segment of the saphenous vein carries blood from the aorta to a part of the right coronary artery that is distal to an occlusion. **(B)** The mammary artery is used to bypass an obstruction in the left anterior descending (LAD) coronary artery. (Porth CM: Pathophysiology, 3rd ed, p 343. Philadelphia: JB Lippincott, 1990.)

(continued)

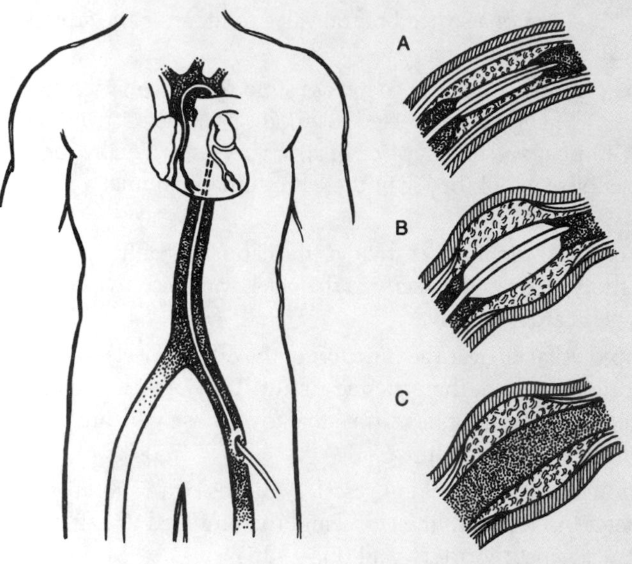

FIGURE 9-15. Coronary angioplasty. **(A)** A balloon catheter is inserted in the femoral artery and advanced to the narrowed coronary artery. **(B)** The balloon is inflated to dilate the central opening (lumen) of the vessel. **(C)** The vessel after angioplasty. (Underhill SL, Woods SL, Froelicher ESS, Halpenny CJ: Cardiac Nursing, 2nd ed, p 532. Philadelphia: JB Lippincott, 1989.)

antiarrhythmic agent	A drug that regulates the rate and rhythm of the heartbeat (*eg,* quinidine)
beta-adrenergic blocking agent	Drug that decreases the rate and strength of heart contractions (*eg,* propranolol)
calcium channel blocker	Drug that controls the rate and force of heart contraction by regulating calcium entrance into the cells
digitalis *(dij-i-TAL-is)*	A drug that slows and strengthens heart muscle contractions
diuretic *(dī-ū-RET-ik)*	Drug that eliminates fluid by increasing the output of urine by the kidneys
hypolipidemic agent *(hī-pō-lip-i-DĒ-mik)*	Drug that lowers serum cholesterol
lidocaine *(LĪ-dō-kān)*	A local anesthetic that is used intravenously to treat cardiac arrhythmias
nitroglycerin *(nī-trō-GLIS-er-in)*	A drug used in the treatment of angina pectoris to dilate coronary vessels
streptokinase (SK) *(strep-tō-KĪ-nas)*	An enzyme used to dissolve blood clots
tissue plasminogen activator (tPA)	A drug used to dissolve blood clots. It activates production of a substance (plasmin) in the blood that normally dissolves clots.
vasodilator *(vas-ō-dī-LA-tor)*	A drug that widens blood vessels and improves blood flow

ABBREVIATIONS

ACE angiotensin converting enzyme
AF atrial fibrillation
ALT alanine aminotransferase (SGPT)
AMI acute myocardial infarction
APC atrial premature complex
AR aortic regurgitation
AS aortic stenosis; arteriosclerosis
ASCVD arteriosclerotic cardiovascular disease
ASD atrial septal defect
ASHD arteriosclerotic heart disease
AST aspartate aminotransferase (SGOT)
AT atrial tachycardia
AV atrioventricular
BBB bundle branch block (left or right)
BP blood pressure
CABG coronary artery bypass graft
CAD coronary artery disease
CCU coronary care unit
CHD coronary heart disease
CHF congestive heart failure
C(P)K creatine (phospho)kinase
CPR cardiopulmonary resuscitation
CVP central venous pressure
DOE dyspnea on exertion
DVT deep vein thrombosis
EKG (ECG) electrocardiogram
HDL high density lipoprotein
HTN hypertension
IVCD intraventricular conduction delay
JVP jugular venous pulse
LAD left anterior descending (coronary artery)
LAHB left anterior hemiblock
LDH lactic dehydrogenase
LDL low density lipoprotein
LV left ventricle
LVAD left ventricular assist device
LVEDP left ventricular end-diastolic pressure
MI myocardial infarction
mm Hg millimeters mercury
MR mitral regurgitation, reflux
MS mitral stenosis
MUGA multigated acquisition (scan)
MVP mitral valve prolapse
NSR normal sinus rhythm
P pulse
PAP pulmonary arterial pressure
PMI point of maximal impulse
PSVT paroxysmal supraventricular tachycardia
PTCA percutaneous transluminal coronary angioplasty
PVC premature ventricular contraction
PVD peripheral vascular disease
PWP pulmonary (artery) wedge pressure
PYP pyrophosphate (scan)
S_1 the first heart sound
S_2 the second heart sound
SA sinoatrial
SBE subacute bacterial endocarditis
SGOT serum glutamic oxaloacetic transaminase (AST)
SK streptokinase
SVT supraventricular tachycardia
^{99m}Tc technetium-99m
tPA tissue plasminogen activator
VF ventricular fibrillation
VLDL very low density lipoprotein
VPC ventricular premature complex
VSD ventricular septal defect
VT ventricular tachycardia
WPW Wolff-Parkinson-White syndrome

Chapter 9

Labeling Exercise

Write the name of each numbered part on the corresponding line of the answer sheet.

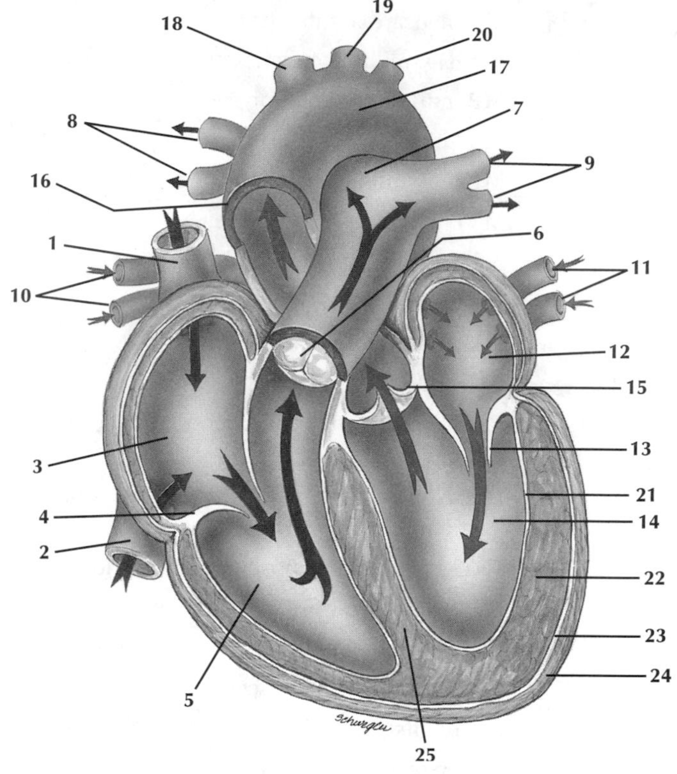

Heart and great vessels

aortic arch
aortic valve
apex
ascending aorta
brachiocephalic artery
endocardium
epicardium
inferior vena cava
interventricular septum
left atrium
left common carotid artery
left pulmonary artery (branches)
left pulmonary veins
left subclavian artery
left ventricle
mitral (bicuspid) valve
myocardium
pulmonary artery
pulmonic (pulmonary) valve
right atrium
right pulmonary artery (branches)
right pulmonary veins
right ventricle
superior vena cava
tricuspid valve

1. ____________________
2. ____________________
3. ____________________
4. ____________________
5. ____________________
6. ____________________
7. ____________________
8. ____________________
9. ____________________
10. ____________________
11. ____________________
12. ____________________
13. ____________________
14. ____________________
15. ____________________
16. ____________________
17. ____________________
18. ____________________
19. ____________________
20. ____________________
21. ____________________
22. ____________________
23. ____________________
24. ____________________
25. ____________________

CHAPTER REVIEW 9-1

Matching. Match the terms in each of the sets below with their definitions and write the appropriate letter (a–e) to the left of each number:

_____ 1. SA node	a. membrane that lines the heart
_____ 2. pericardium	b. the right atrioventricular valve
_____ 3. vena cava	c. fibrous sac around the heart
_____ 4. endocardium	d. pacemaker of the heart
_____ 5. tricuspid	e. vessel that empties into the right atrium
_____ 6. atherosclerosis	a. abnormal heartbeat
_____ 7. aneurysm	b. formation of a blood clot in a vessel
_____ 8. ischemia	c. localized dilatation of a blood vessel
_____ 9. thrombosis	d. accumulation of fatty deposits in the lining of a blood vessel
_____ 10. arrhythmia	e. local deficiency of blood
_____ 11. infarction	a. twisted and swollen vessel
_____ 12. fibrillation	b. interruption in the heart's conduction system
_____ 13. varix	c. part of the heart's conduction system
_____ 14. heart block	d. ineffective quivering of muscle
_____ 15. Purkinje fibers	e. localized death of tissue

Fill in the blanks:

16. Each upper receiving chamber of the heart is a(n) ______________________
17. The heart muscle is the ______________________
18. The microscopic vessels through which materials are exchanged between the blood and the tissues are the ______________________
19. The largest artery is the ______________________
20. The lymphoid organ in the chest is the ______________________
21. The large artery that supplies the head is the (see Figure 9-5) ______________________
22. The large vein that drains the head is the (see Figure 9-6) ______________________
23. Polyarteritis (*pol-ē-ar-te-RĪ-tis*) is inflammation of many ______________________
24. Phlebostasis (*fleb-OS-ta-sis*) is stoppage of blood flow in a(n) ______________________
25. The term *varicoid* pertains to a(n) ______________________

True-False. Examine each of the following statements. If the statement is true, write T in the first blank. If the statement is false, write F in the first blank and correct the statement by replacing the *underlined* word in the second blank.

26. The systemic circuit pumps blood to the lungs. _____ ______________________

27. A <u>vein</u> is a vessel that carries blood back to the heart. ____ ____________

28. <u>Systole</u> is the relaxation phase of the heart cycle. ____ ____________

29. The <u>right ventricle</u> pumps blood into the aorta. ____ ____________

30. The femoral artery supplies blood to the <u>arm</u>. ____ ____________

31. The <u>bicuspid valve</u> is also called the mitral valve. ____ ____________

Definitions. Write the meaning of each of the following terms:

32. Intracardiac *(in-tra-KAR-dē-ak)* ____________
33. Perivascular *(per-i-VAS-kū-lar)* ____________
34. Atriotomy *(ā-trē-OT-ō-mē)* ____________
35. Venospasm *(VĒ-nō-spazm)* ____________
36. Asplenia *(ā-SPLĒ-nē-a)* ____________
37. Lymphangitis *(lim-fan-JĪ-tis)* ____________

Word building. Write a word for each of the following definitions:

38. Any disease of the heart muscle ____________
39. Suture (-rhaphy) of an artery ____________
40. Originating (-genic) in the heart ____________
41. Spasm of an artery ____________
42. Radiographic study (-graphy) of blood vessels ____________
43. Around (peri-) the ventricles ____________
44. Incision of a lymph node ____________
45. Surgical fixation (-pexy) of the spleen ____________

Use the root *aort/o* for the remaining words:

46. Radiograph (-gram) of the aorta ____________
47. Around (peri-) the aorta ____________
48. Narrowing (-stenosis) of the aorta ____________
49. Any disease (-pathy) of the aorta ____________
50. Downward displacement (-ptosis) of the aorta ____________

Adjectives. Write the adjective form of each of the following words:

51. artery ______________________
52. septum ______________________
53. atrium ______________________
54. apex ______________________
55. spleen ______________________

Write the meaning of the following abbreviations as they apply to the carciovascular system:

56. BBB ______________________
57. CHF ______________________
58. CCU ______________________
59. NSR ______________________
60. CAD ______________________
61. CVP ______________________

Word analysis. Define each of the following words and give the meaning of the word parts in each. Use a dictionary if necessary.

62. Hemangioma *(hē-man-jē-Ō-ma)* ______________________
    a. hem/o ______________________
    b. angi/o ______________________
    c. -oma ______________________
63. Endarterectomy *(end-ar-ter-EK-tō-mē)* ______________________
    a. end/o- ______________________
    b. arteri/o ______________________
    c. ecto- ______________________
    d. -tomy ______________________
64. Lymphangiophlebitis *(lim-fan-jē-ō-fle-BĪ-tis)* ______________________
    a. lymph/o ______________________
    b. angi/o ______________________
    c. phleb/o ______________________
    d. -itis ______________________

CHAPTER REVIEW 9-2

Matching. Match the terms in each of these sets with their definitions and write the appropriate letter (a–e) to the left of each number:

____	1. cardioversion	a. a mass carried in the circulation
____	2. lumen	b. area over the heart
____	3. embolus	c. removal of plaque from a vessel
____	4. atherectomy	d. correction of an abnormal heart rhythm
____	5. precordium	e. central opening, as of a vessel
____	6. Hodgkin's disease	a. dissolving of a blood clot
____	7. varicotomy	b. malignant disease of lymphoid tissue
____	8. thrombolysis	c. swelling of tissue due to lymph blockage
____	9. lymphadenopathy	d. any disease of lymph nodes
____	10. lymphedema	e. incision of a varicose vein
____	11. CABG	a. sudden damage to heart tissue
____	12. ECG	b. surgery to bypass a blocked artery in the heart
____	13. AST	c. chronic infection of heart valves
____	14. SBE	d. enzyme released from damaged heart tissue
____	15. AMI	e. record of the electrical activity of the heart

Fill in the blanks:

16. Thrombophlebitis *(throm-bō-fle-BĪ-tis)* is inflammation of a vein associated with formation of a(n) ____________________

17. Blood returning to the heart from the lungs enters the chamber of the heart named the ____________________

18. A small vein is called a(n) ____________________

19. The unit in which blood pressure is measured is ____________________

20. The adjective *ischemic (is-KEM-ik)* means lacking in ____________________

21. The large lymphoid organ in the upper left abdomen is the ____________________

22. At its lower end the aorta divides into a pair of arteries called the (see Figure 9-5) ____________________

23. The longest vein in the body, which runs the length of the leg is the (see Figure 9-6) ____________________

24. A phlebotomist *(fle-BOT-ō-mist)* is one who drains blood from a(n) ____________________

25. Atriotomy (*ā-trē-OT-ō-mē*) is incision of a(n) ____________________

26. A lymphangiogram (*lim-FAN-jē-ō-gram*) is an x-ray of ____________________

Definitions. Write the meaning of each of the following terms:

27. Supravalvular (*sū-pra-VAL-vū-lar*) ____________________

28. Interatrial (*in-ter-Ā-trē-al*) ____________________

29. Avascular (*ā-VAS-kū-lar*) ____________________

30. Thymectomy (*thī-MEK-tō-mē*) ____________________

31. Angiostenosis (*an-jē-ō-ste-NŌ-sis*) ____________________

Word building. Write a word for each of the following definitions:

32. Suture (-rhaphy) of an artery ____________________

33. Study of the heart ____________________

34. Before or in front of (pre-) the aorta ____________________

35. Pertaining to the heart and blood vessels ____________________

36. Radiographic study of the ventricles ____________________

37. An instrument for incising (-tome) a valve ____________________

38. Stoppage (-stasis) of lymph flow ____________________

39. Cell (-cyte) found in the lymphatic system ____________________

40. Inflammation of the spleen ____________________

Opposites. Write a word that means the opposite of each of the following words:

41. diastole ____________________

42. tachycardia ____________________

43. vasodilation ____________________

44. hypertension ____________________

Adjectives. Write the adjective form of each of the following words:

45. ventricle ____________________

46. arteriole ____________________

47. sclerosis ____________________

48. vein ____________________

49. varix ____________________

50. aorta ____________________

Plurals. Write the plural form of each of the following words:

51. thrombus ______________________
52. stenosis ______________________
53. apex ______________________
54. varix ______________________
55. septum ______________________

Unscrambles. Form a word from each of the following groups of letters and write it in the blank:

56. yremusan ______________________
57. etsloadi ______________________
58. hytsmu ______________________
59. rtnfaci ______________________
60. hpyml ______________________

Word analysis. Define each of the following words and give the meaning of the word parts in each. Use a dictionary if necessary.

61. Telangiectasia *(tel-an-jē-ĕk-TĀ-zē-a)* ______________________
    a. tel- ______________________
    b. angi/o ______________________
    c. -ectasia ______________________
62. Bradyarrhythmia *(brad-ē-a-RITH-mē-a)* ______________________
    a. brady- ______________________
    b. a- ______________________
    c. rhythm ______________________
    d. -ia ______________________

Chapter 9

Case Studies

1. Percutaneous transluminal coronary angioplasty (PTCA)

This 45-year-old female was admitted on 29 July complaining of chest pain which had increased in frequency over the previous 3 months. These episodes were accompanied by nausea and diaphoresis and were relieved with sublingual nitroglycerin. A previous stress test and thallium scan showed some abnormalities.

Family history was positive for myocardial infarction in both her mother and grandmother. Review of systems and physical examination were noncontributory. EKG on admission showed normal sinus rhythm with inverted T waves.

A cardiac catheterization performed on 30 July revealed significant stenosis of the LAD (left anterior descending) coronary artery with normal LV (left ventricular) function. She had a PTCA performed on 31 July which relieved the stenosis.

The patient was discharged on 4 August with prescriptions for Procardia 10 mg qid, Persantine 75 mg tid, aspirin 5 gr po qd, nitroglycerin sublingual 0.3 mg q 5 min times three prn. She was placed on a low cholesterol diet and allowed activity as tolerated. A follow-up visit with a stress test was scheduled with Dr. _____ in 4 weeks.

2. Echocardiogram

Echocardiogram shows the right and left ventricular cavities to be of normal size. The mitral valve has normal amplitude of motion. The anterior and posterior leaflets move in the opposite direction in diastole. There is a late systolic prolapse of the mitral leaflet at rest and with provocation. This is mild in nature. The left atrium is not enlarged. The aortic cusps were seen. They have normal thickness and normal amplitude of motion. The tricuspid valve is seen and appears normal. The interventricular septum and posterior myocardium have normal thickness and normal amplitude of motion.

Impression: Mild mitral leaflet prolapse. No echographic evidence of mitral regurgitation.

3. Aortogram and Bilateral Femoral Arteriogram

This is a 72-year-old male with known coronary disease and an anginal syndrome who has had progressive lower extremity intermittent claudication for the past 6 months. On 4 April he had an aortogram and bifemoral arteriogram which showed the following:

1) generalized atherosclerosis; 2) stenosis of both renal arteries, mild; 3) aneurysmal dilatation of the infrarenal abdominal aorta, minimal; 4) critical stenosis just beyond the origin of the right superficial femoral artery; 5) run-off on the right principally through a peroneal artery which is, itself, stenotic in its midportion, but which can be traced to the ankle; and 6) occlusion of the left popliteal artery above the knee with reconstitution (revisualization) at the knee and principal run-off through a widely patent peroneal artery to the ankle.

Flow from the aorta through the feet was extraordinarily slow with contrast arriving at about 40 seconds following the onset of injection. Based on the patient's history, physical examination, and angiographic findings, it was decided that he should be treated nonsurgically at this time. He was discharged on 5 April. Follow up in one week; aspirin, 325 mg a day.

Chapter 9
Case Study Questions

Multiple choice. Select the best answer and write the letter of your choice to the left of each number:

_____ 1. The word transluminal pertains to the lumen of a vessel, which is the

a. wall
b. branch
c. outer layer
d. central opening
e. valve

_____ 2. In Case 1, the patient's nitroglycerin was administered

a. into a vein
b. into the skin
c. under the skin
d. into a muscle
e. under the tongue

_____ 3. The term that means a backflow of blood is

a. infarction
b. regurgitation
c. amplitude
d. prolapse
e. tourniquet

_____ 4. The interventricular septum is the

a. cavity of the ventricle
b. wall between the atrium and ventricle

c. valve between the atrium and ventricle
d. wall between the ventricles
e. vessel that carries blood out of the ventricle

_____ 5. The phrase *anginal syndrome* refers to

a. difficulty in breathing
b. swelling of body tissues
c. feeling of discomfort around the heart
d. an abnormal heart sound
e. inflammation of the heart valves

_____ 6. The occlusion of the left popliteal artery is

a. dilatation of the artery
b. weakening of the artery wall
c. rapid blood flow through the artery
d. x-ray of the artery
e. closing of the artery

_____ 7. The peroneal artery is in the

a. upper arm
b. lower leg
c. thigh
d. abdomen
e. neck

Fill in the blanks:

8. A sinus rhythm is a normal heart rhythm that originates at the ____________________
9. Another term for the leaflet of a valve is the ____________________
10. The adjective form of the word *stenosis* is ____________________

Find the word or phrase in the case studies that means each of the following:

11. Through the skin ____________________
12. Pain in a muscle during exercise due to inadequate blood flow ____________________
13. Below the kidney ____________________
14. Open ____________________

Give the meaning of the following abbreviations:

15. qid ____________________
16. tid ____________________
17. po ____________________
18. q 5 min ____________________
19. prn ____________________

Define the following terms:

20. diaphoresis ____________________
21. stenosis ____________________
22. aortogram ____________________
23. diastole ____________________
24. superficial ____________________

CIRCULATION

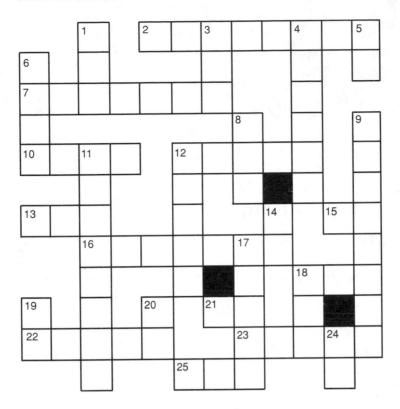

ACROSS

2. the circuit into which the left side of the heart pumps
7. a mass that occludes a vessel
10. a small mass of lymphoid tissue
12. the upper receiving chambers of the heart
13. profuse sweating: ____ phoresis
15. an enzyme used to dissolve blood clots (abbr.)
16. contraction of the heart
18. high blood pressure (abbr.)
21. unit used to describe blood pressure: ____ Hg
22. a structure that keeps blood moving in a forward direction
23. a wave of increased pressure produced in the vessels by contraction of the ventricles
25. an enzyme released from damaged heart tissue (abbr.)

DOWN

1. a form of heart block (abbr.)
3. suffix: condition of
4. the valve between the left chambers of the heart
5. an enzyme released from damaged heart tissue (abbr.)
6. a vessel that carries blood back to the heart
8. prefix: before, in front of
9. fibers that are part of the conduction system of the heart
11. the relaxation phase of the heartbeat
12. the artery that receives blood from the left ventricle
14. prefix: down, without, removal, loss
17. the fluid that circulates in the lymphatic system
18. a type of lipoprotein (abbr.)
19. part of the conduction system of the heart: ____ node (abbr.)
20. prefix: again, back
24. the pacemaker of the heart

Chapter 9
Answer Section

Answers to Chapter Exercises

Exercise 9-1

1. heart
2. atria
3. ventricle
4. valve
5. cardiac *(KAR-dē-ak)*
6. myocardial *(mī-ō-KAR-dē-al)*
7. atrial *(Ā-trē-al)*
8. pericardial *(per-i-KAR-dē-al)*
9. ventricular *(ven-TRIK-ū-lar)*
10. valvular *(VAL-vū-lar);* also valvar *(VAL-var)*
11. endocarditis *(en-dō-kar-DĪ-tis)*
12. myocarditis *(mī-ō-kar-DĪ-tis)*
13. pericarditis *(per-i-kar-DĪ-tis)*
14. cardiology *(kar-dē-OL-ō-jē)*
15. cardioptosis *(kar-dē-op-TŌ-sis)*
16. supraventricular *(sū-pra-ven-TRIK-ū-lar)*
17. atrioventricular *(ā-trē-ō-ven-TRIK-ū-lar)*
18. valvotomy *(val-VOT-ō-mē)*; also valvulotomy *(val-vū-LOT-ō-mē)*

Exercise 9-2

1. vessel
2. artery
3. arteriole
4. inflammation of a vessel
5. pertaining to the heart and blood vessels
6. rupture of an artery
7. downward displacement
8. inflammation of a vein
9. angiectomy *(an-jē-EK-tō-mē)*
10. angiectasis *(an-jē-EK-tā-sis)*; also hemangiectasis *(hē-man-jē-EK-tā-sis)*
11. angiogenesis *(an-jē-ō-JEN-e-sis)*
12. angioplasty *(AN-jē-ō-plas-tē)*
13. aortostenosis *(ā-or-tō-ste-NŌ-sis)*
14. arteritis *(ar-te-RĪ-tis)*
15. intravenous *(in-tra-VĒ-nus)*
16. venography *(vē-NOG-ra-fē)*
17. phlebotomy *(fle-BOT-o-mē);* also venotomy *(vē-NOT-o-mē);* venisection *(ven-i-SEK-shun)*

Exercise 9-3

1. lymph
2. lymph node
3. lymphatic vessels
4. spleen
5. thymus gland
6. tonsils
7. lymphangi/o; lymphatic vessel
8. lymphaden/o; lymph node
9. splen/o; spleen
10. thym/o; thymus gland
11. tonsill/o; tonsil
12. lymphangitis *(lim-fan-JĪ-tis);* also lymphangiitis *(lim-fan-jē-Ī-tis)*
13. lymphoma *(lim-FŌ-ma)*
14. lymphadenopathy *(lim-fad-e-NOP-a-thē)*
15. splenalgia *(splē-NAL-jē-a)*
16. tonsillitis *(ton-si-LĪ-tis)*

Answers to Labeling Exercise

Heart and Great Vessels

1. superior vena cava
2. inferior vena cava
3. right atrium
4. tricuspid valve
5. right ventricle
6. pulmonic (pulmonary) valve
7. pulmonary artery
8. right pulmonary artery (branches)
9. left pulmonary artery (branches)
10. right pulmonary veins
11. left pulmonary veins
12. left atrium
13. mitral (bicuspid) valve
14. left ventricle
15. aortic valve
16. ascending aorta
17. aortic arch
18. brachiocephalic artery
19. left common carotid artery
20. left subclavian artery
21. endocardium
22. myocardium
23. epicardium
24. apex
25. interventricular septum

Answers to Chapter Review 9-1

1. d
2. c
3. e
4. a
5. b
6. d
7. c
8. e
9. b
10. a
11. e
12. d
13. a
14. b
15. c
16. atrium
17. myocardium
18. capillaries
19. aorta
20. thymus
21. common carotid (*ka-ROT-id*)
22. jugular (*JUG-ū-lar*)
23. arteries
24. vein
25. varicose vein, varix
26. F; pulmonary circuit
27. T
28. F; diastole
29. F; left ventricle
30. F; leg
31. T
32. within the heart
33. around the vessels
34. incision of an atrium
35. spasm of a vein
36. absence of a spleen
37. inflammation of lymphatic vessels
38. cardiomyopathy;
    also myocardiopathy
39. arteriorrhaphy
40. cardiogenic
41. arteriospasm
42. angiography
43. periventricular
44. lymphadenotomy
45. splenopexy
46. aortogram
47. periaortic
48. aortostenosis
49. aortopathy
50. aortoptosis
51. arterial
52. septal
53. atrial
54. apical
55. splenic; also splenetic
56. bundle branch block
57. congestive heart failure
58. coronary care unit
59. normal sinus rhythm
60. coronary artery disease
61. central venous pressure
62. A benign tumor of dilated blood vessels
    a. blood
    b. vessel
    c. tumor

63. Excision of the inner layer of an artery thickened by atherosclerosis
    a. within
    b. artery
    c. gout
    d. to cut

64. Inflammation of lymphatic vessels and veins
    a. lymphatic system
    b. vessel
    c. vein
    d. inflammation

Chapter Review 9-2

1. d
2. e
3. a
4. c
5. b
6. b
7. e
8. a
9. d
10. c
11. b
12. e
13. d
14. c
15. a
16. thrombus, blood clot
17. left atrium
18. venule
19. mm Hg; millimeters mercury
20. blood
21. spleen
22. common iliac *(IL-e-ak)*
23. saphenous *(sa-FE-nus)*
24. vein
25. atrium
26. lymphatic vessels
27. above a valve
28. between the atria
29. without vessels
30. surgical removal of the thymus
31. narrowing of a blood vessel
32. arteriorrhaphy
33. cardiology
34. preaortic
35. cardiovascular
36. ventriculography
37. valvotome; also valvulotome
38. lymphostasis *(lim-FOS-ta-sis)*
39. lymphocyte
40. splenitis
41. systole
42. bradycardia
43. vasoconstriction
44. hypotension
45. ventricular
46. arteriolar
47. sclerotic
48. venous
49. varicose
50. aortic
51. thrombi *(THROM-bī)*
52. stenoses *(ste-NŌ-sēz)*
53. apices *(Ā-pi-sēz)*
54. varices *(VAR-i-sēz)*
55. septa
56. aneurysm
57. diastole
58. thymus
59. infarct
60. lymph
61. Permanent dilation of small blood vessels causing small, local red lesions
    a. end
    b. vessel
    c. dilation
62. An excessively slow and irregular heartbeat
    a. slow
    b. without
    c. rhythm, pattern
    d. condition of

Answers to Case Study Questions

1. d
2. e
3. b
4. d
5. c
6. e
7. b
8. sinoatrial (SA) node
9. cusp, flap
10. stenotic
11. percutaneous
12. intermittent claudication
13. infrarenal
14. patent

15. four times a day
16. three times a day
17. by mouth
18. every 5 minutes
19. as needed
20. profuse sweating
21. narrowing
22. radiograph (x-ray) of the aorta
23. relaxation phase of the heart cycle
24. close to the surface

Answers to Crossword Puzzle

CIRCULATION

		1 B		2 S	Y	3 S	T	E	4 M	I	5 C
6 V		B				I			I		K
7 E	M	B	O	L	U	S			T		
I							8 P		R		9 P
10 N	O	11 D	E		12 A	T	R	I	A		U
		I			O		E		L		R
13 D	I	A			R			14 D		15 S	K
		16 S	Y	S	T	O	17 L	E			I
		T			A		Y		18 H	T	N
19 A		O		20 R		21 M	M		D		J
22 V	A	L	V	E			23 P	U	L	24 S	E
		E			25 L	D	H			A	

10 Blood and Immunity

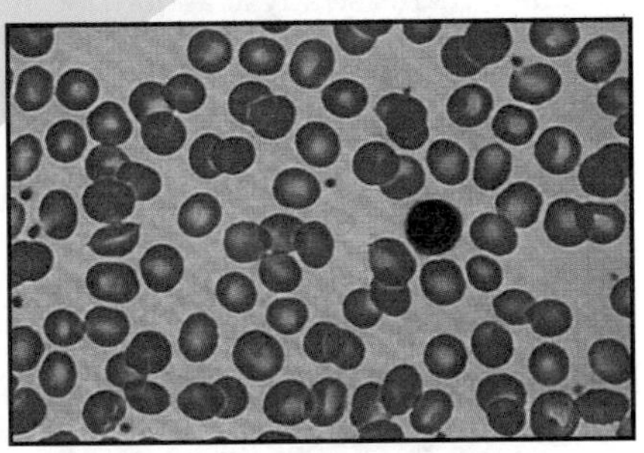

Chapter Contents

Objectives

After study of this chapter you should be able to:

1. Describe the composition of the blood plasma
2. Describe and give the functions of the three types of blood cells
3. Label pictures of the blood cells
4. Explain the basis of blood types
5. Define *immunity*
6. Identify and use roots and suffixes pertaining to the blood and immunity
7. Identify and use roots pertaining to the chemistry of the blood and other body tissues
8. List and describe the major disorders of the blood
9. List and describe the major disorders of the immune system
10. Describe the major tests used to study blood
11. Interpret abbreviations used in blood studies
12. Analyze several case studies involving the blood

Blood circulates through the vessels bringing oxygen and nourishment to all cells and carrying away waste products. The total adult blood volume is about 5 liters (5.2 quarts). Whole blood can be divided into two main components: the liquid portion or **plasma** (55%) and **formed elements** or blood cells (45%).

Plasma is about 90% water. The remaining 10% contains nutrients, **electrolytes** (dissolved salts), gases, albumin (a protein), clotting factors, antibodies, wastes, enzymes, and hormones. A host of these substances are tested for in blood chemistry tests. The pH (relative acidity) of the plasma remains steady at about 7.4.

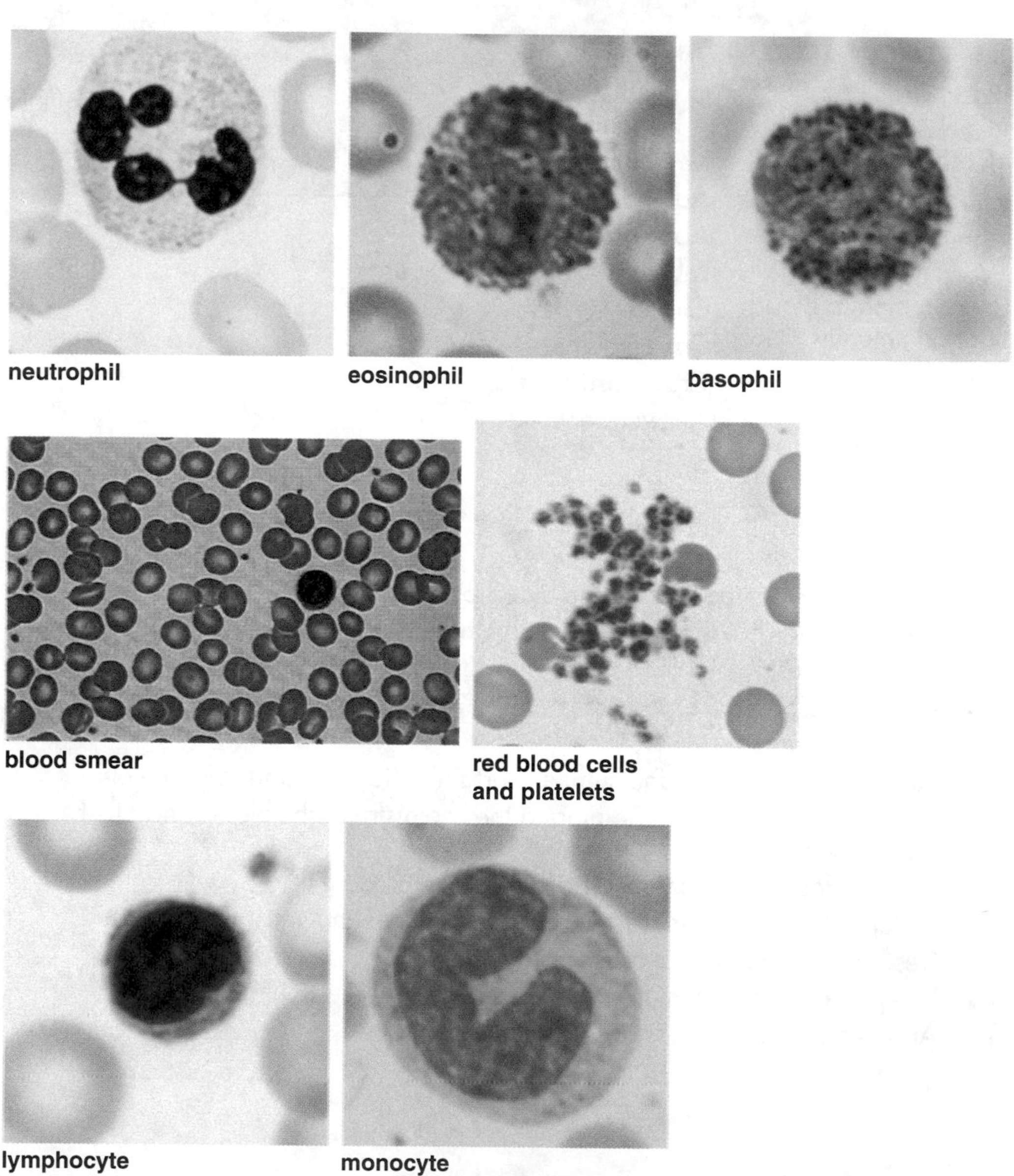

FIGURE 10-1. Normal blood smear and close-up view of individual blood cells.

Blood Cells

The blood cells (Fig. 10-1) are 1) **erythrocytes**, or red blood cells; 2) **leukocytes**, or white blood cells; and 3) **platelets**, also called **thrombocytes**. All blood cells are produced in red bone marrow. Some white blood cells multiply in lymphoid tissue as well.

Erythrocytes

The major function of erythrocytes is to carry oxygen to cells. This oxygen is bound to an iron-containing pigment within the cells called **hemoglobin**. Erythrocytes are small, disk-shaped cells with no nucleus. Their concentration of about 5 million per cubic millimeter (µL) of blood makes them by far the most numerous of the blood cells. The hemoglobin that they carry averages 15 g per dL (100 mL) of blood.

Leukocytes

White blood cells all show prominent nuclei when stained. They total about 5,000 to 10,000 per cubic millimeter, but their number may increase during infection. There are five different types of leukocytes which are identified by the size and appearance of the nucleus and by their staining properties. Granular leukocytes or **granulocytes** have visible granules in the cytoplasm when stained; there are three types of granulocytes: neutrophils, eosinophils, and basophils, named for the kind of stain they take up. **Agranulocytes** do not have visible granules when stained; there are two types of agranulocytes: lymphocytes and monocytes. Characteristics of the different types of cells are given in Table 10-1.

White blood cells protect against foreign substances. Some engulf foreign material by the process of **phagocytosis**; others function as part of the immune system. In diagnosis it is important to know not only the total number of leukocytes but also the relative number of each type. The most numerous white blood cells, neutrophils, are called *polymorphs* because of their various-shaped nuclei. They are also referred to as *segs, polys, or PMNs* (polymorphonuclear leukocytes).

TABLE 10-1 White Blood Cells (Leukocytes)

Type of Cell	Relative Percentage (Adult)	Function
Granulocytes		
neutrophils (*NŪ-trō-fils*)	54%–62%	phagocytosis
eosinophils (*ē-ō-SIN-ō-fils*)	1%–3%	allergic reactions; defense against parasites
basophils (*BĀ-sō-fils*)	less than 1%	allergic reactions
Agranulocytes		
lymphocytes (*LIM-Fō-sītz*)	25%–38%	immunity
monocytes (*MON-ō-sitz*)	3%–7%	phagocytosis

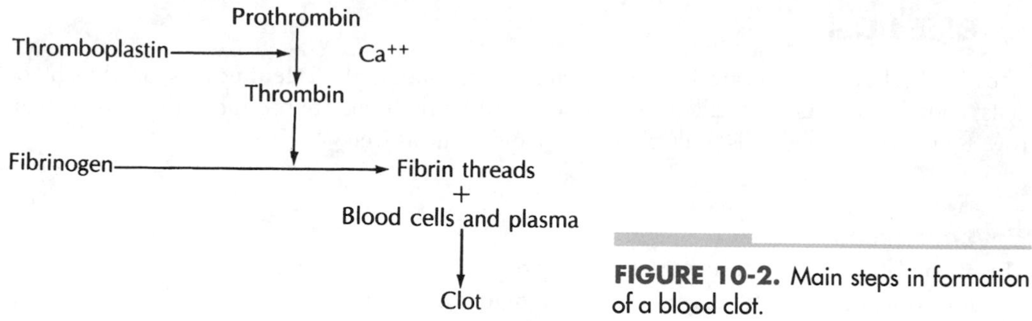

FIGURE 10-2. Main steps in formation of a blood clot.

Platelets

The blood platelets (thrombocytes) are fragments of larger cells formed in the bone marrow. They number from 200,000–400,000 per cubic millimeter of blood. Platelets are important in **hemostasis**, the prevention of blood loss, a component of which is the process of blood clotting, also known as **coagulation**.

When a vessel is injured, platelets stick together to form a plug at the site. Substances released from the platelets and from damaged tissue then interact with clotting factors in the plasma to produce a wound-sealing clot. Clotting factors are inactive in the blood until an injury occurs. To protect against unwanted clot formation, 12 different factors must interact before blood coagulates. The final reaction is the conversion of **fibrinogen** to threads of **fibrin** that trap blood cells and plasma to produce the clot (Fig. 10-2). What remains of the plasma after blood coagulates is **serum**.

Blood Types

Genetically inherited proteins on the surface of red blood cells determine blood type. More than 20 groups of these proteins have now been identified, but the most familiar are the ABO and Rh blood groups. The ABO system includes types A, B, AB, and O. The Rh types are Rh^+ and Rh^-. In giving blood transfusions it is important to give blood of the same type as the recipient's blood or of a type to which the recipient will not show an immune reaction. Compatible blood types are determined by crossmatching. Whole blood may be used to replace a large volume of blood lost, but in most cases requiring blood transfusion, a blood fraction such as packed red cells, platelets, plasma, or specific clotting factors, is administered.

The Immune System

Our bodies have an array of defenses against foreign matter. Some of these defenses are non-specific, that is, they protect against any intruder. Such defenses include the unbroken skin, blood-filtering lymphoid tissue, cilia and mucus that trap foreign material, bactericidal body secretions, and reflexes, such as coughing and sneezing.

Specific attacks on disease organisms are mounted by the immune system. The immune response involves complex interactions between components of the lymphatic system and the blood. Any foreign particle may act as an **antigen**, that is, a substance that provokes a response by the immune system. This response comes from two types of lymphocytes that circulate in the blood and lymphatic system. One type, the **T cells** (T lymphocytes), mature in the thymus gland. They are capable of attacking a foreign cell directly, producing *cell mediated immunity*. The **B cells** (B lymphocytes) mature in lymphoid tissue. When they meet a foreign antigen they multiply rapidly and produce **antibodies** that inactivate the antigen. Antibodies remain in the blood, often providing long-term immunity to the specific organism against which they were formed. Antibody based immunity is referred to as *humoral immunity*.

Types of Immunity

Passive immunity involves the transfer of antibodies to an individual, either naturally through the placenta or mother's milk, or artificially by the administration of an immune serum. Active immunity involves the individual's own response to a disease organism, either through natural contact with the organism or by the administration of an artificially prepared vaccine.

Immunology is one of the most active areas of current research. The above description is only the barest outline of the events that occur in the immune response, and there is much still to be discovered. Some of the areas of research include the autoimmune diseases, in which an individual produces antibodies to his or her own body tissues; hereditary and acquired immune deficiency diseases; the relationship between cancer and immunity; and the development of techniques for avoiding rejection of transplanted tissue.

KEY TERMS: NORMAL STRUCTURE AND FUNCTION

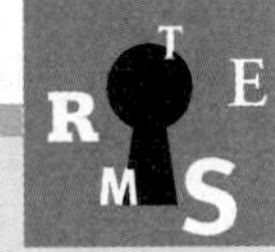

albumin *(al-BŪ-min)*	A simple protein found in blood plasma
antibody *(AN-ti-bod-ē)*	A protein produced in response to, and interacting specifically with, an antigen
antigen *(AN-ti-jen)*	A substance that induces the formation of antibodies
B cell	A lymphocyte that matures in lymphoid tissue and is active in producing antibodies; B lymphocyte *(LIM-fō-sīt)*
blood	The fluid that circulates in the cardiovascular system (root hem/o, hemat/o)
coagulation *(kō-ag-ū-LĀ-shun)*	The process of clot formation
electrolyte *(ē-LEK-trō-līt)*	A substance that separates into charged particles (ions) in solution; a salt. Also refers to ions in body fluids.
erythrocyte *(e-RITH-rō-sīt)*	A red blood cell (root erythr/o, erythrocyt/o)
fibrin *(FĪ-brin)*	The protein that forms a clot in the process of blood coagulation
fibrinogen (fi-BRIN-ō-jen)	The inactive precursor of fibrin
formed elements	The cellular components of blood
hemoglobin (Hb, Hgb) *(HĒ-mō-glō-bin)*	The iron-containing pigment in red blood cells that transports oxygen
hemostasis *(hē-mō-STĀ-sis)*	The stoppage of bleeding
immunity *(i-MŪ-ni-tē)*	The state of being protected against a specific disease (root immun/o)
leukocyte *(LŪ-kō-sīt)*	A white blood cell (root leuk/o, leukocyt/o)

(continued)

lymphocyte
(LIM-fō-sīt) — A lymphatic cell; a type of agranular leukocyte (root lymph/o, lymphocyt/o)

phagocytosis
(fag-ō-sī-TŌ-sis) — The engulfing of foreign material by white blood cells

plasma
(PLAZ-ma) — The liquid portion of the blood

platelet
(PLĀT-let) — A formed element of the blood that is active in hemostasis; a thrombocyte (root thrombocyte/o)

serum
(SĒR-um) — The fraction of the plasma that remains after blood coagulation; it is the equivalent of plasma without its clotting factors

T cell — A lymphocyte that matures in the thymus gland and attacks foreign cells directly; T lymphocyte

thrombocyte — A blood platelet (root thrombocyt/o)

Word Parts Pertaining to Blood and Immunity

Suffixes for Blood

Suffix	Meaning	Example	Definition of Example
-emia,* -hemia	condition of blood	pachyemia *pak-ē-Ē-mē-a*	thickness (pachy-) of the blood
-penia	decrease in, deficiency of	neutropenia *nū-trō-PĒ-nē-a*	deficiency of neutrophils in the blood
-poiesis	formation, production	hemopoiesis *hē-mō-poy-Ē-sis*	production of blood cells

*A shortened form of the root *hem* plus the suffix *-ia*.

Exercise 10-1

Define the following terms:

1. hyperalbuminemia *(hī-per-al-bū-mi-NĒ-mē-a)* Excess albumin in the blood.
2. hypoproteinemia *(hī-pō-prō-tēn-Ē-mē-a)* ____________
3. cytopenia *(sī-tō-PĒ-nē-a)* ____________
4. leukopenia *(lū-kō-PĒ-nē-a)* ____________
5. lymphocytopoiesis *(lim-fō-sī-tō-poy-Ē-sis)* ____________

Word Building. Use the suffix *-emia* to write a word for each of the following definitions:

6. Presence of pus in the blood ________________
7. Presence of viruses in the blood ________________
8. Presence of toxins in the blood ________________
9. Overgrowth of white cells in the blood ________________

Many of the words relating to blood cells can be formed either with or without including the root *cyt/o*, as in erythropenia or erythrocytopenia, leukopoiesis or leukocytopoiesis.

Roots for Blood and Immunity

Root	Meaning	Example	Definition of Example
myel/o	bone marrow	myelogenous *mi-e-LOJ-e-nus*	originating in bone marrow
hem/o, hemat/o	blood	hemorrhage *HEM-or-ij*	profuse flow of blood
erythr/o, erythrocyt/o	red blood cell	erythrocytosis *e-rith-RŌ-sī-TŌ-sis*	condition of increased red blood cells
leuk/o, leukocyt/o	white blood cell	leukoblast *LŪ-kō-blast*	immature white blood cell
lymph/o, lymphocyt/o	lymphocyte	lymphopoiesis *lim-fō-poy-Ē-sis*	production of lymphocytes in the blood
thromb/o	blood clot	thrombotic *throm-BOT-ik*	pertaining to a blood clot
thrombocyt/o	platelet, thrombocyte	thrombocythemia *throm-bō-si-THĒ-mē-a*	increase in the number of platelets in the blood
immun/o	immunity, immune system	immunize *IM-ū-niz*	to render immune

The remaining types of blood cells are designated by easily recognized roots such as agranulocyt/o, monocyt/o, granul/o, etc.

Exercise 10-2

Identity and define the root in each of the following words.

	Root	Meaning of Root
1. panmyeloid *(pan-MĪ-e-loyd)*	myel/o	bone marrow
2. prothrombin *(prō-THROM-bin)*		
3. preimmunization *(prē-im-ū-ni-ZĀ-shun)*		
4. hematic *(hē-MAT-ik)*		

Fill in the blanks:

5. Erythroclasis *(er-i-THROK-la-sis)* is the breaking (-clasis) of ________________.
6. A myeloblast *(MĪ-e-lō-blast)* is an immature cell found in ________________.
7. The term *thrombogenesis (throm-bō-JEN-e-sis)* refers to the formation of a(n) ________________.
8. Leukocytosis *(lū-kō-sī-TŌ-sis)* is an increase in the number of ________________.
9. An immunocyte *(im-u-nō-SĪT)* is a cell active in ________________.
10. A hemocytometer *(hē-mō-sī-TOM-e-ter)* is a device for counting ________________.
11. Lymphokines *(LIM-fō-kīnz)* are chemicals active in immunity that are produced by ________________.

Word building. Write a word for each of the following definitions:

12. Tumor of bone marrow ________________
13. Immature lymphocyte ________________
14. Decrease in red blood cells ________________
15. Study of blood ________________
16. Dissolving (-lysis) of a blood clot ________________
17. Formation (-poiesis) of bone marrow ________________

The suffix *-osis* added to a root for a type of cell means an increase in that type of cell in the blood. Following the example, write a word that means:

18. Increase in red blood cells erythrocytosis
19. Increase in monocytes in the blood ________________
20. Increase platelets in the blood ________________
21. Increase in granulocytes in the blood ________________
22. Increase in lymphocytes in the blood ________________

Roots for Chemistry

Root	Meaning	Example	Definition of Example
azot/o	nitrogen compounds	azoturia *az-ō-TŪ-rē-a*	increased nitrogen compounds in the urine (-uria)
calc/i	calcium (symbol Ca)	calcipenia *kal-si-PĒ-nē-a*	deficiency of calcium in the blood
ferr/o, ferr/i	iron (symbol Fe)	ferric *FER-ik*	pertaining to or containing iron

(continued)

Roots for Chemistry (Continued)

Root	Meaning	Example	Definition of Example
sider/o	iron	sideroblast *SID-er-ō-blast*	an immature red blood cell containing iron granules
kali	potassium (symbol K)	hyperkalemia* *hi-per-ka-LĒ-mē-a*	excess potassium in the blood
natri	sodium (symbol Na)	natriuresis *nā-trē-ū-RĒ-sis*	excretion of sodium in the urine (ur/o)
ox/y	oxygen (symbol O)	hypoxemia *hi-pok-SĒ-mē-a*	deficiency of oxygen in the blood

*The *i* in the root is dropped.

Exercise 10-3

Fill in the blanks:

1. Sideroderma *(sid-er-ō-DER-ma)* is the deposit of ______________________ into the skin.
2. The term *normokalemia (nor-mō-ka-LĒ-mē-a)* refers to a normal amount of ______________________ in the blood.
3. An oxide *(OKS-īd)* is a compound that contains ______________________.
4. Ferritin *(FER-i-tin)* is a compound that contains ______________________.

Word building. Use the suffix *-emia* to form words with the following meanings:

5. Presence of sodium in the blood ______________________
6. Presence of nitrogen compounds in the blood ______________________
7. Presence of calcium in the blood ______________________

Clinical Aspects: Blood

Anemia

Anemia is defined as a decrease in the amount of hemoglobin in the blood. It may result from too few red blood cells, cells that are too small, or too little hemoglobin in the cells. Cells may be normal in size (normocytic), or abnormal (micro- or macrocytic); they may be normal in hemoglobin (normochromic) or have too little (hypochromic). Key tests in diagnosing anemia are MCV (mean corpuscular volume) and MCHC (mean corpuscular hemoglobin concentration) (Table 10-2). The general symptoms of anemia include fatigue, shortness of breath, heart palpitations, pallor, and irritability. There are many different types of anemia, some of which are caused by underproduction of red cells, others by loss or destruction of cells.

Aplastic anemia results from destruction of the bone marrow and affects all blood cells (pancytopenia). It may be caused by drugs, toxins, viruses, radiation, or bone marrow cancer. It has been treated successfully with bone marrow transplants.

infarction
(in-FARK-shun)
Localized necrosis (death) of tissue resulting from a blockage or a narrowing of the artery that supplies the area. A myocardial infarction (MI) occurs in cardiac muscle and usually results from formation of a thrombus (clot) in a coronary artery (see Figure 9-9).

ischemia
(is-KĒ-mē-a)
Local deficiency of blood supply due to obstruction of the circulation

murmur
An abnormal heart sound. A *functional murmur* is generated by normal heart function and does not indicate a defect.

occlusion
(ō-KLŪ-zhun)
A closing off or obstruction, as of a vessel

phlebitis
(fle-BĪ-tis)
Inflammation of a vein

rheumatic heart disease
(rū-MAT-ik)
Damage to heart valves following infection with a type of streptococcus (group A hemolytic streptococcus). The antibodies produced in response to the infection produce scarring of the valves, usually the mitral valve.

shock
Circulatory failure resulting in inadequate supply of blood to the heart. Cardiogenic shock is due to heart failure; hypovolemic shock is due to a loss of blood volume; septic shock is due to bacterial infection.

stenosis
(ste-NŌ-sis)
Constriction or narrowing of an opening

stroke
See cerebrovascular accident

syncope
(SIN-kō-pē)
A temporary loss of consciousness due to inadequate blood flow to the brain; fainting

thrombosis
(throm-BŌ-sis)
Development of a blood clot within a vessel

thrombus
(THROM-bus)
A blood clot that forms within a blood vessel (root thromb/o)

varicose vein
(VAR-i-kōs)
A twisted and swollen vein resulting from breakdown of the valves, pooling of blood, and chronic dilatation of the vessel (root varic/o); also called varix (VAR-iks) or varicosity (var-i-KOS-i-tē)

Diagnosis and Treatment

cardioversion
(KAR-dē-ō-ver-zhun)
Correction of an abnormal cardiac rhythm. May be accomplished pharmacologically, with antiarrhythmic drugs, or electrically, by application of direct current to the chest wall or by means of an implanted device. This device, called a cardioverter-defibrillator controls heart rhythm by automatically delivering shocks directly to the myocardium.

echocardiography
(ek-ō-kar-dē-OG-ra-fē)
A noninvasive method that uses ultrasound to visualize internal cardiac structures

TABLE 10-2 Common Blood Tests

Test	Abbreviation	Measurement Given
red blood count	RBC	number of red blood cells per cubic millimeter of blood
white blood count	WBC	number of white blood cells per cubic millimeter of blood
differential count	Diff	relative percentage of the different types of leukocytes
hematocrit (Fig. 10-3)	Ht, Hct, crit	relative percentage of packed red cells in a given volume of blood
packed cell volume	PCV	hematocrit
hemoglobin	Hb, Hgb	amount of hemoglobin in g/dL (100 mL) of blood
mean corpuscular volume	MCV	volume of an average red cell
mean corpuscular hemoglobin	MCH	average weight of hemoglobin in red cells
mean corpuscular hemoglobin concentration	MCHC	average percent concentration of hemoglobin in red cells
erythrocyte sedimentation rate	ESR	rate of settling of erythrocytes per unit of time
activated partial thromboplastin time	APPT	test of coagulation
bleeding time	BT	test of coagulation
partial thromboplastin time	PTT	test of coagulation
prothrombin time	PT, Pro Time	test of coagulation
thrombin time	TT	test of coagulation
complete blood count	CBC	series of tests including cell counts, hematocrit, hemoglobin, and cell volume measurements

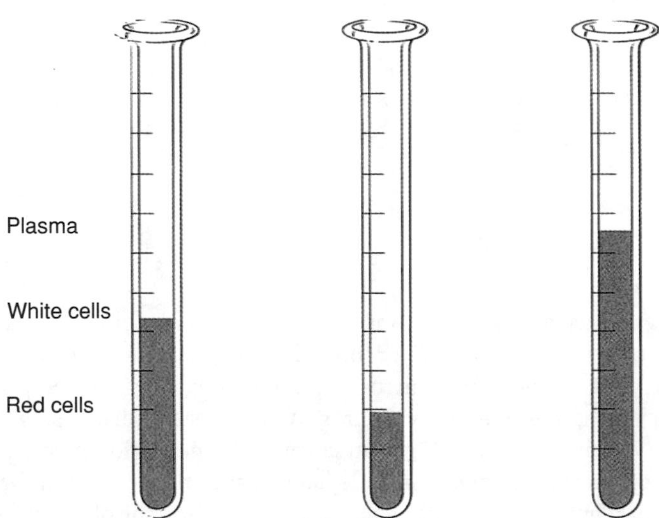

FIGURE 10-3. Hematocrit. The tube on the left shows a normal hematocrit. The middle tube shows the percentage of red blood cells is low, indicating anemia. The tube on the right shows an excessively high percentage of red blood cells, as in polycythemia.

Nutritional anemia may result from a deficiency of vitamin B_{12}, folic acid, or most commonly, iron. A specific form of B_{12} deficiency is **pernicious anemia**. This results from the lack of a substance, **intrinsic factor** (IF), produced in the stomach, that aids in the absorption of this vitamin from the intestine. Pernicious anemia must be treated with regular injections of B_{12}.

Hemorrhagic anemia results from blood loss. This may be a sudden loss, as from injury, or loss from chronic internal bleeding, as from the digestive tract in cases of ulcers or cancer.

Several hereditary diseases cause **hemolysis** (rupture) of red cells resulting in anemia. **Thalassemia** appears in Mediterranean populations. It affects the production of hemoglobin and is designated as α (alpha) or β (beta), according to the part of the molecule affected. Severe β thalassemia is also called **Cooley's anemia**. In **sickle cell anemia**, a mutation alters the hemoglobin molecule so that it precipitates when it gives up oxygen. The altered cells block small blood vessels and deprive tissues of oxygen. The misshapen cells are also readily destroyed (hemolyzed). The disease predominates in black populations. Genetic carriers of the defect, those with one normal and one abnormal gene, show sickle cell trait. They usually have no symptoms, except when oxygen is low, such as at high altitudes. They can, however, pass the defective gene to offspring. Sickle cell anemia, as well as many other genetic diseases, can be diagnosed in carriers and in the fetus before birth.

Reticulocyte counts are useful in diagnosing the causes of anemia. **Reticulocytes** are immature red blood cells that normally appear in small percentage in the blood. A rise in the number of reticulocytes indicates increased red blood cell formation, as in response to hemorrhage or destruction of red cells. A decrease indicates a failure in red blood cell production, as caused by nutritional deficiency or aplastic anemia.

Coagulation Disorders

The most common cause of coagulation problems is a deficiency in the number of circulating platelets, a condition termed **thrombocytopenia**. Possible causes include aplastic anemia, infections, cancer of the bone marrow, or agents that destroy bone marrow, such as x-rays or certain drugs. This disorder results in bleeding into the skin and mucous membranes, variously described as **petechiae, ecchymoses**, and **purpura**.

In **disseminated intravascular coagulation** (DIC) there is widespread clotting in the vessels that obstructs circulation to the tissues. This is followed by diffuse hemorrhages as clotting factors are removed and the coagulation process is impaired. DIC may be caused by infection, cancer, hemorrhage, or allergy.

Hemophilia is a hereditary deficiency of a specific clotting factor. It is a sex-linked disease that is passed from mother to son. There is bleeding into the tissues, especially into the joints (hemarthrosis). Hemophilia must be treated with transfusions of the necessary clotting factor.

Neoplasms

Leukemia is a neoplasm of white blood cells. The symptoms of leukemia include anemia, fatigue, easy bleeding, splenomegaly, and sometimes hepatomegaly (enlargement of the liver). Myelogenous leukemia originates in the bone marrow and involves mainly the granular leukocytes. Lymphocytic leukemia affects B cells and the lymphatic system, causing lymphadenopathy and adverse effects on the immune system. Leukemias are further differentiated as acute or chronic based on clinical progress. Treatment of leukemia includes chemotherapy, radiation therapy, and bone marrow transplantation. A recent advance in transplantation is the use of umbilical cord blood to replace blood-forming cells in bone marrow. This is more readily available than bone marrow and does not have to match as closely to avoid rejection.

Hodgkin's disease is a disease of the lymphatic system which may spread to other tissues. It begins with enlarged but painless lymph nodes in the cervical (neck) region and then progresses to other nodes. There are fever, night sweats, weight loss and itching of the skin (pruritis). Persons of any age may be affected, but the disease predominates in young adults and those over 50. Most cases can be cured with radiation and chemotherapy.

Non-Hodgkin's lymphoma is also a malignant enlargement of lymph nodes, but does not show the giant Reed-Sternberg cells that characterizes Hodgkin's disease. It is more common than Hodgkin's disease and has a higher mortality rate. Cases vary in severity and prognosis. It is most prevalent in the older adult population and those with immunodeficiency. Non-Hodgkin's lymphoma involves the T or B lymphocytes, and some cases may be related to infection with certain viruses. It requires systemic chemotherapy and, sometimes, bone marrow transplantation.

Multiple myeloma is a cancer of the blood forming cells in bone marrow, mainly the plasma cells that produce antibodies. The disease causes anemia, bone pain, and weakening of the bones. There is a greater susceptibility to infection because of immune deficiency. Abnormally high levels of calcium and protein in the blood often lead to kidney failure. Multiple myeloma is treated with radiation and chemotherapy, but the prognosis is generally poor.

Clinical Aspects: Immunity

Hypersensitivity is a harmful overreaction of the immune system, commonly known as **allergy**. In cases of allergy, a person is more sensitive to a particular antigen than the average individual. Common **allergens** are pollen, animal dander, dust, and foods, but there are many more. Responses may include itching, redness or tearing of the eyes, skin rash, asthma, sneezing, and **urticaria** (hives). An **anaphylactic reaction** is a severe generalized allergic response that can lead rapidly to death as a result of shock and interference with breathing. It must be treated by immediate administration of adrenaline, maintenance of open airways, and antihistamines.

The term **immunodeficiency** refers to any failure in the immune system. This may be congenital (present at birth) or acquired, and may involve any components of the system. The deficiency may vary in severity, but is always evidenced by an increased susceptibility to disease. **AIDS** is acquired by infection with **HIV** (human immunodeficiency virus), which attacks certain T cells. These cells have a specific surface attachment site, the CD4 receptor, for the virus. The disease is spread by sexual contact, use of contaminated needles, blood transfusions, and by passage from an infected mother to a fetus. It leaves the host susceptible to opportunistic infections such as pneumonia caused by the protozoon *Pneumocystis carinii*, thrush, a fungal infection of the mouth caused by *Candida albicans*, and infection with *Cryptosporidium*, a protozoon that causes cramps and diarrhea. It also predisposes to Kaposi's sarcoma, a previously rare form of skin cancer. At present there is no vaccine or cure for AIDS, but some drugs can delay progress of the disease.

A disease that results from an immune response to one's own tissues is classified as an **autoimmune disorder**. The cause may be a reaction to body cells that have been slightly altered by mutation or disease. The list of diseases that are believed to be caused, at least in part, by autoimmunity is long. It includes pernicious anemia, systemic lupus erythematosus (see Chapter 21), rheumatoid arthritis, Graves' disease (of the thyroid), myasthenia gravis (a muscle disease), rheumatic heart disease, glomerulonephritis (a kidney disease), and scleroderma (see Chapter 21).

KEY CLINICAL TERMS

Disorders

Term	Definition
AIDS	Acquired immunodeficiency syndrome. Failure of the immune system caused by infection with human immunodeficiency virus (HIV). The virus infects certain T cells and thus interferes with immunity.
allergen *(AL-er-jen)*	A substance that causes an allergic response
allergy *(AL-er-jē)*	Hypersensitivity
anaphylactic reaction *(an-a-fi-LAK-tic)*	An exaggerated allergic reaction to a foreign substance (G. root *phylaxis* means "protection")
anemia *(a-NĒ-mē-a)*	A decrease in the number or size of red blood cells or in the amount of hemoglobin in the blood. May result from blood loss, malnutrition, a hereditary defect, environmental factors, and other causes.
aplastic anemia *(a-PLAS-tik)*	Anemia caused by bone marrow failure resulting in deficient blood cell production, especially that of red cells
autoimmune disorder	A condition in which the immune system produces antibodies against an individual's own tissues
Cooley's anemia	A form of thalassemia (hereditary anemia) in which the B (beta) chain of hemoglobin is abnormal
disseminated intravascular coagulation (DIC)	Widespread formation of clots in the microscopic vessels; may be followed by bleeding as a result of depletion of clotting factors
ecchymosis *(ek-i-MŌ-sis)*	A collection of blood under the skin caused by leakage from small vessels (root *chym* means "juice")
hemolysis *(hē-MOL-i-sis)*	The rupture of red blood cells and the release of hemoglobin (adj. hemolytic)
hemophilia *(hē-mō-FIL-ē-a)*	A hereditary blood disease caused by lack of a clotting factor and resulting in abnormal bleeding
HIV	Human immunodeficiency virus. The virus that causes AIDS.
Hodgkin's disease	A neoplastic disease of unknown cause that involves the lymph nodes, spleen, liver, and other tissues; characterized by the presence of giant Reed-Sternberg cells
hypersensitivity	An immunologic reaction to a substance that is harmless to most people; allergy
immunodeficiency *(im-ū-nō-de-FISH-en-sē)*	A congenital or acquired failure in the immune system to protect against disease
leukemia *(lū-KĒ-mē-a)*	Malignant overgrowth of immature white blood cells. May be chronic or acute; may affect bone marrow (myelogenous leukemia) or lymphoid tissue (lymphocytic leukemia).

(continued)

lymphadenopathy *(lim-fad-e-NOP-a-thē)* — Any disease of the lymph nodes

lymphoma *(lim-FŌ-ma)* — Any malignant disease of lymphoid tissue, such as Hodgkin's disease, Burkitt's disease, and others

multiple myeloma *(mī-e-LŌ-ma)* — A tumor of the blood forming tissue in bone marrow

non-Hodgkin's lymphoma — A widespread malignant disease of lymph nodes that involves lymphocytes. It differs from Hodgkin's disease in the absence of giant Reed-Sternberg cells.

pernicious anemia *(per-NISH-us)* — Anemia caused by failure of the stomach to produce intrinsic factor, a substance needed for the absorption of vitamin B_{12}. This vitamin is required for the formation of erythrocytes.

petechiae *(pē-TĒ-kē-ē)* — Pinpoint, flat, purplish-red spots caused by bleeding within the skin or mucous membrane (s. petechia)

purpura *(PUR-pū-ra)* — A condition characterized by hemorrhages into the skin, mucous membranes, internal organs, and other tissues (from G. word meaning "purple"). Thrombocytopenic purpura is caused by a deficiency of platelets.

sickle cell anemia — A hereditary anemia caused by the presence of abnormal hemoglobin. Red blood cells become sickle-shaped and interfere with normal blood flow to the tissues. Most common in Mediterranean and African populations.

splenomegaly *(splē-nō-MEG-a-lē)* — Enlargement of the spleen

thalassemia *(thal-a-SĒ-mē-a)* — A group of hereditary anemias mostly found in Mediterranean populations (the name comes from the Greek word for "sea")

thrombocytopenia *(throm-bō-sī-tō-PĒ-nē-a)* — A deficiency of thrombocytes (platelets) in the blood

urticaria *(ur-ti-KAR-ē-a)* — A skin reaction consisting of round, raised eruptions with itching; hives

Diagnosis and Treatment

band cell — An immature neutrophil with a nucleus in the shape of a band. Also called a stab or staff cell.

CD4+ T-lymphocyte count — A count of the T cells that have the CD4 receptors for the AIDS virus (HIV). A count of less than 200/µL of blood signifies severe immunodeficiency. Direct counts of virus in the blood also are used in tracking the disease.

intrinsic factor — A substance produced in the stomach that aids in the absorption of vitamin B_{12} necessary for the manufacture of red blood cells

reticulocyte *(re-TIK-ū-lō-sīt)* — An immature red blood cell; counts are useful in diagnosis

Reed-Sternberg cells — Giant cells that are characteristic of Hodgkin's disease. They usually have two large nuclei and are surrounded by a halo.

ADDITIONAL TERMS

Normal Structure and Function

agglutination (*a-glū-ti-NĀ-shun*) — The clumping of cells or particles in the presence of specific antibodies

bilirubin (*bil-i-RŪ-bin*) — A pigment derived from the breakdown of hemoglobin. It is eliminated by the liver in bile.

complement (*COM-ple-ment*) — A group of plasma enzymes that interacts with antibody to destroy foreign cells

corpuscle (*KOR-pus-l*) — A small mass or body. A blood corpuscle is a blood cell.

gamma globulin — The fraction of the blood plasma that contains antibodies

heparin (*HEP-a-rin*) — A substance found throughout the body that inhibits blood coagulation; an anticoagulant

immunoglobulin (Ig) (*im-ū-nō-GLOB-ū-lin*) — An antibody. Immunoglobulins fall into 5 classes, each abbreviated with a capital letter: IgG, IgM, IgA, IgD, IgE.

macrophage (*MAK-rō-faj*) — A phagocytic cell derived from a monocyte; usually found within the tissues. Macrophages work with T cells in immunity.

megakaryocyte (*meg-a-KAR-ē-ō-sīt*) — A large bone marrow cell that fragments to release platelets

plasmin (*PLAZ-min*) — An enzyme that dissolves clots; also called fibrinolysin

thrombin (*THROM-bin*) — The enzyme derived from prothrombin that converts fibrinogen to fibrin

stem cell — A primitive bone marrow cell that gives rise to all varieties of blood cells

Symptoms and Conditions

agranulocytosis (*ā-gran-ū-lō-sī-TŌ-sis*) — A condition involving decrease in the number of granulocytes in the blood; also called granulocytopenia

acute lymphoblastic leukemia (ALL) — A malignant disease of lymphoblasts, the cells that give rise to lymphocytes. Eighty-five percent of cases occur in children, more than half of which can now be cured.

delayed hypersensitivity reaction — An allergic reaction involving T cells that takes at least 12 hours to develop. Examples are various types of contact dermatitis, such as poison ivy or poison oak, the tuberculin reaction (test for TB), and rejections of transplanted tissue.

erythrocytosis (*e-rith-rō-sī-TŌ-sis*) — Increase in the number of red cells in the blood. May be normal, such as to compensate for life at high altitudes, or abnormal, such as in cases of pulmonary or cardiac disease.

graft-versus-host-reaction (GVHR) — An immunological reaction of transplanted lymphocytes against tissues of the host. A common complication of bone marrow transplantation.

hairy cell leukemia — A form of leukemia in which cells have filaments making them look "hairy"

hematoma (*hē-ma-TŌ-ma*) — A localized collection of blood, usually clotted, caused by a break in a blood vessel

hemosiderosis (*hē-mō-sid-er-Ō-sis*) — A condition involving the deposition of an iron-containing pigment (hemosiderin) mainly in the liver and the spleen. The pigment comes from hemoglobin released from disintegrated red blood cells.

idiopathic thrombocytopenic purpura (ITP) — A clotting disorder due to destruction of platelets that usually follows a viral illness. Causes petechiae and hemorrhages into the skin and mucous membranes.

infectious mononucleosis (*mon-ō-nū-klē-Ō-sis*) — An acute infectious disease caused by Epstein-Barr virus (EBV). Characterized by fever, weakness, lymphadenopathy, hepatosplenomegaly, and atypical lymphocytes (resembling monocytes).

lymphocytosis (*lim-fō-sī-TŌ-sis*) — An increase in the number of circulating lymphocytes. Usually a result of infection.

myelofibrosis (*mī-ē-lō-fī-BRŌ-sis*) — Condition in which bone marrow is replaced with fibrous tissue

neutropenia (*nū-trō-PĒ-nē-a*) — A decrease in the number of neutrophils with increased susceptibility to infection. Causes include drugs, irradiation, and infection. May be a side effect of treatment for malignancy.

pancytopenia (*pan-sī-tō-PĒ-nē-a*) — A decrease in all cells of the blood, as in aplastic anemia

polycythemia vera (*pol-ē-sī-THĒ-mē-a VĒ-ra*) — A condition in which overactive bone marrow produces too many red blood cells. These interfere with circulation and promote thrombosis and hemorrhage. Treated by blood removal. Also called erythremia.

spherocytic anemia (*sfēr-ō-SIT-ik*) — Hereditary anemia in which red blood cells are round instead of disk-shaped and rupture (hemolyze) excessively

systemic lupus erythematosus (SLE) — An autoimmune disease of connective tissue that affects skin, joints, blood, and other tissues

thrombotic thrombocytopenic purpura (TTP) — An often fatal disorder in which multiple clots form in blood vessels

von Willebrand's disease — A hereditary bleeding disease caused by lack of von Willebrand's factor, a substance necessary for blood clotting

Diagnosis (See also Table 10-2)

Bence Jones protein — A protein that appears in the urine of patients with multiple myeloma

Coombs' test — A test for detection of antibodies to red blood cells, such as appear in cases of autoimmune hemolytic anemias

electrophoresis (*ē-lek-trō-fo-RĒ-sis*) — Separation of particles in a liquid by application of an electrical field. Used to separate components of blood.

ELISA — Enzyme-linked immunoabsorbent assay. A highly sensitive immunologic test used to diagnose HIV infection, hepatitis, and Lyme disease, among others.

monoclonal antibody *(mon-ō-KLŌ-nal)* — A pure antibody produced in the laboratory; used for diagnosis and treatment

pH — A scale that measures the relative acidity or alkalinity of a solution. Represents the amount of hydrogen ion in the solution.

Philadelphia chromosome (Ph) — An abnormal chromosome found in the cells of most individuals with chronic myelogenous leukemia

seroconversion *(sē-rō-con-VER-zhun)* — The appearance of antibodies in the serum in response to a disease or an immunization

Western blot assay — A very sensitive test used to detect small amounts of antibodies in the blood

Wright's stain — A commonly used blood stain

Treatment

adrenaline *(a-DREN-a-lin)* — A powerful stimulant naturally produced by the adrenal gland and sympathetic nervous system. Activates the cardiovascular, respiratory, and other systems needed to meet stress. Used as a drug to treat severe allergic reactions and shock. Also called epinephrine.

anticoagulant *(an-ti-kō-AG-ū-lant)* — An agent that prevents or delays blood coagulation

antihistamine *(an-ti-HIS-ta-mēn)* — A drug that counteracts the effects of histamine and is used to treat allergic reactions

apheresis *(af-e-RĒ-sis)* — A procedure in which blood is withdrawn, a portion is separated and retained, and the remainder is returned to the donor. Apheresis may be used as a suffix with a root meaning the fraction retained, such as plasmapheresis, leukapheresis.

autologous blood *(aw-TOL-ō-gus)* — A person's own blood. May be donated in advance of surgery and transfused if needed.

cryoprecipitate *(krī-ō-prē-SIP-i-tāt)* — A sediment obtained by cooling. The fraction obtained by freezing blood plasma contains clotting factors.

desensitization *(dē-sen-si-ti-ZĀ-shun)* — Treatment of allergy by small injections of the offending allergen. This causes an increase of antibody to destroy the antigen rapidly on contact.

immunosuppression *(im-ū-nō-sū-PRESH-un)* — Depression of the immune response. May be correlated with disease, but also may be induced therapeutically to prevent rejection in cases of tissue transplantation.

protease inhibitor *(PRŌ-tē-ās)* — An anti-HIV drug that acts by inhibiting an enzyme the virus needs to multiply

ABBREVIATIONS*

Ab antibody
Ag antigen
AIDS acquired immunodeficiency syndrome
ALL acute lymphocytic leukemia
AML acute myelogenous leukemia
CLL chronic lymphocytic leukemia
CML chronic myelogenous leukemia
DIC disseminated intravascular coagulation
EBV Epstein-Barr virus
ELISA enzyme-linked immunoabsorbent assay
HIV human immunodeficiency virus
IF intrinsic factor
Ig immunoglobulin
ITP idiopathic thrombocytopenic purpura

*See also blood tests, Table 10-2

lytes electrolytes
mEq milliequivalent
pH scale for measuring hydrogen ion concentration (acidity)
Ph Philadelphia chromosome
PMN polymorphonuclear (neutrophil)
poly neutrophil
polymorph neutrophil
RBC red blood cell; red blood (cell) count
seg neutrophil
SLE systemic lupus erythematosus
TTP thrombotic thrombocytopenic purpura
vWF von Willebrand's factor
WBC white blood cell; white blood (cell) count

CHAPTER REVIEW 10-1

Matching. Match the terms in each of the sets below with their definitions and write the appropriate letter (a–e) to the left of each number:

_____ 1. hematocrit	a. lymphocyte
_____ 2. T cell	b. type of blood test
_____ 3. albumin	c. plasma protein
_____ 4. hemostasis	d. engulfing of foreign particles
_____ 5. phagocytosis	e. stoppage of blood flow
_____ 6. leukopoiesis	a. malignant overgrowth of white blood cells
_____ 7. leukemia	b. separation of white blood cells from whole blood
_____ 8. leukapheresis	c. deficiency of white blood cells
_____ 9. leukoblast	d. immature white blood cell
_____ 10. leukopenia	e. formation of white blood cells
_____ 11. azoturia	a. decreased sodium in the blood
_____ 12. sideropenia	b. containing iron
_____ 13. hyponatremia	c. increased nitrogen compounds in the urine
_____ 14. calcareous	d. containing calcium

Chapter 10
Labeling Exercise

Write the name of each numbered part on the corresponding line of the answer sheet.

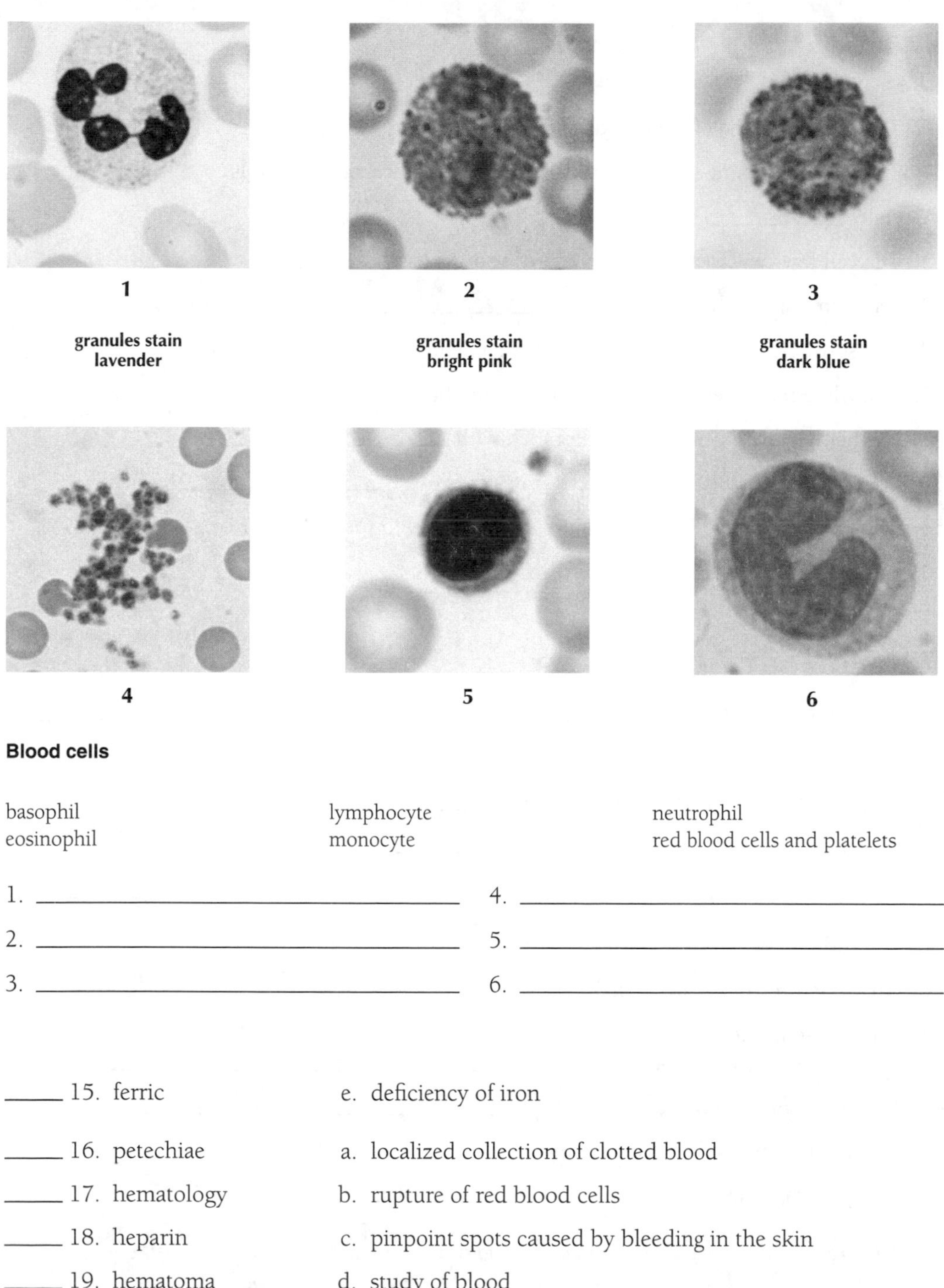

Blood cells

basophil
eosinophil
lymphocyte
monocyte
neutrophil
red blood cells and platelets

1. ______________________
2. ______________________
3. ______________________
4. ______________________
5. ______________________
6. ______________________

_____ 15. ferric — e. deficiency of iron

_____ 16. petechiae — a. localized collection of clotted blood

_____ 17. hematology — b. rupture of red blood cells

_____ 18. heparin — c. pinpoint spots caused by bleeding in the skin

_____ 19. hematoma — d. study of blood

_____ 20. hemolysis — e. anticoagulant

_____ 21. PMN a. a form of leukemia

_____ 22. ABO b. virus that causes infectious mononucleosis

_____ 23. ALL c. antibody

_____ 24. Ig d. neutrophil

_____ 25. EBV e. blood type group

Fill in the blanks:

26. The liquid fraction of the blood is called _____________________.
27. The iron-containing pigment in red blood cells that carries oxygen is called _____________________.
28. The cell fragments active in blood clotting are the _____________________.
29. The term for all white blood cells is _____________________.
30. The substance that forms a blood clot is named _____________________.
31. The white blood cells active in immunity are the _____________________.
32. Oxyhemglobin is hemoglobin combined with _____________________.
33. When bone tissue calcifies it incorporates salts of _____________________.
34. Natriuretic factor acts on the urinary system (ur/o) to promote the release of _____________________.

The suffixes *-ia, -osis*, and *-hemia* all denote an increase in the type of cell indicated by the word root. Define the following terms:

35. eosinophilia *(ē-ō-sin-ō-FIL-ē-a)* _____________________.
36. erythrocytosis *(e-rith-rō-sī-TŌ-sis)* _____________________.
37. thrombocythemia *(throm-bō-sī-THĒ-mē-a)* _____________________.
38. neutrophilia *(nū-trō-FIL-ē-a)* _____________________.
39. monocytosis *(mon-ō-sī-TŌ-sis)* _____________________.

Word building. Write a word for each of the following definitions:

40. An immature bone marrow cell _____________________
41. A decrease in the number of platelets (thrombocytes) in the blood _____________________
42. Formation of red blood cells _____________________
43. Specialist in the study of blood _____________________
44. Study of immunity _____________________

Use the ending *-ic* to write the adjective form of each of the following words:

45. basophil ______________________
46. lymphocyte ______________________
47. hemorrhage ______________________
48. leukemia ______________________
49. hemolysis ______________________

Plurals. Write the plural form of each of the following words.

50. allergy ______________________
51. petechia ______________________
52. ecchymosis ______________________
53. serum ______________________

Word analysis. Define each of the following words and give the meaning of the word parts in each. Use a dictionary if necessary.

54. Anemia ______________________

    a. an- ______________
    b. (h)em ______________
    c. -ia ______________

55. Hemocytometer ______________________

    a. hem/o ______________
    b. cyt/o ______________
    c. -meter ______________

56. Anisocytosis *(an-ī-sō-sī-TŌ-sis)* ______________________

    a. an- ______________
    b. iso- ______________
    c. cyt/o ______________
    d. -osis ______________

57. Polycythemia *(pol-ē-sī-THĒ-mē-a)* ______________________

    a. poly- ______________
    b. cyt/o ______________
    c. hem ______________
    d. -ia ______________

CHAPTER REVIEW 10-2

Matching. Match the terms in each of the sets below with their definitions and write the appropriate letter (a–e) to the left of each number:

Term	Definition
_____ 1. anaphylaxis	a. group of enzymes that aids in destroying foreign cells
_____ 2. complement	b. substance that dissolves blood clots
_____ 3. cryoprecipitate	c. exaggerated allergic reaction
_____ 4. gamma globulin	d. fraction of the blood plasma that contains antibodies
_____ 5. fibrinolysin	e. blood fraction obtained by cooling

Term	Definition
_____ 6. thrombocyte	a. pigment derived from hemoglobin
_____ 7. hemostat	b. blood platelet
_____ 8. band cell	c. immature red blood cell
_____ 9. bilirubin	d. instrument used to stop blood flow
_____ 10. reticulocyte	e. immature neutrophil

Term	Definition
_____ 11. septicemia	a. hereditary anemia
_____ 12. ecchymosis	b. hives
_____ 13. hyperemia	c. collection of blood under the skin
_____ 14. thalassemia	d. excess blood in a part
_____ 15. urticaria	e. presence of disease organisms in the blood

Term	Definition
_____ 16. PTT	a. hematocrit
_____ 17. diff	b. clotting test
_____ 18. CBC	c. measurement of the relative percentages of leukocytes
_____ 19. Hb	d. hemoglobin
_____ 20. PCV	e. series of tests on blood

Fill in the blanks:

21. The portion of plasma that remains after clotting factors have been removed is called _____________________.
22. Lymphocytes and monocytes do not show visible granules when stained and so together they are called _____________________.
23. Any substance that induces the formation of antibodies is termed a(n) _____________________.
24. The inactive form of fibrin is called _____________________.
25. The most numerous of the leukocytes are the _____________________.

26. Prothrombin is a blood factor involved in ________________.
27. A myelotoxin is a substance that destroys ________________.
28. Siderosis is a condition involving an excess of ________________.

Definitions. Write the meaning of each of the following terms:

29. neutropenia ________________
30. hypoxemia ________________
31. myeloma ________________
32. granulocytosis ________________
33. lymphoblast ________________
34. azotemia ________________

Word building. Write a word for each of the following definitions:

35. An immature leukocyte ________________
36. Formation of thrombocytes ________________
37. Specialist in study of the immune system ________________
38. Immunity to one's own tissues ________________
39. Profuse flow of blood ________________

Unscrambles. Form a word from each of the following groups of letters and write it in the blank:

40. gitnane ________________
41. ribnif ________________
42. lodiyem ________________
43. tlealtpe ________________
44. irapneh ________________

Word analysis. Define each of the following words and give the meaning of the word parts in each. Use a dictionary if necessary.

45. Pancytopenia *(pan-sī-tō-PĒ-nē-a)* ________________

____

a. pan- ________________

b. cyt/o ________________

c. -penia ________________

46. Hemophilia ________________

____

a. hem/o- __________

b. phil- __________

c. -ia __________

47. Ischemia __________

a. isch- suppression

b. (h)em __________

c. -ia __________

48. Poikilocytosis *(poy-kil-ō-sī-TŌ-sis)* __________

a. poikil/o- __________

b. cyt/o __________

c. -osis __________

49. Hemochromatosis *(hē-mō-krō-ma-TŌ-sis)* __________

a. hem/o __________

b. chromat/o __________

c. -osis __________

Chapter 10

Case Studies

1. *Salmonella* Infection Complicated by Thrombocytopenia

This patient, a 38-year-old female, came to the emergency room with a urinary tract infection and a temperature of 101°F. She had a previously diagnosed lymphoma stabilized with chemotherapeutic agents. On admission, her hemoglobin was 7.9, white count 3,700 with 62% polys and 11% bands. Platelet count was 72,000. Urine cultures were positive for gram-negative rods.

The patient was started on combined antibiotics. When blood cultures showed *Salmonella* sensitive to Ampicillin, this alone was continued at 2 grams IV every 6 hours. During treatment, her platelet count fell to about 40,000, probably due to the chemotherapy in combination with infection. Septra was added to treatment in case of platelet destruction by Ampicillin.

The patient was discharged with an appointment for a follow-up in 1 week.

2. Sickle Cell Anemia

The patient is a 31-year-old male with sickle cell anemia. He presents with pain in the lower extremities which is more severe than the usual crisis pain. The patient does not report any other recent illness, shortness of breath, joint swelling, or dysuria. When last admitted he was found to be positive for HIV, presumably due to repeated transfusions. Physical examination shows cervical, axillary, and inguinal lymph node adenopathy. There is also splenomegaly.

Demerol was administered for pain at the time of admission. Based on hemoglobin 8.5 and hematocrit 27.0, a blood transfusion was given. The patient was discharged with Rx for Tylox analgesic 1–2 tabs po q 4 prn and folate 1 mg po qd.

3. Thrombosis Complicated by Anemia

This patient is a 52-year-old female with a history of multiple pulmonary emboli currently treated with Coumadin (anticoagulant). Her chief complaint is increasing dyspnea on exertion. Physical examination is noncontributory except for fine crackles at the base of the right lung and a soft systolic heart murmur. Laboratory data show a low hemoglobin of 8.0, suggesting gastrointestinal or retroperitoneal bleeding as a result of anticoagulation therapy. A lung scan is consistent with multiple pulmonary embolizations.

Studies of the lower extremities for thrombosis proved normal. CT scan of the abdomen showed no hematoma or other abnormalities. Tranfusion produced marked improvement in clinical symptoms. The patient was discharged with instructions to continue her previous therapy. She will be followed by the Pulmonary Service.

Chapter 10
Case Study Questions

Multiple choice. Select the best answer and write the letter of your choice to the left of each number:

_____ 1. Polys and bands are

a. neutrophils
b. platelets
c. proteins
d. red blood cells
e. sera

_____ 2. The patient in Case 1 had a hemoglobin of 7.9 g per dL of blood. An average value for hemoglobin is

a. 100
b. 30
c. 15
d. 45
e. 300

_____ 3. A hematocrit measures

a. average red cell volume
b. coagulation time
c. erythrocyte sedimentation rate
d. percentage of packed cells in whole blood
e. total leukocytes

_____ 4. Multiple pulmonary emboli are

a. sounds heard in the lungs
b. blood clots in the lungs
c. blood clots in the spleen
d. sounds heard when the coronary vessels fill
e. viral infections of the liver

_____ 5. A systolic heart murmur is

a. an abnormal sound heard when the heart relaxes
b. a normal sound made as the heart beats
c. prolapse of the mitral valve
d. an abnormal sound heard when the heart contracts
e. heart block

_____ 6. Inguinal lymph nodes are located in the

a. armpit
b. leg
c. groin
d. neck
e. brain

_____ 7. Retroperitoneal bleeding occurs

a. under the peritoneum
b. behind the peritoneum
c. into the thorax
d. into the peritoneum
e. above the pelvis

Give the meaning of the following abbreviations:

8. HIV _______________
9. dL _______________
10. IV _______________
11. q6h _______________

Define the following terms:

12. chemotherapeutic _______________
13. dyspnea _______________
14. lymphoma _______________
15. adenopathy _______________
16. splenomegaly _______________

BLOUD AND IMMUNITY

ACROSS

3. the fraction of the blood plasma that contains antibodies: ____ globulin
6. a deficiency in the amount of hemoglobin in the blood
8. a coagulation test that involves prothrombin (abbr.)
9. a fraction obtained by freezing blood plasma: ____ precipitate
10. root (with combining vowel): blood
12. antigen (abbr.)
13. a type of granulocyte
15. a coagulation test that measures bleeding (abbr.)
16. prefix: before, in front of
17. prefix: not
18. the liquid portion of the blood
19. the pigment in red blood cells that carries oxygen: hemo ____
20. a sensitive immunologic test (abbr.)

DOWN

1. a thrombocyte
2. root (with combining vowel): bone marrow
4. a type of agranular leukocyte: ____ cyte
5. the substance in blood that produces a clot
7. a red blood cell: _____ cyte
8. a scale for measuring acidity
11. immunoglobulin (abbr.)
12. a simple protein found in blood plasma
14. prevention of blood loss: hemo ______
18. prefix: before, in front of

Chapter 10 Answer Section

Answers to Chapter Exercises

Exercise 10-1

1. excess albumin in the blood
2. decreased amount of protein in the blood
3. deficiency of cells in the blood
4. deficiency of leukocytes in the blood
5. production of lymphocytes
6. pyemia *(pī-Ē-mē-a)*
7. viremia *(vī-RĒ-mē-a)*
8. toxemia *(tok-SĒ-mē-a)*
9. leukemia *(lū-KĒ-mē-a)*

Exercise 10-2

1. myel/o; bone marrow
2. thromb/o; blood clot
3. immun/o; immunity
4. hem/o; blood
5. erythrocytes; red blood cells
6. bone marrow
7. blood clot
8. leukocytes; white blood cells
9. immunity
10. blood cells
11. lymphocytes
12. myeloma *(mī-e-LŌ-ma)*
13. lymphoblast *(LIM-fō-blast)*
14. erythropenia *(e-rith-rō-PĒ-nē-a)*; also erythrocytopenia
15. hematology *(hē-ma-TOL-ō-jē)*
16. thrombolysis *(throm-BOL-i-sis)*
17. myelopoiesis *(mī-e-lō-poy-Ē-sis)*
18. erythrocytosis *(e-rith-rō-sī-TŌ-sis)*
19. monocytosis *(mon-ō-sī-TŌ-sis)*
20. thrombocytosis *(throm-bō-sī-TŌ-sis)*
21. granulocytosis *(gran-ū-lō-sī-TŌ-sis)*
22. lymphocytosis *(lim-fō-sī-TŌ-sis)*

Exercise 10-3

1. iron
2. potassium
3. oxygen
4. iron
5. natremia *(na-TRĒ-mē-a)*
6. azotemia *(az-ō-TĒ-mē-a)*
7. calcemia *(KAL-sē-mĒ-a)*

Labeling Exercise

Blood Cells

1. neutrophil
2. eosinophil
3. basophil
4. red blood cells (erythrocytes) and platelets (thrombocytes)
5. lymphocyte
6. monocyte

Answers to Chapter Review 10-1

1. b
2. a
3. c
4. e
5. d
6. e
7. a
8. b
9. d
10. c
11. c
12. e
13. a
14. d
15. b
16. c
17. d
18. e
19. a
20. b
21. d
22. e
23. a
24. c
25. b
26. plasma
27. hemoglobin
28. platelets (thrombocytes)
29. leukocytes
30. fibrin
31. lymphocytes
32. oxygen
33. calcium
34. sodium
35. increase in the number of eosinophils in the blood
36. increase in the number of erythrocytes (red blood cells) in the blood
37. increase in the number of thrombocytes (platelets) in the blood
38. increase in the number of neutrophils in the blood
39. increase in the number of monocytes in the blood
40. myeloblast
41. thrombocytopenia
42. erythropoiesis
43. hematologist
44. immunology
45. basophilic *(bā-sō-FIL-ik)*
46. lymphocytic *(lim-fō-SIT-ik)*
47. hemorrhagic *(hem-ō-RAJ-ik)*
48. leukemic *(lū-KĒ-mik)*
49. hemolytic *(hē-mō-LIT-ik)*
50. allergies
51. petechiae *(pe-TĒ-kē-ē)*
52. ecchymoses *(ek-i-MŌ-sēz)*
53. sera *(SĒ-ra)*; also serums
54. Decrease in the number or size of red cells or in the amount of hemoglobin in the blood
    a. lack, absence
    b. blood
    c. condition of
55. Device used to count blood cells
    a. blood
    b. cell
    c. instrument for measuring
56. Presence in the blood of erythrocytes showing excessive variation in size
    a. not
    b. equal
    c. cell
    d. condition of
57. An increase in the red blood cells
    a. many
    b. cell
    c. blood
    d. condition of

Answers to Chapter Review 10-2

1. c
2. a
3. e
4. d
5. b
6. b
7. d
8. e
9. a
10. c
11. e
12. c
13. d
14. a
15. b
16. b
17. c
18. e

19. d
20. a
21. serum
22. agranulocytes
23. antigen
24. fibrinogen
25. neutrophils
26. clotting
27. bone marrow
28. iron
29. decrease in the number of neutrophils in the blood
30. deficiency of oxygen in the blood
31. tumor of bone marrow
32. increase in the number of granulocytes in the blood
33. an immature lymphocyte
34. presence of nitrogen compounds in the blood
35. leukoblast
36. thrombocytopoiesis; also thrombopoiesis, thrombogenesis
37. immunologist
38. autoimmunity
39. hemorrhage
40. antigen
41. fibrin
42. myeloid
43. platelet
44. heparin
45. Deficiency of all blood cells; aplastic anemia
    a. all
    b. cell
    c. deficiency of
46. Hereditary blood disease caused by a lack of a clotting factor and resulting in abnormal bleeding
    a. blood
    b. attract, absorb
    c. condition of
47. A local deficiency of blood supply due to obstruction of the circulation
    a. suppression
    b. blood
    c. condition of
48. Presence in the blood of erythrocytes showing abnormal variation in shape
    a. varied, irregular
    b. cell
    c. condition of
49. A disease of iron metabolism in which iron is deposited in the tissues
    a. blood
    b. color
    c. condition of

Answers to Case Study Questions

1. a
2. c
3. d
4. b
5. d
6. c
7. b
8. human immunodeficiency virus
9. deciliter
10. intravenous
11. every 6 hours
12. treatment by use of drugs
13. difficulty in breathing
14. tumor of lymphoid tissue
15. any disease of the lymph nodes
16. enlargement of the spleen

Answers to Crossword Puzzle

BLOOD AND IMMUNITY

	1 P		2 M				3 G	A	M	4 M	A
	L		Y		5 F					O	
	6 A	N	E	M	I	A		7 E		N	
8 P	T	■	L		B		9 C	R	Y	O	
10 H	E	M	O		R			Y			11 I
	L				I			T		12 A	G
	13 E	O	14 S	I	N	O	P	H	I	L	
15 B	T		T					R		B	
			A			16 P	R	O		17 U	N
18 P	L	A	S	M	A					M	
R			I			19 G	L	O	B	I	N
20 E	L	I	S	A						N	

11 Respiration

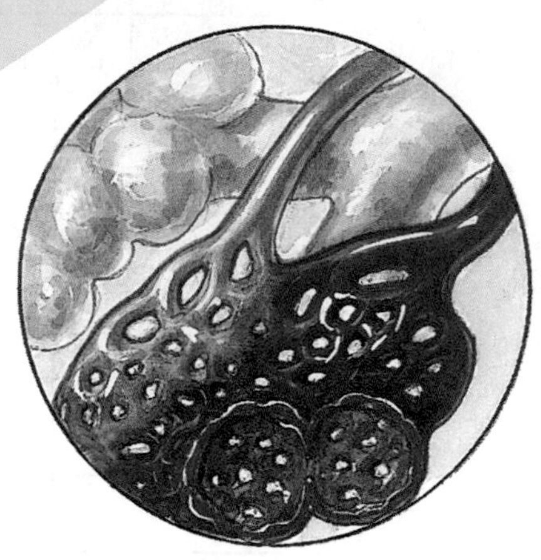

Chapter Contents

Objectives

After study of this chapter you should be able to:

1. Explain the roles of oxygen and carbon dioxide in the body and describe how each is carried in the blood
2. Label a diagram of the respiratory tract and briefly explain the function of each part
3. Describe the mechanism of breathing, including the roles of the diaphragm and phrenic nerve
4. Identify and use word parts pertaining to respiration
5. Discuss the major disorders of the respiratory tract
6. Define medical terms related to breathing and diseases of the respiratory tract
7. List and define eight volumes and capacities commonly used to measure pulmonary function
8. Interpret abbreviations commonly used in referring to respiration
9. Analyze case studies pertaining to diseases that affect respiration

The main function of the respiratory system is to provide **oxygen** to body cells for energy metabolism and to eliminate **carbon dioxide**, a by-product of metabolism. Because these gases must be carried to and from the cells in the blood, the respiratory system works closely with the cardiovascular system to accomplish gas exchange.

Exchange of gases between the atmosphere and the blood takes place in the **lungs**, two cone-shaped organs located in the thoracic cavity. A double membrane, the **pleura**, covers the lungs and the lines the thoracic cavity. The very thin, fluid-filled space between the two layers of the pleura is the **pleural space**.

Upper Respiratory Passageways

Air is carried to and from the lungs in a series of tubes in which no gas exchange occurs. Refer to Figure 11-1 as you read the following description of the respiratory tract. Air enters through the **nose** where it is warmed, filtered, and moistened as it passes over the hair-covered mucous membranes of the nasal cavity. Cilia, microscopic hairlike projections from the cells that line the nose, sweep dirt and foreign material toward the throat for elimination. Receptors for the sense of smell are located within bony side projections called **turbinate bones** or conchae.

Inhaled air passes into the throat, or **pharynx**, where it mixes with air that enters through the mouth and also with food destined for the digestive tract. The pharynx is divided into three regions: 1) an upper portion, the **nasopharynx**, behind the nasal cavity; 2) a middle portion, the **oropharynx**, behind the mouth; 3) a lower portion, the **laryngeal pharynx**, behind the larynx. The palatine tonsils are on either side of the soft palate in the oropharynx; the pharyngeal tonsils, or **adenoids**, are in the nasopharynx.

Lower Respiratory Passageways and Lungs

The pharynx conducts air into the **trachea**, a tube reinforced with C-shaped rings of cartilage to prevent its collapse (you can feel these rings if you press your fingers gently against the front of your throat). At the top of the trachea is the **larynx** containing the vocal cords. These mark the point of division between the upper and the lower respiratory tract. The larynx is shaped by nine cartilages, the most prominent of which is the thyroid cartilage at the front that forms the "Adam's apple." The opening between the vocal cords is the **glottis**. The small leaf-shaped cartilage at the top of the larynx is called the **epiglottis**. When one swallows, the epiglottis covers the opening of the larynx and helps to prevent food from entering the respiratory tract.

At its lower end, the trachea divides into two main stem **bronchi** that enter the lungs. The right bronchus is shorter and wider; it divides into three secondary bronchi that enter the three lobes of the right lung. The left divides into two branches that supply the two lobes of the left lung. Further divisions produce an increasing number of smaller tubes that supply air to smaller subdivisions of lung tissue. As the air passageways progress through the lungs, the cartilage in the walls gradually disappears and is replaced by smooth (involuntary) muscle.

The smallest of the conducting tubes, the **bronchioles**, carry air into the microscopic air sacs, the **alveoli**, through which gases are exchanged between the lungs and the blood. It is through the ultra-thin walls of the alveoli and the surrounding capillaries that oxygen diffuses into the blood and carbon dioxide diffuses out of the blood for elimination.

Breathing

Air is moved into and out of the lungs by the process of breathing, technically called **ventilation**. This consists of a steady cycle of **inspiration** (inhalation) and **expiration** (exhalation), separated by a period of rest. The cycle begins when the **phrenic nerve** stimulates the **diaphragm** to contract

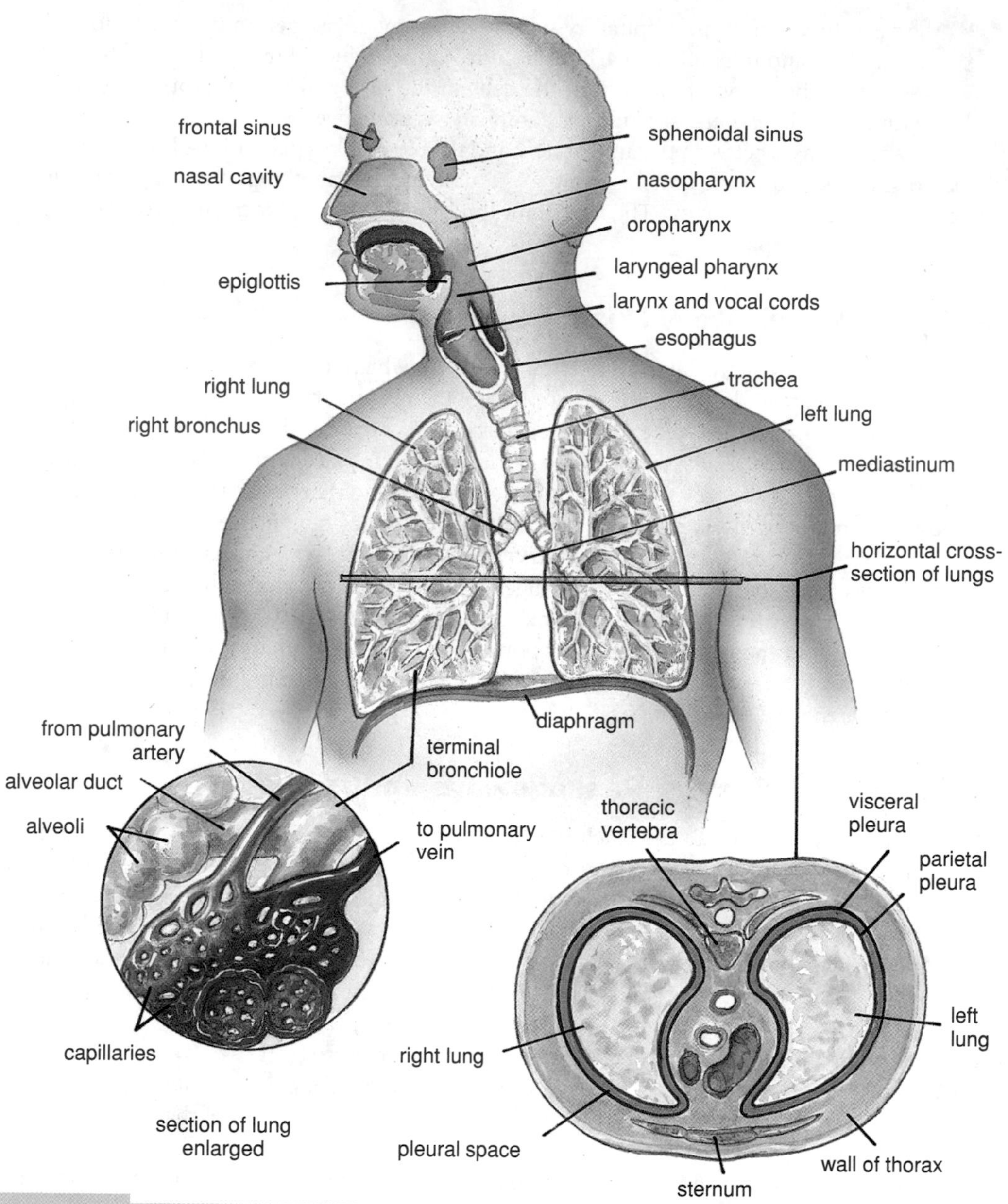

FIGURE 11-1. Respiratory system.

and flatten, thus enlarging the chest cavity. The resulting decrease in pressure within the thorax causes air to be pulled into the lungs. The intercostal muscles between the ribs also aid in inspiration by pulling the ribs up and out. The measure of how easily the lungs expand under pressure is **compliance**. Expiration occurs as the breathing muscles relax, the lungs spring back to their original size, and air is forced out.

Breathing is normally regulated unconsciously by centers in the brainstem. These centers adjust the rate and rhythm of breathing according to changes in the composition of the blood, especially the concentration of carbon dioxide.

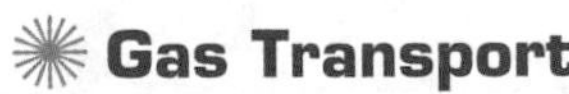

Gas Transport

Oxygen is carried in the blood bound to **hemoglobin** in red blood cells. The oxygen is released to the cells as needed. Carbon dioxide is carried in several ways, but is mostly converted to an acid called **carbonic acid**. The amount of carbon dioxide that is exhaled is important in regulating the acidity or alkalinity of the blood. If too much carbon dioxide is exhaled by **hyperventilation**, body fluids tend to become more alkaline, a condition termed **alkalosis**. If too little carbon dioxide is exhaled as a result of **hypoventilation**, body fluids tend to become more acid, a condition termed **acidosis**.

KEY TERMS: NORMAL STRUCTURE AND FUNCTION

Term	Definition
adenoids *(AD-e-noyds)*	Lymphoid tissue located in the nasopharynx; the pharyngeal tonsils
alveolus *(al-VĒ-ō-lus)*	A tiny air sac in the lungs through which gases are exchanged between the atmosphere and the blood in respiration (pl. alveoli)
bronchiole *(BRONG-kē-ōl)*	One of the smaller subdivisions of the bronchial tubes (root bronchiol)
bronchus *(BRONG-kus)*	One of the larger air passageways in the lungs. The bronchi begin as two branches of the trachea and then subdivide within the lungs (pl. bronchi) (root bronch)
carbon dioxide (CO_2)	A gas produced by energy metabolism in cells and eliminated through the lungs
compliance *(kom-PLĪ-ans)*	A measure of how easily the lungs expand under pressure. Compliance is reduced in many types of respiratory disorders.
diaphragm *(DĪ-a-fram)*	The dome-shaped muscle under the lungs that flattens during inspiration (root phren/o)
epiglottis *(ep-i-GLOT-is)*	A leaf-shaped cartilage that covers the larynx during swallowing to prevent food from entering the trachea
expiration *(ek-spi-RĀ-shun)*	The act of breathing out or expelling air from the lungs; exhalation
glottis *(GLOT-is)*	The opening between the vocal cords
inspiration *(in-spi-RĀ-shun)*	The act of drawing air into the lungs; inhalation
larynx *(LAR-inks)*	The enlarged upper end of the trachea that contains the vocal cords (root laryng/o)
lung	A cone-shaped spongy organ of respiration contained within the thorax (root pneum, pulm)
mediastinum *(mē-dē-as-TĪ-num)*	The space and organs between the lungs

(continued)

nose *(NŌZ)*	The organ of the face used for breathing and for housing receptors for the sense of smell. Includes an external portion and an internal nasal cavity (root nas/o, rhin/o)
oxygen (O_2) *(OK-si-jen)*	The gas needed by cells to release energy from food in metabolism
pharynx *(FAR-inks)*	The throat; a common passageway for food entering the esophagus and air entering the larynx (root pharyng/o)
phrenic nerve *(FREN-ik)*	The nerve that activates the diaphragm (root phrenic/o)
pleura *(PLŪR-a)*	A double-layered membrane that covers the lungs (visceral pleura and lines the thoracic cavity (parietal pleura) (root pleur/o)
pleural space	The thin, fluid-filled space between the two layers of the pleura; pleural cavity
sputum *(SPŪ-tum)*	The substance released by coughing or clearing the throat. It may contain a variety of material from the respiratory tract.
trachea *(TRĀ-kē-a)*	The air passageway that extends from the larynx to the bronchi (root trache/o)
turbinate bones	The bony projections in the nasal cavity that contain receptors for the sense of smell. Also called conchae (KON-kē).
ventilation	The movement of air into and out of the lungs

Word Parts Pertaining to Respiration

Suffixes for Respiration

Suffix	Meaning	Example	Definition of Example
-pnea	breathing	orthopnea *or-THOP-nē-a*	difficulty in breathing except in an upright (-ortho) position
-oxia	level of oxygen	anoxia *an-OK-sē-a*	absence of oxygen
-capnia	level of carbon dioxide	hypocapnia *hi-pō-KAP-nē-a*	decrease of carbon dioxide in the tissues
-phonia	voice	dysphonia *dis-FŌ-nē-a*	difficulty in speaking

Exercise 11-1

Using the suffix *-pnea* write a word that fits each of the following definitions:

1. Easy, normal (eu-) breathing ____eupnea____
2. Painful or difficult breathing ________
3. Lack of (a-) of breathing ________
4. Decreased (hypo-) depth and rate of breathing ________

Write the adjective form of each of the above words using the ending *-pneic*:

5. eupneic
6. ______
7. ______
8. ______

Using the suffixes in the previous chart, write a word that fits each of the following definitions:

9. Decreased amount of oxygen in the tissues ______
10. Increased carbon dioxide in the tissues ______
11. Normal levels (eu-) of carbon dioxide in the tissues ______
12. Lack of voice ______

Roots for the Respiratory Passageways

Root	Meaning	Example	Definition of Example
nas/o	nose	paranasal *par-a-NĀ-zal*	near the nose
rhin/o	nose	rhinitis *rī-NĪ-tis*	inflammation of the nasal passageways
pharyng/o	pharynx	pharyngeal* *fa-RIN-jē-al*	pertaining to the pharynx
laryng/o	larynx	laryngoscopy *lar-ing-GOS-kō-pē*	endoscopic examination of the larynx
trache/o	trachea	tracheotome *trā-kē-ō-TŌM*	instrument used to incise the trachea
bronch/o, bronch/i	bronchus	bronchiectasis *brong-kē-EK-ta-sis*	chronic dilatation of the bronchi
bronchiol	bronchiole	bronchiolitis *brong-kē-ō-LĪ-tis*	inflammation of the bronchioles

*Note addition of *e* before adjective ending *-al*.

Exercise 11-2

Write a word for each of the following definitions:

1. Discharge from the nose rhinorrhea
2. Inflammation of the pharynx ______
3. Inflammation of a bronchus ______
4. Endoscopic examination of the larynx ______

5. Endoscopic examination of a bronchus ____________
6. Plastic repair of the trachea ____________
7. Surgical removal of the larynx ____________
8. Surgical incision of the trachea ____________

Define the following terms. Note the adjective endings:

9. intranasal (*in-tra-NĀ-zal*) within the nose
10. laryngeal (*la-RIN-jē-al*) (note spelling) ____________
11. bronchiolar (*brong-KĒ-ō-lar*) ____________
12. peribronchial (*per-i-BRONG-kē-al*) ____________
13. laryngotracheal (*la-ring-gō-TRĀ-kē-al*) ____________
14. nasopharyngeal (*nā-zō-fa-RIN-jē-al*) ____________

Roots for the Lungs and Breathing

Root	Meaning	Example	Definition of Example
pleur/o	pleura	pleurocentesis *plūr-ō-sen-TĒ-sis*	surgical puncture of the pleural space
phren/o	diaphragm	phrenic *FREN-ik*	pertaining to the diaphragm
phrenic/o	phrenic nerve	phrenicectomy *fren-i-SEK-tō-mē*	surgical resection of the phrenic nerve
pneumon/o	lung	pneumonitis *nū-mō-NĪ-tis*	inflammation of the lung
pneum/o, pneumat/o	air, gas; also respiration, lung	pneumothorax *nū-mō-THOR-aks*	accumulation of air or gas in the pleural space
pulm/o, pulmon/o	lungs	subpulmonary *sub-PUL-mō-ner-ē*	below the lungs
spir/o	breathing	spirogram *SPĪ-rō-gram*	record of breathing movements

Exercise 11-3

Define the following words:

1. pleuropulmonary (*plūr-ō-PUL-mō-ner-ē*) ____________
2. pleuralgia (*plū-RAL-jē-a*) ____________
3. pulmonology (*pul-mō-NOL-ō-jē*) ____________
4. pneumonopathy (*nū-mō-NOP-a-thē*) ____________

Write a word for each of the following definitions:

5. Within (intra-) the pleura ________________
6. Below the diaphragm ________________
7. Surgical incision of the phrenic nerve ________________
8. Surgical removal of the lung or lung tissue ________________
9. Instrument (-meter) for measuring breathing movements ________________

Clinical Aspects of Respiration

Pulmonary function is affected by conditions that cause resistance to air flow through the respiratory tract or that limit expansion of the chest. These may be conditions that affect the respiratory system directly, such as infection, injury, allergy, **aspiration** (inhalation) of foreign bodies, or cancer. They also may be conditions that result from disturbances in other systems, such as in the skeletal, muscular, cardiovascular, or nervous systems.

Infections

Influenza is a viral disease of the respiratory tract. Different strains of the influenza virus have caused serious epidemics throughout history.

Pneumonia is caused by several different microorganisms, most commonly bacteria and viruses. Bronchopneumonia (bronchial pneumonia) begins in terminal bronchioles, which become clogged with exudate and form consolidated (solidified) patches. Lobar pneumonia is an acute infectious disease caused by *Streptococcus pneumoniae* and involves one or more lobes of the lung. The term *pneumonia* is applied as well to inflammation of the lungs due to non-infectious causes, such as asthma, allergy, or inhalation of irritants. In these cases, however, the more general term *pneumonitis* is often used.

Tuberculosis (TB) has increased in recent years along with the rise of AIDS and the appearance of resistance to antibiotics in the organism that causes the disease, *M. tuberculosis* (MTB). (This organism, because of its staining properties, also is referred to as AFB meaning *acid-fast bacillus*.) The name tuberculosis comes from the small lesions, or tubercles, that appear with the infection. The symptoms of TB include fever, weight loss, weakness, cough, and as a result of damage to blood vessels in the lungs, **hemoptysis**, the coughing up of sputum containing blood. Accumulation of exudate in the alveoli may result in consolidation of lung tissue. The **tuberculin test** is used to test for tuberculosis infection. PPD (purified protein derivative) is the form of tuberculin commonly used.

Emphysema

Emphysema is a chronic disease associated with overexpansion and destruction of the alveoli. Common causes are exposure to cigarette smoke and other forms of pollution as well as chronic infection. Emphysema is the main disorder included under the heading of **chronic obstructive pulmonary disease** (COPD). (Also COLD, chronic obstructuve lung disease.) Other conditions included in this category are **asthma**, chronic **bronchitis**, and **bronchiectasis** (chronic dilation of the bronchi).

Asthma

Attacks of asthma result from narrowing of the bronchial tubes. This constriction, along with edema (swelling) of the bronchial linings and accumulation of mucus results in wheezing, extreme

dyspnea (difficulty in breathing), and **cyanosis**. Although the causes of asthma are uncertain, a main factor is irritation caused by allergy. Treatment of asthma includes removal of allergens, administration of **bronchodilators** to widen the airways, and administration of steroids.

Pneumoconiosis

Chronic irritation and inflammation caused by inhalation of dust particles is termed **pneumoconiosis**. This is an occupational hazard seen mainly in mining and stoneworking industries. Different forms are named for the specific type of dust inhaled: silicosis (silica or quartz), anthracosis (coal dust), asbestosis (asbestos fibers).

Pneumothorax

As a result of injury, infection, or weakness in the pleural membrane, substances may accumulate between the layers of the pleura. When air or gas collects in this space, the condition is termed **pneumothorax** (Fig. 11-2). Compression may result in collapse of the lung, termed **atelectasis**. Other substances that may accumulate in the pleural space include pus (pyothorax or empyema), blood (hemothorax), and fluid (hydrothorax).

Lung Cancer

Lung cancer is the leading cause of cancer-related deaths in both men and women. The incidence of this form of cancer has increased steadily over the past 50 years, especially in females. Cigarette smoking is a major risk factor in this as well as other forms of cancer. The most common form of lung cancer is squamous carcinoma, originating in the lining of the bronchi (bronchogenic). Lung cancer usually cannot be detected early and it metastasizes rapidly. The overall survival rate is low.

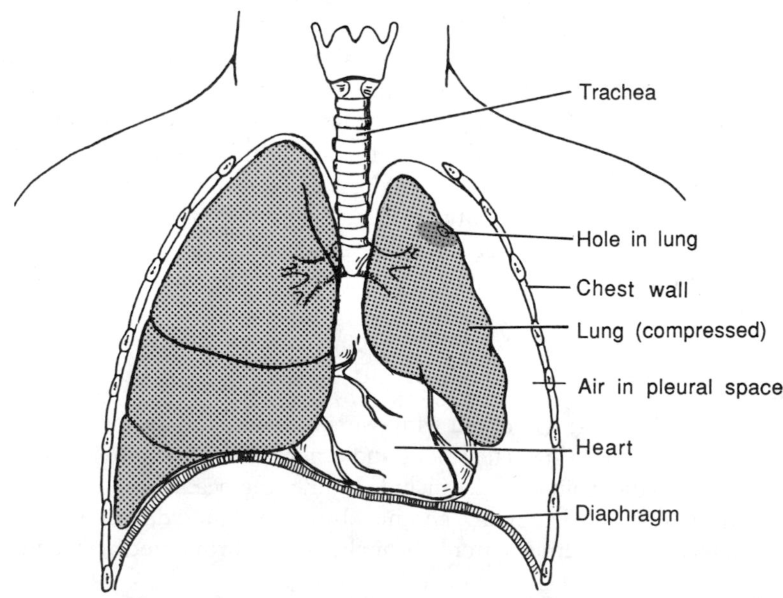

FIGURE 11-2. Pneumothorax. Injury to lung tissue allows air to leak into the pleural space and put pressure on the lung. (Jones SA, Weigel A, White RD, McSwain NE Jr, Breiter M: Advanced Emergency Care for Paramedic Practice, p 331. Philadelphia: JB Lippincott, 1992.)

Methods used to diagnose lung cancer include x-ray studies, CT scans, and examination of sputum for cancer cells. A bronchoscope can be used to examine the airways and to collect tissue samples for study. Surgical or needle biopsies may also be taken.

KEY CLINICAL TERMS

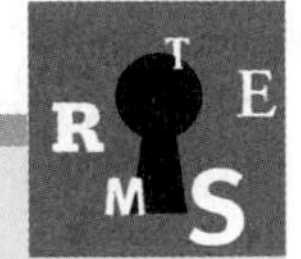

acidosis *(as-i-DŌ-sis)*	Abnormal acidity of body fluids. Respiratory acidosis is caused by abnormally high levels of carbon dioxide in the body.
alkalosis *(al-ka-LŌ-sis)*	Abnormal alkalinity of body fluids. Respiratory alkalosis is caused by abnormally low levels of carbon dioxide in the body.
aspiration *(as-pi-RĀ-shun)*	The withdrawing of fluid from a cavity by suction; the accidental inhalation of food or other foreign material into the lungs
asthma *(AZ-ma)*	A disease characterized by dyspnea and wheezing caused by spasm of the bronchial tubes or swelling of their mucous membranes
atelectasis *(at-e-LEK-ta-sis)*	Incomplete expansion of a lung or part of a lung; lung collapse. May be present at birth or be caused by obstruction or compression of lung tissue (prefix *atel/o* means "imperfect")
bronchiectasis *(brong-kē-EK-ta-sis)*	Chronic dilatation of a bronchus or bronchi
bronchitis *(brong-KĪ-tis)*	Inflammation of the bronchi
cyanosis *(sī-a-NŌ-sis)*	Bluish discoloration of the skin due to lack of oxygen in the blood (adj. cyanotic)
dyspnea *(dysp-NĒ-a)*	Difficult or labored breathing, sometimes with pain; "air hunger"
emphysema *(em-fi-SĒ-ma)*	A chronic pulmonary disease characterized by enlargement and destruction of the alveoli
hemoptysis *(hē-MOP-ti-sis)*	The spitting of blood from the mouth or respiratory tract (*ptysis* means "spitting")
hyperventilation	Increased rate and depth of breathing; increase in the amount of air entering the alveoli
hypoventilation	Decreased rate and depth of breathing; decrease in the amount of air entering the alveoli
influenza *(in-flū-EN-za)*	An acute, contagious respiratory infection causing fever, chills, headache, and muscle pain
pleurisy *(PLŪR-i-sē)*	Inflammation of the pleura; pleuritis. A symptom of pleuritis is sharp pain on inhalation.
pneumoconiosis *(nū-mō-kō-nē-Ō-sis)*	Disease of the respiratory tract caused by inhalation of dust particles. Named more specifically by the type of dust inhaled, such as silicosis, anthracosis, asbestosis

(continued)

pneumonia
(nū-MŌ-nē-a)
Inflammation of the lungs generally caused by infection. May involve the bronchioles and alveoli (bronchopneumonia) or one or more lobes of the lung (lobar pneumonia)

pneumonitis
(nū-mō-NĪ-tis)
Inflammation of the lungs; may follow infection or be caused by asthma, allergy, or inhalation of irritants

pneumothorax
(nū-mō-THOR-aks)
Accumulation of air or gas in the pleural space. May result from injury or disease or may be produced artificially to collapse a lung.

tuberculosis
(tū-ber-kū-LŌ-sis)
An infectious disease caused by the tubercle bacillus, *Mycobacterium tuberculosis*. Often involves the lungs but may involve other parts of the body as well.

ADDITIONAL TERMS

Normal Structure and Function

expectoration
(ek-spek-to-RĀ-shun)
The act of coughing up material from the respiratory tract. Also the material thus released; sputum.

hilum
(HĪ-lum)
A depression in an organ where vessels and nerves enter. Also called hilus.

nares
(NĀ-rēz)
The external openings of the nose; the nostrils (s. naris)

nasal septum
The partition that divides the nasal cavity into two parts (root *sept/o* means "septum")

sinus
A cavity or channel. The paranasal sinuses are air-filled cavities in the bones of the face and skull that drain into the nasal cavity. They are named for the bones in which they are located, such as the sphenoid, ethmoid, and maxillary sinuses.

surfactant
(sur-FAK-tant)
A substance that decreases surface tension within the alveoli and eases expansion of the lungs

Symptoms and Conditions

anoxia
(an-OK-sē-a)
Lack or absence of oxygen in the tissues. Often used incorrectly to mean hypoxia.

apnea
(AP-nē-a)
Cessation of breathing

asphyxia
(as-FIK-sē-a)
Condition caused by inadequate intake of oxygen; suffocation (literally "lack of pulse")

bronchospasm
(BRONG-kō-spazm)
Narrowing of the bronchi due to spasm of the smooth muscle in their walls. Common in cases of asthma and bronchitis.

Cheyne-Stokes respiration
(chān-stokes)
A repeating cycle of gradually increased then decreased respiration followed by a period of apnea. Due to depression of the breathing centers of the nervous system.

cor pulmonale *(kor pul-mō-NĀ-lē)*	Enlargement of the right ventricle of the heart due to disease of the lungs or their blood vessels
coryza *(kō-RĪ-za)*	Acute inflammation of the nasal passages with profuse nasal discharge
croup *(krūp)*	A childhood disease characterized by a barking cough, difficult breathing, and laryngeal spasm
deviated septum	A shifted nasal septum; may require surgical correction
empyema *(em-pī-Ē-ma)*	Accumulation of pus in a body cavity, especially the pleural space; pyothorax
epistaxis *(ep-i-STAK-sis)*	Hemorrhage from the nose; nosebleed (G. *-staxis* means "dripping")
fremitus *(FREM-i-tus)*	A vibration, especially as felt through the chest wall on palpation
hemothorax *(hē-mō-THOR-aks)*	Presence of blood in the pleural space
hypercapnemia *(hī-per-cap-NĒ-mē-a)*	Excess carbon dioxide in the blood
hyperpnea *(hī-PERP-nē-a)*	An increase in the rate and depth of breathing that may occur normally, as after exercise
hypoxia *(hī-POK-sē-a)*	Insufficient oxygen in the tissues
Kussmaul breathing *(KOOS-mawl)*	Rapid and deep gasping respiration without pause; characteristic of severe acidosis
pleural effusion	Accumulation of fluid in the pleural space. The fluid may contain blood (hemothorax) or pus (pyothorax).
pleural friction rub	A sound heard on auscultation produced by the rubbing together of the two layers of the pleura. A common sign of pleurisy.
rale *(rāl)*	Abnormal chest sounds heard when air enters small airways or alveoli containing fluid. Usually heard during inspiration (pl. rales)
rhonchi *(RONG-kī)*	Abnormal chest sounds produced in airways with accumulated fluids. More noticeable during expiration (s. rhonchus).
stridor *(STRĪ-dor)*	A harsh, high-pitched sound caused by obstruction of an upper air passageway
tachypnea *(tak-IP-nē-a)*	Abnormal increase in the rate of respiration
tussis *(TUS-is)*	A cough. An antitussive drug is one that relieves or prevents coughing.
wheeze	A whistling or sighing sound caused by narrowing of a respiratory passageway

(continued)

Disorders

adult respiratory distress syndrome (ARDS)
A serious pulmonary complication that follows trauma or severe infection in young and previously healthy individuals. There is respiratory failure with hypoxemia and radiographic opacity ("white out") in both lungs. Also called shock lung.

cystic fibrosis (CF) *(SIS-tik fi-BRŌ-sis)*
An inherited disease that affects the pancreas, respiratory system, and sweat glands. Thick mucus accumulates in the bronchi causing obstruction and leading to infection. CF is diagnosed by the increased amounts of sodium and chloride in the sweat. Treatment includes postural drainage, use of aerosol mists, bronchodilators, antibiotics, and mucolytic agents that dissolve mucus.

miliary tuberculosis *(MIL-ē-ar-ē)*
Acute generalized form of tuberculosis with formation of minute tubercles that resemble millet seeds

pertussis *(per-TUS-is)*
An acute, infectious disease characterized by a cough ending in a whooping inspiration; whooping cough.

respiratory distress syndrome (RDS) **of the newborn**
A respiratory condition of unknown cause seen most often in premature newborns; involves a lack of surfactant in the alveoli that reduces compliance. Surfactants are now available to treat this disease. It was originally called hyaline membrane disease because of the material that collects within the lungs.

small-cell carcinoma
A highly malignant type of bronchial tumor involving small, undifferentiated cells; "oat cell" carcinoma

sudden infant death syndrome (SIDS)
The sudden and unexplained death of an apparently healthy infant; crib death

Diagnosis

arterial blood gases (ABGs)
The concentrations of gases, specifically oxygen and carbon dioxide, in arterial blood. Reported as the partial pressure (P) of the gas in arterial (A) blood, such as PAO_2 or $PACO_2$. These measurements are important in measuring acid–base balance.

bronchoscope *(BRONG-kō-skōp)*
An endoscope used to examine the tracheobronchial passageways. Also allows access for biopsy of tissue to removal of a foreign object (see Figure 7–3).

forced expiratory volume (FEV)
Volume of gas exhaled with maximum force within a given interval of time. The time interval is shown as a subscript, such as FEV_1 (1 second), FEV_3 (3 seconds).

forced vital capacity (FVC)
The volume of gas exhaled as rapidly and completely as possible after a complete inhalation

lung scan
Study based on the accumulation of radioactive isotope in lung tissue. A *ventilation scan* measures ventilation following inhalation of radioactive material. A *perfusion scan* measures blood supply to the lungs following injection of radioactive material. Also called a pulmonary scintiscan.

Mantoux test *(man-TOO)*
A test for tuberculosis, in which PPD (tuberculin) is injected into the skin. The test does not differentiate active from inactive cases.

pulse oximetry *(ok-SIM-e-trē)* — Determination of the oxygen saturation of arterial blood by means of a photoelectric apparatus (oximeter), usually placed on a thin part of the body such as the ear or the finger; reported as SpO_2

plethysmograph *(ple-THIZ-mō-graf)* — An instrument that measures changes in gas volume and pressure during respiration

pneumotachometer *(nū-mō-tak-OM-e-ter)* — A device for measuring air flow

pulmonary function tests — Tests done to assess breathing, usually by spirometry. The main volumes and capacities measured in these tests are given in Table 11-1.

TABLE 11-1 Volumes and Capacities (Sums of Volumes) Used in Pulmonary Function Tests

Volume or Capacity	Definition
tidal volume (TV)	amount of air breathed into or out of the lungs in quiet, relaxed breathing
residual volume (RV)	amount of air that remains in the lungs after maximum exhalation
expiratory reserve volume (ERV)	amount of air that can be exhaled after a normal exhalation
inspiratory reserve volume (IRV)	amount of air that can be inhaled above a normal inspiration
total lung capacity (TLC)	total amount of air that can be contained in the lungs after maximum inhalation
inspiratory capacity (IC)	amount of air that can be inhaled after normal exhalation
vital capacity (VC)	amount of air that can be expelled from the lungs by maximum exhalation following maximum inhalation
functional residual capacity (FRC)	amount of air remaining in the lungs after normal exhalation

spirometer — An apparatus used to measure breathing volumes and capacities; record of test is a spirogram

tine test — A test for tuberculosis in which PPD (tuberculin) is introduced into the skin with a multi-pronged device. The test does not differentiate active from inactive cases.

Treatment

aerosol therapy — Treatment by inhalation of a drug or water in spray form

continuous positive airway pressure (CPAP) — Use of a mechanical respirator to maintain pressure throughout the respiratory cycle in a patient who is breathing spontaneously

extubation — Removal of a previously inserted tube

intermittent positive pressure breathing (IPPB) — Use of a ventilator to inflate the lungs at intervals under positive pressure during inhalation

(continued)

intermittent positive pressure ventilation (IPPV) — Use of a mechanical ventilator to force air into the lungs while allowing for passive exhalation

intubation *(in-tū-BĀ-shun)* — Insertion of a tube into a hollow organ, such as into the larynx or trachea for entrance of air (Fig. 11-3)

nasal cannula *(KAN-ū-la)* — A two-pronged plastic device inserted into the nostrils for delivery of oxygen (Fig. 11-4)

orthopneic position *(or-thop-NĒ-ik)* — An upright or semi-upright position that aids breathing

positive end-expiratory pressure (PEEP) — Use of a mechanical ventilator to increase the volume of gas in the lungs at the end of exhalation, thus improving gas exchange

thoracic gas volume (TGV, V_{TG}) — The volume of gas in the thoracic cavity calculated from measurements made with a body plethysmograph

Surgery

adenoidectomy *(ad-e-noyd-EK-tō-mē)* — Surgical removal of the adenoids

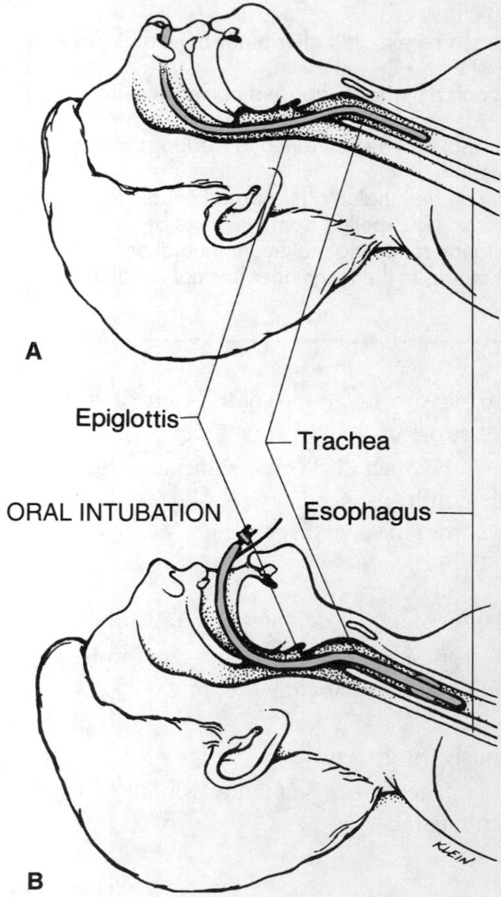

FIGURE 11-3. Intubation. An endotracheal tube is inserted **(A)** through the nose (intranasal intubation) or **(B)** through the mouth (oral intubation). (Smeltzer SC, Bare BG: Brunner and Suddarth's Textbook of Medical-Surgical Nursing, 7th ed, p 425. Philadelphia: JB Lippincott, 1992.)

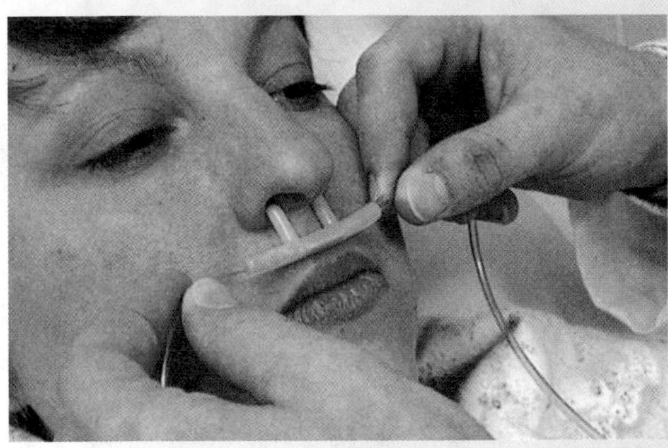

FIGURE 11-4. A nasal cannula. (Taylor C, Lillis CA, LeMone P: Fundamentals of Nursing, 2nd ed, p 921. Philadelphia: JB Lippincott, 1993.)

lobectomy
(lō-BEK-tō-mē)
Surgical removal of a lobe of the lung or of another organ

thoracentesis
(thor-a-sen-TĒ-sis)
Surgical puncture of the chest for removal of air or fluids, such as may accumulate following surgery. Also called thoracocentesis (Fig. 11-5).

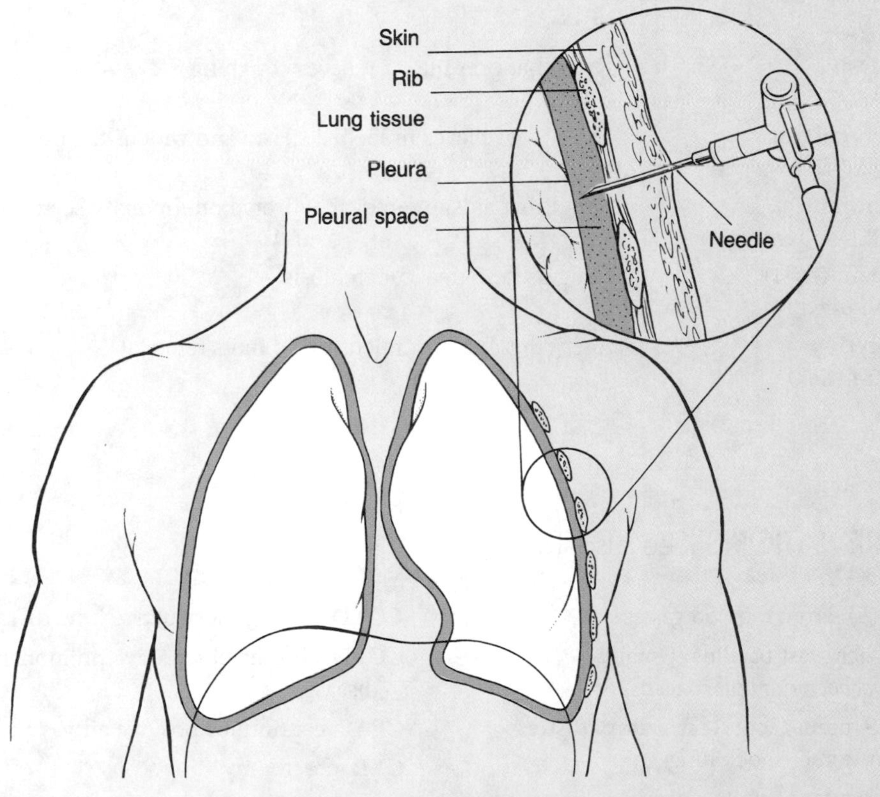

FIGURE 11-5. Thoracentesis. A needle is inserted into the pleural space.

(continued)

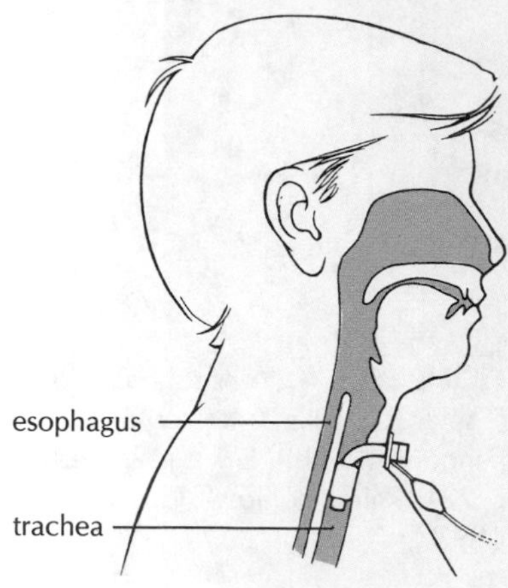

FIGURE 11-6. A tracheostomy tube. (Smeltzer SC, Bare BG: Brunner and Suddarth's Textbook of Medical-Surgical Nursing, 7th ed, p 533. Philadelphia: JB Lippincott, 1992.)

tracheotomy Incision of the trachea through the neck, usually to establish an airway in cases of tracheal obstruction

tracheostomy Surgical creation of an opening into the trachea to form an airway or to prepare for the insertion of a tube for ventilation (Fig. 11-6). Also the opening thus created.

Drugs

antitussive *(an-ti-TUS-iv)* Drug that prevents or relieves coughing

bronchodilator *(brong-kō-DĪ-lā-tor)* Drug that relieves bronchial spasm and widens the bronchi

expectorant *(ek-SPEK-tō-rant)* Agent that aids in removal of bronchopulmonary secretions

isoniazid (INH) *(ī-sō-NĪ-a-zid)* Drug used to treat tuberculosis

mucolytic *(mū-kō-LIT-ik)* Agent that loosens mucus to aid in its removal

ABBREVIATIONS (See also Table 11-1)

ABG(s) arterial blood gas(es)

AFB acid-fast bacillus (Usually *Mycobacterium tuberculosis)*

ARDS adult (acute) respiratory distress syndrome; shock lung

ARF acute respiratory failure

C compliance

CO_2 carbon dioxide

COLD chronic obstructive lung disease

COPD chronic obstructive pulmonary disease

CPAP continuous positive airway pressure

CXR chest x-ray

FEV forced expiratory volume

FVC forced vital capacity

INH isoniazid

IPPB intermittent positive pressure breathing

IPPV intermittent positive pressure ventilation

LLL left lower lobe (of lung)

LUL left upper lobe (of lung)

MEFR maximal expiratory flow rate

MMFR maximum midexpiratory flow rate

O_2 oxygen

$PACO_2$ arterial partial pressure of carbon dioxide

PAO_2 arterial partial pressure of oxygen

PCP *Pneumocystis carinii* pneumonia

PEEP positive end-expiratory pressure

PEFR peak expiratory flow rate

PFT pulmonary function test(s)

PIP peak inspiratory pressure

PPD purified protein derivative (tuberculin)

R respiration

RDS respiratory distress syndrome

RLL right lower lobe (of lung)

RML right middle lobe (of lung)

RUL right upper lobe (of lung)

SIDS sudden infant death syndrome

SpO_2 oxygen percent saturation

TB tuberculosis

T & A tonsils and adenoids; tonsillectomy and adenoidectomy

TGV thoracic gas volume

URI upper respiratory infection

V_{TG} thoracic gas volume

CHAPTER REVIEW 11-1

Matching. Match the words in each of the sets below with their definitions and write the appropriate letter (a–e) to the left of each number:

_____ 1. aspiration — a. rapid rate of respiration
_____ 2. tachypnea — b. accidental inhalation of foreign material
_____ 3. rale — c. cessation of breathing
_____ 4. septum — d. abnormal chest sound
_____ 5. apnea — e. partition

_____ 6. surfactant — a. nosebleed
_____ 7. asphyxia — b. a measure of how easily the lungs expand
_____ 8. compliance — c. incomplete expansion of lung tissue
_____ 9. atelectasis — d. substance that reduces surface tension
_____ 10. epistaxis — e. suffocation

_____ 11. concha — a. nostril
_____ 12. glottis — b. turbinate bone
_____ 13. hilum — c. space and organs between the lungs
_____ 14. mediastinum — d. depression in an organ where vessels enter
_____ 15. naris — e. opening between the vocal cords

Chapter 11
Labeling Exercise

Write the name of each numbered part on the corresponding line of the answer sheet.

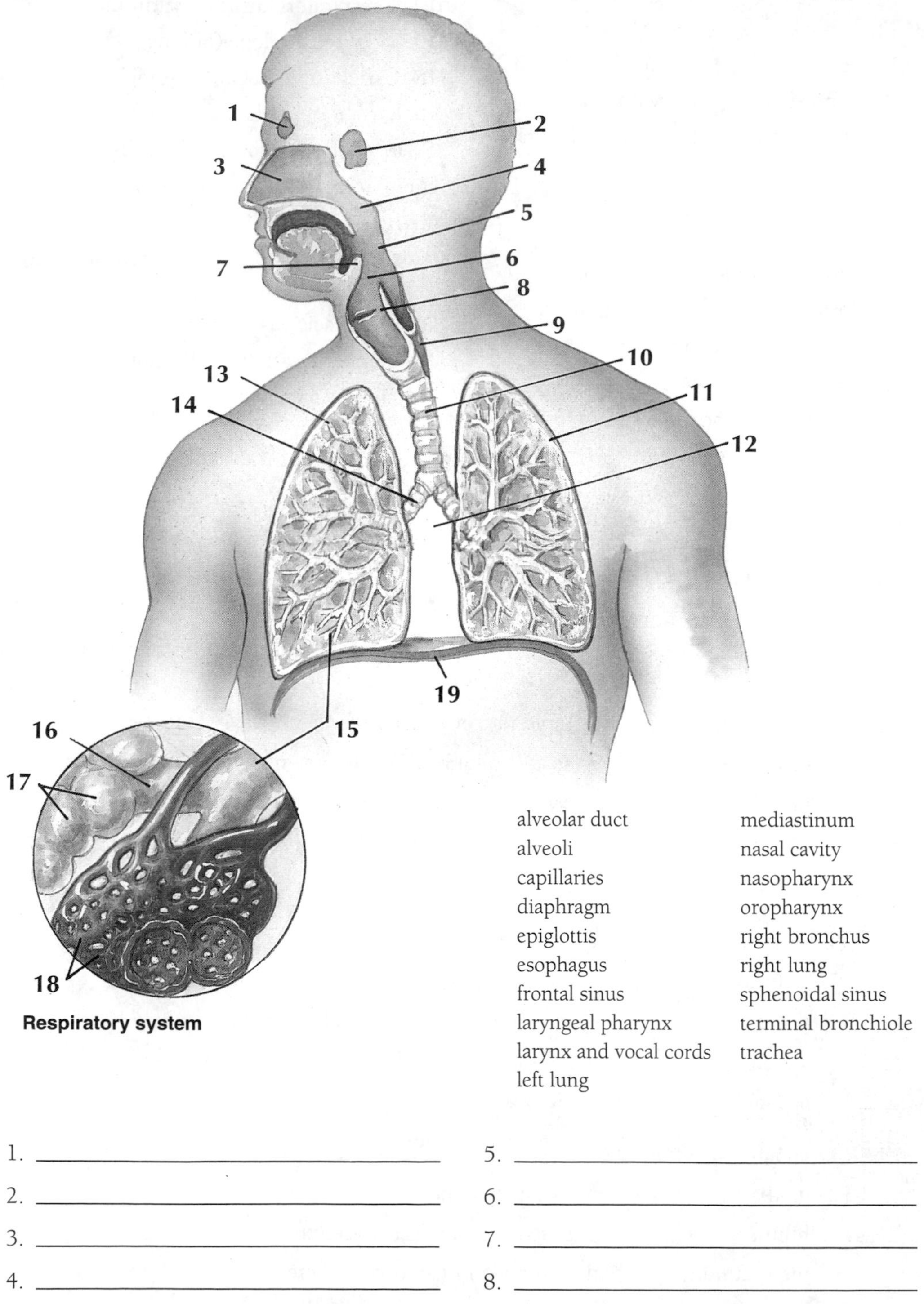

Respiratory system

alveolar duct	mediastinum
alveoli	nasal cavity
capillaries	nasopharynx
diaphragm	oropharynx
epiglottis	right bronchus
esophagus	right lung
frontal sinus	sphenoidal sinus
laryngeal pharynx	terminal bronchiole
larynx and vocal cords	trachea
left lung	

1. ______________________
2. ______________________
3. ______________________
4. ______________________
5. ______________________
6. ______________________
7. ______________________
8. ______________________

9. ______________________
10. ______________________
11. ______________________
12. ______________________
13. ______________________
14. ______________________
15. ______________________
16. ______________________
17. ______________________
18. ______________________
19. ______________________

Fill in the blanks:

16. The dome-shaped muscle under the lungs that flattens during inspiration is the ______________.
17. The turbinate bones contain receptors for the sense of ______________.
18. The double membrane that covers the lungs and lines the thoracic cavity is the ______________.
19. The pigment that carries oxygen in red blood cells is ______________.
20. The adjective *hypoxic* refers to a deficiency of ______________.
21. The scientific name for the throat is the ______________.
22. A small air sac in the lung through which gases are exchanged between the atmosphere and the blood is a(n) ______________.
23. Pneumococci are round bacteria (cocci) so named because they infect the ______________.
24. The amount of air moved into or out of the lungs in quiet breathing is the ______________.
25. The tonsils located in the nasopharyx are commonly called ______________.
26. Phrenicotripsy (*fren-i-kō-TRIP-sē*) is crushing of the ______________.
27. A mucolytic agent dissolves ______________.

Word building. Write a word for each of the following definitions:

28. Binding or fusion (-desis) of the pleurae ______________
29. Incision into the trachea ______________
30. Inflammation of the throat ______________
31. Surgical removal of the larynx ______________
32. Inflammation of the bronchioles ______________
33. Spasm of a bronchus ______________

The word *thorax* (chest) is used as an ending in compound words that mean the accumulation of substances in the pleural space. Define the following terms:

34. pneumothorax ______accumulation of air or gas in the pleural space______
35. hemothorax ______________________
36. pyothorax ______________________
37. hydrothorax ______________________

Definitions. Write the meaning of each of the following words:

38. adenoidectomy ______________________
39. bradypnea *(brad-IP-nē-a)* ______________________
40. endotracheal ______________________
41. pneumonitis ______________________
42. bronchostenosis ______________________
43. pleuralgia ______________________
44. subphrenic ______________________

Identify and define the root in each of the following words:

	Root	Meaning of Root
45. respiration	________	________
46. intrapulmonary	________	________
47. empyema	________	________
48. phrenodynia	________	________
49. apneumia	________	________

Plurals. Write the plural form of each of the following words:

50. naris ______________________
51. bronchiole ______________________
52. alveolus ______________________
53. concha ______________________
54. bronchus ______________________

Word analysis. Define each of the following words and then give the meaning of the words parts of each. Use a dictionary if necessary.

55. Thoracentesis ______________________

____

a. thorac/o ______________________

b. -centesis ______________________

56. Hemoptysis ____

____

a. hem/o ____________________

b. ptysis ____________________

57. Pharyngoxerosis ____

____

a. pharyng/o ____________________

b. xer/o ____________________

c. -osis ____________________

CHAPTER REVIEW 11-2

Matching. Match the words in each of the sets below with their definitions and write the appropriate letter (a–e) to the left of each number.

_____ 1. sinus — a. profuse nasal discharge
_____ 2. expectoration — b. behind the nose
_____ 3. paranasal — c. a cavity or channel
_____ 4. postnasal — d. sputum
_____ 5. rhinorrhea — e. near the nose

_____ 6. coryza — a. cough
_____ 7. fremitus — b. pus in the pleural space
_____ 8. empyema — c. inflammation of the nose with profuse discharge
_____ 9. tussis — d. bluish discoloration
_____ 10. cyanosis — e. vibration

_____ 11. COPD — a. breathing measurement
_____ 12. ARDS — b. chronic lung disease
_____ 13. FVC — c. infection of the upper air passages
_____ 14. URI — d. shock lung
_____ 15. RLL — e. lobe of the lung

Fill in the blanks:

16. The nerve that activates the diaphragm is the ____________________.

17. The term *acid-fast bacillus* (AFB) is commonly applied to the organism that causes ____________________.

18. The scientific name for nosebleed is ______________________.
19. A person suffering from orthopnea can breathe comfortably only in a(n) ______________________ postion.
20. The adjective *hypocapnic* refers to a deficiency of ______________________.
21. The trachea divides into a right and left ______________________.
22. The amount of air that can be expelled from the lungs by maximum exhalation following maximum inhalation is the ______________________.
23. The vocal cords are located in the ______________________.
24. Pleuropneumonia is inflammation of the pleura and the ______________________.
25. The portion of the pharynx that is behind the mouth is the ______________________.
26. Sleep apnea is a sudden lack of ______________________ during sleep.
27. A bronchodilator is a drug that causes the bronchi to ______________________.

Word building. Write a word for each of the following definitions:

28. Surgical creation of an opening in the trachea ______________________
29. Originating in a bronchus ______________________
30. An instrument for examining a bronchus is a(n) ______________________
31. Hernia of the pleura ______________________
32. Incision of the phrenic nerve ______________________

Definitions. Write the meaning of each of the following terms:

33. bronchiectasis ______________________
34. laryngocentesis ______________________
35. spirometry ______________________
36. pulmonology ______________________
37. bronchorrhea ______________________
38. pneumonopathy ______________________
39. rhinoplasty ______________________

Opposites. Write a word that means the opposite of each of the following:

40. hypocapnia ______________________
41. inspiration ______________________
42. bradypnea ______________________
43. hypoxia ______________________
44. extubation ______________________
45. hyperpnea ______________________

Adjectives. Write the adjective form of each of the following words:

46. alveolus ______________________
47. pharynx ______________________
48. pleura ______________________
49. nose ______________________
50. trachea ______________________
51. bronchus ______________________

Unscrambles. Form a word from each of the following groups of letters and write it in the blank:

52. sndeioad ______________________
53. nrayxl ______________________
54. ypendas ______________________
55. tipaesixs ______________________
56. uporc ______________________
57. smtaha ______________________

Word analysis. Define each of the following words and give the meaning of the word parts in each. Use a dictionary if necessary.

58. Atelectasis ______________________

____

    a. atel/o- ______________________

    b. -ectasis ______________________

59. Epiglottis ______________________

____

    a. epi- ______________________

    b. glottis ______________________

Chapter 11

Case Studies

1. AIDS-Related *Pneumocytsis carinii* Pneumonia (PCP)

Mr. S. is a 29-year-old homosexual male. For the last 4–6 weeks he has experienced shortness of breath and a nonproductive cough. He finally presented to his family physician and was referred to this hospital for further evaluation. Arterial blood gas (ABG) revealed hypoxemia with a PO_2 of 60. A chest x-ray showed a mixed interstial and alveolar pattern. Bronchial lavage was performed and was positive for *Pneumocystis carinii*. He was treated with Trimethoprim-Sulfamethoxazole but developed a rash and fever. He was therefore switched to pentamidine. He was treated for 4 weeks with relief of his symptoms.

2. Chronic Obstructive Pulmonary Disease (COPD)

This is a 50-year-old male with a long history of COPD. He has had multiple admissions to this hospital for CHF, atherosclerotic heart disease, and hypertension. Four days ago he began to experience shortness of breath and general discomfort. At the time of admission he was in acute respiratory distress. Vital signs: BP 160/90, pulse 104, respiratory rate: 21 and labored, breath sounds: audible wheezing with prolonged expiratory phase. ABGs: pH 7.28, P_{CO_2} 62, P_{O_2} 40, HCO_3 21.

Treatment consisted of oxygen, Keflex IV, and IPPB with the bronchodilator Alupent 0.3 mL qid. Subsequent improvement led to discharge after 2 days on his standard regimen of medication with additional antibiotic therapy.

3. Giant Cell Sarcoma of the Left Lung

The patient is a 65-year-old male with a history of primary giant cell sarcoma in the left lung. Resection was done 3 months prior to admission. At this time he presented with pain, dyspnea, and diaphoresis. Social history was negative for alcohol use. He had smoked 1 1/2 packs a day for 40 years, but had stopped 3 months ago.

Physical examination was unremarkable except for a thoracotomy scar in the left hemithorax, decreased breath sounds, and dullness to percussion of the left base. There was no hemoptysis. Radionuclide bone scan showed increased activity in the left upper posterior hemithorax. Chest and upper abdomen CT scan showed findings compatible with recurrent sarcoma of the left hemithorax. Abnormal mediastinal nodes were evident. Thoracentesis was attempted, but did not yield fluid. Patient will be seen by Dr. ____________________ for possible radiation therapy or chemotherapy as an outpatient.

Chapter 11
Case Study Questions

Multiple choice. Select the best answer and write the letter of your choice to the left of each number.

_____ 1. Bronchial lavage is

a. washing of the bronchi
b. inflation of the bronchi
c. constriction of the bronchioles
d. coughing
e. inhalation of an aerosol

_____ 2. Hemoptysis is

a. anemia
b. hemorrhage
c. leukemia
d. spitting blood
e. discoloration of the skin

_____ 3. Mediastinal nodes are

a. lymph nodes in the space between the lungs
b. lymph nodes in the groin
c. adenoids
d. palatine tonsils
e. lymph nodes in the armpits

_____ 4. Sarcoma is a tumor of

a. blood
b. epithelial tissue
c. muscle
d. nerve cells
e. connective tissue

Fill in the blanks:

5. The word in the case histories that means "partial excision" is ____________.
6. The word that means "profuse sweating" is ____________.
7. The word that means "surgical puncture of the chest" is ____________.
8. The word that means "half of the chest" is ____________.

Write the meaning of the following abbreviations.

9. ABGs ____________
10. PAO_2 ____________
11. $PACO_2$ ____________
12. IPPB ____________
13. CHF ____________

Define the following words:

14. hypoxemia ____________
15. bronchodilator ____________
16. dyspnea ____________
17. thoracotomy ____________

RESPIRATION

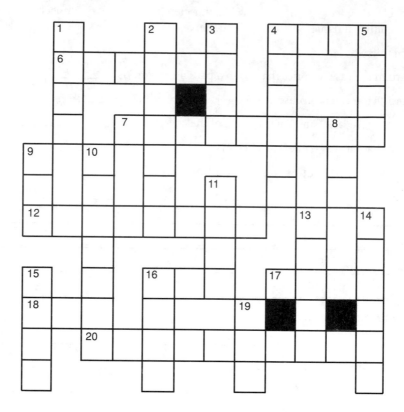

ACROSS

4. suffix: breathing
6. a common respiratory disease caused by spasm of the bronchial tubes
7. an infectious disease also called whooping cough
12. a large air passageway in the lungs
16. one measure of blood gas (abbr.)
17. an abnormal chest sound usually heard during inspiration
18. nose bleed: ____ staxis
20. an apparatus used to measure breathing volumes and capacities

DOWN

1. root (with combining vowel): nose
2. the nerve that activates the diaphragm
3. describing the tuburculosis organism: acid ____
4. the coughing up of sputum containing blood: hemo____
5. acute respiratory distress; shock lung (abbr.)
8. drug used to treat tuberculosis (abbr.)
9. one name for the tuberculosis organism (abbr.)
10. the opening between the vocal cords
11. an organ of respiration
13. the organ involved in cor pulmonale
14. the membrane that covers the lung
15. presence of blood in the pleural space: ____ thorax
16. produced as a result of hypo-ventilation
19. suffix: tumor

Chapter 11 Answer Section

Answers to Chapter Exercises

Exercise 11-1

1. eupnea (*ŪP-nē-a*)
2. dyspnea (*DISP-nē-a*)
3. apnea (*AP-nē-a*)
4. hypopnea (*hī-POP-nē-a*)
5. eupneic (*ūp-NĒ-ik*)
6. dyspneic (*disp-NĒ-ik*)
7. apneic (*AP-nē-ik*)
8. hypopneic (*hī-pop-NĒ-ik*)
9. hypoxia (*hī-POK-sē-a*)
10. hypercapnia (*hī-per-KAP-nē-a*)
11. eucapnia (*ū-KAP-nē-a*)
12. aphonia (*a-FŌ-nē-a*)

Exercise 11-2

1. rhinorrhea (*rī-nō-RĒ-a*)
2. pharyngitis (*far-in-JĪ-tis*)
3. bronchitis (*brong-KĪ tis*)
4. laryngoscopy i(*lar-ing-GOS-kō-pē*)
5. bronchoscopy (*brong-KOS-kō-pē*)
6. tracheoplasty (*trā-kē-ō-PLAS-tē*)
7. laryngectomy (*lar-in-JEK-tō-mē*)
8. tracheotomy (*trā-kē-OT-ō-mē*)
9. within the nose
10. pertaining to the larynx
11. pertaining to a bronchiole
12. around the bronchi
13. pertaining to the larynx and trachea
14. pertaining to the nose and pharynx

Exercise 11-3

1. pertaining to the pleura and lung
2. pain in the pleura
3. study of the lungs
4. any disease of the lung
5. intrapleural (*in-tra-PLŪR-al*)
6. subphrenic (*sub-FREN-ik*); also subdiaphragmatic
7. phrenicotomy (*fren-i-KOT-ō-mē*)
8. pneumonectomy (*nū-mō-NEK-tō-mē*); also pneumectomy, pulmonectomy
9. spirometer (*spi-ROM-e-ter*)

Labeling Exercise

The Respiratory System

1. frontal sinus
2. sphenoidal sinus
3. nasal cavity
4. nasopharynx
5. oropharynx
6. laryngeal pharynx
7. epiglottis
8. larynx and vocal cords
9. esophagus
10. trachea
11. left lung
12. mediastinum
13. right lung
14. right bronchus
15. terminal bronchiole
16. alveolar duct
17. alveoli
18. capillaries
19. diaphragm

Answers to Chapter Review

Chapter Review 11-1

1. b
2. a
3. d
4. e
5. c
6. d
7. e
8. b
9. c
10. a
11. b
12. e
13. d
14. c
15. a
16. diaphragm
17. smell
18. pleura
19. hemoglobin
20. oxygen
21. pharynx
22. alveolus
23. lungs
24. tidal volume
25. adenoids
26. phrenic nerve
27. mucus
28. pleurodesis *(plū-ROD-e-sis)*
29. tracheotomy *(trā-kē-OT-ō-mē)*
30. Pharyngitis *(far-in-JĪ-tis)*
31. laryngectomy *(lar-in-JEK-tō-mē)*
32. bronchiolitis *(brong-kē-ō-LĪ-tis)*
33. bronchospasm
34. accumulation of air or gas in the pleural space
35. accumulation of blood in the pleural space
36. accumulation in the pus in the pleural space
37. accumulation of fluid in the pleural space
38. excision of the adenoids
39. slow rate of respiration
40. within the trachea
41. inflammation of the lungs
42. narrowing or constriction of a bronchus
43. pain in the pleura
44. under the diaphragm
45. lack of voice
46. spir/o; breathing
47. pulmon/o; lung
48. py/o; pus
49. phren/o; diaphragm
50. pneum/o; lung
51. nares
52. bronchioles
53. alveoli
54. conchae
55. bronchi
56. Surgical puncture of the thoracic cavity
    a. chest; thorax
    b. surgical puncture
57. spitting blood
    a. blood
    b. spitting
58. Dryness of the throat
    a. pharynx; throat
    b. dry
    c. condition of

Chapter Review 11-2

1. c
2. d
3. e
4. b
5. a
6. c
7. e
8. b
9. a
10. d
11. b
12. d
13. a
14. c
15. e
16. phrenic nerve
17. tuberculosis
18. epistaxis
19. upright
20. carbon dioxide
21. bronchus
22. vital capacity
23. larynx
24. lungs
25. oropharynx
26. breathing
27. widen or dilate
28. tracheostomy
29. bronchogenic
30. bronchoscope

31. pleurocele
32. phrenicotomy
33. chronic dilatation of the bronchi
34. surgical puncture of the larynx
35. measurement of breathing
36. study of the lungs
37. discharge from the bronchi
38. any disease of the lungs
39. plastic repair of the nose
40. hypercapnia
41. expiration
42. tachypnea (tak-IP-ne-a)
43. hyperoxia
44. intubation
45. hypopnea
46. alveolar
47. pharyngeal
48. pleural
49. nasal
50. tracheal
51. bronchial
52. adenoids
53. larynx
54. dyspnea
55. epistaxis
56. croup
57. asthma
58. incomplete expansion of the alveoli
    a. incomplete
    b. expansion; dilation
59. The cartilage that covers the larynx during swallowing
    a. over, upon
    b. the space between the vocal cords

Answers to Case Study Questions

1. a
2. d
3. a
4. e
5. resection
6. diaphoresis
7. thoracentesis
8. hemithorax
9. arterial blood gases
10. arterial partial pressure of oxygen
11. arterial partial pressure of carbon dioxide
12. intermittent positive pressure breathing
13. congestive heart failure
14. deficiency of oxygen in the blood
15. drug that widens the bronchi
16. pain or difficulty in breathing
17. incision into the thorax (chest)

Answers to Crossword Puzzle

RESPIRATION

	1 N			2 P		3 F		4 P	N	E	5 A
	6 A	S	T	H	M	A		T			R
	S			R	■	S		Y			D
	O		7 P	E	R	T	U	S	S	8 I	S
9 A		10 G		N				I		N	
F		L		I		11 L		S		H	
12 B	R	O	N	C	H	U	S		13 H		14 P
		T				N			E		L
15 H		T		16 A	B	G		17 R	A	L	E
18 E	P	I		C			19 O	■	R	■	U
M		20 S	P	I	R	O	M	E	T	E	R
O				D			A				A

12 Digestion

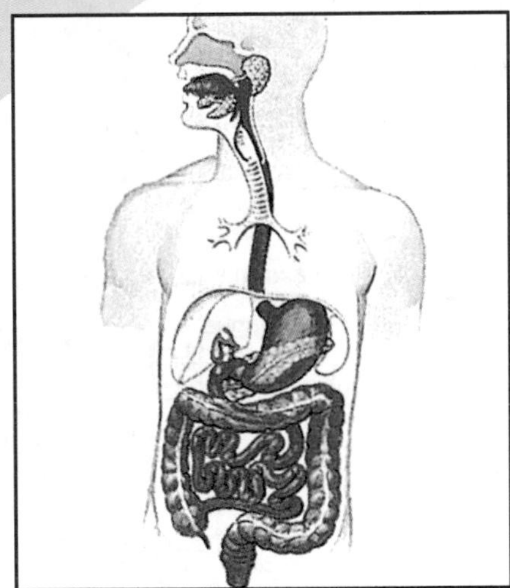

Chapter Contents

Objectives

After study of this chapter you should be able to:

1. Explain the function of the digestive system
2. Label a diagram of the digestive tract and describe the function of each part
3. Label a diagram of the accessory organs and explain the role of each in digestion
4. Identify and use the roots pertaining to the digestive system
5. Describe the major disorders of the digestive system
6. Define medical terms used in reference to the digestive system
7. Interpret abbreviations used in referring to the gastrointestinal system
8. Analyze case studies concerning gastroenterology

The function of the digestive system (Fig. 12-1) is to prepare food for intake by body cells. Nutrients must be broken down by mechanical and chemical means into molecules that are small enough to be absorbed into the circulation. Within cells the nutrients are used for energy and for rebuilding vital cell components. Digestion takes place in the digestive tract proper, also called the alimentary canal or gastrointestinal (GI) tract. Also contributing to the di-

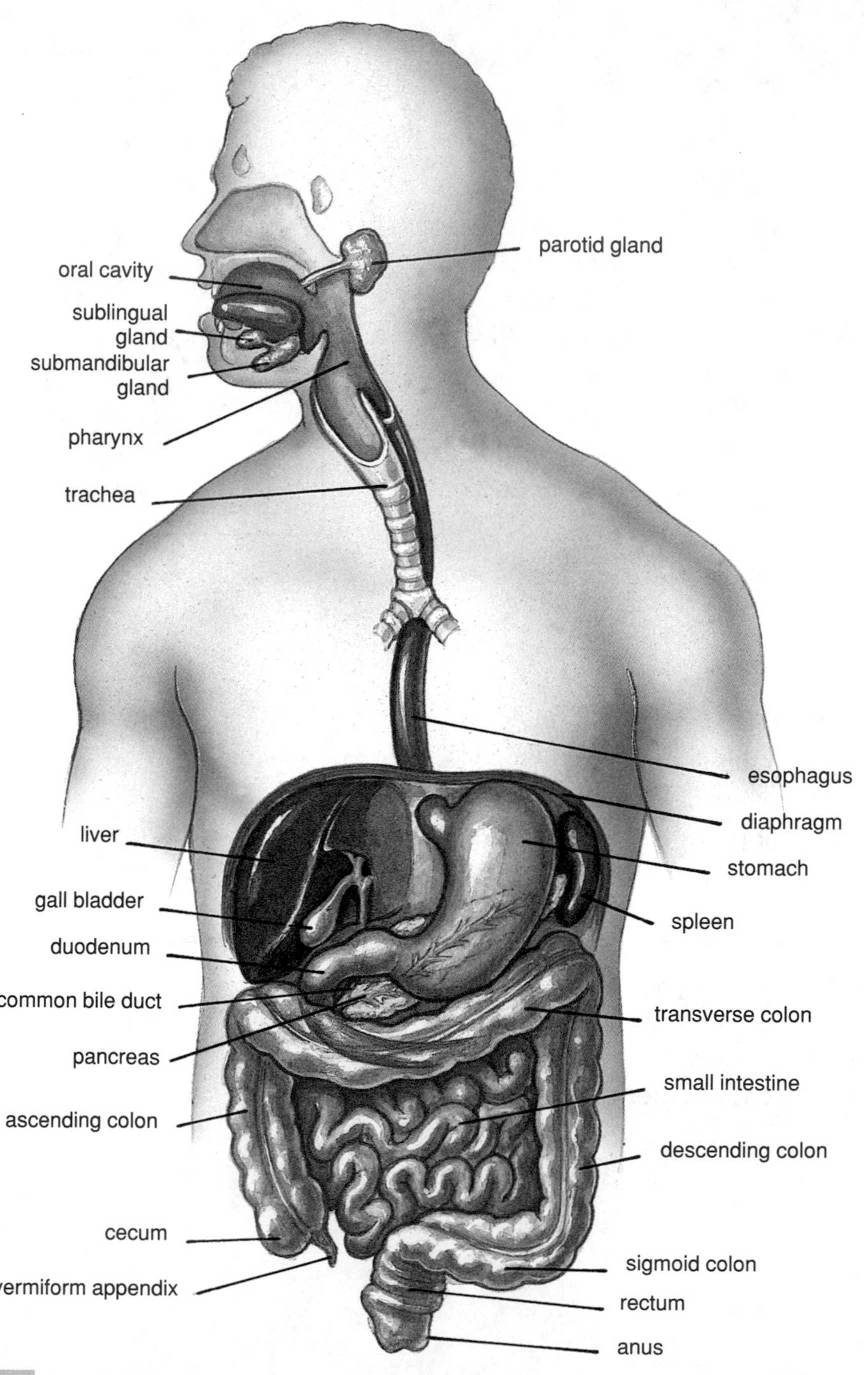

FIGURE 12-1. Digestive system.

gestive process are several accessory organs which release secretions into the small intestine. Food is moved through the digestive tract by **peristalsis**, wavelike contractions of the organ walls. Peristalsis also moves undigested waste material out of the body.

The Mouth to the Small Intestine

Digestion begins in the **mouth** (Fig. 12-2) where food is chewed by the teeth (Fig. 12-3) into small bits and mixed with **saliva**, which contains an enzyme that breaks down starch. The moistened food is then passed into the pharynx (throat) and through the **esophagus** into the **stomach**. Here it is further broken down by churning of the stomach as it is mixed with the enzyme pepsin and with powerful hydrochloric acid (HCl), both of which break down proteins.

The partially digested food passes through the **pylorus** of the stomach into the first part of the small intestine, the **duodenum**. As the food continues through the **jejunum** and **ileum**, the remaining sections of the small intestine, digestion is completed. The digested nutrients, as well as water, minerals, and vitamins are absorbed into the circulation. The substances active in digestion in the small intestine include enzymes from the intestine itself and secretions from the accessory organs of digestion.

The Accessory Organs

The accessory organs of digestion are illustrated in Figure 12-4.

The **liver** is a large gland with many functions. A large part of its activity is to process blood brought to it by a special circulatory pathway called the **hepatic portal system**. Its role in

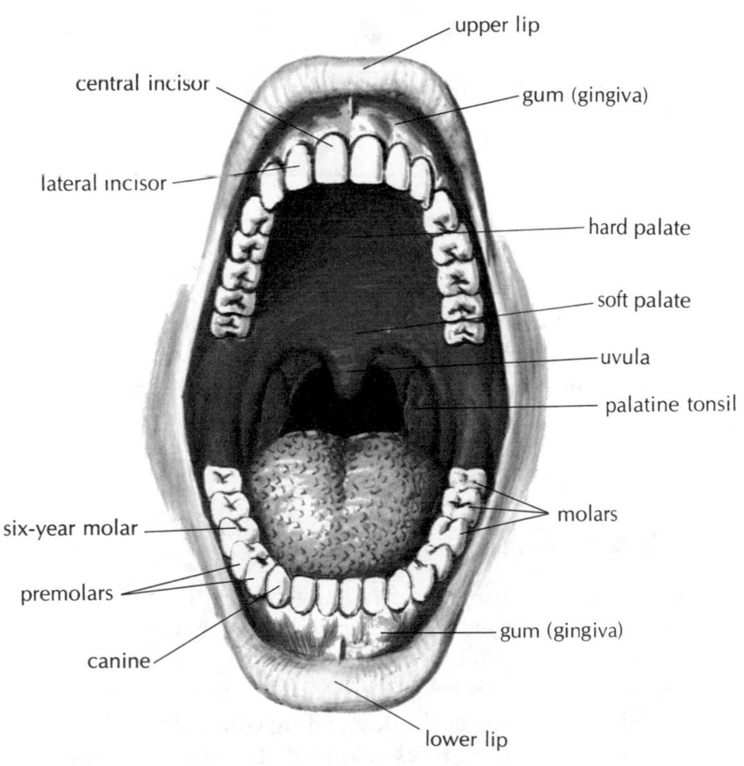

FIGURE 12-2. The mouth, showing the teeth and tonsils.

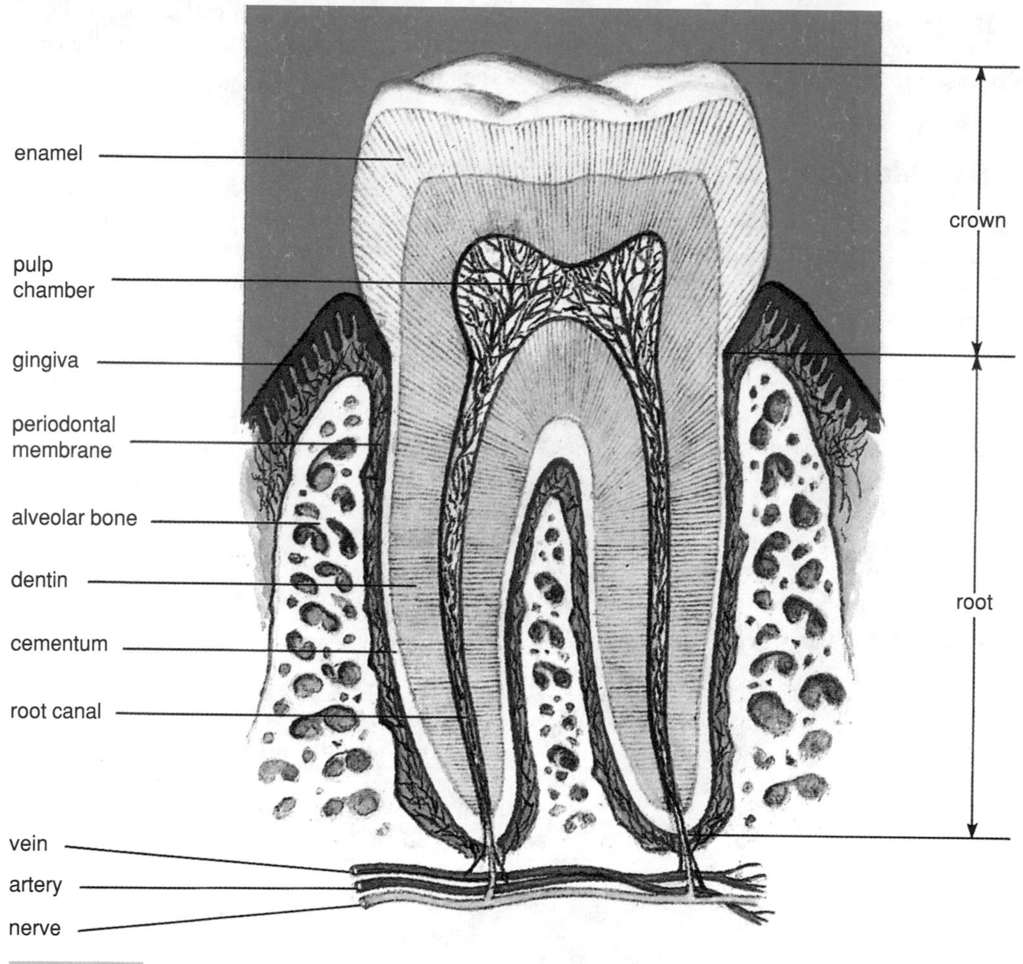

FIGURE 12-3. Tooth.

digestion is the secretion of **bile**, which breaks down fats. Bile is stored in the **gallbladder** until needed. The common hepatic duct from the liver and the cystic duct from the gallbladder merge to form the **common bile duct** which empties into the duodenum. The **pancreas** produces a mixture of digestive enzymes which is delivered into the duodenum through the pancreatic duct.

The Large Intestine

Undigested food, water, and digestive juices pass into the large intestine. This part of the digestive tract begins in the lower right region of the abdomen with a small pouch, the **cecum**, to which the **appendix** is attached. The large intestine continues upward along the right side of the abdomen as the **ascending colon**, crosses below the stomach as the **transverse colon**, then continues down the left side of the abdomen as the **descending colon**. As food is pushed through the colon, water is reabsorbed and stool or **feces** is formed. This waste material passes into the S-shaped **sigmoid colon** and is stored in the **rectum** until eliminated through the **anus**.

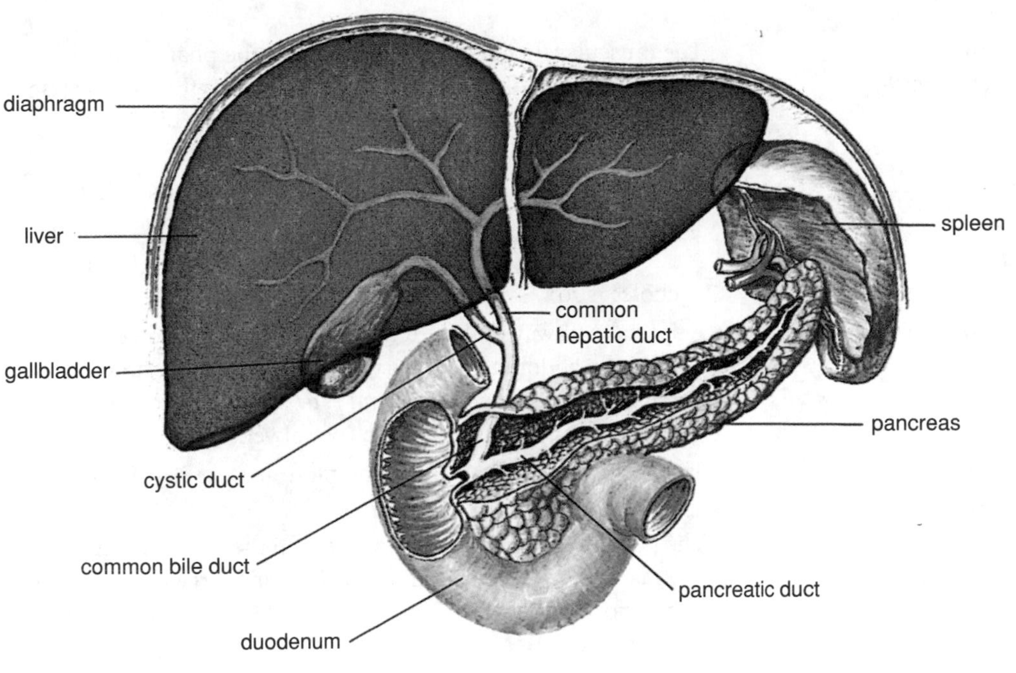

FIGURE 12-4. The accessory organs of digestion.

KEY TERMS

Normal Structure and Function

anus (*Ā-nus*) — The distal opening of the digestive tract (root an/o)

appendix — An appendage; usually means the vermiform (wormlike) appendix attached to the cecum

bile — The fluid secreted by the liver which aids in the digestion and absorption of fats (root chol, bili)

cecum (*SĒ-kum*) — A blind pouch at the beginning of the large intestine (root cec/o)

colon (*KŌ-lon*) — The major portion of the large intestine; extends from the cecum to the rectum (root col/o, colon/o)

common bile duct — The duct that carries bile into the duodenum; formed by the union of the cystic duct and the common hepatic duct (root choledoch/o)

duodenum (*dū-ō-DĒ-num*) — The first portion of the small intestine (root duoden/o)

(continued)

esophagus *(e-SOF-a-gus)*	The muscular tube that carries food from the pharynx to the stomach. The opening of the esophagus into the stomach is controlled by the lower esophageal sphincter (LES). (root esphag/o)
feces *(FĒ-sēz)*	The waste material eliminated from the intestine (adj. *fecal*); stool
gallbladder	A sac on the undersurface of the liver that stores bile (root cholecyst/o)
hepatic portal system	A special pathway of the circulation that brings blood directly from the abdominal organs to the liver for processing (also called simply the *portal system*). The vessel that enters the liver is the hepatic portal vein (portal vein).
ileum *(IL-ē-um)*	The terminal portion of the small intestine (root ile/o)
intestine *(in-TES-tin)*	The portion of the digestive tract betwen the stomach and the anus. It consists of the small intestine and large intestine. It functions in digestion, absorption, and elimination of waste (root enter/o).
jejunum *(je-JŪ-num)*	The middle portion of the small intestine (root jejun/o)
liver	A large gland in the upper right part of the abdomen. In addition to many other functions it secretes bile for digestion of fats (root hepat/o).
pancreas *(PAN-krē-as)*	A large, elongated gland behind the stomach. It produces hormones that regulate sugar metabolism and also produces digestive enzymes (root pancreat/o).
palate *(PAL-at)*	The roof of the mouth; the partition between the mouth and nasal cavity (root palat/o)
peristalsis *(per-i-STAL-sis)*	Wavelike contractions of the walls of an organ
pylorus *(pī-LOR-us)*	The distal opening of the stomach into the duodenum. The opening is controlled by a ring of muscle, the pyloric sphincter (root pylor/o).
rectum *(REK-tum)*	The distal portion of the large intestine. It stores and eliminates undigested waste (root rect/o, proct/o).
saliva *(sa-LĪ-va)*	The clear secretion released into the mouth that moistens food and contains an enzyme that digests starch. It is produced by three pairs of glands: the parotid, submandibular, and sublingual glands (see Figure 12-1) (root sial/o).
stomach	A muscular saclike organ below the diaphragm that stores food and secretes juices that digest proteins (root gastr/o)
villi *(VIL-ī)*	Tiny projections in the lining of the small intestine that absorb digested foods into the circulation (s. villus)

Roots Pertaining to Digestion

Roots for the Mouth

Root	Meaning	Example	Definition of Example
or/o	mouth	oronasal *or-ō-NĀ-zal*	pertaining to the mouth and nose
stoma, stomat/o	mouth	stomatosis *stō-ma-TŌ-sis*	any disease condition of the mouth
gnath/o	jaw	prognathous *PROG-na-thus*	having a projecting jaw
cheil/o	lip	cheilorrhaphy *kī-LOR-a-fē*	suture of the lip
labi/o	lip	glossolabial *glos-ō-LĀ-bē-al*	pertaining to the tongue (gloss/o) and lip
bucc/o	cheek	intrabuccal *in-tra-BUK-al*	within the cheek
dent/o, dent/i	tooth	dentifrice *DEN-ti-fris*	a substance used to clean the teeth
odont/o	tooth	periodontist *per-ē-ō-DON-tist*	dentist who treats the tissues around the teeth
gingiv/o	gum (gingiva)	gingivitis *jin-ji-VĪ-tis*	inflammation of the gums
lingu/o	tongue	sublingual *sub-LING-gwal*	under the tongue
gloss/o	tongue	hemiglossal *hem-i-GLOS-al*	pertaining to one half of the tongue
sial/o	saliva, salivary gland, salivary duct	sialography *sī-a-LOG-ra-fē*	radiographic study of the salivary glands and ducts
palat/o	palate	palatine *PAL-a-tīn*	pertaining to the palate

Exercise 12-1

Using the adjective suffix *-al* write a word for each of the following definitions:

1. Pertaining to the mouth ____oral____
2. Pertaining to the teeth ________
3. Pertaining to the gums ________
4. Pertaining to the tongue ________
5. Pertaining to the cheek ________
6. Pertaining to the lip (labi/o) ________

Fill in the blanks:

7. Micrognathia *(mī-krō-NĀ-thē-a)* is excessive smallness of the ____________________.
8. Glossorrhaphy *(glos-OR-a-fē)* is suture of the ____________________.
9. The oropharynx is the part of the pharynx that is located behind the ____________________.
10. A sialolith *(sī-AL-ō-lith)* is a stone formed in a ____________________ gland or duct.
11. Orthodontics *(or-thō-DON-tiks)* is the branch of dentistry the deals with straightening (orotho-) of the ____________________.
12. Cheiloplasty *(kī-lō-PLAS-tē)* is plastic surgery of the ____________________.
13. Xerostomia *(zē-rō-STŌ-mē-a)* is dryness of the ____________________.

Define the following words:

14. orolingual *(or-o-LING-gwal)* ____________________
15. palatorrhaphy *(pal-at-OR-a-fē)* ____________________
16. gingivectomy *(jin-ji-VEK-tō-mē)* ____________________
17. labiodental *(lā-bē-ō-DEN-tal)* ____________________
18. stomatitis *(stō-ma-TĪ-tis)* ____________________

Roots for the Digestive Tract (except the mouth)

Root	Meaning	Example	Definition of Example
esophag/o	esophagus	esophageal* *e-sof-a-JĒ-al*	pertaining to the esophagus
gastr/o	stomach	epigastrium *ep-i-GAS-trē-um*	the region of the abdomen over the stomach
pylor/o	pylorus	pyloroplasty *pī-LOR-ō-plas-tē*	plastic repair of the pylorus
enter/o	intestine	enterovirus *EN-ter-ō-vī-rus*	virus that infects the intestinal tract
duoden/o	duodenum	duodenoscopy *dū-ō-den-OS-kō-pē*	endoscopic examination of the duodenum
jejun/o	jejunum	jejunostomy *je-jū-NOS-tō-mē*	surgical creation of an opening into the jejunum
ile/o	ileum	ileectomy *il-ē-EK-tō-mē*	excision of the ileum
cec/o	cecum	cecoptosis *sē-kop-TŌ-sis*	downward displacement of the cecum

(continued)

Roots for the Digestive Tract (Continued)

Root	Meaning	Example	Definition of Example
col/o, colon/o	colon	coloclysis *kō-lō-KLĪ-sis*	irrigation of the colon
sigmoid/o	sigmoid	sigmoidoscope *sig-MOY-dō-skōp*	an endoscope for examining the sigmoid colon (Fig. 12-5)
rect/o	rectum	rectocele *REK-tō-sēl*	hernia of the rectum
proct/o	rectum	proctopexy *PROK-tō-pek-sē*	surgical fixation of the rectum
an/o	anus	anorectal *ā-nō-REK-tal*	pertaining to the anus and rectum

*Note addition of *e* before *-al*.

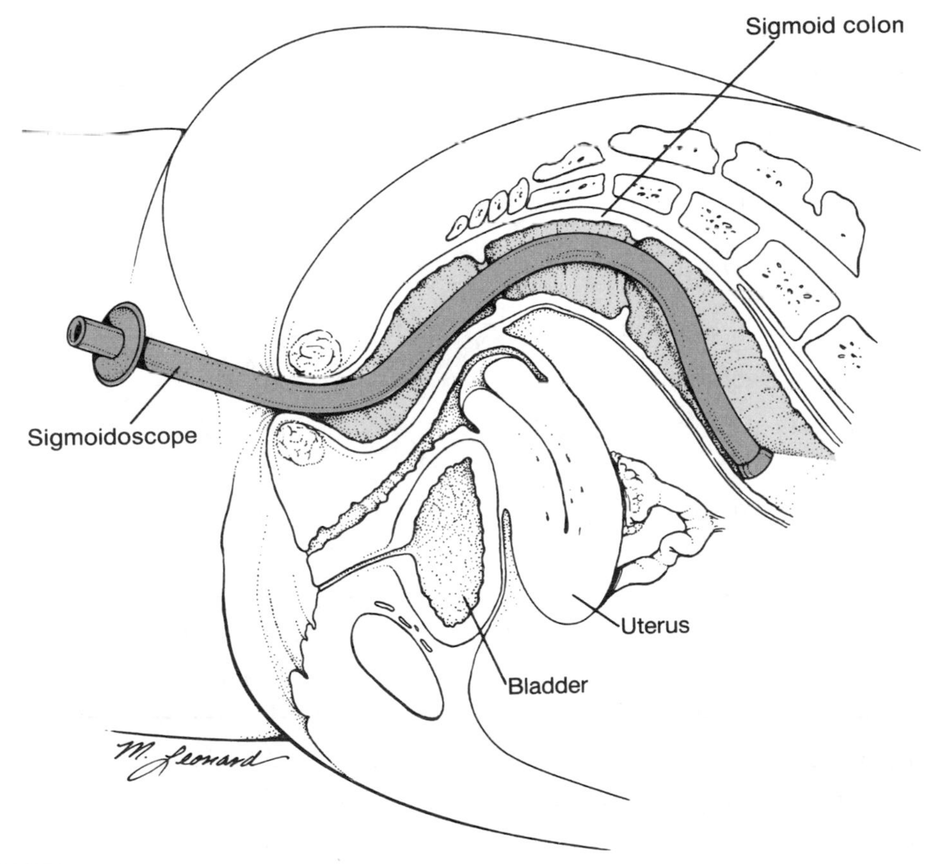

FIGURE 12-5. Sigmoidoscopy. The endoscope is advanced through the sigmoid colon and into the descending colon. (Smeltzer SC, Bare BG: Brunner and Suddarth's Textbook of Medical-Surgical Nursing, 7th ed, p 836. Philadelphia: JB Lippincott, 1992.)

Exercise 12-2

Using the adjective ending *-ic* write a word for each of the following definitions:

1. Pertaining to the intestine ____enteric____
2. Pertaining to the stomach ________
3. Pertaining to the colon ________
4. Pertaining to the pylorus ________
5. Pertaining to the epigastrium ________

Using the adjective ending *-al* write a word for each of the following definitions:

6. Pertaining to the duodenum ____duodenal____
7. Pertaining to the cecum ________
8. Pertaining to the jejunum ________
9. Pertaining to the ileum ________
10. Pertaining to the rectum ________
11. Pertaining to the anus ________

Write a word for each of the following definitions:

12. Excision of the stomach (or part of the stomach) ________
13. Plastic repair of the esophagus ________
14. Inflammation of the ileum ________
15. Surgical creation of an opening into the duodenum ________
16. Surgical creation of an opening into the ileum ________
17. Study of the stomach and intestines ________

Use the root *col/o* for the next three words:

18. Inflammation of the colon ________
19. Surgical fixation of the colon ________
20. Surgical creation of an opening into the colon ________

Use the root *colon/o* for the next two words:

21. Any disease of the colon ________
22. Endoscopic examination of the colon ________

Two organs of the digestive tract or even two parts of the same organ may be surgically connected by a passage (anastomosis) following removal of damaged tissue. Such a procedure is named for the connected organs plus the ending *-stomy*. Use two roots plus the suffix *-stomy* for the following words:

23. Surgical creation of a passage between the esophagus and stomach ___esophagogastrostomy___
24. Surgical creation of a passage between the stomach and intestine ______________________
25. Surgical creation of a passage between the stomach and the jejunum ______________________
26. Surgical creation of a passage between the duodenum and the ileum ______________________
27. Surgical creation of a passage between the sigmoid colon and the rectum (proct/o) ______________________

Roots for the Accessory Organs

Root	Meaning	Example	Definition of Example
hepat/o	liver	hepatomegaly *hep-a-tō-MEG-a-lē*	enlargement of the liver
bili	bile	biliary *BIL-ē-ar-ē*	pertaining to the bile or bile ducts
chol/e, chol/o	bile, gall	cholelith *KŌ-lē-lith*	gallstone, biliary calculus
cholecyst/o	gallbladder	cholecystorrhaphy *kō-lē-sis-tor-a-fē*	suture of the gallbladder
cholangi/o	bile duct	cholangiogram *kō-LAN-jē-ō-gram*	x-ray of the bile ducts
choledoch/o	common bile duct	choledochal *kō-LED-o-kal*	pertaining to the common bile duct
pancreat/o	pancreas	pancreatolysis *pan-krē-a-TOL-i-sis*	dissolving of the pancreas

Exercise 12-3

Use the suffix *-ic* write a word for each of the following definitions:

1. Pertaining to the liver ______________________
2. Pertaining to the gallbladder ______________________
3. Pertaining to the pancreas ______________________

Use the ending *-graphy* for the next four words:

4. Radiographic study of the bile ducts ____________________
5. Radiographic study of the liver ____________________
6. Radiographic study of the gallbladder ____________________
7. Radiographic study of the pancreas ____________________

Use the ending *-lithiasis* for the next two words:

8. Condition of having a stone in the common bile duct ____________________
9. Condition of having a stone in the pancreas ____________________

Fill in the blanks:

10. The word *biligenesis (bil-i-JEN-e-sis)* means the formation of ____________________.
11. Choledochotomy *(kō-led-o-KOT-o-mē)* is incision of the ____________________.
12. A hepatocyte *(HEP-a-tō-sīt)* is a cell in the ____________________.
13. A word that means inflammation of the liver is ____________________.
14. A pancreatotropic *(pan-krē-at-ō-TROP-ik)* substance acts on the ____________________.
15. Cholangitis is inflammation of a(n) ____________________.

Clinical Aspects of Digestion

Gastrointestinal Tract

Infection

A variety of organisms can infect the gastrointestinal tract, from viruses and bacteria to protozoa and worms. Some produce short-lived upsets with **gastroenteritis, nausea, diarrhea**, and **emesis** (vomiting). Others, such as typhoid, cholera, and dysentery, are more serious, even fatal.

Ulcers

Ulcers caused by the damaging action of digestive, or peptic, juices on the lining of the GI tract are termed **peptic ulcers**. The origins of such ulcers are not completely known, although infection with a bacterium, *H. pylori*, has been identified as a major cause. Heredity and stress may be factors, as well as chronic inflammation and exposure to damaging drugs, such as aspirin, or to irritants in food and drink. Current treatment includes the administration of antibiotics to eliminate *H. pylori* infection and use of drugs that block the action of histamine, which stimulates gastric secretion. Ulcers may lead to hemorrhage or to perforation of the wall of the digestive tract. They can be diagnosed by endoscopy and by radiographic study of the upper GI tract using a contrast medium, usually barium sulfate.

Cancer

The most common sites for cancer of the GI tract are the colon and rectum. Together these colorectal cancers rank among the most frequent causes of cancer deaths in the United States in both men and women. A diet low in fiber and calcium and high in fat is a major risk factor in colorectal cancer. Heredity is also a factor, as is chronic inflammation of the colon (colitis). **Polyps** (growths) in the intestine often become cancerous and should be removed. Often this can be ac-

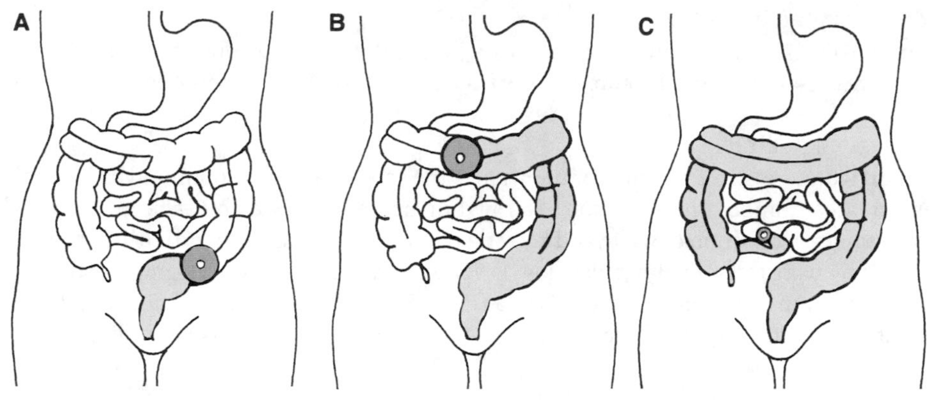

FIGURE 12-6. Several ostomy locations. **(A)** Sigmoid colostomy. **(B)** Transverse colostomy. **(C)** Ileostomy. (Taylor C, Lillis CA, LeMone P: Fundamentals of Nursing, 2nd ed, p 930. Philadelphia: JB Lippincott, 1993.)

complished by endoscopy. Bleeding into the intestine is a sign of cancer and can be tested for in the stool. Because this blood may be present in very small amounts it is described as **occult** ("hidden") **blood**. Colorectal cancers are staged according to **Dukes' classification**, ranging from A to D according to severity. The interior of the intestine can be observed with various endoscopes named for the specific area in which they are used (Fig. 12-5), such as proctoscope (rectum), sigmoidoscope (sigmoid colon), colonoscope (colon).

In some cases of cancer, and for other reasons as well, it may be necessary to surgically remove a portion of the GI tract and create a **stoma** (opening) on the abdominal wall for elimination of waste. Such **ostomy** surgery (Fig. 12-6) is named for the organ involved, such as ileostomy (ileum) or colostomy (colon). When a connection (anastomosis) is formed between two organs of the tract, both are included in naming: gastroduodenostomy (stomach and duodenum), coloproctostomy (colon and rectum).

Obstructions

A **hernia** is the protrusion of an organ through an abnormal opening. The most common type is an inguinal hernia, described in Chapter 14 (Fig. 14-4). In a **hiatal hernia**, part of the stomach moves upward into the chest cavity through the space (hiatus) in the diaphragm where the esophagus passes through (see Figure 6-1). Often this condition produces no symptoms, but it may result in chest pain, **dysphagia** (difficulty in swallowing), or reflux of stomach contents into the esophagus.

In **pyloric stenosis** the opening between the stomach and small intestine is too narrow. This usually appears in infants, and in males more than females. A sign of this condition is projectile vomiting. Surgery may be needed to correct it.

Other types of obstruction include **intussusception** (Fig. 12-7), **volvulus**, and **ileus**, all of which are defined in the Key Terms.

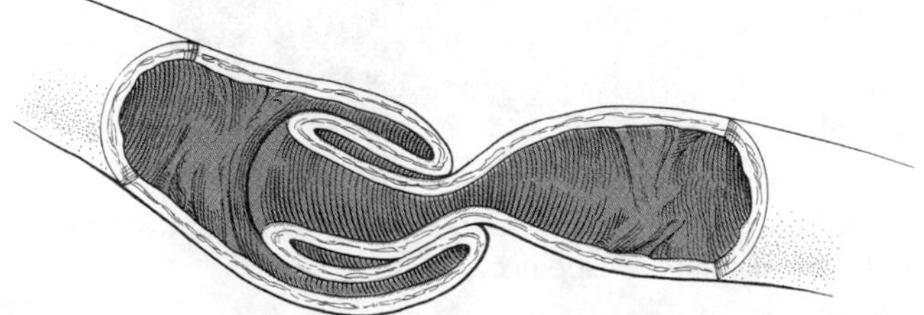

FIGURE 12-7. Intussusception.

Appendicitis

Appendicitis results from infection of the appendix, often secondary to its obstruction. Surgery is necessary to avoid rupture and **peritonitis**, infection of the peritoneal cavity.

Diverticulitis

Diverticula are small pouches in the wall of the intestine, most commonly in the colon. If present in large number, the condition is termed **diverticulosis**, which has been attributed to a diet low in fiber. Collection of waste and bacteria in these sacs leads to **diverticulitis**, which is accompanied by pain and sometimes bleeding. Diverticula can be seen by radiographic studies using a contrast medium, a so-called barium enema (Fig. 12-8). Although there is no cure, diverticulitis is treated with diet, stool softeners, and drugs to reduce motility (antispasmodics).

Inflammatory Bowel Disease (IBD)

Two similar diseases are included under the heading of IBD: **Crohn's disease** and **ulcerative colitis**, both of which occur mainly in adolescents and young adults. The first is a chronic inflammation of segments of the intestinal wall causing pain, diarrhea, abscess, and often **fistula** for-

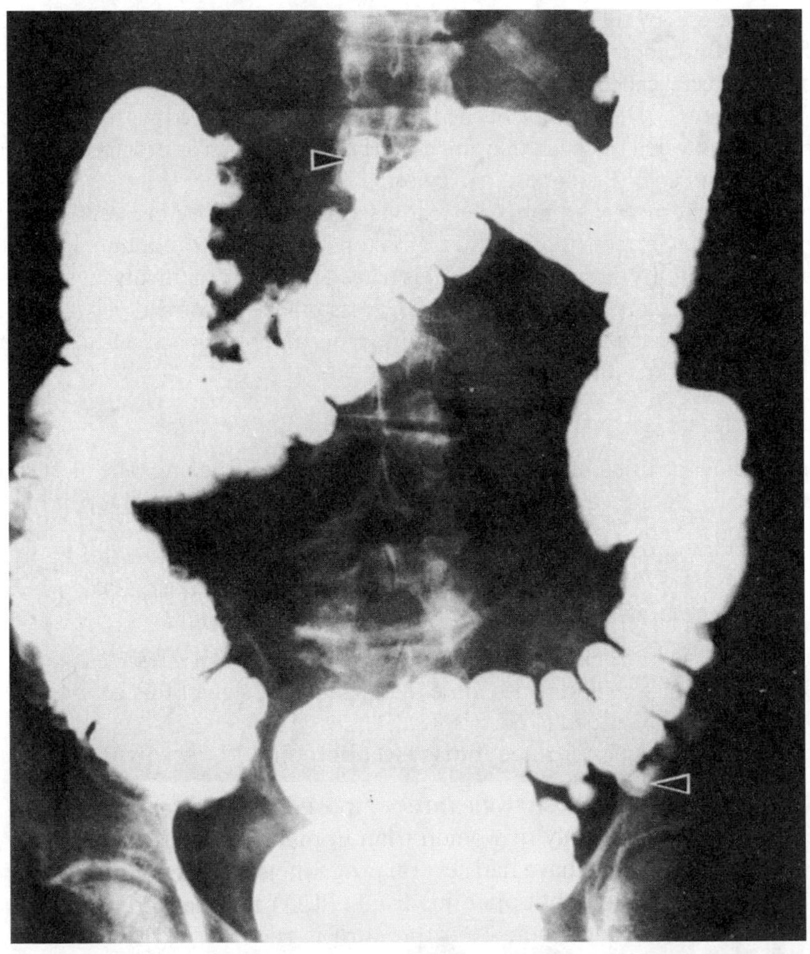

FIGURE 12-8. Barium enema x-ray study of the colon showing diverticula *(arrows)*. (Eastwood GL: Core Textbook of Gastroenterology, p 181. Philadelphia: JB Lippincott, 1984.)

mation. Ulcerative colitis involves a continuous inflammation of the lining of the colon and usually the rectum.

Hemorrhoids are varicose veins in the rectum associated with pain, bleeding, and in some cases, prolapse of the rectum.

Accessory Organs

Hepatitis

In the US and other industrialized countries, **hepatitis** is most often caused by viral infection. More than five types of hepatitis virus have now been identified. The most common is hepatitis A virus (HAV), which is spread by fecal–oral contamination, often by food handlers and in crowded, unsanitary conditions. It may also be acquired by eating contaminated food. Hepatitis B virus (HBV) is spread by blood and other body fluids. It may be transmitted sexually, by sharing needles used for injection, and by close interpersonal contact. Infected individuals may become carriers of the disease. Most patients recover, but the disease may be serious, even fatal, and may lead to liver cancer. Hepatitis C is spread through blood and blood products or by close contact with an infected person. Hepatitis D, the delta virus, is highly pathogenic, but only infects those already infected with hepatitis B. Hepatitis E, like HAV, is spread by contaminated food and water. It has caused epidemics in Asia, Africa, and Mexico. Vaccines are available for hepatitis A and B.

The name *hepatitis* simply means "inflammation of the liver," but this disease also causes necrosis (death) of liver cells. Hepatitis may be caused in addition by other infections and by drugs and toxins. Serum tests of liver function are important in diagnosis.

Jaundice, or icterus, is a symptom of hepatitis and other diseases of the liver and biliary system. It is a condition of yellowness of the skin, whites of the eyes, and mucous membranes due to the presence of bile pigments, mainly **bilirubin**, in the blood.

Cirrhosis

Cirrhosis is a chronic liver disease characterized by hepatomegaly, edema, ascites, and jaundice. As the disease progresses there is splenomegaly, internal bleeding, and brain damage caused by changes in the composition of the blood. A complication of cirrhosis is increased pressure in the portal system that brings blood from the abdominal organs to the liver, a condition called **portal hypertension**. The main cause of cirrhosis is the excess consumption of alcohol.

Gallstones

Cholelithiasis refers to the presence of stones in the gallbladder or bile ducts, which is usually associated with **cholecystitis**, inflammation of the gallbladder. Most of these stones are composed of cholesterol, an ingredient of bile. Gallstones form more commonly in women than in men, especially in women on oral contraceptives and those who have had several pregnancies. The condition is characterized by biliary **colic** (pain) in the right upper quadrant (RUQ), nausea, and vomiting. Drugs may be used to dissolve gallstones, but often the cure is removal of the gallbladder. Such a **cholecystectomy** is traditionally performed through a major abdominal incision, but a newer method for removing the gallbladder with a laparoscope through a small incision in the abdomen is now in use.

Ultrasonography and radiography are used for diagnosis of gallstones. **ERCP** (endoscopic retrograde cholangiopancreatography) (Fig. 12-9) is a technique for viewing the pancreatic and bile ducts and for performing certain techniques to relieve obstructions. Contrast medium is injected into the biliary system from the duodenum and x-rays are taken.

Pancreatitis

Inflammation of the pancreas may result from alcohol abuse, drug toxicity, bile obstruction, infections, and other causes. Often the disease subsides with only treatment of the symptoms.

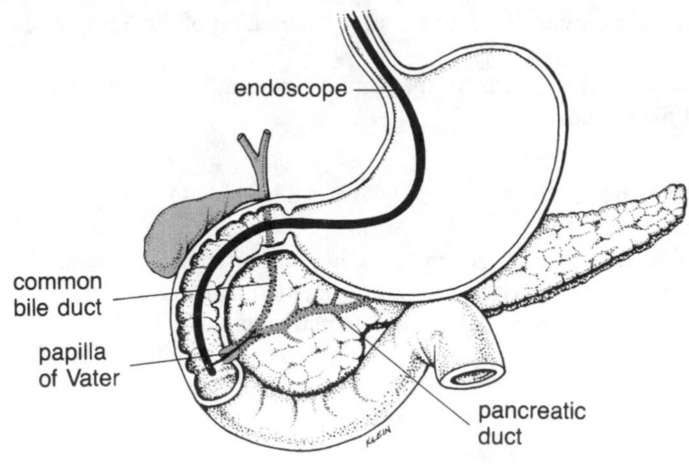

FIGURE 12-9. Endoscopic retrograde cholangiopancreatography (ERCP). A contrast medium is injected into the pancreatic and bile ducts in preparation for radiography. (© 1982 Redrawn from Hospital Medicine, February 1982, with permission of Cahners Publishing Company.)

KEY CLINICAL TERMS

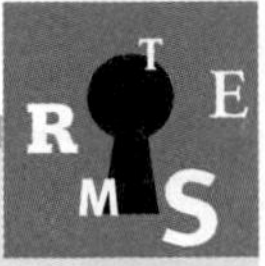

Disorders

appendicitis *(a-pen-di-SĪ-tis)* — Inflammation of the appendix

ascites *(a-SĪ-tēz)* — Accumulation of fluid in the abdominal cavity; a form of edema. May be caused by heart disease, lymphatic or venous obstruction, cirrhosis, or changes in plasma composition.

cholecystitis *(kō-lē-sis-TĪ-tis)* — Inflammation of the gallbladder

cholelithiasis *(kō-lē-li-THĪ-a-sis)* — The condition of having stones in the gallbladder; also used to refer to stones in the common bile duct

cirrhosis *(sir-RŌ-sis)* — Chronic liver disease with degeneration of liver tissue

colic *(KOL-ik)* — Acute abdominal pain, such as biliary colic caused by gallstones in the bile ducts

Crohn's disease *(krōnz)* — A chronic inflammatory disease of the gastrointestinal tract usually involving the ileum

diarrhea *(dī-a-RĒ-a)* — The frequent passage of watery bowel movements

diverticulitis *(dī-ver-tik-ū-LĪ-tis)* — Inflammation of diverticula (small pouches) in the wall of the digestive tract, especially in the colon

diverticulosis *(dī-ver-tik-ū-LŌ-sis)* — The presence of diverticula, especially in the colon

dysphagia *(dis-FĀ-jē-a)*	Difficulty in swallowing
emesis *(EM-e-sis)*	Vomiting
fistula *(FIS-tū-la)*	An abnormal passageway between two organs or from an organ to the body surface, such as between the rectum and anus (anorectal fistula)
gastroenteritis *(gas-trō-en-ter-Ī-tis)*	Inflammation of the stomach and intestine
hepatitis *(hep-a-TĪ-tis)*	Inflammation of the liver; commonly caused by a viral infection
hepatomegaly *(hep-a-tō-MEG-a-lē)*	Enlargement of the liver
hiatal hernia *(hī-Ā-tal)*	A protrusion of the stomach through the opening (hiatus) in the diaphragm through which the esophagus passes (see Figure 6-1)
icterus *(IK-ter-us)*	Jaundice
ileus *(IL-ē-us)*	Intestinal obstruction. May be caused by lack of peristalsis (adynamic, paralytic ileus) or by contraction (dynamic ileus). Intestinal matter and gas may be relieved by passage of a tube for drainage.
intussusception *(in-tu-su-SEP-shun)*	Slipping of one part of the intestine into another part below it. Occurs mainly in children in the ileocecal region (see Figure 12-7).
jaundice *(JAWN-dis)*	A yellowish color of the skin, mucous membranes, and whites of the eye caused by bile pigments in the blood (from French *jaune* meaning "yellow"). The main pigment is bilirubin, a byproduct of the breakdown of red blood cells.
nausea *(NAW-zha)*	An unpleasant sensation in the upper abdomen that often precedes vomiting. Typically occurs in digestive upset, motion sickness, and sometimes early pregnancy.
occult blood	Blood present in such small amounts that it can be detected only microscopically or chemically; in the feces, a sign of intestinal bleeding (*occult* means "hidden")
pancreatitis *(pan-krē-a-TĪ-tis)*	Inflammation of the pancreas
peritonitis *(per-i-tō-NĪ-tis)*	Inflammation of the peritoneum, the membrane that lines the abdominal cavity and covers the abdominal organs. May result from perforation of an ulcer, rupture of the appendix, or infection of the reproductive tract, among other causes.
polyp *(POL-ip)*	A tumor that grows on a stalk and bleeds easily
portal hypertension	An abnormal increase in pressure in the hepatic portal system. May be caused by cirrhosis, infection, thrombosis, or tumors.

(continued)

pyloric stenosis — Narrowing of the opening between the stomach and the duodenum

splenomegaly *(splē-nō-MEG-a-lē)* — Enlargement of the spleen

ulcer *(UL-ser)* — A sore or lesion of the skin or mucous membrane. A peptic ulcer is caused by the action of digestive (peptic) juice, as in the stomach or duodenum.

volvulus *(VOL-vū-lus)* — Twisting of the intestine resulting in obstruction. Usually involves the sigmoid colon and occurs most often in children and in the elderly.

Diagnosis and Treatment

anastomosis *(a-nas-to-MŌ-sis)* — A passage or communication between two vessels or organs. May be normal or pathologic or may be created surgically.

barium studies — Use of barium sulfate as a liquid contrast medium for fluoroscopic and radiographic study of the digestive tract. Included are studies of the esophagus (barium swallow), upper GI series of the esophagus, stomach, and duodenum (barium meal), and lower GI series of the colon (barium enema).

cholecystectomy *(kō-lē-sis-TEK-tō-mē)* — Surgical removal of the gallbladder

ERCP — Endoscopic retrograde cholangiopancreatography; a technique for viewing the pancreatic and bile ducts and for performing certain techniques to relieve obstructions. Contrast medium is injected into the biliary system from the duodenum and x-rays are taken.

ostomy *(OS-tō-mē)* — An opening into the body; generally refers to an opening created for elimination of body waste. Also refers to the operation done to create such an opening. (See stoma.)

stoma *(STŌ-ma)* — A surgically created opening to the body surface or between two organs (literally "mouth")

ADDITIONAL TERMS

Normal Structure and Function

bolus *(BŌ-lus)* — A mass, such as the rounded mass of food that is swallowed.

cardia *(KAR-dē-a)* — The part of the stomach near the esophagus. Named for its closeness to the heart.

chyme *(kīm)* — The semiliquid partially digested food that moves from the stomach into the small intestine

defecation *(def-e-KĀ-shun)*	The evacuation of feces from the rectum
deglutition *(deg-lū-TISH-un)*	Swallowing
diverticulum *(dī-ver-TIK-ū-lum)*	A pouch in the lining of an organ occurring normally or by herniation through a defect in the organ wall (pl. diverticula)
duodenal bulb	The part of the duodenum near the pylorus. The first bend (flexure) of the duodenum
greater omentum *(ō-MEN-tum)*	A fold of the peritoneum that extends from the stomach over the abdominal organs
hepatic flexure	The right bend of the colon, forming the junction between the ascending colon and the transverse colon (see Figure 12-1)
mastication *(mas-ti-KĀ-shun)*	Chewing
mesentery *(MES-en-ter-ē)*	The portion of the peritoneum that folds over and supports the intestine
mesocolon *(mes-ō-KŌ-lon)*	The portion of the peritoneum that folds over and supports the colon
peritoneum *(per-i-tō-NĒ-um)*	The serous membrane that lines the abdominal cavity and supports the abdominal organs
papilla of Vater *(FĀ-ter)*	The raised area where the common bile duct and pancreatic duct enter the duodenum (see Figure 12-4); the duodenal papilla
peptic *(PEP-tik)*	Pertaining to digestion or gastric juices
rugae *(RŪ-jē)*	The large folds in the lining of the stomach seen when the stomach is empty
sphincter of Oddi *(OD-ē)*	The ring of muscle at the opening of the common bile duct into the duodenum
splenic flexure	The left bend of the colon, forming the junction between the transverse colon and the descending colon (see Figure 12-1)
uvula *(Ū-vū-la)*	A hanging fleshy mass. Usually means the mass that hangs from the soft palate (see Figure 12-2).

Disorders

achalasia *(ak-a-LĀ-zē-a)*	Failure of a smooth muscle to relax, especially the lower esophageal sphincter, so that food is retained in the esophagus
achlorhydria *(ā-klor-HĪ-drē-a)*	Lack of hydrochloric acid in the stomach. Opposite is hyperchlorhydria.
anorexia *(an-ō-REK-sē-a)*	Loss of appetite. Anorexia nervosa is refusal or inability to eat due to psychological causes. (adj. anorectic, anorexic)

(continued)

aphagia *(a-FĀ-jē-a)*	Refusal or inability to eat
aphthous ulcer *(AF-thus)*	A small ulcer in the mucous membrane of the mouth
bulimia *(bū-LIM-ē-a)*	Excessive, insatiable appetite. A disorder characterized by overeating followed by induced vomiting, diarrhea, or fasting.
cachexia *(ka-KEK-sē-a)*	Profound ill health, malnutrition, and wasting
caries *(KA-rēz)*	Tooth decay
celiac disease *(SĒ-lē-ak)*	A disease characterized by the inability to absorb foods containing gluten
cheilosis *(kī-LŌ-sis)*	Cracking at the corners of the mouth, often due to B vitamin deficiency
cholangitis *(kō-lan-JĪ-tis)*	Inflammation of the bile ducts
cholestasis *(kō-lē-STA-sis)*	Stoppage of bile flow
constipation *(con-sti-PĀ-shun)*	Infrequency or difficulty in defecation and the passage of hard, dry feces
dyspepsia *(dis-PEP-sē-a)*	Poor or painful digestion
eructation *(e-ruk-TĀ-shun)*	Belching
familial adenomatous polyposis (FAP)	A heredity condition in which multiple polyps form in the colon and rectum, predisposing to colorectal cancer
flatus *(FLĀ-tus)*	Gas or air in the gastrointestinal tract; gas or air expelled through the anus
irritable bowel syndrome (IBS)	A chronic stress-related disease characterized by diarrhea, constipation, and pain associated with rhythmic contractions of the intestine. Mucous colitis; spastic colon.
megacolon *(meg-a-KŌ-lon)*	An extremely dilated colon. Usually congenital, but may occur in acute ulcerative colitis.
melena *(MEL-ē-na)*	Black tarry feces resulting from blood in the intestines. Common in newborns. May also be a sign of gastrointestinal bleeding.
obstipation *(ob-sti-PĀ-shun)*	Extreme constipation
pernicious anemia *(per-NISH-us)*	A form of anemia caused by failure of the stomach to secrete a substance (intrinsic factor) needed for the absorption of vitamin B_{12}
pilonidal cyst *(pī-lō-NĪ-dal)*	A dermal cyst in the region of the sacrum, usually at the top of the cleft between the buttocks. May become infected and begin to drain.
pylorospasm *(pī-LOR-ō-spazm)*	Spasmodic contraction of the pyloric opening

regurgitation *(rē-gur-ji-TĀ-shun)* — A backward flowing, such as the backflow of undigested food

Diagnosis and Treatment

appendectomy *(ap-en-DEK-tō-mē)* — Surgical removal of the appendix

Billroth's operations(s) — Gastrectomy with anastomosis of the stomach to the duodenum (Billroth I) or to the jejunum (Billroth II). Used for the treatment of peptic ulcers.

gavage *(ga-VAHZH)* — Process of feeding through a nasogastric tube into the stomach

Murphy's sign — Inability to take a deep breath when fingers are pressed firmly below the right arch of the ribs (below the liver). Signifies gallbladder disease.

nasogastric (NG) **tube** — Tube that is passed through the nose into the stomach (Fig. 12-10). May be used for emptying the stomach, administering medication, giving liquids, or sampling stomach contents.

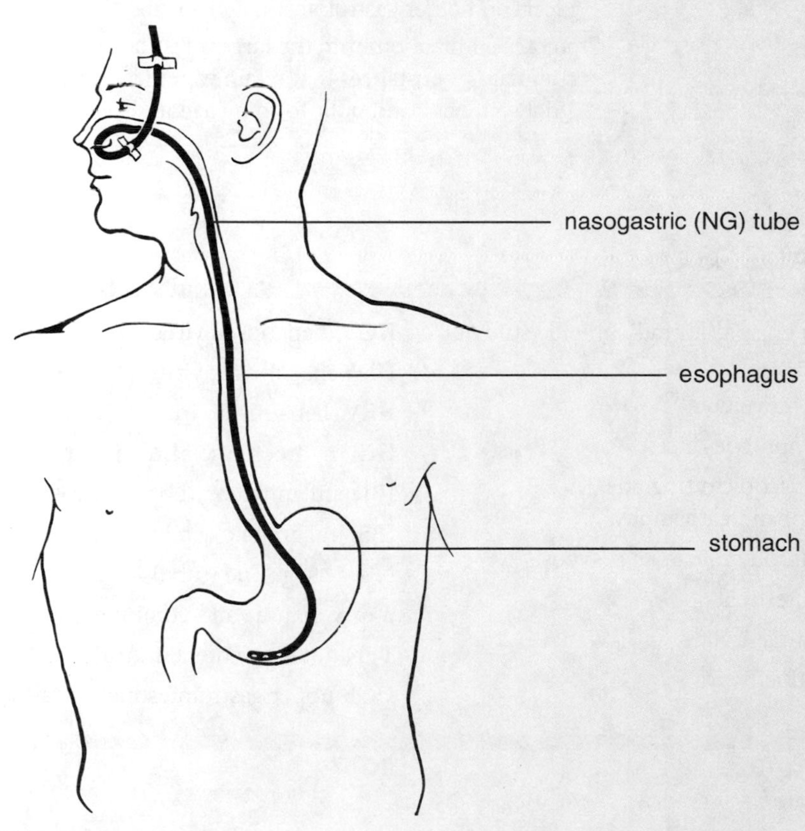

FIGURE 12-10. A nasogastric (NG) tube in place. (Scherer JC: Introductory Medical-Surgical Nursing, 5th ed, p 532. Philadelphia: JB Lippincott, 1991.)

(continued)

parenteral hyperalimentation Complete intravenous feeding for one who cannot take in food. Total parenteral nutrition (TPN).

vagotomy *(vā-GOT-ō-mē)* Interruption of impulses from the vagus nerve to reduce stomach secretions in the treatment of gastric ulcer. Originally done surgically, but may also be done with drugs.

Drugs

antidiarrheal *(an-ti-dī-a-RĒ-al)* Treats or prevents diarrhea by reducing intestinal motility or absorbing irritants and soothing the intestinal lining

antiemetic *(an-tē-e-MET-ik)* Agent that relieves or prevents nausea and vomiting

antispasmodic *(an-ti-spas-MOD-ik)* Agent that relieves spasm, usually of smooth muscle

emetic *(e-MET-ik)* An agent that causes vomiting

histamine H_2 antagonist Drug that decreases secretion of stomach acid by interfering with the action of histamine at H_2 receptors. Used to treat ulcers and other gastrointestinal problems.

laxative *(LAK-sa-tiv)* Promotes elimination from the large intestine. Types include stimulants, substances that retain water (hyperosmotics), stool softeners, and bulk-forming agents.

ABBREVIATIONS

BE barium enema (for radiographic study of the colon)

BM bowel movement

CBD common bile duct

ERCP endoscopic retrograde cholangiopancreatography

FAP familial adenomatous polyposis

GI gastrointestinal

HAV hepatitis A virus

HBV hepatitis B virus

HCV hepatitis C virus

HDV hepatitis D virus

HEV hepatitis E virus

HCl hydrochloric acid

IBD inflammatory bowel disease

IBS inflammatory bowel syndrome

NG nasogastric (tube)

n & v nausea and vomiting

TPN total parenteral nutrition

UGI upper gastrointestinal (x-ray series)

Chapter 12

Labeling Exercise

Write the name of each numbered part on the corresponding line of the answer sheet.

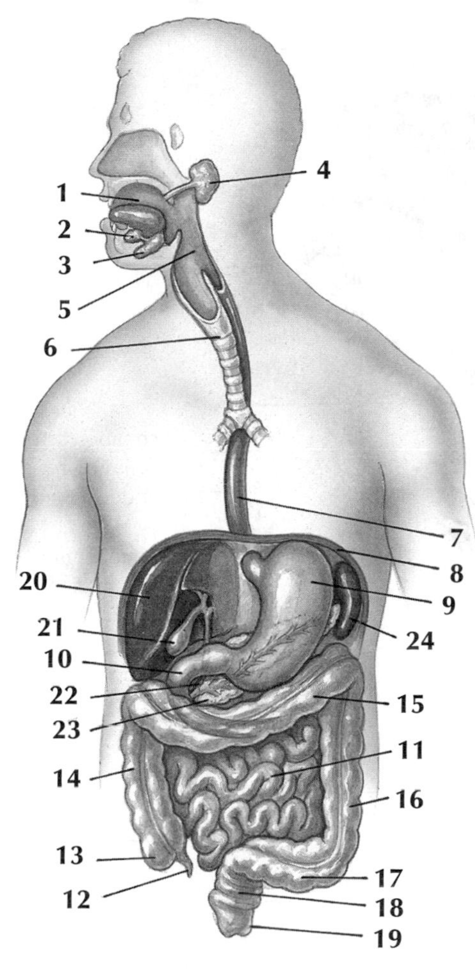

The digestive system

anus
ascending colon
cecum
common bile duct
descending colon
diaphragm
duodenum
esophagus
gall bladder
liver
oral cavity
pancreas
parotid gland
pharynx
rectum
sigmoid colon
small intestine
spleen
stomach
sublingual gland
submandibular gland
trachea
transverse colon
vermiform appendix

1. ____________________
2. ____________________
3. ____________________
4. ____________________
5. ____________________
6. ____________________
7. ____________________
8. ____________________
9. ____________________
10. ____________________
11. ____________________
12. ____________________
13. ____________________
14. ____________________
15. ____________________
16. ____________________
17. ____________________
18. ____________________
19. ____________________
20. ____________________
21. ____________________
22. ____________________
23. ____________________
24. ____________________

Write the name of each numbered part on the corresponding line of the answer sheet.

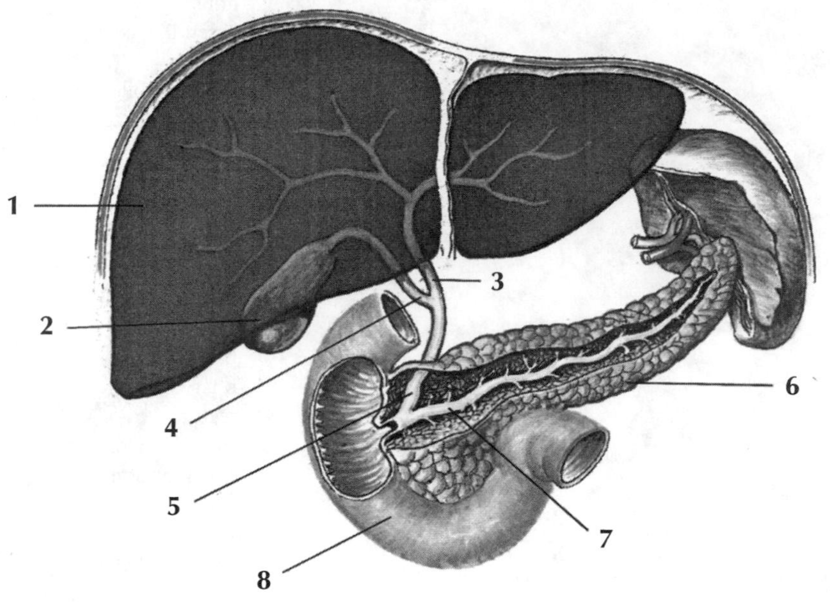

common bile duct
common hepatic duct
cystic duct
duodenum
gallbladder
liver
pancreas
pancreatic duct

Accessory organs of digestion

1. ______________________
2. ______________________
3. ______________________
4. ______________________
5. ______________________
6. ______________________
7. ______________________
8. ______________________

CHAPTER REVIEW 12-1

Matching. Match the words in each of the sets below with their definitions and write the appropriate letter (a–e) to the left of each number:

_____	1. sialolith	a. tooth decay
_____	2. gingiva	b. gum
_____	3. pylorus	c. distal opening of the stomach
_____	4. hypoglossal	d. salivary calculus
_____	5. caries	e. sublingual
_____	6. choledochal	a. jaundice

_____ 7. emesis	b. pertaining to the common bile duct
_____ 8. acholia	c. crushing of a biliary calculus
_____ 9. icterus	d. vomiting
_____ 10. cholelithotripsy	e. absence of bile

_____ 11. gastropathy	a. narrowing of the pylorus
_____ 12. pylorostenosis	b. feeding through a tube
_____ 13. gastrocele	c. hernia of the stomach
_____ 14. pylorospasm	d. any disease of the stomach
_____ 15. gavage	e. contraction of the pylorus

_____ 16. cecopexy	a. inflammation of the cecum
_____ 17. protocele	b. hernia of the rectum
_____ 18. cecitis	c. surgical fixation of the cecum
_____ 19. proctorrhaphy	d. surgical puncture of the colon
_____ 20. colocentesis	e. surgical repair of the rectum

_____ 21. anorexia	a. liver disease
_____ 22. lithiasis	b. chewing
_____ 23. deglutition	c. condition of having stones
_____ 24. cirrhosis	d. swallowing
_____ 25. mastication	e. loss of appetite

Fill in the blanks:

26. The palatine tonsils are located on either side of the ____________________.
27. Dentin is the main substance of the ____________________.
28. From its name you might guess that the buccinator muscle is in the ____________________.
29. An enterotoxin is a bacterial poison produced in or acting on the ____________________.
30. Wavelike contractions of organ walls, such as the contractions that move material through the digestive tract, is called ____________________.
31. The blind pouch at the beginning of the colon is the ____________________.
32. The anticoagulant heparin is found throughout the body, but it is named for its presence in the ____________________.
33. The substance cholesterol is named for its chemical composition (sterol) and for its presence in ____________________.
34. The organ that produces bile is the ____________________.
35. The organ that stores bile is the ____________________.

True-False. Examine each of the following statements. If the statement is true, write T in the first blank. If the statement is false, write F in the first blank and correct the statement by replacing the underlined word in the second blank.

36. The term *hypogastric* means below the stomach. ____ ____________
37. The first portion of the small intestine is the jejunum. ____ ____________
38. Aphagia is an inability to sleep. ____ ____________
39. The term *gnathic* pertains to the jaw. ____ ____________
40. Cheiloplasty is plastic repair of the tongue. ____ ____________
41. The common hepatic duct and the cystic duct merge to form the common bile duct. ____ ____________
42. Enteropathy is any disease of the esophagus. ____ ____________
43. The hepatic portal system carries blood to the spleen. ____ ____________

Word building. Write a word for each of the following definitions:

44. A dentist who specializes in straightening of the teeth is a(n) ____________
45. Narrowing (-stenosis) of a salivary duct ____________
46. Pain in the stomach ____________
47. Inflammation of the pancreas ____________
48. Pertaining to the ileum and cecum ____________
49. Suture of the cecum ____________
50. Surgical creation of a passage between the stomach and the duodenum ____________
51. Surgical creation of an opening into the colon ____________
52. Inflammation of the ileum ____________

Plurals. Write the plural form of each of the following words:

53. diverticulum ____________
54. gingiva ____________
55. calculus ____________
56. anastomosis ____________

Word analysis. Define each of the following words and give the meaning of the word parts in each. Use a dicitionary if necessary.

57. Myenteric *(mī-en-TER-ik)* ____________

____

a. my/o ____________________

b. enter/o ____________________

c. -ic ____________________

58. Cholecystectomy ____

____

a. chol/e ____________________

b. cyst/o ____________________

c. ec- ____________________

d. -tomy ____________________

59. Diarrhea ____

____

a. dia- ____________________

b. -rhea ____________________

CHAPTER REVIEW 12-2

Matching. Match the words in each of the sets below with their definitions and write the appropriate letter (a–e) to the left of each number:

_____ 1. agnathia — a. excision of gum tissue

_____ 2. gingivectomy — b. x-ray of the salivary ducts

_____ 3. anastomosis — c. absence of the jaw

_____ 4. perioral — d. around the mouth

_____ 5. sialogram — e. passage between two organs

_____ 6. cholemia — a. presence of bile in the blood

_____ 7. cholemesis — b. dilatation of bile ducts

_____ 8. cholestasis — c. x-ray study of bile ducts

_____ 9. cholangiectasis — d. stoppage of bile flow

_____ 10. cholangiography — e. vomiting of bile

_____ 11. hepatopexy — a. tumor of the liver

_____ 12. hepatectomy — b. excision of the liver

_____ 13. hepatotropic — c. enlargement of the liver

_____ 14. hepatoma — d. acting on the liver

_____ 15. hepatomegaly — e. surgical fixation of the liver

_____ 16. regurgitation — a. pertaining to gastric juices

_____ 17. diverticulum	b. pouch or sac in the lining of an organ
_____ 18. sphincter	c. ring of muscle that regulates a body opening
_____ 19. bolus	d. backward flow
_____ 20. peptic	e. a mass

Fill in the blanks:

21. The large membrane that lines the abdominal cavity and supports the abdominal organs is the _____________________.
22. The word *dentition* refers to the number and arrangement of the _____________________.
23. The hormone gastrin, which is active in digestion, is so named because it is produced in the _____________________.
24. The pigment bilirubin is named for its presence in _____________________.
25. A hepatocyte is a cell found in the _____________________.
26. Appendicitis is inflammation of the _____________________.
27. The distal opening of the stomach is the _____________________.
28. The part of the large intestine between the descending colon and the rectum is the _____________________.
29. The cystic duct carries bile to and from the _____________________.
30. The word *polysialia* means excessive secretion of _____________________.
31. The epigastrium is the region of the abdomen above the _____________________.

Word building. Write a word that fits each of the following definitions:

32. Surgical repair of the palate _____________________
33. Hernia of the rectum _____________________
34. Surgical creation of a passage between the common bile duct and the duodenum _____________________
35. Specialist who treats diseases of the stomach and intestine _____________________
36. Surgical removal of the cecum _____________________
37. Inflammation of the esophagus _____________________

Write the meaning of the following abbreviations:

38. HCl _____________________
39. TPN _____________________
40. HBV _____________________

41. ERCP ____________________

42. GI ____________________

Unscrambles. Form a word from each of the following groups of letters and write it in the blank.

43. eippct ____________________

44. auluv ____________________

45. chntrpies ____________________

46. hsrisroic ____________________

47. noetirumpe ____________________

Word analysis. Define each of the following words and give the meaning of the word parts in each. Use a dictionary if necessary.

48. Dysentery *(DIS-en-ter-ē)* ____________________

____

a. dys- ____________________

b. enter/o ____________________

c. -y ____________________

49. Parenteral *(par-EN-ter-al)* ____________________

____

a. par(a)- ____________________

b. enter/o ____________________

c. -al - ____________________

Chapter 12

Case Studies

1. Cholecystectomy

This 57-year-old female entered the hospital with nausea and vomiting, temperature of 100.5°F, and continuous pain in the right upper quadrant of the abdomen. Examination revealed rebound tenderness in the RUQ with a positive Murphy's sign. Her skin, nails, and conjunctivae were yellowish and she complained of clay-colored stools. Leukocyte count was 16,000. Ultrasonography indicated cholelithiasis.

A cholecystectomy was performed with ligation of the cystic duct. Bile ducts were free of stones. Postop treatment included respiratory therapy, IM meperidine prn for pain, an antiemetic IM, and IV fluid therapy. The NG tube, which had been inserted preoperatively, was removed on the second postop day.

The patient was discharged, without complications, 1 week after surgery. Instruction pertaining to diet, activity level, and possible adverse reactions were given, and the patient understood them well. She was to make an appointment with her physician for postoperative care.

2. Surgical Pathology Report

Gross Description: The specimen is received in formalin labeled "ruptured duodenal diverticula" and consists of a segment of enteric tissue measuring approximately 6.3 cm × 2.8 cm × 0.7 cm. The serosal surface is markedly dull in appearance and fibrotic. The mucosal surface is hemorrhagic. Representative sections are taken for microscopic examination.

Microscopic Description: Sectioned slide shows segments of duodenal tissues with areas of gangrenous change in the bowel wall with acute and chronic inflammatory cell infiltrates. There are chronic and focal acute inflammatory cell infiltrates with hemorrhage in the mesenteric fatty tissue. There are areas of acute inflammatory exudate noted in the fatty tissue. Histopathologic changes are consistent with ruptured duodenal diverticula.

3. Colonoscopy With Biopsy

The fiberoptic colonoscope was passed with minimal difficulty to the distal right colon-cecum region. Random biopsies of the distal right colon and sigmoid colon were obtained. There was no evidence of swelling or ulceration in any region of the colon. A colon secretion was aspirated for bacteriologic study.

This patient had been complaining of abdominal pain within 2 hours after a meal. There was also a change in bowel movements. A previous proctosigmoidoscopy showed some irregularities in the sigmoid and rectal region.

A tentative diagnosis of irritable bowel syndrome was made. The patient was placed on a lactose-free, low residue diet. Imodium was prescribed to reduce intestinal motility.

Chapter 12
Case Study Questions

Multiple Choice. Select the best answer and write the letter of your choice to the left of each number.

_____ 1. The conjunctivae are membranes located in the

a. eyes
b. nose
c. mouth
d. vagina
e. rectum

_____ 2. The average leukocyte count (per cubic millimeter) is

a. 100–200
b. 15,000–20,000
c. 5,000–10,000
d. 1,000–2,000
e. 50,000–100,000

_____ 3. Enteric tissue is found in the

a. gallbladder
b. stomach
c. esophagus
d. liver
e. intestine

_____ 4. The mucosal surface of a digestive organ is the

a. outer surface
b. medulla
c. cortex
d. inner surface
e. central opening

_____ 5. Diverticula are

a. small pouches in the wall of the colon
b. communications between two organs
c. ducts in the liver
d. intestinal obstructions
e. polyps in the intestine

_____ 6. Murphy's sign is tested for

a. under the ribs on the left
b. near the spleen
c. in the lower right abdomen
d. under the ribs on the right
e. in the lower left abdomen

_____ 7. A tentative diagnosis is

a. preliminary
b. final
c. partial
d. definitive
e. complete

Give the meaning of the following abbreviations:

8. NG _______________
9. RUQ _______________
10. IM _______________
11. postop _______________
12. cm _______________

Give the word in the case studies that means each of the following:

13. Pertaining to the first part of the small intestine _______________
14. Pertaining to the membrane that supports the intestine _______________
15. Localized _______________
16. Fluid that escapes from blood vessels as a result of inflammation _______________
17. Withdrawn by suction _______________

Define the following words:

18. antiemetic _______________
19. cholelithiasis _______________
20. motility _______________
21. chronic _______________

DIGESTION

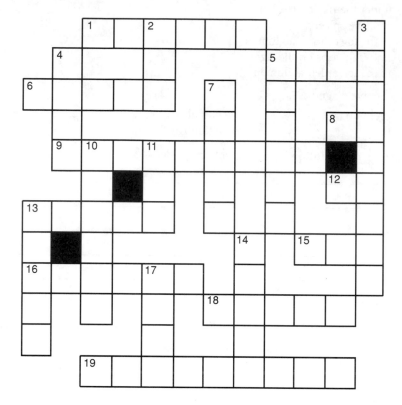

ACROSS

1. root (with combining vowel): liver
5. pertaining to the mouth
6. organ that secretes bile
8. mouth; body opening
9. the tube that carries food from the pharynx to the stomach
12. pertaining to the stomach and intestine (abbr.)
13. the major portion of the large intestine
15. prefix: one
16. a type of tooth
18. the terminal portion of the small intestine
19. root: gallbladder

DOWN

2. prefix: through
3. inflammation of the tongue
4. fluid that aids in the digestion and absorption of fats
5. describing blood that may appear in the stool as a result of intestinal bleeding
7. root (with combining vowel): eat; ingest
10. enlargement of the spleen: _____ megaly
11. prefix: all
13. a blind pouch at the beginning of the large intestine
14. acute abdominal pain
17. tube that is passed into the stomach: _____ gastric tube

Chapter 12 Answer Section

Answers to Chapter Exercises

Exercise 12-1

1. oral *(OR-al)*; stomal *(STŌ-mal)*
2. dental *(DEN-tal)*
3. gingival *(JIN-ji-val)*
4. lingual *(LING-gwal)*; glossal *(GLOS-sal)*
5. buccal *(BUK-kal)*
6. labial *(LĀ-bē-al)*
7. jaw
8. tongue
9. mouth
10. salivary
11. teeth
12. lip
13. mouth
14. pertaining to the mouth and tongue
15. suture of the palate
16. excision of gum tissue
17. pertaining to the lips and teeth
18. inflammation of the mouth

Exercise 12-2

1. enteric *(en-TER-ik)*
2. gastric *(GAS-trik)*
3. colic *(KOL-ik)*; also colonic *(kō-LON-ik)*
4. pyloric *(pī-LOR-ik)*
5. epigastric *(ep-i-GAS-trik)*
6. duodenal *(dū-ō-DĒ-nal)*
7. cecal *(SĒ-kal)*
8. jejunal *(je-JUN-al)*
9. ileal *(IL-ē-al)*; also ileac *(IL-ē-ak)*
10. rectal *(REK-tal)*
11. anal *(Ā-nal)*
12. gasrectomy *(gas-TREK-tō-mē)*
13. esophagoplasty *(e-sof-a-gō-PLAS-tē)*
14. ileitis *(il-ē-Ī-tis)*
15. duodenostomy *(dū-ō-de-NOS-tō-mē)*
16. ileostomy *(il-ē-OS-tō-mē)*
17. gastroenterology *(gas-trō-en-ter-OL-ō-jē)*
18. colitis *(kō-LĪ-tis)*
19. colopexy *(KŌ-lō-pek-sē)*
20. colostomy *(kō-LOS-tō-mē)*
21. colonopathy *(kō-lō-NOP-a-thē)*
22. colonoscopy *(kō-lon-OS-kō-pē)*
23. esophagogastrostomy *(e-sof-a-gō-gas-TROS-tō-mē)*
24. gastroenterostomy *(gas-trō-en-ter-OS-tō-mē)*
25. gastrojejunostomy *(gas-trō-je-jū-NOS-tō-mē)*
26. duodenoileostomy *(dū-ō-dē-nō-il-ē-OS-tō-mē)*
27. sigmoidoproctostomy *(sig-moy-dō-prok-TOS-tō-mē)*

Exercise 12-3

1. hepatic *(he-PAT-ik)*
2. cholecystic *(kō-lē-SIS-tik)*
3. pancreatic *(pan-krē-AT-ik)*
4. cholangiography *(kō-lan-jē-OG-ra-fē)*
5. hepatography *(hep-a-TOG-ra-fē)*
6. cholecystography *(kō-lē-sis-TOG-ra-fē)*
7. pancreatography *(pan-krē-a-TOG-ra-fē)*
8. choledocholithiasis *(kō-led-o-kō-li-THI-a-sis)*
9. pancreatolithiasis *(pan-krē-a-tō-li-THĪ-a-sis)*
10. bile
11. common bile duct
12. liver
13. hepatitis
14. pancreas
15. bile duct

Labeling Exercise

Digestive System

1. oral cavity
2. sublingual gland
3. submandibular gland
4. parotid gland
5. pharynx
6. trachea
7. esophagus
8. diaphragm
9. stomach
10. duodenum
11. small intestine
12. vermiform appendix
13. cecum
14. ascending colon
15. transverse colon
16. descending colon
17. sigmoid colon
18. rectum
19. anus
20. liver
21. gallbladder
22. common bile duct
23. pancreas
24. spleen

Accessory Organs of Digestion

1. liver
2. gallbladder
3. common hepatic duct
4. cystic duct
5. common bile duct
6. pancreas
7. pancreatic duct
8. duodenum

Chapter Review 12-1

1. d
2. b
3. c
4. e
5. a
6. b
7. d
8. e
9. a
10. c
11. d
12. a
13. c
14. e
15. b
16. c
17. b
18. a
19. e
20. d
21. e
22. c
23. d
24. a
25. b
26. palate
27. teeth
28. cheek
29. intestine
30. peristalsis
31. cecum
32. liver
33. bile
34. liver
35. gallbladder
36. T
37. F duodenum
38. F eat
39. T
40. F lip
41. T
42. F intestine
43. liver
44. orthodontist
45. sialostenosis
46. gastralgia
47. pancreatitis
48. ileocecal
49. cecorrhaphy
50. gastroduodenostomy
51. colostomy
52. ileitis
53. diverticula
54. gingivae
55. calculi
56. anastomoses
57. Pertaining to the muscular coat of the intestine
    a. muscle
    b. intestine
    c. pertaining to

58. Surgical removal of the gallbladder
    a. gall, bile
    b. bladder
    d. out
    e. to cut
59. Frequent passage of watery bowel movements
    a. through
    b. discharge, flow

Chapter Review 12-2

1. c
2. a
3. e
4. d
5. b
6. a
7. e
8. d
9. b
10. c
11. e
12. b
13. d
14. a
15. c
16. d
17. b
18. c
19. e
20. a
21. peritoneum
22. teeth
23. stomach
24. bile
25. liver
26. appendix
27. pylorus
28. sigmoid colon
29. gallbladder
30. saliva
31. stomach
32. palatorrhaphy
33. rectocele; proctocele
34. choledochoduodenostomy
35. gastroenterologist
36. cecectomy *(sē-SEK-tō-mē)*
37. esophagitis
38. hydrochloric acid
39. total parenteral nutrition
40. hepatitis B virus
41. endoscopic retrograde cholangiopancreatography
42. gastrointestinal
43. peptic
44. uvula
45. sphincter
46. cirrhosis
47. peritoneum
48. A general term for inflammatory disease of the intestinal tract, especially of the colon
    a. painful or difficult
    b. intestine
    c. condition of
49. Referring to any route other than the alimentary canal
    a. beside
    b. intestine
    c. pertaining to

Answers to Case Study Questions

1. a
2. c
3. e
4. d
5. a
6. d
7. a
8. nasogastric
9. right upper quadrant
10. intramuscular(ly)
11. postoperative
12. centimeter
13. duodenal
14. mesenteric
15. focal
16. exudate
17. aspirated
18. agent that relieves or prevents nausea and vomiting
19. condition of having gallstones
20. movement
21. occurring over a long period of time

Answers to Crossword Puzzle

DIGESTION

		1 H	E	2 P	A	T	O				3 G
	4 B			E				5 O	R	A	L
6 L	I	V	E	R		7 P		C			O
	L					H		C		8 O	S
	9 E	10 S	O	11 P	H	A	G	U	S	■	S
		P	■	A		G		L		12 G	I
13 C	O	L	O	N		O		T			T
E	■	E					14 C		15 U	N	I
16 C	A	N	I	17 N	E		O				S
U		O		A		18 I	L	E	U	M	
M				S			I				
		19 C	H	O	L	E	C	Y	S	T	

13 The Urinary System

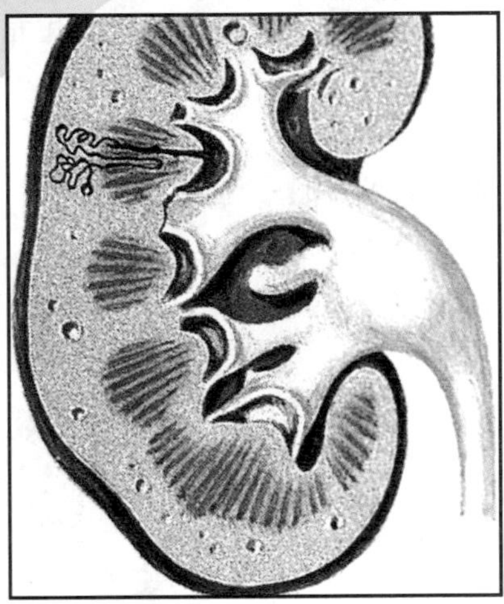

Chapter Contents

Objectives

After study of this chapter you should be able to:

1. Label a diagram of the urinary tract and follow the flow of urine through the body
2. Label a diagram of the kidney
3. Identify the portions of the nephron and explain how each functions in urine formation
4. Explain the relationship between the kidney and the blood circulation
5. Identify and use the roots pertaining to the urinary system
6. Describe the major disorders of the urinary system
7. Define medical terms commonly used in reference to the urinary system.
8. Interpret abbreviations used in reference to the urinary system
9. Analyze several case studies pertaining to urinary disorders

The urinary system consists of two kidneys, two ureters, the urinary bladder, and a urethra (Fig. 13-1). This system forms and eliminates urine, which contains metabolic waste products., The kidneys, the organs of excretion, also regulate the composition, volume, and acid–base balance (pH) of body fluids. Thus they are of critical importance in maintaining the state of internal balance known as homeostasis. In addition, they produce two substances that act on the circulatory system. **Erythropoietin** (EPO) is a hormone that stimulates the production of red blood cells in the bone marrow. **Renin** is an enzyme that functions to raise blood pressure. It does so by activating a blood component called **angiotensin**, which causes constriction of the blood vessels. The drugs known as ACE inhibitors (angiotensin converting enzyme inhibitors) lower blood pressure by interfering with the production of angiotensin.

The Kidneys

The **kidneys** are located behind the peritoneum in the lumbar region. On the top of each kidney rests an adrenal gland. Each kidney is encased in a capsule of fibrous connective tissue

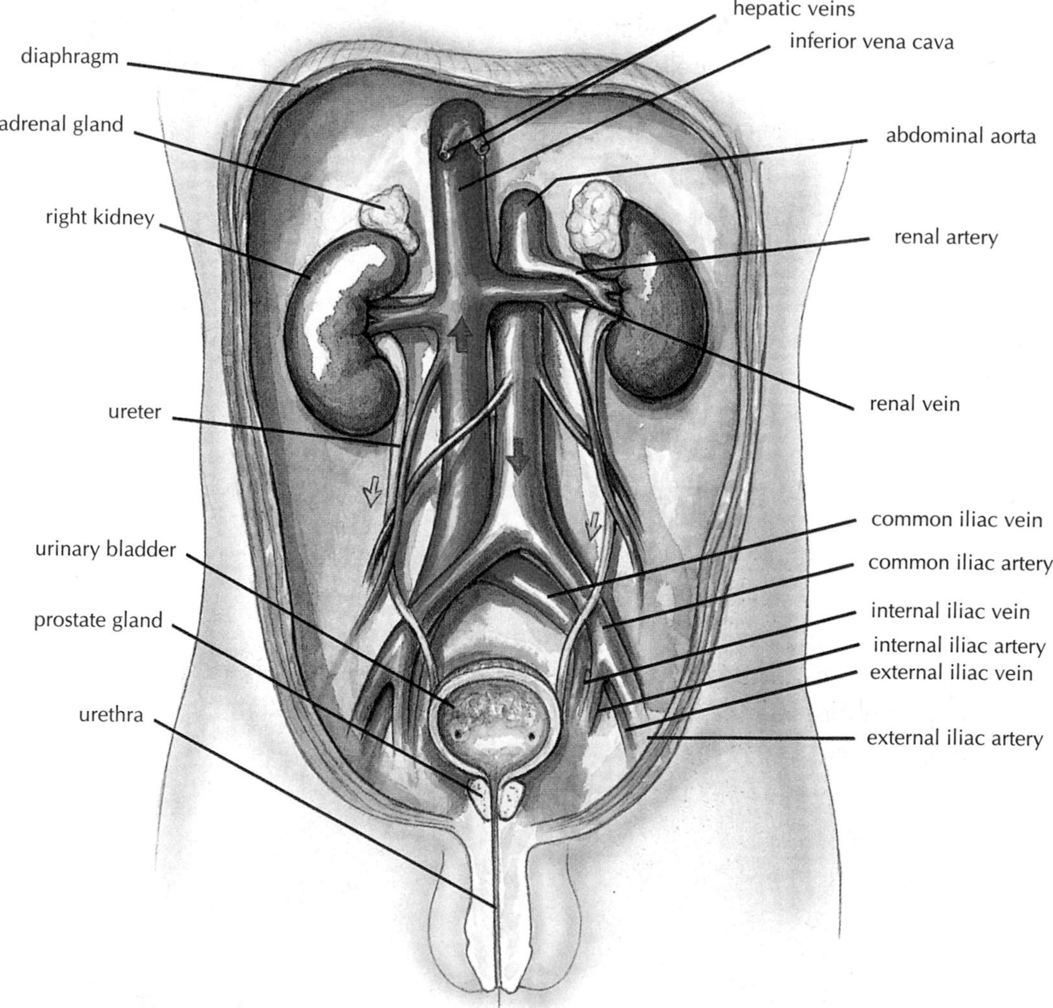

FIGURE 13-1. Male urinary system, with blood vessels.

overlaid with fat. An outermost layer of connective tissue supports the kidney and anchors it to the body wall.

If you look inside the kidney you can see that it has an outer region, the **cortex**, and an inner region, the **medulla** (Fig. 13-2). The medulla is divided into triangular sections called **pyramids**. The pyramids have a lined appearance because they are made up of the loops and collecting tubules of the nephrons, the functional units of the kidney. Each collecting tubule empties into a urine collecting area called a **calyx** (from the Latin word meaning *cup*). Several of these smaller minor calyces merge to form a major calyx. The major calyces then unite to form the **renal pelvis**, the main collecting area for urine.

The Nephrons

The tiny working units of the kidneys are the **nephrons** (Fig. 13-3). Each of these microscopic structures is basically a single tubule coiled and folded into various shapes. At the beginning of the tubule is the cup-shaped **Bowman's capsule** which is part of the blood-filtering device of the nephron. The tubule then folds into the **proximal convoluted tubule**, straightens out to form the **loop of Henle**, coils again into the **distal convoluted tubule**, and then finally straightens out to form a **collecting tubule**.

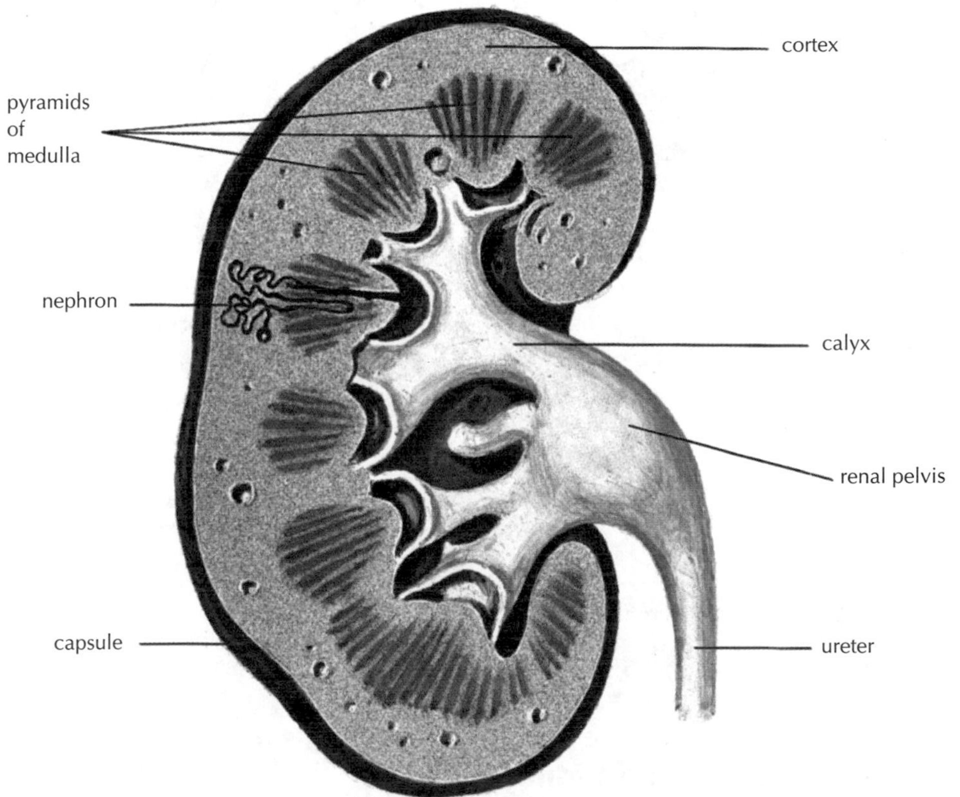

FIGURE 13-2. Longitudinal section through the kidney showing its internal structure and a much enlarged diagram of a nephron. There are more than 1 million nephrons in each kidney.

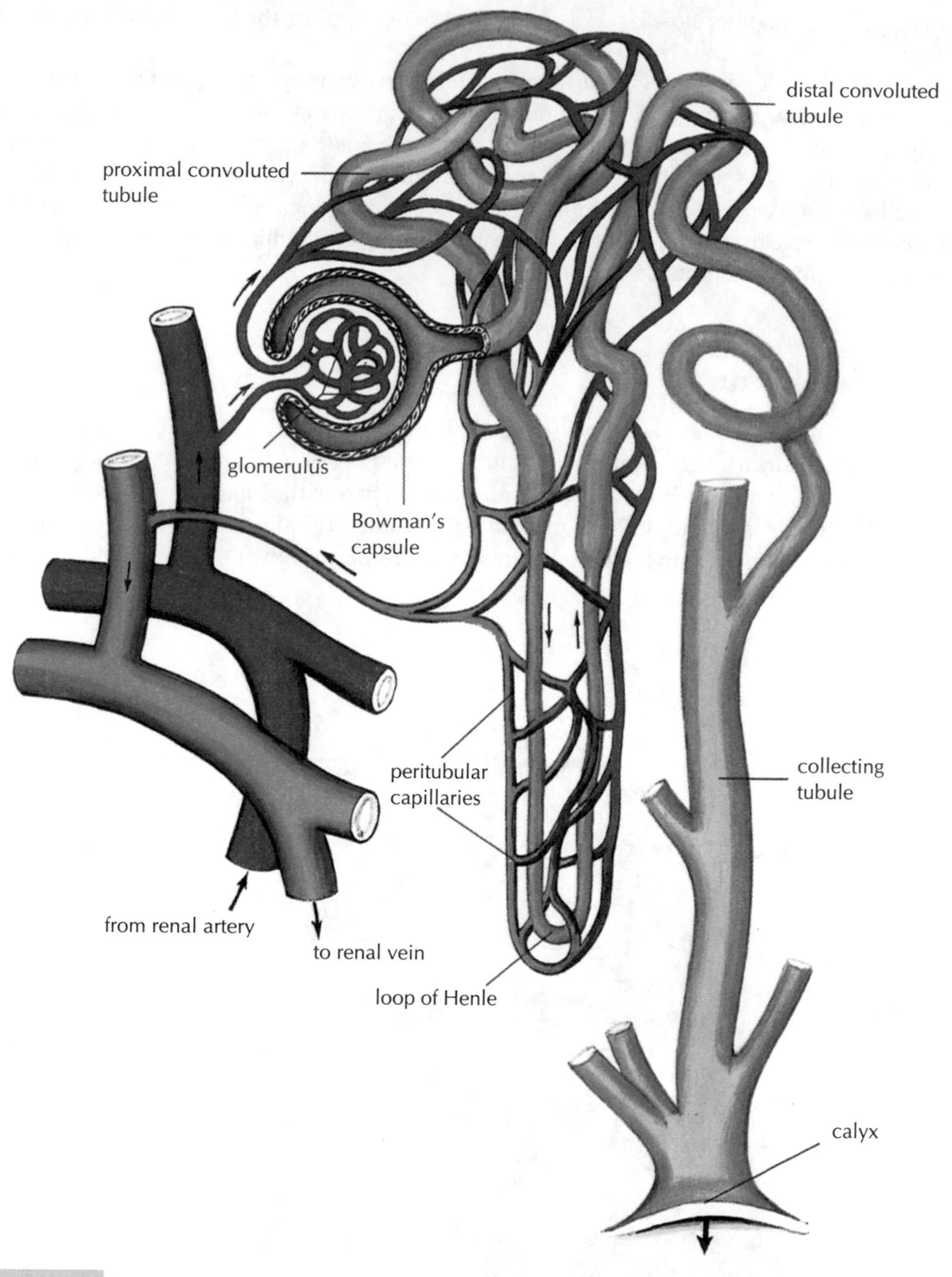

FIGURE 13-3. Simplified nephron.

Blood Supply to the Kidney

Blood enters the kidney through a renal artery, a short branch of the abdominal aorta. This vessel subdivides into smaller vessels as it branches throughout the kidney tissue until, finally, blood is brought into Bowman's capsule and circulated through a cluster of capillaries called a **glomerulus** within the capsule.

Urine Formation

As blood flows through the glomerulus, blood pressure forces materials through the glomerular wall and through the wall of Bowman's capsule into the nephron. The fluid that enters the nephron, the **glomerular filtrate**, consists mainly of water, electrolytes, soluble wastes, nutrients, and toxins. It should not contain any cells or proteins, such as albumin. The waste material and the toxins must be eliminated, but most of the water, electrolytes, and nutrients must be returned to the blood or we would rapidly starve and dehydrate. This return process, termed **tubular reabsorption**, occurs through the peritubular capillaries that surround the nephron. As the filtrate flows through the nephron, other processes further regulate its composition and pH. The concentration of the filtrate is also adjusted under the effects of the pituitary hormone **ADH** (antidiuretic hormone). Finally, the filtrate, now called **urine**, flows into the collecting tubules to be eliminated.

Blood leaves the kidney by a series of vessels that finally merge to form the renal vein, which empties into the inferior vena cava.

Removal of Urine

Urine is drained from the renal pelvis and carried by the **ureter** to the **urinary bladder** (Fig. 13-4). Urine is stored in the bladder until fullness stimulates a reflex contraction of the bladder muscle and expulsion of urine through the **urethra**. The female urethra is short (4 cm; 1.5 in) and carries only urine. The male urethra is longer (20 cm; 8 in) and carries both urine and semen.

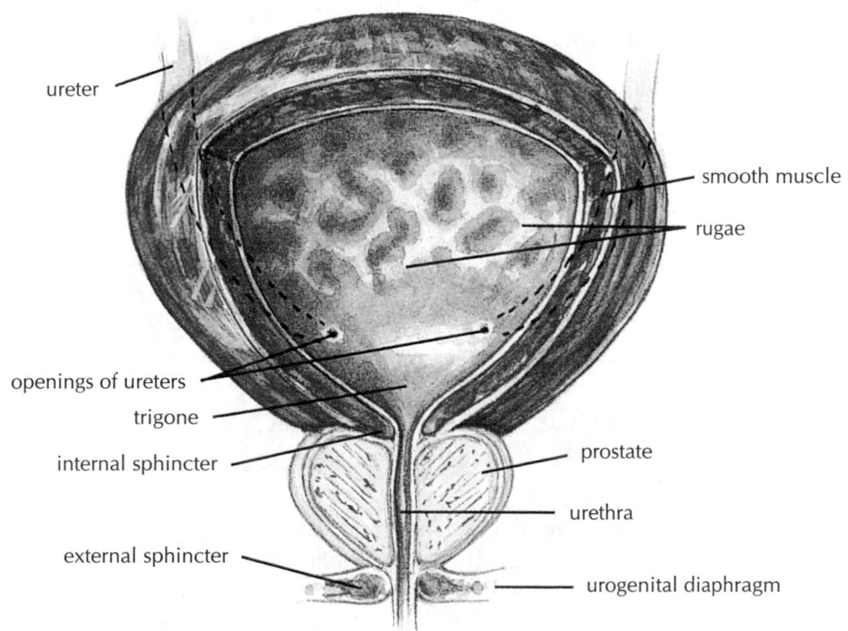

FIGURE 13-4. Interior of the urinary bladder, shown in the male. The trigone is a triangle in the floor of the bladder marked by the openings of the ureters and the urethra.

The voiding (release) of urine, technically called **urination** or **micturition**, is regulated by two sphincters (circular muscles) that surround the urethra. The upper sphincter, just below the bladder, functions involuntarily; the lower sphincter is under conscious control.

KEY TERMS

Normal Structure and Function

ADH	A hormone released from the pituitary gland that causes reabsorption of water in the kidneys, thus concentrating the urine; antidiuretic *(an-ti-dī-ū-RET-ik)* hormone
angiotensin *(an-jē-ō-TEN-sin)*	A substance that raises blood pressure; activated in the blood by renin, an enzyme produced by the kidneys
Bowman's capsule	The cup-shaped structure at the beginning of the nephron that surrounds the glomerulus
calyx *(KĀ-liks)*	A cuplike cavity in the pelvis of the kidney; also calix (pl. calyces) (root cali, calic)
erythropoietin (EPO) *(e-rith-rō-POY-e-tin)*	A hormone produced by the kidneys that stimulates red blood cell production
glomerular filtration	The passage of fluid and dissolved materials from the blood into the nephron
glomerulus *(glō-MER-ū-lus)*	The cluster of capillaries within Bowman's capsule (pl. glomeruli) (root glomerul/o)
kidney	An organ of excretion (root ren/o, nephr/o)
micturition *(mik-tū-RISH-un)*	The voiding of urine; urination
nephron *(NEF-ron)*	A microscopic functional unit of the kidney
renal cortex	The outer portion of the kidney
renal medulla *(me-DUL-la)*	The inner portion of the kidney
renal pelvis	The expanded upper end of the ureter that receives urine from the kidney (root pyel/o)
renal pyramid *(PIR-a-mid)*	A triangular structure in the medulla of the kidney composed of the loops and collecting tubules of the nephrons
renal tubule	The tubular portion of the nephron
renin *(RĒ-nin)*	An enzyme produced by the kidneys that activates angiotensin in the blood
tubular reabsorption	The return of substances from the glomerular filtrate to the blood through the peritubular capillaries
urea *(ū-RĒ-a)*	The main nitrogen waste product in the urine
ureter *(Ū-rē-ter)*	The tube that carries urine from the kidney to the bladder (root ureter/o)

urethra
(*ū-RĒ-thra*)
The tube that carries urine from the bladder to the outside (root urethr/o)

urinary bladder
Organ organ that stores and eliminates urine excreted by the kidneys (root cyst/o, vesic/o)

urine
The fluid excreted by the kidneys. It consists of water, electrolytes, urea, other metabolic wastes, and pigment. A variety of other substances may appear in urine in cases of disease. (root ur/o)

Roots Pertaining to the Urinary System

Roots for the Kidney

Root	Meaning	Example	Definition of Example
ren/o	kidney	renal *RĒ-nal*	pertaining to the kidney
nephr/o	kidney	nephritis *nef-RĪ-tis*	inflammation of the kidney
glomerul/o	glomerulus	juxtaglomerular *juks-ta-glō-MER-ū-lar*	near the glomerulus
pyel/o	renal pelvis	pyelectasis *pi-e-LEK-ta-sis*	dilatation of the renal pelvis
cali-, calic-	calyx	caliceal *kal-i-SĒ-al*	pertaining to a calyx

Exercise 13-1

Use the root *ren/o* to write a word that means:

1. Between the kidneys ___interrenal___
2. Above (supra-) the kidney ______
3. Behind (post-) the kidney ______
4. Around the kidneys ______
5. Near (para-) the kidney ______

Use the root *nephr/o* to write a word that means:

6. Any disease of the kidney ______
7. Surgical removal of the kidney ______
8. Any noninflammatory disease condition (-sis) of the kidney ______

9. Softening of the kidney ______
10. Study of the kidney ______

Use the appropriate root to write a word that means each of the following:

11. Radiograph of the renal pelvis ______
12. Plastic repair of the renal pelvis ______
13. Dilatation of the renal calyx ______
14. Inflammation of a glomerulus ______
15. Hardening of a glomerulus ______
16. Radiographic study (-graphy) of the kidney ______
17. Inflammation of the renal pelvis and kidney ______

Roots for the Urinary Tract (Except the Kidney)

Root	Meaning	Example	Definition of Example
ur/o	urine, urinary tract	oliguria *ol-i-GŪ-rē-a*	excretion of a decreased amount of urine
urin/o	urine	urination *ū-ri-NĀ-shun*	discharge of urine
ureter/o	ureter	hydroureter *hi-drō-ū-RĒ-ter*	distention of the ureter with fluid
cyst/o	urinary bladder	cystostomy *sis-TOS-tō-mē*	surgical creation of an opening into the bladder
vesic/o	urinary bladder	vesical *VES-i-kal*	pertaining to the urinary bladder
urethr/o	urethra	urethrotome *ū-RĒ-thrō-tōm*	instrument for incising the urethra

Exercise 13-2

Use the root *ur/o* to write a word that means:

1. A urinary calculus ______
2. Radiography of the urinary tract ______
3. Presence of urinary waste products in the blood (-emia) ______
4. Study of the urinary tract ______

The root *ur/o-* is used in the suffix *-uria* which means "condition of urine or of urination." Use *-uria* for words with the following meanings:

5. Presence of proteins in the urine ______proteinurea______
6. Painful or difficult urination ____________
7. Urination during the night (noct/i) ____________
8. Lack of urine ____________
9. Presence of pus in the urine ____________
10. Presence of blood (hemat/o) in the urine ____________
11. Presence of cells in the urine ____________

The suffix *-uresis* means "urination." Use *-uresis* to write words with the following meanings:

12. Increased excretion of urine ______diuresis______
13. Lack of urination ____________
14. Excretion of sodium (natri-) in the urine ____________
15. Excretion of potassium (kali-) in the urine ____________

The adjective endings for the above words is *-uretic* as in *diuretic* (pertaining to diuresis) and *natriuretic* (pertaining to the excretion of sodium in the urine).

Fill in the blanks:

16. Urinalysis *(ū-ri-NAL-i-sis)* is the laboratory study of ____________.
17. Ureterostenosis *(ū-rē-ter-ō-ste-NŌ-sis)* is narrowing of the ____________.
18. Urethroscopy *(ū-rē-THROS-kō-pē)* is endoscopic examination of the ____________.
19. The word *cystic (SIS-tik)* pertains to the ____________.
20. *Intravesical (in-tra-VES-i-kal)* means within the ____________.

Using the appropriate root, write a word for each of the following definitions:

21. A ureteral stone ____________
22. Surgical creation of an opening in the ureter ____________
23. Surgical fixation of the urethra ____________
24. Inflammation of the urethra ____________

Use the root *cyst/o* for the next four words:

25. Inflammation of the urinary bladder ____________
26. Surgical fixation of the urinary bladder ____________

27. An instrument for examining the inside of the bladder (also used for removing foreign objects, surgery, and other forms of treatment) ____________

28. Hernia of the bladder ____________

Use the root *vesic/o* for the next two words:

29. In front of (pre-) the bladder ____________

30. Pertaining to the urethra and bladder ____________

Define the following terms:

31. ureterotomy
(*ū-rē-ter-OT-ō-mē*) ____________

32. uropoiesis
(*ū-rō-poy-Ē-sis*) ____________

33. cystalgia
(*sis-TAL-jē-a*) ____________

34. cystotomy
(*sis-TOT-ō-mē*) ____________

35. transurethral
(*trans-ū-RĒ-thral*) ____________

Clinical Aspects of the Urinary System

Infections

Organisms that infect the urinary tract generally enter through the urethra and ascend toward the bladder. Infection of the urinary bladder produces **cystitis**. The infecting organisms are usually colon bacteria carried in feces. Cystitis is more common in females than in males because the female urethra is shorter than the male urethra and the opening is closer to the anus. Poor toilet habits and **urinary stasis** are contributing factors. In the hospital, urinary tract infections may complicate **catheterization** for the withdrawal of urine from the bladder (Fig. 13-5).

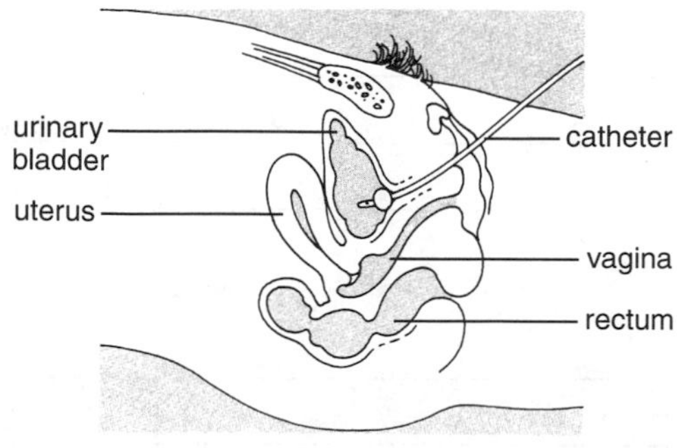

FIGURE 13-5. An indwelling (Foley) catheter in place in the female bladder. (Taylor C, Lillis CA, LeMone P: Fundamentals of Nursing, 2nd ed, p 871. Philadelphia: JB Lippincott, 1993.)

An infection that involves the kidney and renal pelvis is termed **pyelonephritis**. As in cystitis, signs of this condition include **dysuria**, painful or difficult urination, and the presence of bacteria and pus in the urine, **bacteriuria** and **pyuria** respectively.

Urethritis is inflammation of the urethra, generally associated with sexually transmitted diseases such as gonorrhea and chlamydia infections (Chapter 14).

Glomerulonephritis

Although the name simply means inflammation of the kidney and glomeruli, **glomerulonephritis** is a specific disorder that follows an immunologic reaction. It is usually a response to infection in another system, commonly a streptococcal infection of the respiratory tract. It may also accompany autoimmune diseases such as lupus erythematosus. The symptoms are hypertension, edema, and **oliguria**, the passage of small amounts of urine. This urine is highly concentrated. Because of damage to kidney tissue, blood and proteins escape into the nephrons causing **hematuria**, blood in the urine, and **proteinuria**, protein in the urine. Blood cells may also form into small molds of the kidney tubule called **casts** which can be found in the urine.

Glomerulonephritis is one of the most common causes of **chronic renal failure** (CRF), or end-stage renal disease (ESRD), in which urea and other nitrogen-containing compounds accumulate in the blood, a condition termed **uremia**. These compounds affect the central nervous system, causing irritability, loss of appetite, stupor, and other symptoms. There is also electrolyte imbalance and **acidosis**.

Acute Renal Failure

Injury, shock, exposure to toxins, infections, and other renal disorders may cause damage to the nephrons, resulting in **acute renal failure** (ARF). There is rapid loss of kidney function with oliguria and accumulation of nitrogen wastes in the blood. Failure of the kidneys to eliminate potassium leads to **hyperkalemia**, along with other electrolyte imbalances and acidosis. When there is destruction (necrosis) of kidney tubules the condition may be referred to as **acute tubular necrosis** (ATN).

Renal failure may lead to a need for kidney **dialysis** or kidney **transplantation**. Dialysis refers to the movement of substances across a semipermeable membrane. In **hemodialysis**, blood is cleansed by passage over a membrane surrounded by fluid (dialysate) that draws out unwanted substances. In **peritoneal dialysis**, fluid is introduced into the peritoneal cavity. The fluid is periodically withdrawn along with waste products and replaced. The exchange may be done at intervals throughout the day in **continuous ambulatory peritoneal dialysis** (CAPD) or during night in **continuous cyclic peritoneal dialysis** (CCPD).

Urinary Stones

Urinary lithiasis (condition of having stones) may be related to infection, irritation, diet, or hormone imbalances that lead to increased calcium in the blood. Most urinary stones, or calculi, are formed of calcium salts, but they may be composed of other materials as well. The stones generally form in the kidney and may move to the bladder. This results in great pain, termed **renal colic**, and obstruction that can promote infection and cause **hydronephrosis** (collection of urine in the renal pelvis). Because they are radiopaque, stones can usually be seen on simple x-rays of the abdomen. Stones may dissolve and pass out of the body on their own. If not, they may be removed surgically, in a **lithotomy**, or by using an endoscope. External shock waves are used to crush stones in the urinary tract in a procedure called extracorporeal (outside the body) shock wave **lithotripsy** (crushing of stones).

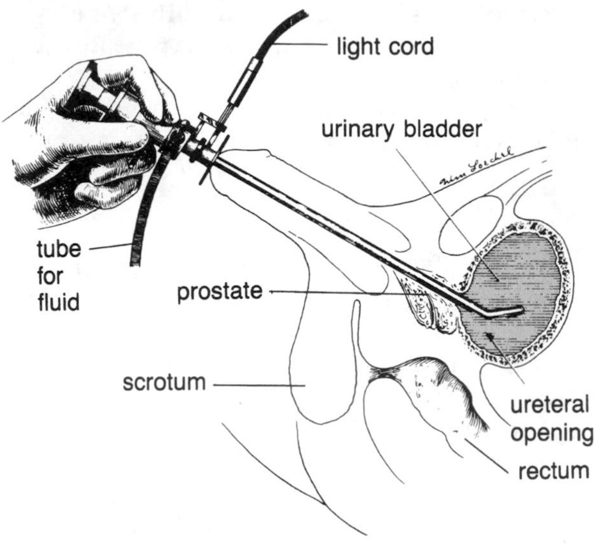

FIGURE 13-6. Cystoscopy. A lighted cystoscope is introduced into the bladder of a male. Sterile fluid is used to wash the bladder and improve visualization. (Smeltzer SC, Bare BG: Brunner and Suddarth's Textbook of Medical-Surgical Nursing, 7th ed, p 1143. Philadelphia: JB Lippincott, 1992.)

Cancer

Carcinoma of the bladder has been linked to occupational exposure to chemicals, parasitic infections, and cigarette smoking. A key symptom is sudden, painless hematuria. Often the cancer can be seen by viewing the lining of the bladder with a **cystoscope** (Fig. 13-6). This instrument can also be used to biopsy tissue for study. If treatment is not effective in permanently removing the tumor a **cystectomy** (removal of the bladder) may be necessary. In this case, the ureters must be vented elsewhere, such as directly to the surface of the body, through the ileum in an **ileal conduit** (Fig. 13-7), or to some other portion of the intestine.

Cancer may also involve the kidney and renal pelvis. Additional means for diagnosing cancer and other disorders of the urinary tract include ultrasound, CT scans, and radiographic studies: **intravenous urography** and **retrograde pyelography**.

Urinalysis

Urinalysis (UA) is a simple and widely used method for diagnosing disorders of the urinary tract. It may also reveal disturbances in other systems when abnormal byproducts are eliminated in the

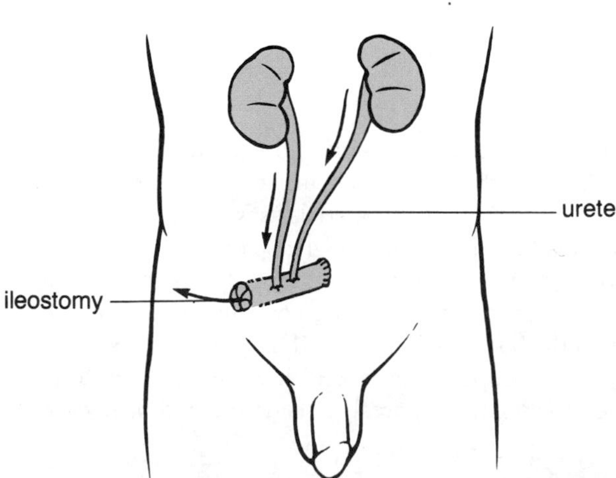

FIGURE 13-7. Ileal conduit. (Smeltzer SC, Bare BG: Brunner and Suddarth's Textbook of Medical-Surgical Nursing, 7th ed, p 1209. Philadelphia: JB Lippincott, 1992.)

urine. In a routine urinalysis, the urine is grossly examined for color and turbidity (a sign of bacteria); **specific gravity** (a measure of concentration) and pH are recorded; chemical components, such as glucose, ketones, and hemoglobin are tested for; and the urine is examined microscopically for cells, crystals, or casts. In more detailed tests, drugs, enzymes, hormones, and other metabolites may be analyzed and bacterial cultures may be done.

KEY CLINICAL TERMS

Disorders

acidosis *(as-i-DŌ-sis)*	Excessive acidity of body fluids
bacteriuria *(bak-tē-rē-Ū-rē-a)*	Presence of bacteria in the urine
cast	A solid mold of a renal tubule found in the urine
cystitis *(sis-TĪ-tis)*	Inflammation of the urinary bladder, usually as a result of infection
dysuria *(dis-Ū-rē-a)*	Painful or difficult urination
glomerulonephritis *(glō-mer-ū-lō-nef-RĪ-tis)*	Inflammation of the kidney primarily involving the glomeruli. The acute form usually follows an infection elsewhere in the body; the chronic form varies in cause and usually leads to renal failure.
hematuria *(hē-mat-Ū-rē-a)*	Presence of blood in the urine
hydronephrosis *(hī-drō-nef-RŌ-sis)*	Collection of urine in the renal pelvis due to obstruction; causes distention and atrophy of renal tissue. Also called nephrohydrosis or nephrydrosis.
hyperkalemia *(hī-per-ka-LĒ-mē-a)*	Excess amount of potassium in the blood
oliguria *(ol-ig-Ū-rē-a)*	Elimination of small amounts of urine
peritoneal dialysis	Removal of unwanted substances from the body by introduction of a dialyzing fluid into the peritoneal cavity, followed by its removal
proteinuria *(prō-tē-NŪ-rē-ā)*	Presence of protein, mainly albumin, in the urine
pyelonephritis *(pī-e-lō-ne-FRĪ-tis)*	Inflammation of the renal pelvis and kidney, usually as a result of infection
pyuria *(pī-Ū-rē-a)*	Presence of pus in the urine
renal colic *(KOL-ik)*	Radiating pain in the region of the kidney associated with the passage of a stone
uremia *(ū-RĒ-mē-a)*	Presence in the blood of toxic levels of nitrogen-containing substances, mainly urea, as a result of renal insufficiency

(continued)

urethritis (*ū-rē-THRĪ-tis*) — Inflammation of the urethra, usually as a result of infection

urinary stasis (*STĀ-sis*) — Stoppage or stagnation of the flow of urine

Diagnosis and Treatment

catherization (*kath-e-ter-i-ZĀ-shun*) — Introduction of a tube into a passage, such as through the urethra into the bladder for withdrawal or urine

hemodialysis (*hē-mō-dī-AL-i-sis*) — Removal of unwanted substances from the blood by passage through a semipermeable membrane; used to substitute for kidney function when these organs are impaired or missing

intravenous pyelography (IVP) — Intravenous urography

intravenous urography (IVU) — Radiographic visualization of the urinary tract after intravenous administration of a contrast medium that is excreted in the urine; also called excretory urography or intravenous pyelography, although the latter is less accurate because the procedure shows more than just the renal pelvis

lithotripsy (*LITH-ō-trip-sē*) — Crushing of a stone

retrograde pyelography — Pyelography in which the contrast medium is injected into the kidneys from below, by way of the ureters

specific gravity (SG) — The weight of a substance compared with the weight of an equal volume of water. The specific gravity of normal urine ranges from 1.015–1.025. This value may increase or decrease in disease.

urinalysis (*ū-ri-NAL-i-sis*) — Laboratory study of the urine. Physical and chemical properties and microscopic appearance are included.

Surgery

cystectomy (*sis-TEK-tō-mē*) — Surgical removal of all or part of the urinary bladder

ileal conduit (*IL-ē-al KON-dū-it*) — Diversion of urine by connection of the ureters to an isolated segment of the ileum. One end of the segment is sealed and the other drains through an opening in the abdominal wall.

lithotomy (*lith-OT-ō-mē*) — Incision of an organ to remove a stone (calculus)

renal transplantation — Surgical implantation of a donor kidney into a patient

ADDITIONAL TERMS

Normal Structure and Function

aldosterone *(al-DOS-ter-ōn)*	A hormone secreted by the adrenal gland that regulates electrolyte excretion by the kidneys
clearance	The volume of plasma that can be cleared of a substance by the kidneys per unit of time; renal plasma clearance
creatinine *(krē-AT-in-in)*	A nitrogen-containing by-product of muscle metabolism. An increase in creatinine in the blood is a sign of renal failure.
detrusor muscle *(dē-TRŪ-sor)*	The muscle in the bladder wall
diuresis *(dī-ū-RĒ-sis)*	Increased excretion of urine
glomerular filtration rate (GFR)	The amount of filtrate formed per minute by the nephrons of both kidneys
maximal transport capacity (Tm)	The maximum amount of a given substance that can be reabsorbed from the renal tubule
renal corpuscle *(KOR-pus-l)*	Bowman's capsule and the glomerulus considered as a unit; the filtration device of the kidney
trigone *(TRĪ-gōn)*	A triangle at the base of the bladder formed by the openings of the two ureters and the urethra (see Figure 13-4)

Symptoms and Conditions

anuresis *(an-ū-RĒ-sis)*	Lack of urination
anuria *(an-Ū-re-a)*	Lack of urine formation
azotemia *(az-ō-TĒ-mē-a)*	Presence of an increased amount of nitrogen waste, especially urea, in the blood
azoturia *(az-ō-TŪ-rē-a)*	Presence of an increased amount of nitrogen-containing compounds, especially urea, in the urine
cystocele *(SIS-tō-sēl)*	Herniation of the bladder into the vagina (see Figure 14-12); vesicocele
dehydration *(dē-hī-DRĀ-shun)*	Excessive loss of body fluids
diabetes insipidus *(dī-a-BĒ-tēz in-SIP-id-us)*	A condition caused by inadequate production of antidiuretic hormone resulting in excessive excretion of dilute urine and extreme thirst
enuresis *(en-ū-RĒ-sis)*	Involuntary urination, usually at night; bed-wetting
epispadias *(ep-i-SPĀ-dē-as)*	A congenital condition in which the urethra opens on the dorsal surface of the penis as a groove or cleft; anaspadias.

(continued)

glycosuria *(glī-kō-SŪ-rē-a)* — Presence of glucose in the urine, as in cases of diabetes mellitus

horseshoe kidney — A congenital union of the lower poles of the kidneys, resulting in a horseshoe-shaped organ

hydroureter *(hī-drō-ū-RĒ-ter)* — Distention of the ureter with urine due to obstruction

hypoproteinemia *(hī-pō-prō-tē-NĒ-mē-a)* — Decreased amount of protein in the blood; may result from loss of protein due to kidney damage

hypospadias *(hī-pō-SPĀ-dē-as)* — A congenital condition in which the urethra opens on the undersurface of the penis or into the vagina (Fig. 13-8)

hypovolemia *(hī-pō-vō-LĒ-mē-a)* — A decrease in blood volume

incontinence *(in-KON-tin-ens)* — Inability to retain urine (also semen or feces)

neurogenic bladder *(nū-rō-JEN-ik)* — Any bladder dysfunction that results from a central nervous system lesion

nocturia *(nok-TŪ-rē-a)* — Excessive urination at night (noct/o means *night*)

pitting edema — Edema in which the skin, when pressed firmly with the finger, will maintain the depression produced

polycystic kidney disease — A hereditary condition in which the kidneys are enlarged and contain many cysts

polydipsia *(pol-i-DIP-sē-a)* — Excessive thirst

polyuria *(pol-ē-Ū-rē-a)* — Elimination of large amounts of urine, as in diabetes mellitus

retention of urine — Accumulation of urine in the bladder due to inability to urinate

staghorn calculus — A kidney stone that fills the renal pelvis and calyces to give a "staghorn" appearance

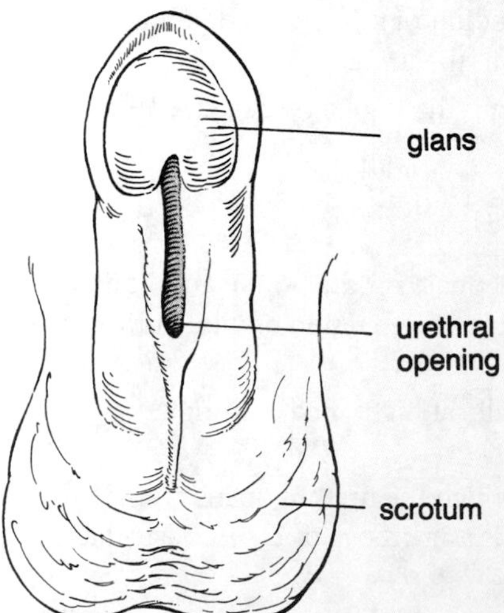

FIGURE 13-8. Hypospadias. Ventral view of penis.

ureterocele *(ū-RĒ-ter-ō-sēl)* — A cystlike dilation of the ureter near its opening into the bladder. Usually results from a congenital narrowing of the ureteral opening.

urinary frequency — A need to urinate often without an increase in average output

urinary urgency — Sudden need to urinate

water intoxication — Excess retention of water and sodium

Wilms tumor — A malignant tumor of the kidney that usually appears in children before the age of 5

Diagnosis

anion gap — A measure of electrolyte imbalance

blood urea nitrogen (BUN) — Nitrogen in the blood in the form of urea. An increase in BUN indicates an increase in nitrogen waste products in the blood and renal failure.

clean-catch specimen — A urine sample obtained after thorough cleansing of the urethral opening and collected in midstream to minimize the chance of contamination

protein electrophoresis (PEP) — Laboratory study of the proteins in urine; used to diagnose multiple myeloma, systemic lupus erythematosus, lymphoid tumor

urinometer *(ū-ri-NOM-e-ter)* — Device for measuring the specific gravity of urine

Treatment

diuretic *(dī-ū-RET-ik)* — A substance that increases the excretion of urine; pertaining to diuresis

indwelling (Foley) catheter — A urinary tract catheter with a balloon at one end that prevents the catheter from leaving the bladder (see Figure 13-5)

lithotrite *(LITH-ō-trīt)* — Instrument for crushing a bladder stone

ABBREVIATIONS

ADH antidiuretic hormone

ARF acute renal failure

ATN acute tubular necrosis

BUN blood urea nitrogen

CAPD continuous ambulatory peritoneal dialysis

CCPD continuous cyclic peritoneal dialysis

CRF chronic renal failure

EPO erythropoietin

ESRD end-stage renal disease

ESWL extracorporeal shock wave lithotripsy

GFR glomerular filtration rate

GU genitourinary

IVP intravenous pyleography

IVU intravenous urography

K potassium

KUB kidney-ureter-bladder (radiography)

Na sodium

PEP protein electrophoresis

SG specific gravity

Tm maximal transport capacity

UA urinalysis

Chapter 13
Labeling Exercise

Write the name of each numbered part on the corresponding line of the answer sheet.

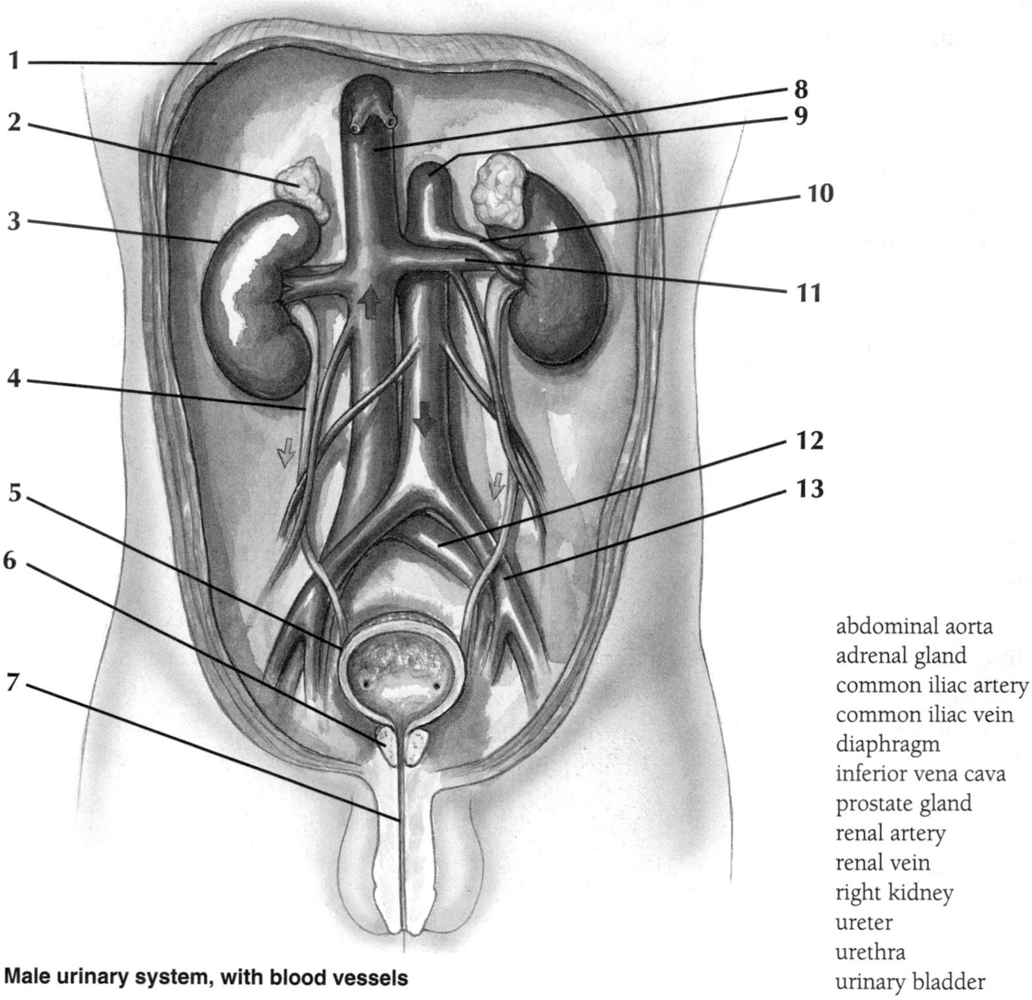

Male urinary system, with blood vessels

abdominal aorta
adrenal gland
common iliac artery
common iliac vein
diaphragm
inferior vena cava
prostate gland
renal artery
renal vein
right kidney
ureter
urethra
urinary bladder

1. ______________________
2. ______________________
3. ______________________
4. ______________________
5. ______________________
6. ______________________
7. ______________________
8. ______________________
9. ______________________
10. ______________________
11. ______________________
12. ______________________
13. ______________________

Write the name of each numbered part on the corresponding line of the answer sheet.

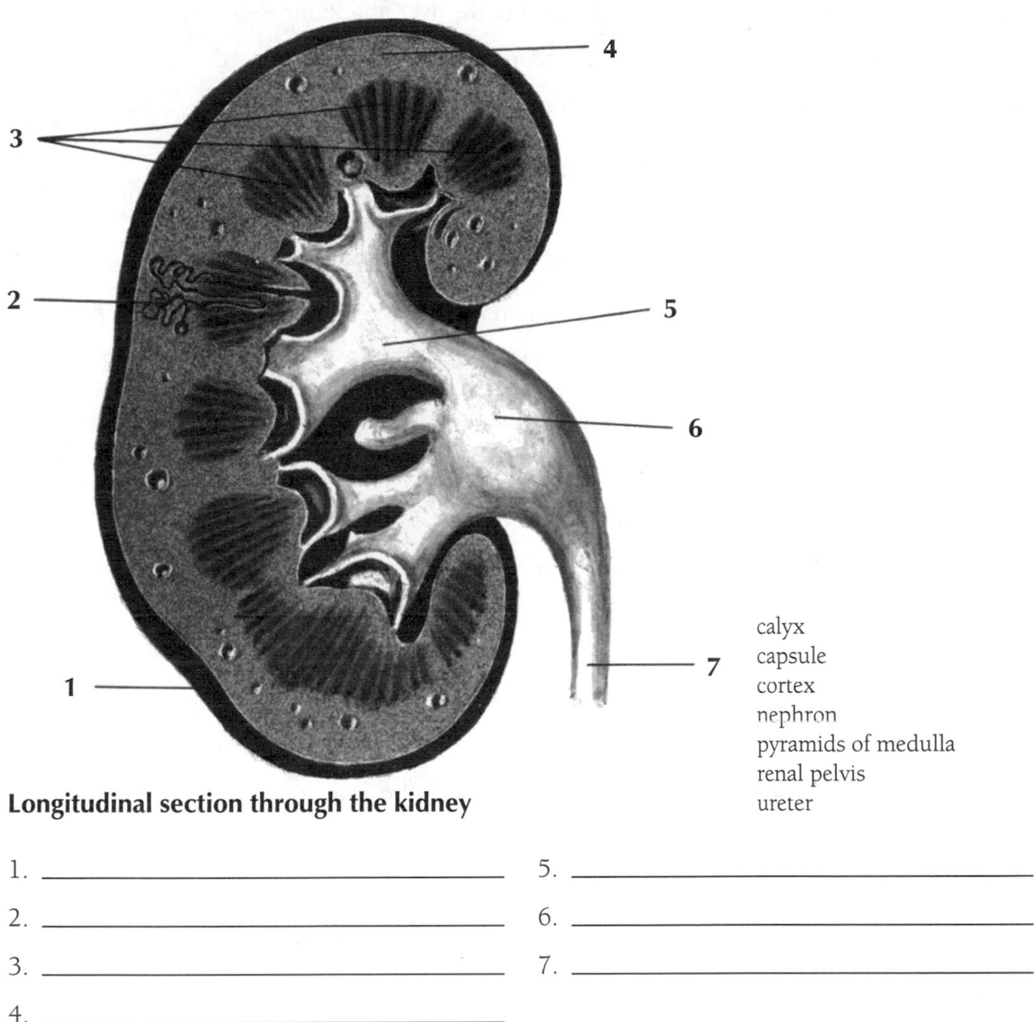

Longitudinal section through the kidney

calyx
capsule
cortex
nephron
pyramids of medulla
renal pelvis
ureter

1. ______________________
2. ______________________
3. ______________________
4. ______________________
5. ______________________
6. ______________________
7. ______________________

CHAPTER REVIEW 13-1

Matching. Match the words in each of the sets below with their definitions and write the appropriate letter (a–e) to the left of each number:

_____	1. albuminuria	a. abnormal color of urine
_____	2. amyluria	b. starch in the urine
_____	3. chromaturia	c. excessive urine formation
_____	4. polyuria	d. blood in the urine
_____	5. hematuria	e. proteinuria

_____	6. adrenal	a. pertaining to the blood vessels of the kidneys
_____	7. intrarenal	b. within the kidneys
_____	8. prerenal	c. pertaining to the liver and kidneys
_____	9. renovascular	d. before or in front of the kidneys
_____	10. hepatorenal	e. near the kidney

_____	11. micturition	a. congenital absence of the bladder
_____	12. cystocele	b. urination
_____	13. acystia	c. instrument for incising the bladder
_____	14. cystotome	d. abnormal opening of the urethra
_____	15. hypospadias	e. hernia of the bladder

_____	16. polydipsia	a. inability to retain urine
_____	17. stasis	b. introduction of a tube
_____	18. incontinence	c. incision to remove a stone
_____	19. catheterization	d. excessive thirst
_____	20. lithotomy	e. stagnation, as of urine

Fill in the blanks:

21. A microscopic working unit of the kidney is called a(n) ______________________.
22. The cluster of capillaries within Bowman's capsule is the ______________________.
23. The outer portion of the kidney is the ______________________.
24. Laboratory study of the urine is a(n) ______________________.
25. The tube that carries urine from the kidney to the bladder is the ______________________.

Definitions. Write the meaning of each of the following words:

26. Reniform *(REN-i-form)* ______________________
27. Nephrotropic *(nef-rō-TROP-ik)* ______________________
28. Juxtaglomerular *(juks-ta-glō-MER-ū-lar)* ______________________
29. Cystitis *(sis-TĪ-tis)* ______________________
30. Calicectasis *(kal-i-SEK-ta-sis)* ______________________
31. Paraurethral *(par-a-ū-RĒ-thral)* ______________________

Word building. Write a word for each of the following definitions:

32. Any disease of the kidney (nephr/o) ______________________
33. Painful or difficult urination ______________________
34. X-ray of the bladder (cyst/o) and urethra ______________________

35. Incision of the bladder (cyst/o) ____________________
36. Inflammation of the urethra ____________________
37. Narrowing of the urethra ____________________
38. Inflammation of the renal pelvis and the kidney ____________________
39. Surgical removal of a kidney (nephr/o) ____________________
40. Plastic repair of the ureter ____________________

Write a word that means the opposite of each of the following:

41. hydration ____________________
42. hypovolemia ____________________
43. diuretic ____________________
44. hyperkalemia ____________________
45. uresis ____________________

Write the adjective form of each of the following words:

46. vesica (bladder) ____________________
47. urology ____________________
48. nephrosis ____________________
49. ureter ____________________
50. urethra ____________________

Write the plural form of each of the following words:

51. glomerulus ____________________
52. calyx ____________________
53. pelvis ____________________

CHAPTER REVIEW 13-2

Matching. Match the words in each of these sets with their definitions and write the appropriate letter (a–e) to the left of each number:

_____	1. melanuria	a. glucose in the urine
_____	2. azoturia	b. dark pigments in the urine
_____	3. uropoiesis	c. urination during the night
_____	4. glycosuria	d. formation of urine
_____	5. nocturia	e. increased nitrogen compounds in the urine
_____	6. kaliuresis	a. bed-wetting

_____ 7. pyuria — b. nitrogen waste in the blood

_____ 8. enuresis — c. deficiency of urine

_____ 9. uremia — d. presence of pus in the urine

_____ 10. uropenia — e. excretion of potassium in the urine

_____ 11. transurethral — a. ureteral calculus

_____ 12. hydroureter — b. distention of the ureter with fluid

_____ 13. urethrography — c. narrowing of the ureter

_____ 14. ureterolith — d. through the urethra

_____ 15. ureterostenosis — e. radiographic study of the urethra

_____ 16. renin — a. triangle in the base of the bladder

_____ 17. creatinine — b. bladder muscle

_____ 18. detrusor — c. nitrogen compound in blood and urine

_____ 19. erythropoietin — d. enzyme that raises blood pressure

_____ 20. trigone — e. hormone that increases red blood cell production

Fill in the blanks:

21. The main nitrogen waste product in urine is ____________________.
22. The medulla of the kidney is subdivided into triangular areas called ____________________.
23. Fully formed urine flows from a collecting tubule into a cup-shaped structure called a(n) ____________________.
24. A urocele is a swelling of the scrotum caused by escape of ____________________.
25. Natriuresis means the excretion of excess ____________________ in the urine.
26. A solid mold of the renal tubule found in the urine is a(n) ____________________.

Word building. Write a word for each of the following definitions:

27. Dilatation of the renal pelvis and calices (cali-) ____________________
28. Surgical creation of an opening into the urethra ____________________
29. Pertaining to the ureter and bladder (vesic/o) ____________________
30. Instrument for examining the inside of the bladder (cyst/o) ____________________
31. Surgical creation of an opening between a ureter and the sigmoid colon ____________________
32. Plastic repair of a ureter and renal pelvis ____________________
33. Surgical incision of the renal pelvis to remove a stone ____________________

Write the adjective form of each of the following words:

34. calyx ______________________

35. uremia ______________________

36. diuresis ______________________

37. nephritis ______________________

Unscrambles. Form a word from each of the following groups of letters and write it in the blank.

38. yaxlc ______________________

39. dsocaisi ______________________

40. radmiyp ______________________

41. hoennrp ______________________

Abbreviations. Write the meaning of the following abbreviations:

42. K ______________________

43. IVP ______________________

44. EPO ______________________

45. ADH ______________________

46. BUN ______________________

Word analysis. Define each of the following words and give the meaning of the word parts in each. Use a dictionary if necessary.

47. Diuresis ______________________

____

a. di(a)- ______________________

b. ur/o ______________________

c. -sis (condition of) ______________________

48. Ureteroneocystostomy (*ū-rē-ter-ō-nē-ō-sis-TOS-tō-mē*) ______________________

____

a. ureter/o ______________________

b. neo- ______________________

c. cyst/o ______________________

d. -stomy ______________________

49. Hemodialysis ______________________

____

a. hem/o ______________________

b. dia- ______________________

c. lysis ______________________

Chapter 13

Case Studies

1. Renal Calculi and Nephrolithotomy

This patient is a 48-year-old male with a history of urolithiasis. Three months prior to admission he developed recurrent urinary tract infections. An IV urogram showed a right staghorn calculus.

On admission, a renal ultrasound confirmed the diagnosis. A renal flow scan showed normal perfusion, no obstruction. Kidney function: 37% right; 63% left. The patient complains of some right flank discomfort, no hematuria, dysuria, frequency, nocturia.

On 3 June under local anesthesia, a cystoscopy was performed with placement of a right retrograde ureteral catheter. Following this, a right percutaneous nephrostomy tube was put into place. On 5 June under epidural anesthesia, a right percutaneous nephrolithotomy was performed. Most of the staghorn was removed from the renal pelvis, but there was stone remaining around the renal calices. Lithotripsy was planned to remove the remaining calculi.

2. End-stage Renal Disease With Suspected MI

This patient is a 55-year-old male on hemodialysis because of a history of end-stage renal disease. His complaint the day prior to this admission was chest pain and shortness of breath; therefore, he was admitted to rule out MI. Physical examination shows blood pressure 145/75. HEENT significant for arteriolar narrowing. Chest reveals lung rales. No CVA (costovertebral angle) tenderness. No clubbing, cyanosis, or edema. Hemoglobin 7.8; ABGs on admission: pH 7.40, $PACO_2$ 28, PAO_2 50, bicarbonate 16.

An MI was ruled out by enzymes and serial EKGs. Angina was probably due to anemia and disappeared after transfusion of two units packed red blood cells. Patient was volume overloaded on admission, requiring immediate hemodialysis. Subsequently, lungs were clear and supplemental oxygen was no longer needed.

He was discharged on a renal diet with Isordil 20 mg po q 8 h. He will be followed up at his regular hemodialysis center.

3. Cystourethroscopy for Stress Incontinence

Patient is a 42-year-old female who is being admitted for a total abdominal hysterectomy for suspected fibroids (benign uterine tumors). Suprapubic urethropexy is also scheduled to correct a long history of recurrent urinary stress incontinence. On admission, urethroscopy showed good bladder capacity and no evidence of urethritis. There was no evidence of cystocele or rectocele.

Intraoperative urethropexy: Urethroscope was inserted; bladder neck was identified for the surgeon and demarcated. The urethrovesical angles on both right and left sides were similarly demarcated after they had been identified by use of the urethroscope. Foley catheter was inserted and the bulb inflated. The surgeon placed nonabsorbable sutures at the level of the bladder neck on either side. These were transfixed to the conjoined tendon in the lower abdominal wall. After removing the Foley catheter, the urethroscope was again inserted. It was ascertained that the bladder neck was elevated by independent and then simultaneous traction on both sutures. It was also established that the sutures did not penetrate either the urethra or the bladder wall. The appropriate amount of traction necessary for closure of the urethrovesical angle was established. The urethroscope was removed; Foley catheter inserted for future filling of the bladder with normal saline solution.

Chapter 13
Case Study Questions

Multiple choice. Select the best answer and write the letter of your choice to the left of each number:

_____ 1. The term perfusion means

a. size
b. shape
c. surrounding tissue
d. passage of fluid
e. metabolism

_____ 2. Part of the system for collecting urine in the kidneys are the

a. calculi
b. calices
c. rales
d. staghorns
e. epidurals

_____ 3. A term that means distal enlargement of the fingers and toes is

a. obstruction
b. edema
c. clubbing
d. infarction
e. dialysis

_____ 4. Cystocele is

a. dropping of the bladder
b. hernia of the bladder
c. rupture of the uterus
d. ptosis of the kidney
e. inflammation of the bladder

_____ 5. The urethrovesical angle is between the

a. urethra and vagina
b. uterus and vagina
c. ureter and urethra
d. bladder and ureter
e. urethra and bladder

Write a word from the case histories that means each of the following:

6. A cystlike dilation of the ureter _____
7. A stone _____
8. Presence of blood in the urine _____
9. Urination during the night _____
10. Crushing of stones _____
11. Incision of the kidney to remove a stone _____
12. Inability to retain urine _____
13. Surgical fixation of the urethra _____
14. Performed during a surgical procedure _____
15. Instrument for examining the urethra _____

Write the meaning of the following words:

16. urogram _____
17. urolithiasis _____
18. cystoscopy _____
19. dysuria _____
20. suprapubic _____

URINARY SYSTEM

ACROSS

1. the outer region of the kidney or other organ
5. his name is given to the loop of the nephron
6. prefix: in, within
7. root: origin, formation
8. root (with combining vowel): urine, urinary tract
10. lack of urine formation
12. suffix: sugar
13. prefix: two, twice
16. excessive urine formation
19. prefix: two, twice
20. prefix: true, good, easy, normal
22. urinalysis (abbr.)
23. root (with combining vowel): urinary bladder
24. a measure of electrolyte imbalance: ______ gap

DOWN

1. a urine collecting area in the kidney
2. a triangle at the base of the bladder
3. suffix: surgical creation of an opening
4. the microscopic funtional unit of the kidney
6. involuntary urination, usually night; bed-wetting
9. by mouth: per ____
11. a pituitary hormone that serves to concentrate urine (abbr.)
14. root (with combining vowel): glucose, sugar
15. pertaining to urine
16. root: pus
17. the main nitrogen waste product in the urine
18. prefix: through
19. a measure of nitrogen in the blood (abbr.)
21. prefix: not

Chapter 13
Answer Section

Answers to Chapter Exercises

Exercise 13-1

1. interenal *(in-ter-RĒ-nal)*
2. suprarenal *(sū-pra-RĒ-nal)*
3. postrenal *(post-RĒ-nal)*
4. perirenal *(per-i-RĒ-nal)*; circumrenal *(sir-kum-RĒ-nal)*
5. pararenal *(par-a-RĒ-nal)*
6. nephropathy *(nef-ROP-a-thē)*
7. nephrectomy *(nef-REK-tō-mē)*
8. nephrosis *(nef-RŌ-sis)*
9. nephromalacia *(nef-rō-ma-LĀ-shē-a)*
10. nephrology *(ne-FROL-ō-jē)*
11. pyelogram *(PĪ-e-lō-gram)*
12. pyeloplasty *(PĪ-e-lo-plas-tē)*
13. calicectasis *(kal-i-SEK-ta-sis)*; caliectasis *(kal-ē-EK-ta-sis)*
14. glomerulitis *(glō-mer-ū-LĪ-tis)*
15. glomerulosclerosis *(glo-mer-ū-lō-skle-RŌ-sis)*
16. renography *(rē-NOG-ra-fē)*; nephrography *(nef-ROG-ra-fē)*
17. pyelitis *(pi-e-LĪ-tis)*

Exercise 13-2

1. urolith *(Ū-rō-lith)*
2. urography *(ū-ROG-ra-fē)*
3. uremia *(ū-RĒ-mē-a)*
4. urology *(ū-ROL-ō-jē)*
5. proteinuria *(prō-te-NŪ-rē-a)*
6. dysuria *(dis-Ū-rē-a)*
7. nocturia *(nok-TŪ-rē-a)*; also nycturia *(nik-TŪ-rē-a)*
8. anuria *(an-Ū-rē-a)*
9. pyuria *(pi-Ū-rē-a)*
10. hematuria *(hē-ma-TŪ-rē-a)*
11. cyturia *(si-TŪ-rē-a)*
12. diuresis *(di-ū-RĒ-sis)*
13. anuresis *(an-ū-RĒ-sis)*
14. natriuresis *(nā-trē-ū-RĒ-sis)*
15. kaliuresis *(kā-lē-ū-RĒ-sis)*
16. urine
17. ureter
18. urethra
19. urinary bladder (also gallbladder or cyst)
20. urinary bladder
21. ureterolith *(ū-RĒ-ter-ō-lith)*
22. ureterostomy *(ū-rē-ter-OS-tō-mē)*
23. urethropexy *(ū-RĒ-thrō-pek-sē)*
24. urethritis *(ū-rē-THRĪ-tis)*
25. cystitis (sis-TĪ-tis)
26. cystopexy *(SIS-tō-pek-sē)*
27. cystoscope *(SIS-tō-skōp)*
28. cystocele *(SIS-tō-sēl)*; also vesicocele *(VES-i-kō-sēl)*
29. prevesical *(prē-VES-i-kal)*
30. urethrovesical *(ū-rē-thrō-VES-i-kal)*
31. incision of the ureter
32. formation of urine
33. pain in the urinary bladder
34. incision of the urinary bladder
35. through the urethra

Labeling Exercise

Male Urinary System, With Blood Vessels

1. diaphragm
2. adrenal gland
3. right kidney
4. ureter
5. urinary bladder
6. prostate gland

7. urethra
8. inferior vena cava
9. abdominal aorta
10. renal artery
11. renal vein
12. common iliac vein
13. common iliac artery

Longitudinal Section Through the Kidney

1. capsule
2. nephron
3. pyramids of medulla
4. cortex
5. calyx
6. renal pelvis
7. ureter

Chapter Review 13-1

1. e
2. b
3. a
4. c
5. d
6. e
7. b
8. d
9. a
10. c
11. b
12. e
13. a
14. c
15. d
16. d
17. e
18. a
19. b
20. c
21. nephron
22. glomerulus
23. cortex
24. urinalysis
25. ureter
26. like or resembling a kidney
27. acting on the kidney
28. near the glomerulus
29. inflammation of the bladder
30. dilatation of the calices
31. near the urethra
32. nephropathy
33. dysuria
34. cystourethrogram
35. cystotomy
36. urethritis
37. urethrostenosis
38. pyelonephritis
39. nephrectomy
40. ureteroplasty
41. dehydration
42. hypervolemia
43. antidiuretic
44. hypokalemia
45. anuresis
46. vesical
47. urologic
48. nephrotic
49. ureteral
50. urethral
51. glomeruli
52. calyces
53. pelves

Chapter Review 13-2

1. b
2. e
3. d
4. a
5. c
6. e
7. d
8. a
9. b
10. c
11. d
12. b
13. e
14. a
15. c
16. d
17. c
18. b
19. e
20. a
21. urea
22. pyramids
23. calyx
24. urine

25. sodium
26. cast
27. pyelocaliectasis
28. urethrostomy
29. ureterovesical
30. cystoscope
31. ureterosigmoidostomy
32. ureteropyeloplasty
33. pyelolithotomy
34. caliceal
35. uremic
36. diuretic
37. nephritic
38. calyx
39. acidosis
40. pyramid
41. nephron
42. potassium
43. intravenous pyelography
44. erythropoietin
45. antididuretic hormone
46. blood urea nitrogen
47. Increased excretion of urine
    a. through
    b.urine
    c. condition of
48. Surgical creation of a new passage between a ureter and the bladder
    a. ureter
    b. new
    c. bladder
    d. surgical creation of an opening
49. Removal of unwanted substance from the blood by passage through a semipermeable membrane
    a. blood
    b. through
    c. separation

Answers to Case Study Questions

1. d
2. b
3. c
4. b
5. e
6. ureterocele
7. calculus
8. hematuria
9. nocturia
10. lithotripsy
11. nephrolithotomy
12. incontinence
13. urethropexy
14. intraoperative
15. urethroscope
16. radiograph of the urinary tract
17. condition of having stones in the urinary tract
18. endoscopic examination of the bladder
19. painful or difficult urination

Answers to Crossword Puzzle

URINARY

			[1] C	O	R	[2] T	E	X			[3] S
	[4] N		A			R					T
[5] H	E	N	L	E		I		[6] E	N	D	O
	P		Y			[7] G	E	N			M
	H		X			O		U			Y
[8] U	R	[9] O			[10] A	N	U	R	I	[11] A	
	[12] O	S	E			E		E		[13] D	I
	N			[14] G				S		H	
[15] U		[16] P	O	L	Y	[17] U	R	I	A		[18] D
R		Y		Y		R		S		[19] B	I
I				C		[20] E	[21] U			[22] U	A
[23] C	Y	S	T	O		[24] A	N	I	O	N	

14 The Reproductive System

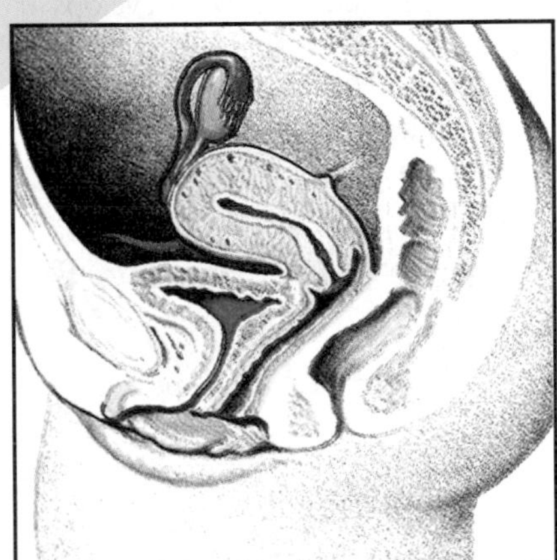

Chapter Contents

Objectives

After careful study of this chapter you should be able to:

1. Label a diagram of the male reproductive tract and describe the function of each part
2. Describe the contents and functions of semen
3. Label a diagram of the female reproductive tract and describe the function of each part
4. Describe the structure and function of the mammary glands
5. Outline the events in the menstrual cycle
6. Identify and use roots pertaining to the male and female reproductive systems
7. Describe the main disorders of the male and female reproductive systems
8. Interpret abbreviations used in referring to the reproductive system
9. Analyze several case studies concerning the male and female reproductive systems

The function of the **gonads** (sex glands) in both males and females is to produce the reproductive cells, the **gametes**, and to produce hormones. The gametes are generated by **meiosis**, a process of cell division that halves the chromosome number from 46 to 23. When male and female gametes unite in fertilization the original chromosome number is restored. The sex hormones aid in the manufacture of the gametes, function in pregnancy and lactation, and also produce the secondary sex characteristics such as the typical size, shape, body hair, and voice which we associate with the male and female genders.

The reproductive tract develops in close association with the urinary tract. In females the two systems become completely separate. In males the reproductive and urinary tracts share a common passage, the urethra. Thus, the two systems are referred to together as the genitourinary (GU) or urogenital (UG) tract, and urologists are called on to treat disorders of the male reproductive system as well as the urinary system.

Male Reproductive System

The Testes

The male germ cells, the **spermatozoa** (sperm cells) are produced in the paired **testes** that are suspended outside the body in the **scrotum** (Fig. 14-1). Although the testes develop in the abdominal cavity, they normally descend through the **inguinal canal** into the scrotum before birth

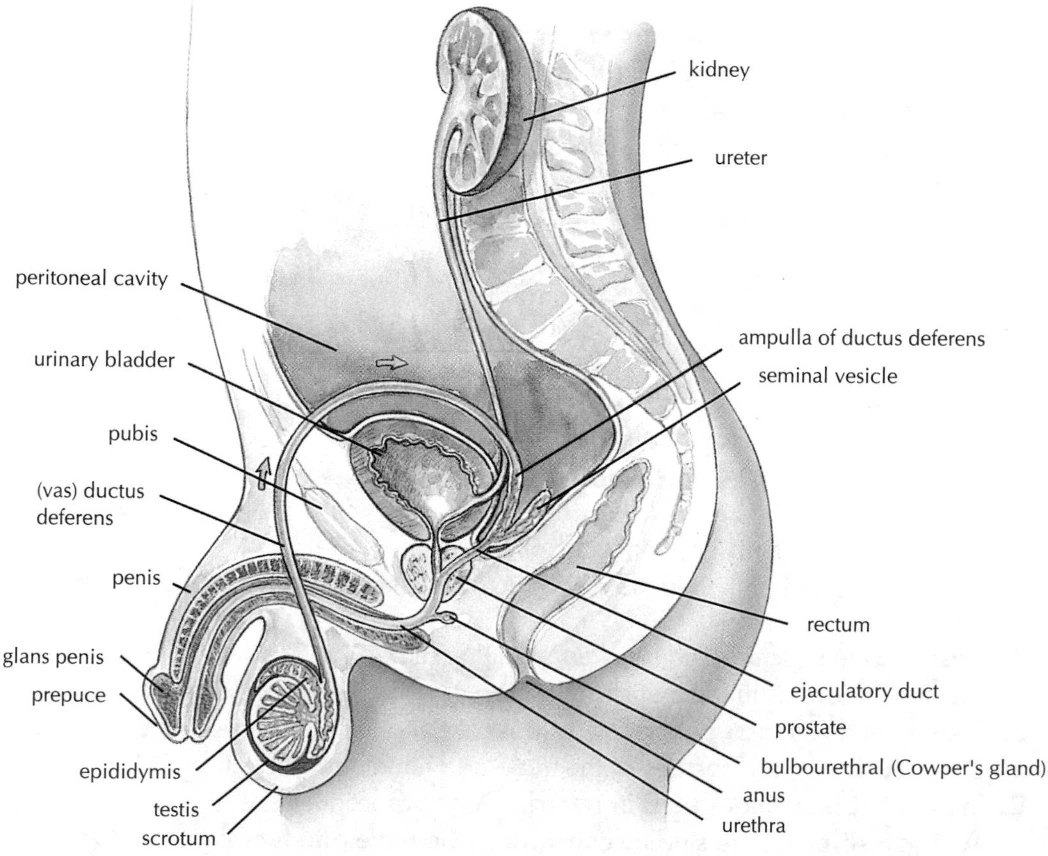

FIGURE 14-1. Male genitourinary system. The arrows indicate the course of sperm cells through the duct system.

or shortly thereafter. From puberty on, spermatozoa form continuously within the testes in coiled **seminiferous tubules** (Fig. 14-2). Their development requires the aid of special **Sertoli's cells** and male sex hormones, or **androgens**, mainly **testosterone**. These hormones are manufactured in **interstitial cells** located between the tubules. In both male and female the gonads are stimulated by the hormones **FSH** (follicle stimulating hormone) and **LH** (luteinizing hormone) released from the anterior pituitary gland beneath the brain. Although it is the same in both males and females, LH is called **ICSH** (interstitial cell-stimulating hormone) in males.

Transport of Spermatozoa

Following their manufacture, sperm cells are stored in a much-coiled tube on the surface of each testis, the **epididymis** (see Figure 14-1). Here they remain until ejaculation propels them into a series of ducts that leads out of the body. The first of these is the **vas (ductus) deferens**. This duct ascends through the inguinal canal into the abdominal cavity and travels behind the bladder. A short continuation, the **ejaculatory duct**, delivers the spermatozoa to the urethra as it passes through the prostate gland below the bladder. Finally, the cells, now mixed with other secretions, travel in the **urethra** through the **penis** to be released. The penis is the male organ that transports both urine and semen. It enlarges at the tip to form the **glans penis** which is covered by loose skin, the **prepuce** or foreskin.

Formation of Semen

Semen is the thick, whitish fluid in which spermatozoa are transported. It contains, in addition to sperm cells, secretions from three types of accessory glands. The first of these, the paired **seminal vesicles**, release their secretions into the ejaculatory duct. The second, the **prostate**, secretes

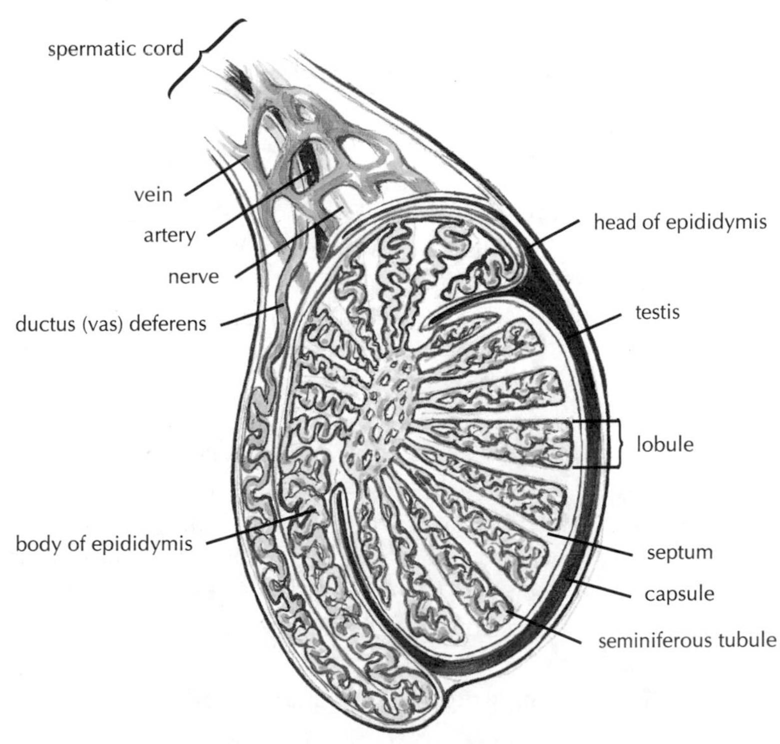

FIGURE 14-2. Structure of the testis, also showing the epididymis and spermatic cord.

into the first part of the urethra beneath the bladder. As men age, enlargement of the prostate may compress the urethra and cause urinary problems. The two **bulbourethral** (Cowper's) **glands** secrete into the urethra just below the prostate. Together these glands produce a slightly alkaline mixture that nourishes and transports the sperm cells and also protects them by neutralizing the acidity of the female vaginal tract.

KEY TERMS

Normal Structure and Function

androgen *(AN-drō-jen)*	Any hormone that produces male characteristics
bulbourethral gland *(bul-bō-ū-RĒ-thral)*	A small gland beside the urethra below the prostate that secretes part of the seminal fluid. Also called Cowper's gland.
ejaculation *(ē-jak-ū-LĀ-shun)*	Ejection of semen from the male urethra
ejaculatory duct *(ē-JAK-ū-la-tō-rē)*	The duct formed by union of the ductus deferens and the duct of the seminal vesicle; it carries spermatozoa and seminal fluid into the urethra
epididymis *(ep-i-DID-i-mis)*	A coiled tube on the surface of the testis that stores sperm until ejaculation (root epididym/o)
***FSH**	A hormone secreted by the anterior pituitary that acts on the gonads; follicle stimulating hormone
***gamete** *(GAM-ēt)*	A mature reproductive cell; spermatozoon or ovum
glans penis (glanz)	The bulbous end of the penis
***gonad** *(GŌ-nad)*	A sex gland; testis or ovary
***inguinal canal** *(ING-gwin-al)*	The channel through which the testes descend in the male; in the female it contains a ligament that extends from the uterus to the vulva
interstitial cells *(in-ter-STISH-al)*	Cells located between the seminiferous tubules of the testes that produce hormones, mainly testosterone. Also called cells of Leydig.
***LH**	A hormone secreted by the anterior pituitary that acts on the gonads; luteinizing *(LŪ-tē-in-ī-zing)* hormone. Called ICSH (interstitial cell-stimulating hormone) in males.
***meiosis** *(mī-Ō-sis)*	The type of cell division that forms the gametes; it results in cells with 23 chromosomes, half the number found in other body cells (from G. word meaning "diminution")
***pituitary gland** *(pi-TŪ-i-tar-ē)*	An endocrine gland at the base of the brain
penis *(PĒ-nis)*	The male organ of copulation and urination

(continued)

prepuce
(PRĒ-pūs)
The fold of skin over the glans penis; the foreskin

prostate gland
(PROS-tāt)
A gland that surrounds the urethra below the bladder in males and contributes secretions to the semen (root prostat/o)

scrotum
(SKRŌ-tum)
A double pouch that contains the testes (root osche/o)

semen
(SĒ-men)
The thick secretion that transports spermatozoa (spelled *semin* when used as a root) (root sperm/i, spermat/o)

seminal vesicle
A saclike structure behind the bladder that contributes to the semen (root vesicul/o)

Sertoli's cells
(ser-TŌ-lēz)
Cells in the seminiferous tubules that aid in the development of spermatozoa

spermatozoon
(sper-ma-tō-zō-on)
The mature male sex cell (pl. spermatozoa) (root sperm/i, spermat/o)

testis
(TES-tis)
The male reproductive gland (pl. testes) (see Figure 14-2); also called testicle (root test/o)

testosterone
(tes-TOS-ter-ōn)
The main male sex hormone

***urethra**
(ū-RĒ-thra)
The duct that carries urine out of the body and also transports semen in the male

vas deferens
(DEF-er-enz)
The duct that conveys spermatozoa from the epididymis to the ejaculatory duct. Also called ductus deferens.

*Term applies to both male and female.

Roots Pertaining to Male Reproduction

Root	Meaning	Example	Definition of Example
test/o	testis, testicle	testicular *tes-TIK-ū-lar*	pertaining to a testicle
orchi/o, orchid/o	testis	orchialgia *or-kē-AL-jē-a*	pain in the testis
sperm/i, spermat/o	semen, spermatozoa	polyspermia *pol-ē-SPER-mē-a*	excess secretion of semen
epididym/o	epididymis	epididymitis *ep-i-did-i-MĪ-tis*	inflammation of the epididymis
vas/o	vessel, vas deferens	vasectomy *va-SEK-tō-mē*	excision of the vas deferens (Fig. 14-3)
vesicul/o	seminal vesicle	vesiculography *ve-sik-ū-LOG-ra-fē*	radiographic study of the seminal vesicles
prostat/o	prostate	prostatometer *pros-ta-TOM-e-ter*	instrument for measuring the prostate
osche/o	scrotum	oscheal *OS-kē-al*	pertaining to the scrotum

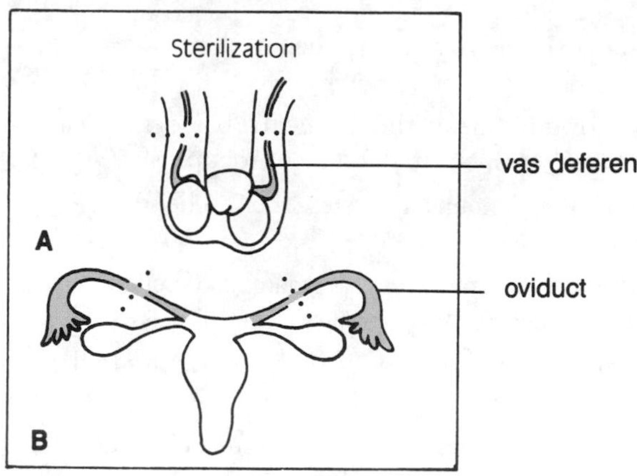

FIGURE 14-3. Sterilization. **(A)** Vasectomy. **(B)** Tubal ligation. (Taylor C, Lillis CA, LeMone P: Fundamentals of Nursing, 2nd ed, p 1086. Philadelphia: JB Lippincott, 1993.)

Exercise 14-1

Define the following terms:

1. Testopathy *(test-TOP-a-thē)* ____________
2. Orchiotomy *(or-kē-OT-ō-mē)* ____________
3. Epididymectomy *(ep-i-did-i-MEK-tō-mē)* ____________
4. Prostatic *(pros-TAT-ik)* ____________
5. Oscheoma *(os-kē-Ō-ma)* ____________
6. Orchiepididymitis *(or-kē-ep-i-did-i-MĪ-tis)* ____________

Use the root *orchi/o* to write words with the following meanings. Each is also written with the root *orchid/o*.

7. Plastic repair of a testis ____________
8. Excision of a testis ____________
9. Surgical fixation of a testis ____________

Use the root spermat/o to write words with the following meanings:

10. A sperm-forming cell ____________
11. Destruction (-lysis) of sperm ____________
12. Formation (-genesis) of spermatozoa ____________
13. Excessive discharge (-rhea) of semen ____________
14. Condition of having sperm in the urine (-uria)____________

The ending *-spermia* means "condition of sperm or semen." Add a prefix to *-spermia* to form words with the following meanings:

15. Presence of blood in the semen ____________
16. Presence of pus in the semen ____________
17. Lack of semen ____________

Write a word for each of the following definitions:

18. X-ray (radiograph) of a seminal vesicle __________
19. Excision of the prostate gland __________
20. Inflammation of a seminal vesicle __________
21. Surgical creation of an opening in the vas deferens __________
22. Suture of the vas deferens __________
23. Incision of the epididymis __________
24. Plastic repair of the scrotum __________

Clinical Aspects of Male Reproduction

Infection

Most infections of the male reproductive tract are **sexually transmitted diseases** (STDs), listed in Table 14-1. Gonorrhea usually centers in the urethra, causing **urethritis** with a purulent discharge and dysuria. Untreated, the disease can spread through the reproductive system. Gonorrhea is treated with antibiotics, but there has been rapid development of resistance to these drugs by the causative organism, the gonococcus (GC).

Mumps is a viral disease that can infect the testes and lead to sterility. Other microorganisms can infect the reproductive tract as well, causing urethritis, **prostatitis, orchitis**, or **epididymitis**.

Benign Prostatic Hyperplasia

As men age, the prostate gland commonly enlarges, a condition known as **benign prostatic hyperplasia** (BPH). While not cancerous, this overgrowth can press on the urethra near the bladder and interfere with urination. Infection often follows. Removal of the prostate, or **prostatectomy**, may be required. When this is performed through the urethra, the procedure is called a transurethral resection of the prostate (TURP).

Cancer of the Prostate

Cancer of the prostate is the most common malignancy in U.S. males. Only lung cancer and colon cancer cause more cancer-related deaths in men past middle age. Prostatic cancer may metastasize rapidly and is difficult to remove surgically. Other methods of treatment include radiation; measures to reduce male hormones (androgens), which stimulate growth; and chemotherapy. In cases of prostatic cancer, a protein produced by prostate cells increases in the blood. This prostate specific antigen (PSA) is used, along with rectal examinations, to screen for prostate cancer and to follow the results of treatment.

Cyptorchidism

It is fairly common that one or both testes will fail to descend into the scrotum by the time of birth. This condition is termed **cryptorchidism**, literally hidden (crypt/o) testis (orchid/o). The condition usually corrects itself within the first year of life. If not, it must be corrected surgically to avoid sterility and an increased risk of cancer.

Infertility

An inability or a diminished ability to reproduce is termed **infertility**. Its causes may be hereditary, hormonal, disease-related, or the result of exposure to chemical or physical agents. The most common causes of infertility are sexually transmitted diseases. A total inability to produce off-

TABLE 14-1 Sexually Transmitted Diseases

Disease	Organism	Description
Bacterial		
gardnerella infection	*Gardnerella vaginalis*	Vaginitis with foul-smelling discharge
chlamydia infection	*Chlamydia trachomatis* types D–K	Ascending infection of reproductive and urinary tracts. May spread to pelvis in females, causing pelvic inflammatory disease (PID)
lymphogranuloma venereum	*Chlamydia trachomatis* type L	General infection with swelling of inguinal lymph nodes; scarring of genital tissue
gonorrhea	*Neisseria gonorrhoeae,* gonococcus (GC)	Inflammation of reproductive and urinary tracts. Urethritis in males. Vaginal discharge and cervicitis in females leading to PID. Possible systemic infection. May spread to newborns. Treated with antibiotics.
syphilis	*Treponema pallidum* (a spirochete)	Primary stage—chancre (lesion); secondary stage—systemic infection and syphilitic warts; tertiary stage—degeneration of other systems. Cause of abortions, stillbirths, and fetal deformities. Treated with antibiotics.
Viral		
genital herpes	herpes simplex type 2	Painful lesions of the genitalia. In females, may be a risk factor in cervical carcinoma. Often fatal infections of newborns. No cure at present.
condyloma acuminatum (genital warts)	human papilloma virus (HPV)	Benign genital warts. In females, predisposes to cervical dysplasia and carcinoma.
Protozoal		
trichomoniasis	*Trichomonas vaginalis*	Vaginitis. Thick, yellowish discharge with itching; pain on intercourse (dyspareunia), and painful urination (dysuria).

spring may be termed **sterility**. Males may be voluntarily sterilized by cutting and sealing the vas deferens on both sides in a **vasectomy** (see Figure 14-3).

Inguinal Hernia

The inguinal canal, through which the testis descends, may represent a weakness in the abdominal wall that can lead to a hernia. In the most common form of **inguinal hernia** (Fig. 14-4), an abdominal organ, usually the intestine, enters the inguinal canal and may extend into the scrotum. This is an indirect or external inguinal hernia. In a direct or internal inguinal hernia, the organ protrudes through the abdominal wall into the scrotum. If blood supply to the organ is cut off, the hernia is said to be *strangulated*. Surgery to correct a hernia is a **herniorrhaphy**.

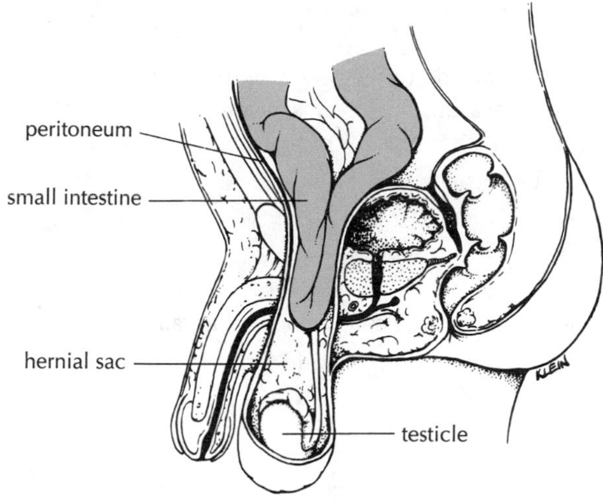

FIGURE 14-4. Inguinal hernia. The hernial sac is a continuation of the peritoneum. The intestine or other abdominal contents can protrude into the hernial sac. (Smeltzer SC, Bare BG: Bruner and Suddarth's Textbook of Medical-Surgical Nursing, 7th ed, p 946, Philadelphia: JB Lippincott, 1992.)

KEY CLINICAL TERMS

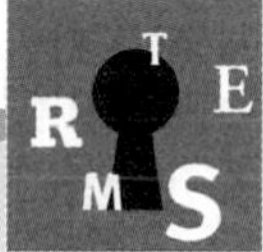

Disorders

benign prostatic hyperplasia (BPH) — Non-malignant enlargement of the prostate; frequently develops with age

cryptorchidism *(krip-TOR-kid-izm)* — Failure of the testis to descend into the scrotum

epididymitis *(ep-i-did-i-MĪ-tis)* — Inflammation of the epididymis. Common causes are urinary tract infections and sexually transmitted diseases.

***infertility** *(in-fer-TIL-i-tē)* — Decreased capacity to produce offspring

***inguinal hernia** *(ING-gwin-al)* — Protrusion of the intestine or other abdominal organ through the inguinal canal (see Figure 14-4) or through the wall of the abdomen into the scrotum

orchitis *(or-KĪ-tis)* — Inflammation of a testis. May be caused by injury, mumps virus, or other infections.

prostatitis *(pros-ta-TĪ-tis)* — Inflammation of the prostate gland. Often appears with urinary tract infection, sexually transmitted disease, and a variety of other stresses.

sexually transmitted disease (STD) — Disease spread through sexual activity (see Table 14-1)

***sterility** — Complete inability to produce offspring

urethritis *(ū-rē-THRĪ-tis)* — Inflammation of the urethra; usually caused by gonorrhea and chlamydia infections

(continued)

Surgery

circumcision
(ser-kum-SI-zhun)
Surgical removal of the end of the prepuce (foreskin); may be done for medical reasons, but is most often performed electively in male infants for reasons of hygiene or religion

herniorrhaphy
(her-nē-OR-a-fē)
Surgical repair of a hernia

prostatectomy
(pros-ta-TEK-tō-mē)
Surgical removal of the prostate

vasectomy
(va-SEK-to-me)
Excision of the vas deferens. Usually done bilaterally to produce sterility. May be accomplished through the urethra (transurethral resection).

*Term applies to both males and females.

ADDITIONAL TERMS

Normal Structure and Function

***coitus**
(KŌ-i-tus)
Sexual intercourse

emission
(ē-MISH-un)
The discharge of semen

***erection**
(e-REK-shun)
The stiffening or hardening of the penis or the clitoris, usually due to sexual excitement

***genitalia**
(jen-i-TĀL-ē-a)
The organs concerned with reproduction, divided into internal and external components

insemination
(in-sem-i-NĀ-shun)
Introduction of semen into the female

***orgasm**
(OR-gazm)
A state of physical and emotional excitement, especially that which occurs at the climax of sexual intercourse

***puberty**
(PŪ-ber-tē)
Period during which the ability for sexual reproduction is attained and secondary sex characteristics begin to develop

spermatic cord
The cord that suspends the testis; composed of the vas deferens, vessels, and nerves

Disorders

balanitis
(bal-a-NĪ-tis)
Inflammation of the glans penis and mucous membrane beneath it (root *balan/o* means "glans penis")

bladder neck obstruction
(BNO)
Blockage of urine flow at the outlet of the bladder. The common cause is benign prostatic hyperplasia.

hydrocele
(HĪ-drō-sēl)
The accumulation of fluid in a saclike cavity, especially within the covering of the testis or spermatic cord (Fig. 14-5)

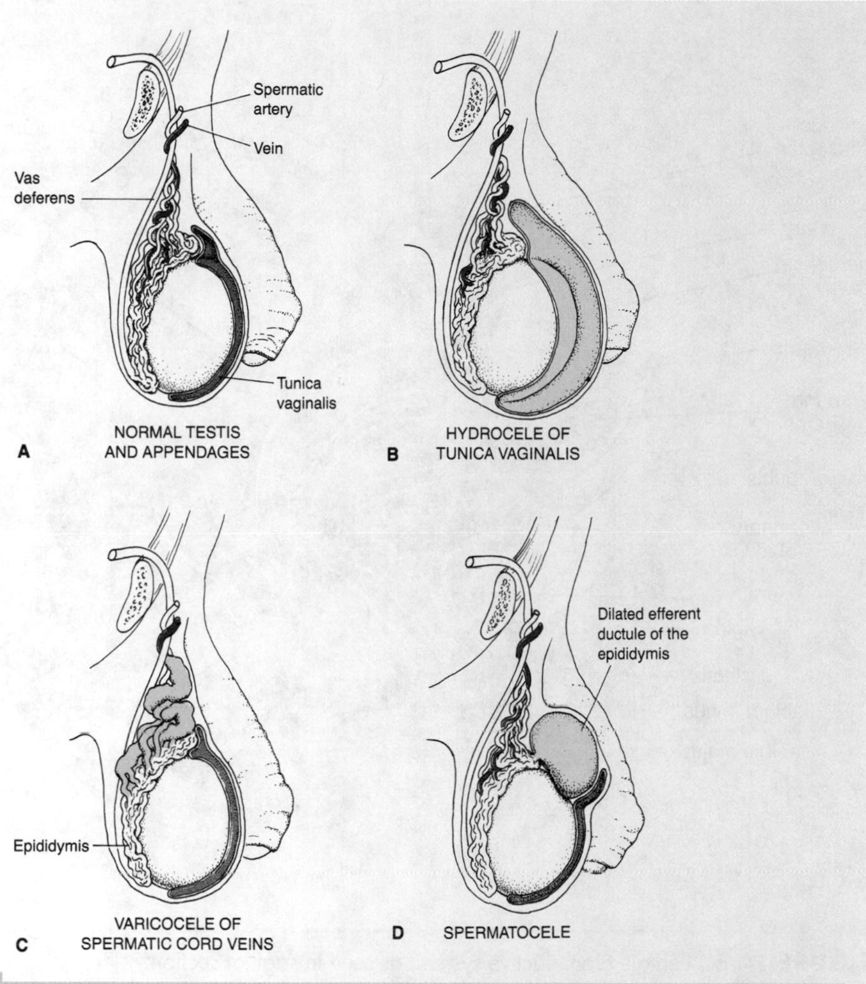

FIGURE 14-5. Scrotal abnormalities. **(A)** Normal. **(B)** Hydrocele. **(C)** Varicocele. **(D)** Spermatocele. (© Dimitri Karetnikov, artist. Rubin E, Farber JL: Essential Pathology, p 925. Philadelphia: JB Lippincott, 1988.)

impotence
(IM-pō-tens)
Weakness, especially inability of the male to achieve or maintain erection

phimosis
(fi-MŌ-sis)
Narrowing of the opening of the prepuce so that the foreskin cannot be pushed back over the glans penis

seminoma
(sem-i-NŌ-ma)
A tumor of the testis

spermatocele
(SPER-ma-tō-sēl)
An epididymal cyst containing spermatozoa (see Figure 14-5)

varicocele
(VAR-i-kō-sēl)
Enlargement of the veins of the spermatic cord (see Figure 14-5)

---

*Term applies to both male and female reproductive systems.

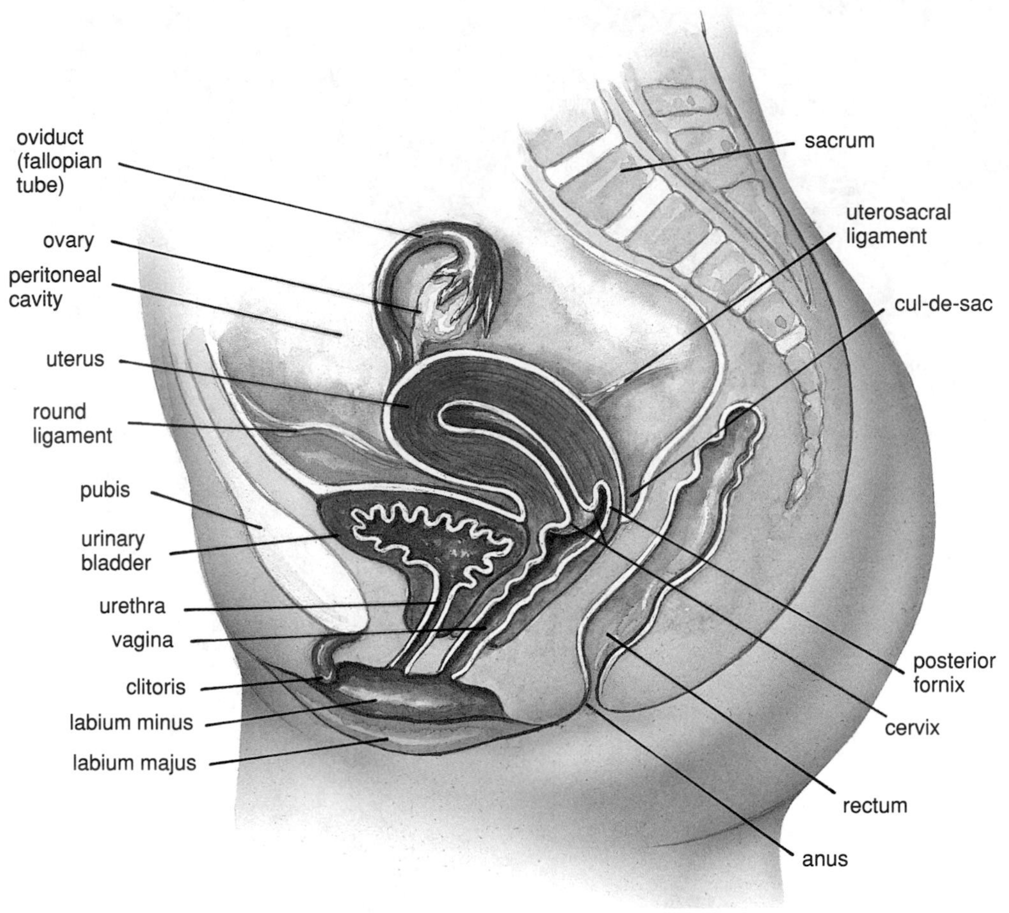

FIGURE 14-6. Female reproductive system, as seen in sagittal section.

Female Reproductive System

The Ovaries

The female gonads are the paired **ovaries** (Fig. 14-6) that are held by ligaments in the pelvic cavity on either side of the uterus. It is within the ovaries that the female gametes, the **ova** (eggs), develop. Every month several ova ripen, each within a cluster of cells called a **graafian follicle**. At the time of ovulation, usually only one ovum is released from the ovary and the remainder of the ripening ova degenerate. The follicle remains behind and continues to function—for about 2 weeks if there is no fertilization of the ovum and for about 2 months if the ovum is fertilized.

The Oviducts and Uterus

Following ovulation, the ovum travels into an **oviduct** (also called the uterine tube or fallopian tube), one of the two tubes attached to the upper lateral portions of the uterus (see Figure 14-6). These tubes arch above the ovaries and have fingerlike projections (fimbriae), that sweep the released ovum into the oviduct. If fertilization occurs, it usually takes place in the oviduct.

The **uterus** is the organ that nourishes the developing offspring. It is pear-shaped with an upper rounded fundus, a triangular cavity, and a lower narrow **cervix** that projects into the vagina. The innermost layer of the uterine wall, the **endometrium**, has a rich blood supply. It receives the fertilized ovum and becomes part of the placenta during pregnancy. The endometrium is shed during the menstrual period if no fertilization occurs. The muscle layer of the uterine wall is the **myometrium**.

The Vagina

The **vagina** is a muscular tube that receives the penis during intercourse, functions as a birth canal, and transports the menstrual flow out of the body (see Figure 14-6).

The External Genital Organs

All of the external female genital organs together are called the **vulva** (Fig. 14-7). This includes the large outer **labia majora** and small inner **labia minora** that enclose the openings of the vagina and the urethra. The **clitoris**, anterior to the urethral opening, is comparable to the penis and responds to sexual stimulation.

The Perineum

In both male and female, the region between the thighs, from the external genital organs to the anus, is the **perineum**. During childbirth, an incision may be made between the vagina and the anus to facilitate birth and prevent the tearing of tissue, a procedure called an *episiotomy*. (This procedure is actually a perineotomy, as the root *episi/o* means "vulva.")

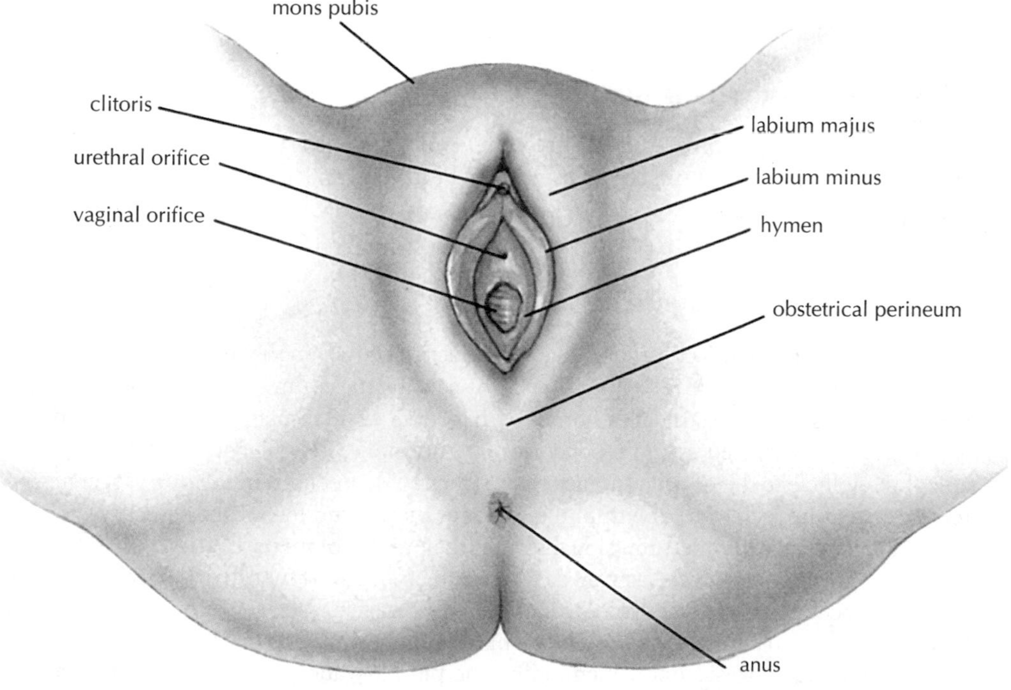

FIGURE 14-7. The external female genitalia.

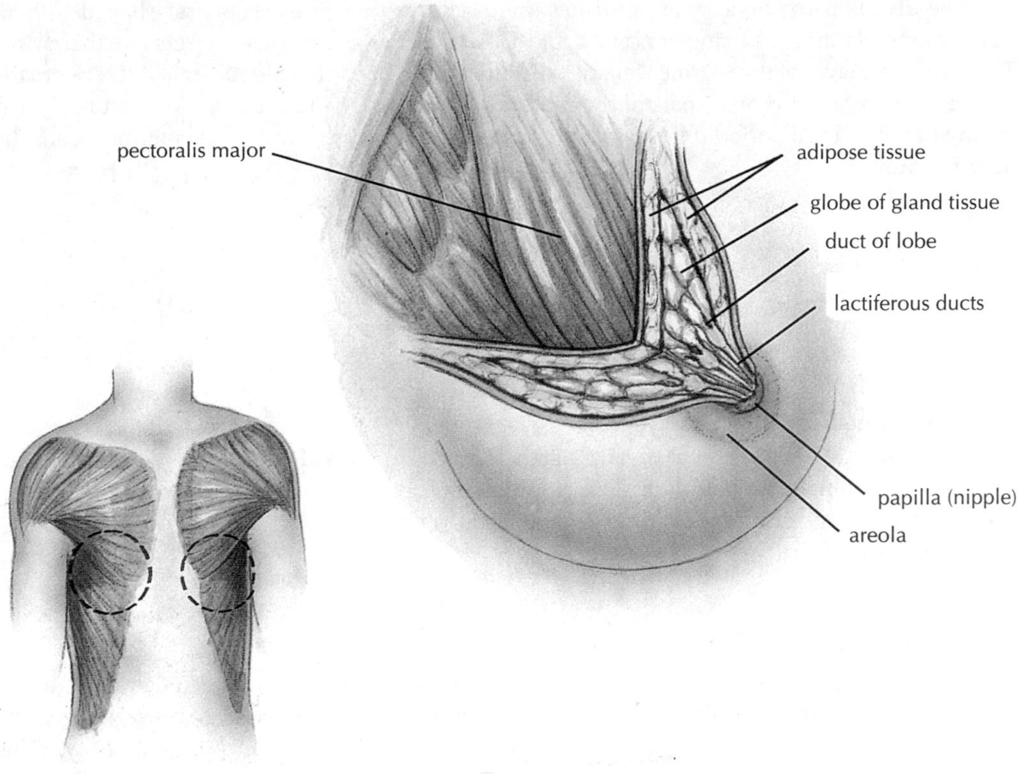

FIGURE 14-8. Section of the breast.

The Mammary Glands

The **mammary glands**, or breasts, are composed mainly of glandular tissue and fat (Fig. 14-8). Their purpose is to provide nourishment for the newborn. The milk secreted by the glands is carried in ducts to the nipple.

The Menstrual Cycle

The female menstrual cycle is controlled, like reproductive activity in the male, by hormones from the anterior pituitary gland. **FSH** begins the cycle by causing the ovum to ripen in the graafian follicle. The follicle secretes **estrogen**, a hormone that starts development of the endometrium in preparation for the fertilized egg. A second pituitary hormone, **LH**, triggers **ovulation** and conversion of the follicle to the **corpus luteum**. This structure, left behind in the ovary, secretes **progesterone** which furthers the growth of the endometrium. If no fertilization occurs, hormone levels decline, and the endometrium sloughs off in the process of **menstruation**.

The average menstrual cycle lasts 28 days, with the first day of menstruation taken as day 1, and ovulation occurring on about day 14. Throughout the cycle, estrogen and progesterone feed back to the pituitary to regulate the production of FSH and LH. The birth control pill acts by supplying estrogen and progesterone which inhibit the pituitary and prevent ovulation, while not interfering with menstruation.

Menopause

Menopause is the cessation of monthly menstrual cycles. This generally occurs between the ages of 45 and 55 years. Levels of reproductive hormones decline and egg cells in the ovaries gradually degenerate. Some women experience unpleasant symptoms, such as hot flashes, headaches, insomnia, and mood swings. There is also some atrophy of the reproductive tract. Decline in estrogen is associated with a higher rate of heart disease and weakening of the bones (osteoporosis). Estrogen replacement therapy (ERT), also known as hormone replacement therapy (HRT), may be recommended to counteract these effects. Exercise and a balanced diet with adequate calcium are also important in maintaining health.

Contraception

Contraception is the use of artificial methods to prevent fertilization of the ovum or its implantation in the uterus. Methods can be used to block sperm penetration of the uterus (condom, diaphragm), prevent implantation (intrauterine device [IUD]), or prevent ovulation (birth control pill). Surgical sterilization for the male is a vasectomy; for the female, surgical sterilization is a **tubal ligation**, in which the fallopian tubes are cut and tied on both sides (see Figure 14-3). The preferred method for performing this surgery is through the abdominal wall with a **laparoscope** (Fig. 14-9).

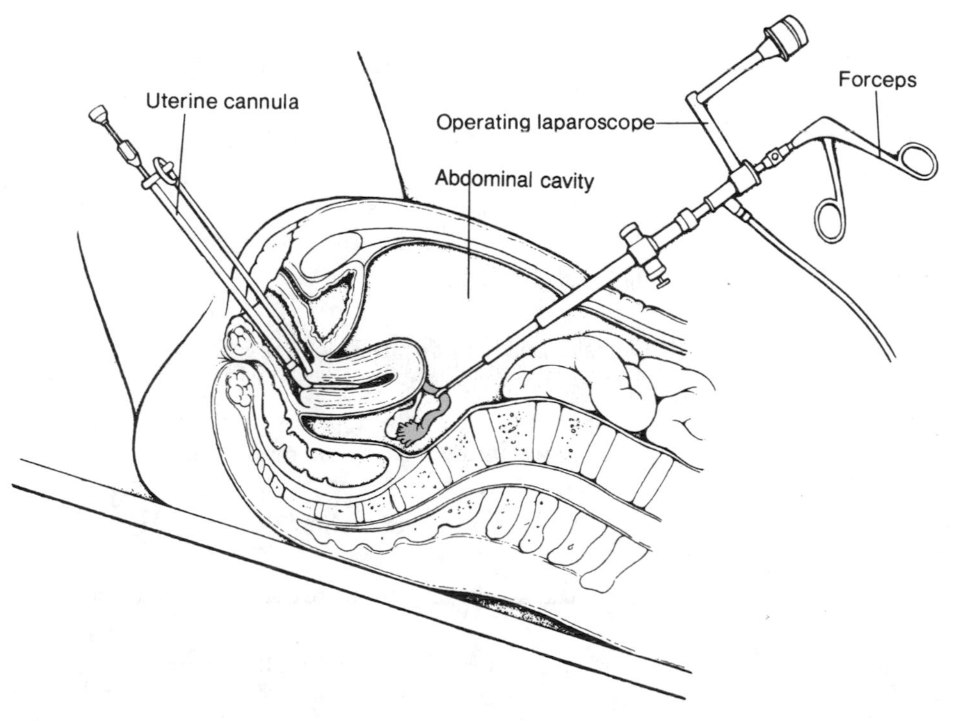

FIGURE 14-9. Laparoscopic sterilization. (Smeltzer SC, Bare BG: Brunner and Suddarth's Textbook of Medical-Surgical Nursing, 7th ed, p 1238. Philadelphia: JB Lippincott, 1992.)

KEY TERMS

Normal Structure and Function

cervix *(SER-viks)*	Neck. Usually means the lower narrow portion (neck) of the uterus; cervix uteri (U-ter-i) (root cervic/o).
clitoris *(KLIT-o-ris)*	A small erectile body in front of the urethral opening that is similar in origin to the penis (root clitor/o, clitorid/o)
***contraception** *(kon-tra-SEP-shun)*	The prevention of pregnancy
endometrium *(en-dō-MĒ-trē-um)*	The inner lining of the uterus
estrogen *(ES-trō-jen)*	A group of hormones that produce female characteristics and prepare the uterus for the fertilized egg. The most active of these is estradiol.
fallopian tube *(fa-LŌ-pē-an)*	See oviduct
graafian follicle *(GRAF-ē-an)*	The cluster of cells in which the ovum ripens in the ovary. Also called ovarian follicle.
labia majora *(LĀ-bē-a ma-JOR-a)*	The two large folds of skin that form the sides of the vulva (root *labi/o* means "lip"); sing. *labium majus*
labia minora *(LĀ-bē-a mī-NOR-a)*	The two small folds of skin within the labia majora; sing. *labium minus*
mammary gland *(MAM-a-rē)*	A specialized gland of the skin capable of secreting milk in the female; the breast (root mamm/o, mast/o)
menopause *(MEN-ō-pawz)*	Cessation of menstrual cycles in the female
menstruation *(men-strū-Ā-shun)*	The cyclic discharge of blood and mucosal tissues from the lining of the nonpregnant uterus (root men/o, mens)
myometrium *(mī-ō-MĒ-trē-um)*	The muscular wall of the uterus
ovary *(Ō-va-rē)*	A female gonad (root ovari/o, oophor/o)
oviduct *(Ō-vi-dukt)*	A tube extending from the upper lateral portion of the uterus that carries the ovum to the uterus. Also called fallopian or uterine tube (root salping/o)
ovulation *(ov-ū-LĀ-shun)*	The release of a mature ovum from the ovary (from *ovule* meaning "little egg")
ovum *(Ō-vum)*	The female gamete or reproductive cell (pl. *ova*) (root oo, ov/o)
***perineum** *(per-i-NĒ-um)*	The region between the thighs from the external genitals to the anus (root perine/o)
progesterone *(prō-JES-ter-ōn)*	A hormone produced by the corpus luteum and the placenta that maintains the endometrium for pregnancy

uterus *(Ū-ter-us)*	The organ that receives the fertilized egg and maintains the developing offspring during pregnancy (root uter/o, metr, hyster/o)
vagina *(va-JĪ-na)*	The muscular tube between the cervix and the vulva (root vagin/o, colp/o)
vulva *(VUL-va)*	The external female genital organs (root vulv/o, episi/o)

*Term applies to both male and female.

Roots Pertaining to the Female Reproductive System

Roots for Female Reproduction and the Ovaries

Root	Meaning	Example	Definition of Example
gyn/o, gynec/o*	woman	gynecology *gi-ne-KOL-ō-jē*	study of diseases of women
men/o, mens	month, menstruation	intermenstrual *in-ter-MEN-strū-al*	between menstrual periods
oo	ovum	oogenesis *ō-ō-JEN-e-sis*	formation of an ovum
ov/o	ovum	ovulatory *OV-ū-la-tō-rē*	pertaining to ovulation
ovari/o	ovary	ovariorrhexis *ō-var-ē-ō-REK-sis*	rupture of the ovary
oophor/o	ovary	oophorectomy *ō-of-ō-REK-tō-mē*	excision of an ovary

*This root may also be pronounced with a soft g as in *jin-e-KOL-ō-jē*.

Exercise 14-2

Define each of the following terms:

1. Anovulatory *(an-OV-ū-la-tō-rē)* ________________
2. Ovariocentesis *(ō-var-ē-ō-sen-TĒ-sis)* ________________
3. Oophoritis *(ō-of-ō-RĪ-tis)* ________________
4. Premenstrual *(prē-MEN-strū-al)* ________________

Write a word for each of the following definitions:

5. A physician who specializes in the study of diseases of women ______________________
6. A cell that gives rise to an ovum (oo-) ______________________
7. Profuse bleeding (-rhagia) at the time of menstruation ______________________

The word *menorrhea* means "menstruation." Add a prefix to *menorrhea* to form words with the following meanings:

8. Absence of menstruation ______________________
9. Painful or difficult menstruation ______________________
10. Scanty menstrual flow ______________________

Use the root *ovari/o* to write the following words:

11. Pertaining to the ovary ______________________
12. Hernia of the ovary ______________________
13. Surgical fixation of the ovary ______________________

Use the root *oophor/o* for the following words:

14. Incision of an ovary ______________________
15. Malignant tumor of the ovary ______________________

Roots for the Oviducts, Uterus, and Vagina

Root	Meaning	Example	Definition of Example
salping/o	tube, oviduct	salpingography *sal-ping-OG-ra-fē*	radiographic study of the oviduct
uter/o	uterus	uterovesical *ū-ter-ō-VES-i-kl*	pertaining to the uterus and bladder
metr/o, metr/i	uterus	metrorrhagia *mē-trō-RĀ-jē-a*	abnormal uterine bleeding
hyster/o	uterus	panhysterectomy *pan-his-ter-EK-tō-mē*	surgical removal of the entire (pan-) uterus
cervic/o	neck, cervix	cervical *SER-vi-kal*	pertaining to the cervix
vagin/o	vagina	transvaginal *trans-VAJ-i-nal*	through the vagina
colp/o	vagina	colpodynia *kol-pō-DĪN-ē-a*	pain in the vagina

Exercise 14-3

Define the following terms:

1. Salpingectomy ______________________
   (sal-pin-JEK-tō-mē)
2. Hysteropexy ______________________
   (his-ter-ō-PEK-sē)
3. Metrostenosis ______________________
   (mē-trō-ste-NŌ-sis)
4. Intrauterine ______________________
   (in-tra-Ū-ter-in)
5. Vaginoplasty ______________________
   (vaj-i-nō-PLAS-tē)
6. Colpectasia ______________________
   (kol-pek-TĀ-sē-a)

Write a word that means each of the following:

7. Surgical fixation of an oviduct ______________________
8. Plastic repair of an oviduct ______________________

The root *salping/o* is taken from the word *salpinx* which means "tube." Add a prefix to salpinx to form words with the following meanings:

9. Presence of pus in an oviduct ______________________
10. Collection of fluid in an oviduct ______________________

Note how the roots *salping/o* and *oophor/o* are combined to form *salpingo-oophoritis* (inflammation of an oviduct and ovary). Write a word that means:

11. Surgical removal of an oviduct and ovary ______________________

Use the roots indicated to write the following words:

12. Behind (retro-) the uterus (uter/o) ______________________
13. Radiograph of the uterus (hyster/o) and oviducts ______________________
14. Surgical incision of the uterus (hyster/o) ______________________
15. Prolapse of the uterus (metr/o) ______________________
16. Softening of the uterus (metr/o) ______________________
17. Inflammation of the cervix (cervic/o) ______________________
18. Within (intra-) the cervix (cervic/o) ______________________
19. Through (trans-) the vagina (vagin/o) ______________________
20. Instrument for measuring the vagina (vagin/o) ______________________
21. Vaginal *(colp/o)* hernia ______________________

Roots for the Female Accessory Structures

Root	Meaning	Example	Definition of Example
vulv/o	vulva	vulvar *VUL-var*	pertaining to the vulva
episi/o	vulva	episiorrhaphy *e-piz-ē-OR-a-fē*	suture of the vulva
perine/o	perineum	perineal *per-i-NĒ-al*	pertaining to the perineum
clitor/o, clitorid/o	clitoris	clitorectomy *kli-tō-REK-tō-mē*	excision of the clitoris
mamm/o	breast, mammary gland	mammoplasty *mam-ō-PLAS-tē*	plastic surgery of the breast
mast/o	breast, mammary gland	amastia *a-MAS-tē-a*	absence of the breasts

Exercise 14-4

Write a word that means each of the following:

1. Any disease of the vulva (vulv/o) ____________
2. Plastic repair of the vulva (episi/o) ____________
3. Pertaining to the vagina (vagin/o) and perineum ____________
4. Inflammation of the clitoris ____________
5. Radiograph of the breast (mamm/o) ____________
6. Excision of the breast ____________
7. Inflammation of the breast (mast/o) ____________

Clinical Aspects of Female Reproduction

Infection

The major organisms that cause sexually transmitted diseases in both males and females are given in Table 14-1. **Pelvic inflammatory disease** (PID) is the spread of infection from the reproductive organs into the pelvic cavity. It is most often caused by the gonorrhea organism or by chlamydia. It is a serious disorder that may result in septicemia or shock. Inflammation of the oviducts (salpingitis) may close off these tubes and cause infertility.

A fungus that infects the vulva and vagina is *Candida albicans*, causing **Candidiasis**. There is **vaginitis**, a thick, cheesy discharge, and itching. Pregnancy, diabetes mellitus, use of antibiotics, steroids, or birth control pills predispose to infection. If recurrent, the patient's partner should be treated to prevent reinfections. Antifungal agents (mycostatics) are used in treatment.

Endometriosis

Growth of endometrial tissue outside the uterus is termed **endometriosis**. Commonly the ovaries, oviducts, peritoneum, and other pelvic organs are involved. Endometriosis causes pain, **dysmenorrhea** (painful or difficult menstruation), and infertility.

Menstrual Disorders

Menstrual abnormalities include flow that is too scanty (oligomenorrhea), too heavy (menorrhagia), or absence of monthly periods (amenorrhea). Together these disorders are classified as dysfunctional uterine bleeding (DUB). These responses may be caused by hormone imbalances, systemic disorders, or uterine problems. They are most common in adolescence or near menopause. At other times they are often related to life changes and emotional upset.

Cancer of the Female Reproductive Tract

Almost all patients with cancer of the cervix have been infected with human papilloma virus (HPV), a virus that causes genital warts. Incidence also is related to high sexual activity and other sexually transmitted viral infections, such as herpes.

In the 1940s and 1950s the synthetic steroid DES (diethylstilbestrol) was given to prevent miscarriages. A small percentage of daughters born to women treated with this drug have shown an increased risk of developing cancer of the cervix and vagina. These women need to be examined regularly.

Cervical carcinoma is often preceded by abnormal growth (dysplasia) of the epithelial cells lining the cervix. Growth is graded as CIN I, II, or III depending on the depth of tissue involved. CIN stands for *cervical intraepithelial neoplasia*. Diagnosis of cervical cancer is by a **Pap** (Papanicolaou) **smear**, examination with a **colposcope**, and biopsy. In a **cone biopsy** (Fig. 14-10), a

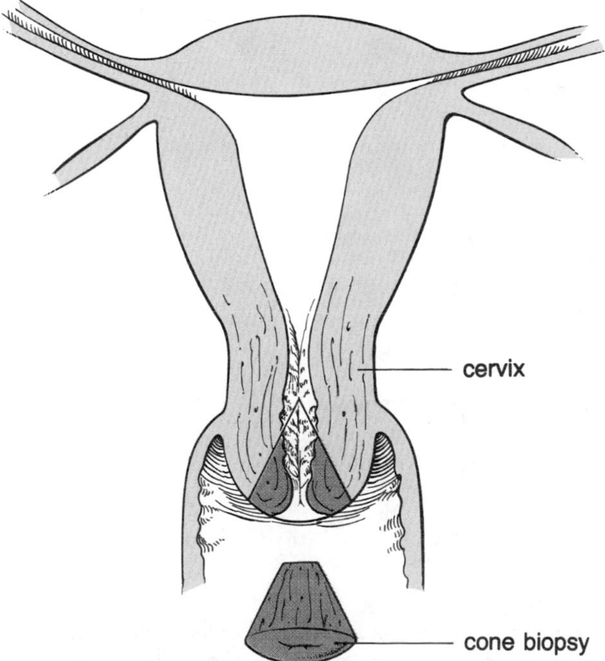

FIGURE 14-10. Cone biopsy of the uterine cervix.

cone-shaped piece of tissue is removed from the lining of the cervix for study. Often in the procedure, all of the abnormal cells are removed as well.

Cancer of the endometrium is the most common cancer of the female reproductive tract. Women at risk should have biopsies taken regularly, as endometrial cancer is not always detected by Pap smear. Treatment consists of **hysterectomy** (removal of the uterus) (Fig. 14-11) and sometimes radiation therapy. A small percentage of cases follows overgrowth (hyperplasia) of the endometrium. This tissue can be removed by **dilation and curettage** (D&C), in which the cervix is widened and the lining of the uterus is scraped with a curette.

Cancer of the ovary has a high mortality rate because it usually causes no early symptoms. Often by the time of diagnosis the tumor has invaded the pelvis and abdomen. Removal of the ovaries (oophorectomy) and oviducts (salpingectomy) along with the uterus is required (see Figure 14-11), in addition to chemotherapy and radiation therapy.

Breast Cancer

Carcinoma of the breast is second only to lung cancer in causing cancer-related deaths among U.S. women. This cancer metastasizes readily through the lymph nodes and blood to other sites such as the lung, liver, bones, and ovaries. Treatment is usually some form of **mastectomy** (removal of the breast). In a radical mastectomy underlying muscle and axillary lymph nodes (in the armpit) also are removed; in a modified radical mastectomy the breast and lymph nodes are removed, but muscles are left in place. Sometimes just the tumor itself is removed surgically in a segmental mas-

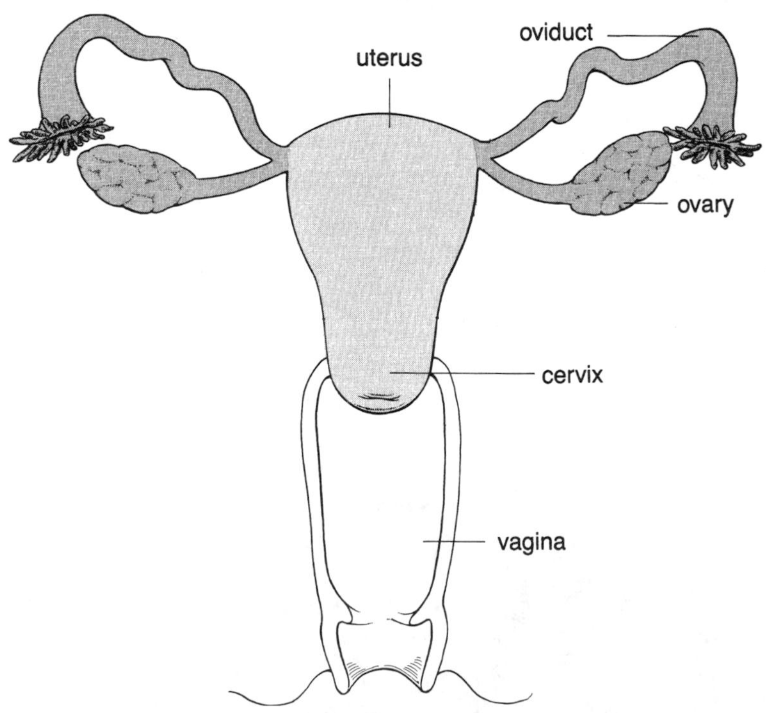

FIGURE 14-11. A hysterectomy is surgical removal of the uterus. Removal of the ovary (oophorectomy) and oviduct (salpingectomy) may also be required either unilaterally or bilaterally.

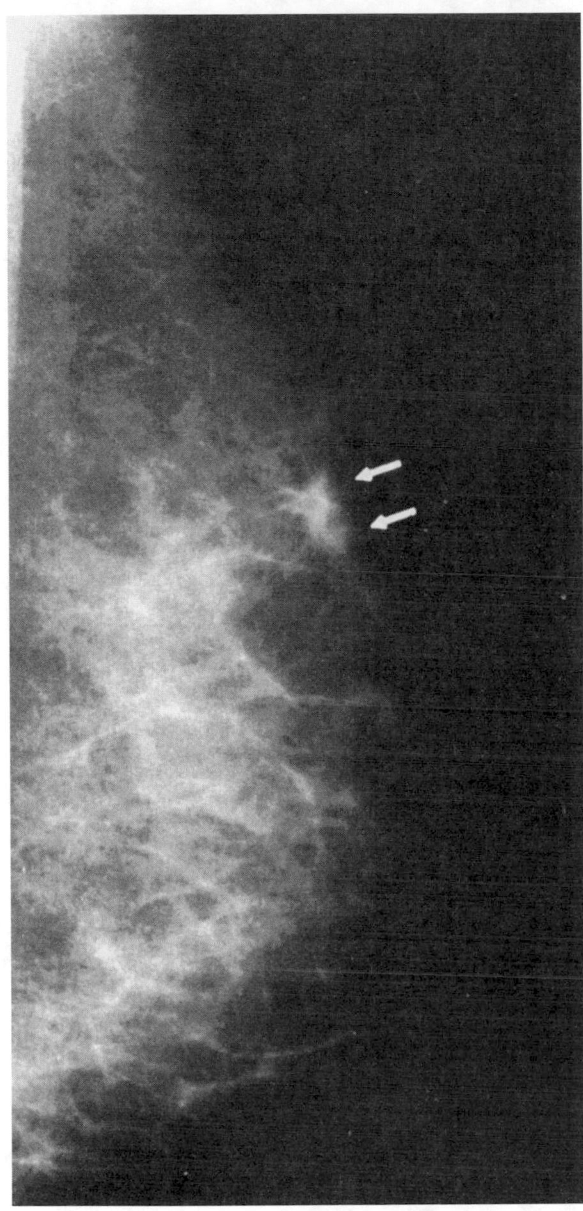

FIGURE 14-12. Mammogram of the breast showing a lesion (arrows). (Andolina VF, Lillé SL, Willison KM: Mammographic Imaging, p 263. Philadelphia: JB Lippincott, 1992.)

tectomy or "lumpectomy." Radiation therapy, chemotherapy, and sometimes hormone therapy are also employed.

Mammography is a method of diagnosing breast cancer by x-ray examination (Fig. 14-12). After the age of 45, women should be examined by this method yearly. Other diagnostic methods include palpation and cytologic study of tissue removed by aspiration or excision. Regular breast self-examination (BSE) is of utmost importance, as the majority of breast cancers are discovered by women themselves.

KEY CLINICAL TERMS

Disorders

candidiasis
(kan-di-DĪ-a-sis)
Infection with the fungus *Candida*; a common cause of vaginitis

dysmenorrhea
(DIS-men-ō-rē-a)
Painful or difficult menstruation. A common disorder that may be caused by infection, use of an IUD, endometriosis, overproduction of prostaglandins, or other factors.

endometriosis
(en-dō-mē-trē-Ō-sis)
Growth of endometrial tissue outside the uterus, usually in the pelvic cavity

pelvic inflammatory disease (PID)
Condition caused by the spread of infection from the reproductive tract into the pelvic cavity. Commonly caused by sexually transmitted gonorrhea and chlamydia infections.

salpingitis
(sal-pin-JĪ-tis)
Inflammation of the oviduct; typically caused by urinary tract or sexually transmitted infection. Chronic salpingitis may lead to infertility or ectopic pregnancy (development of the fertilized egg outside the uterus).

vaginitis
(vaj-i-NĪ-tis)
Inflammation of the vagina

Diagnosis and Treatment

colposcope
(KOL-pō-skōp)
Instrument for examining the vagina and cervix

cone biopsy
Removal of a cone of tissue from the lining of the cervix for cytologic examination; also called conization (see Figure 14-10)

dilation and curettage (D&C)
Procedure in which the cervix is dilated (widened) and the lining of the uterus is scraped with a curette

hysterectomy
(his-ter-EK-tō-mē)
Surgical removal of the uterus. Most commonly done because of tumors. Often the oviducts and ovaries are removed as well (see Figure 14-11).

mammography
(mam-OG-ra-fē)
Radiographic study of the breast for the detection of breast cancer.

mastectomy
(mas-TEK-tō-mē)
Excision of the breast to eliminate malignancy.

oophorectomy
(ō-of-ō-REK-tō-mē)
Excision of an ovary (see Figure 14-11)

Pap smear
Study of cells collected from the cervix and vagina for early detection of cancer. Also called Papanicolaou smear or Pap test.

salpingectomy
(sal-pin-JEK-tō-mē)
Surgical removal of the oviduct (see Figure 14-11)

ADDITIONAL TERMS

Normal Structure and Function

adnexa *(ad-NEK-sa)* — Appendages, such as the adnexa uteri—the ovaries, oviducts, and uterine ligaments

areola *(a-RĒ-ō-la)* — A pigmented ring, such as the dark area around the nipple of the breast

cul-de-sac *(kul-di-SAK)* — A blind pouch, such as the recess between the rectum and the uterus; the rectouterine pouch or pouch of Douglas

fimbriae *(FIM-brē-ē)* — The long fingerlike extensions of the oviduct that wave to capture the released ovum (see Figure 14-6); sing. *fimbria*

fornix *(FOR-niks)* — An archlike space, such as the space between the uppermost wall of the vagina and the cervix (see Figure 14-6)

greater vestibular gland — A small mucus-secreting gland on the side of the vestibule (see below) near the vaginal opening. Also called Bartholin's *(BAR-tō-linz)* gland (see Figure 15-1).

hymen *(HĪ-men)* — A fold of mucous membrane that partially covers the entrance of the vagina

menarche *(men-AR-kē)* — The start of regular monthly periods

menses *(MEN-sēz)* — The monthly flow of bloody discharge from the lining of the uterus

mons pubis *(monz PŪ-bis)* — The rounded, fleshy elevation in front of the pubic joint that is covered with hair after puberty

vestibule *(VES-ti-būl)* — The space between the labia minora that contains the openings of the urethra, vagina, and ducts of the greater vestibular glands

Infections and Conditions

cystocele *(SIS-tō-sēl)* — Herniation of the urinary bladder into the wall of the vagina (Fig. 14-13)

dyspareunia *(dis-par-Ū-nē-a)* — Pain during sexual intercourse

fibrocystic disease of the breast *(fi-brō-SIS-tik)* — A condition in which there are palpable lumps in the breasts, usually associated with pain and tenderness. These lumps or "thickenings" change with the menstrual cycle and must be distinguished from malignant tumors by palpation, mammography, and biopsy.

fibroid *(FĪ-broyd)* — Benign tumor of smooth muscle (see leiomyoma)

leiomyoma *(lī-ō-mī-Ō-ma)* — Benign tumor of smooth muscle. In the uterus, may cause bleeding and pressure on the bladder or rectum. Surgical removal or hysterectomy may be necessary. Also called fibroid.

leukorrhea *(lū-kō-RĒ-a)* — White or yellowish discharge from the vagina. Infection and other disorders may change the amount, color, or odor of the discharge.

(continued)

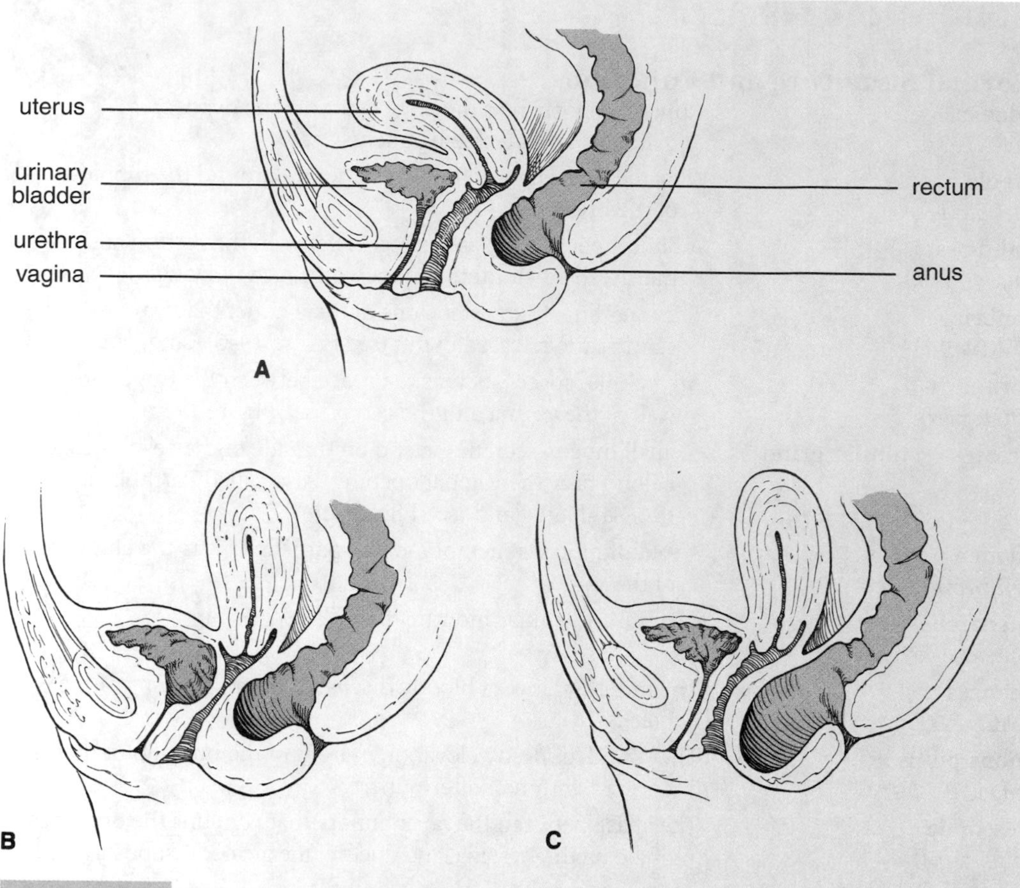

FIGURE 14-13. Herniation into the vagina. **(A)** Normal. **(B)** Cystocele. **(C)** Rectocele.

prolapse of the uterus — Downward displacement of the uterus with the cervix sometimes protruding from the vagina

rectocele *(REK-tō-sēl)* — Herniation of the rectum into the wall of the vagina; also called proctocele (see Figure 14-13)

Diagnosis and Treatment

episiorrhaphy *(e-pis-ē-OR-a-fē)* — Suture of the vulva or suture of the perineum cut in an episiotomy

laparoscopy *(lap-a-ROS-kō-pē)* — Endoscopic examination of the abdomen; may include surgical procedures, such as tubal ligation (see Figure 14-9)

speculum *(SPEK-ū-lum)* — An instrument used to enlarge the opening of a passage or cavity for examination

tubal ligation *(lī-GĀ-shun)* — Surgical constriction of the oviducts to produce sterilization (See Figures 14-3 and 14-9)

ABBREVIATIONS

BNO bladder neck obstruction
BPH benign prostatic hyperplasia
BSE breast self-examination
CIN cervical intraepithelial neoplasia
D&C dilation and curettage
DES diethylstilbestrol
DUB dysfunctional uterine bleeding
ERT estrogen replacement therapy
FSH follicle-stimulating hormone
GC gonococcus (cause of gonorrhea)
GU genitourinary
GYN gynecology
HPV human papilloma virus
HRT hormone replacement therapy
ICSH interstitial cell-stimulating hormone (luteinizing hormone)
IUD intrauterine device
LH luteinizing hormone
NGU nongonococcal urethritis
PID pelvic inflammatory disease
PMS premenstrual syndrome
PSA prostate-specific antigen
STD sexually transmitted disease
TPUR transperineal urethral resection
TSE testicular self examination
TSS toxic shock syndrome
TURP transurethral resection of prostate
VD venereal disease (sexually transmitted disease)
VDRL venereal disease research laboratory (test for syphilis)

Chapter 14
Labeling Exercise

For each of the following illustrations, write the name of each numbered part on the corresponding line of the answer sheet.

anus
bulbourethral (Cowper's) gland
ejaculatory duct
epididymis
glans penis
kidney
penis
peritoneal cavity
prepuce
prostate
rectum
scrotum
seminal vesicle
testis
ureter
urethra
urinary bladder

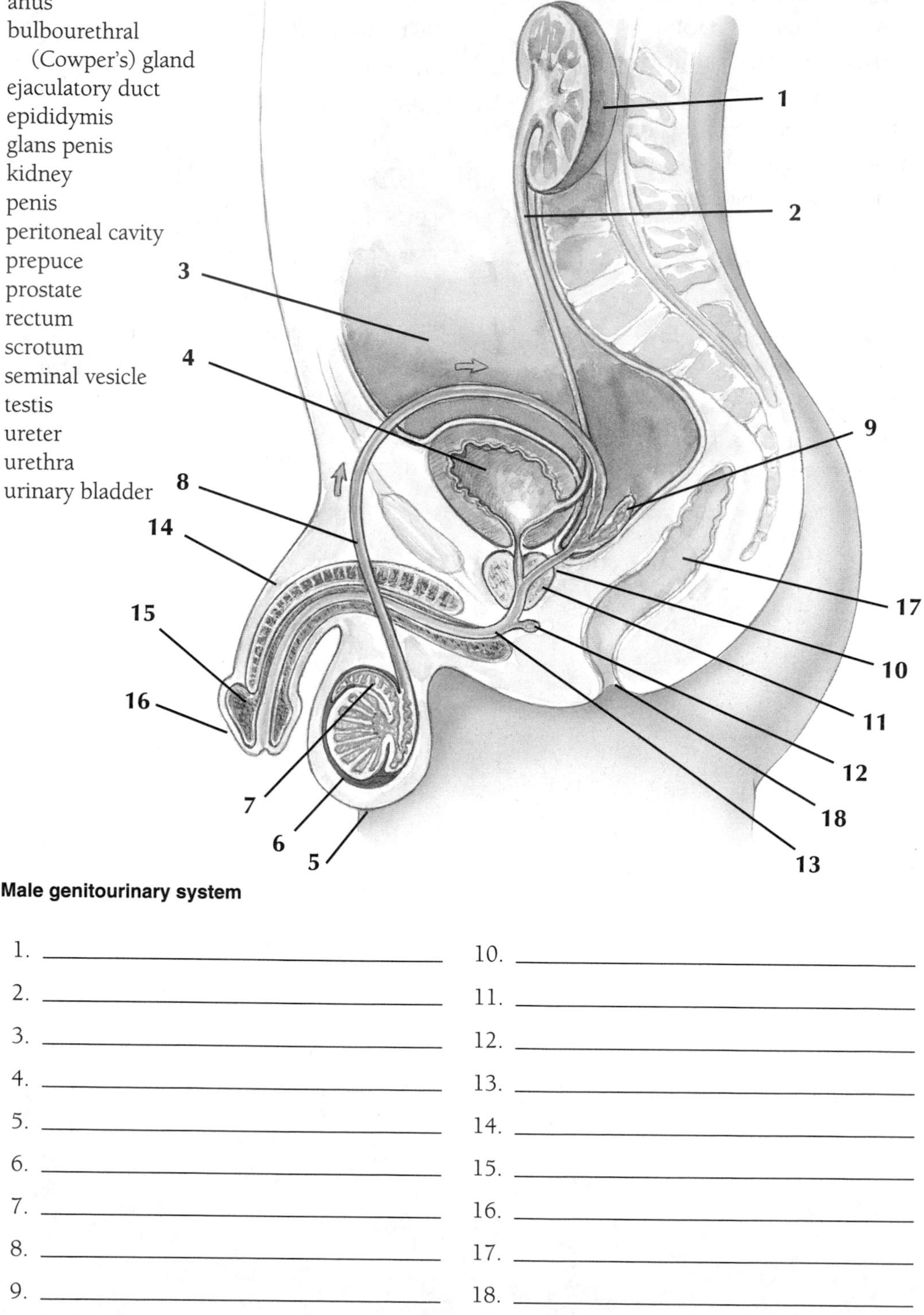

Male genitourinary system

1. ______________________
2. ______________________
3. ______________________
4. ______________________
5. ______________________
6. ______________________
7. ______________________
8. ______________________
9. ______________________
10. ______________________
11. ______________________
12. ______________________
13. ______________________
14. ______________________
15. ______________________
16. ______________________
17. ______________________
18. ______________________

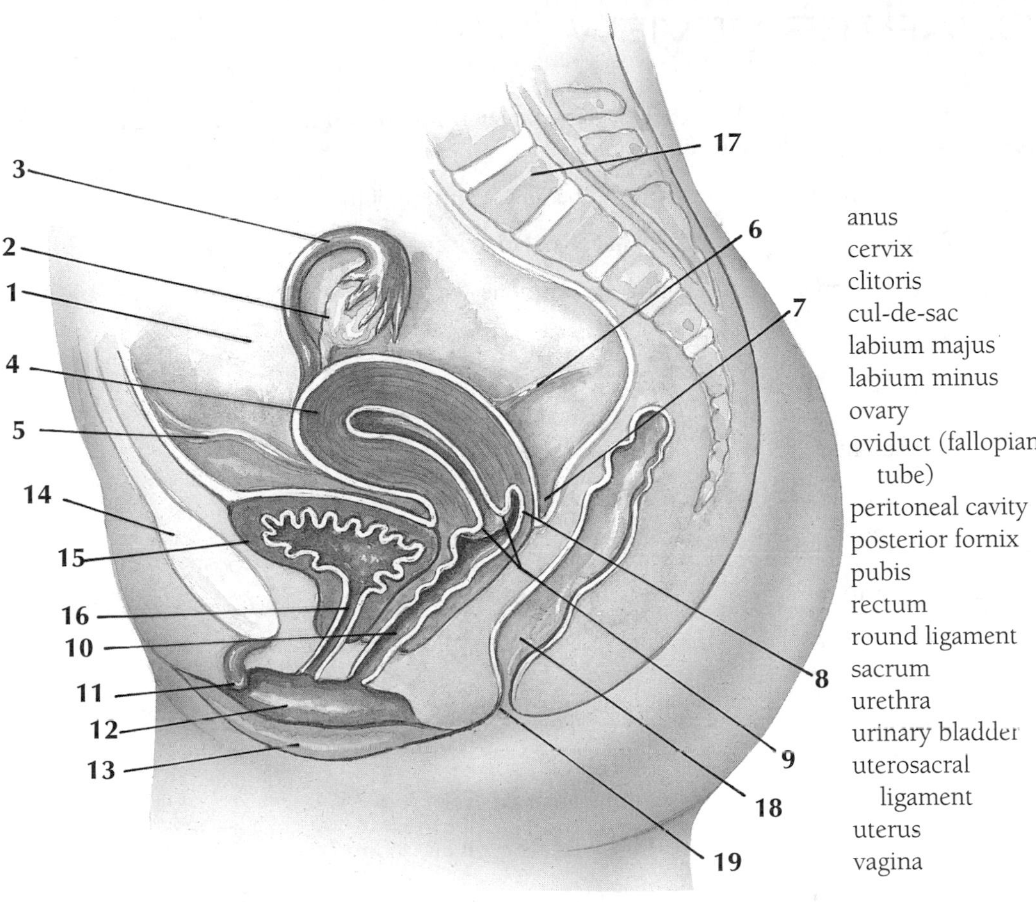

anus
cervix
clitoris
cul-de-sac
labium majus
labium minus
ovary
oviduct (fallopian tube)
peritoneal cavity
posterior fornix
pubis
rectum
round ligament
sacrum
urethra
urinary bladder
uterosacral ligament
uterus
vagina

Female genitourinary system

1. ______________________
2. ______________________
3. ______________________
4. ______________________
5. ______________________
6. ______________________
7. ______________________
8. ______________________
9. ______________________
10. ______________________
11. ______________________
12. ______________________
13. ______________________
14. ______________________
15. ______________________
16. ______________________
17. ______________________
18. ______________________
19. ______________________

CHAPTER REVIEW 14-1

Matching. Match the words in each of these sets with their definitions and write the appropriate letter (a–e) to the left of each number:

_____ 1. gonad	a. coiled tube on the surface of the testis
_____ 2. glans	b. any male sex hormone
_____ 3. epididymis	c. pituitary hormone
_____ 4. androgen	d. end of the penis
_____ 5. FSH	e. sex gland

_____ 6. anorchism	a. excision of the ductus deferens
_____ 7. prostate	b. absence of testes
_____ 8. oligospermia	c. tumor of the scrotum
_____ 9. vasectomy	d. deficiency of spermatozoa
_____ 10. oscheoma	e. gland located below the bladder in the male

_____ 11. clitoris	a. muscle of the uterus
_____ 12. myometrium	b. fallopian tube
_____ 13. oviduct	c. start of menstrual cycles
_____ 14. menarche	d. external female genitalia
_____ 15. vulva	e. female erectile tissue

_____ 16. metrorrhea	a. any disease specific to women
_____ 17. hysterotomy	b. abnormal uterine discharge
_____ 18. metratrophia	c. wasting of uterine tissue
_____ 19. gynecopathy	d. suppression of menstruation
_____ 20. menostasis	e. incision of the uterus

Fill in the blanks:

21. The common passage for urine and semen in the male is the _____________________.
22. The male gonad is the _____________________.
23. The thick fluid that transports spermatozoa is _____________________.
24. The main male sex hormone is _____________________.
25. The neck of the uterus is the _____________________.
26. The inner lining of the uterus is the _____________________.
27. Orchiopexy is surgical fixation of the _____________________.
28. Colpostenosis (*kol-pō-ste-NŌ-sis*) is a narrowing of the _____________________.

Definitions. Write the meaning of each of the following terms:

29. Orchiectomy *(or-kē-EK-tō-mē)* ______
30. Hemospermia *(hē-mō-SPER-mē-a)* ______
31. Prostatitis *(pros-ta-TĪ-tis)* ______
32. Metrorrhagia *(mē-trō-RĀ-jē-a)* ______
33. Hysteropathy *(his-te-ROP-a-thē)* ______
34. Pyosalpinx *(pī-ō-SAL-pinx)* ______

Word building. Write a word for each of the following definitions:

35. Excision of the vas deferens ______
36. Stone in the scrotum ______
37. Surgical incision of the prostate ______
38. Inflammation of a seminal vesicle ______
39. Rupture of the uterus (metr/o) ______
40. Surgical removal of the uterus (hyster/o) and oviducts ______
41. Cell that produces an ovum (oo) ______
42. Radiographic study of the breast (mamm/o) ______

Write the adjective form of each of the following words:

43. semen ______
44. prostate ______
45. cervix ______
46. perineum ______

Write the plural of each of the following words:

47. testis ______
48. spermatozoon ______
49. labium ______
50. fornix ______

CHAPTER REVIEW 14-2

Matching. Match the words in each of these sets with their definitions and write the appropriate letter (a–e) to the left of each number:

______	1. phimosis	a. enlargement of the veins in the spermatic cord
______	2. emission	b. sexual intercourse

_____	3. varicocele	c. narrowing of the prepuce opening
_____	4. coitus	d. inflammation of the glans penis
_____	5. balanitis	e. discharge of semen

_____	6. metrostenosis	a. whitish vaginal discharge
_____	7. menorrhagia	b. benign tumor of smooth muscle
_____	8. leukorrhea	c. excessive menstrual bleeding
_____	9. leiomyoma	d. instrument used to examine the vagina
_____	10. colposcope	e. narrowing of the uterine cavity

_____	11. corpus luteum	a. follicle left in ovary after ovulation
_____	12. hymen	b. recess at the top of the vagina
_____	13. fornix	c. fungal infection
_____	14. candidiasis	d. pain during intercourse
_____	15. dyspareunia	e. membrane over the vagina

Fill in the blanks:

16. The type of cell division that forms the gametes is _____________________.
17. The female gonad is the _____________________.
18. The sac that holds the testes is the _____________________.
19. A vasectomy involves cutting of the _____________________.
20. Release of an ovum from the ovary is called _____________________.
21. Parametritis *(par-a-mē-TRĪ-tis)* means inflammation of the tissue near the _____________________.
22. Polymastia *(pol-ē-MAS-tē-a)* means the presence of more than one pair of _____________________.
23. Hysteropexy is surgical fixation of the _____________________.

Definitions. Write the meaning of each of the following terms:

24. Orchialgia *(or-kē-AL-jē-a)* _____________________
25. Vesiculotomy *(ve-sik-ū-LOT-ō-mē)* _____________________
26. Prostatometer *(pros-ta-TOM-e-ter)* _____________________
27. Amenorrhea *(a-men-ō-RĒ-a)* _____________________
28. Inframmmary *(in-fra-MAM-a-rē)* _____________________
29. Mastectomy *(mas-TEK-tō-mē)* _____________________

Word building. Write a word for each of the following definitions:

30. Inflammation of the testis (orchi/o) and epididymis _____________________
31. Inflammation of the ductus (vas) deferens and seminal vesicle _____________________

32. Surgical creation of an opening between two parts of a cut ductus deferens (done to restore fertility) ____________

33. Plastic repair of the scrotum ____________

34. Hernia of an oviduct ____________

35. Through (-trans) the cervix ____________

36. Plastic repair of the vagina (colp/o) and perineum ____________

37. Radiographic study of the oviduct ____________

Write the adjective form of each of the following words:

38. uterus ____________

39. vagina ____________

40. labium ____________

Write the plural form of each of the following words:

41. cervix ____________

42. fimbria ____________

43. ovum ____________

Write the meaning of the following abbreviations:

44. BPH ____________

45. GC ____________

46. PSA ____________

47. PID ____________

48. D&C ____________

49. STD ____________

50. TURP ____________

Word analysis. Define each of the following words and give the meaning of the word parts in each. Use a dictionary if necessary.

51. Cryptorchidism ____________

____

a. crypt- ____________
b. orchid/o ____________
c. -ism ____________

52. Gynecomastia *(jin-e-kō-MAS-tē-a)* ____________

____

a. gynec/o ____________

b. mast/o ______________

c. -ia ______________

53. Myometrial ______________________________

____

a. my/o ______________

b. metr/i ______________

c. -al ______________

Chapter 14

Case Studies

1. Bilateral Vasectomy

In the supine position, the patient was thoroughly prepped with drapes placed below the scrotal sac as well as the anterior abdominal wall. The right vas was gently palpated and brought to skin level. This area was then injected with 2% Xylocaine anesthesia. After an appropriate period, an incision was made and the area was excised.

The vas was carefully located from its surrounding tissue and grasped with a towel clamp. A curved mosquito hemostat was then clamped on the right vas and on the left vas. 1 cm of the right vas was then removed. Both ends of the vas were then coagulated and tied independently using 2-0 chromic material. The same procedure was performed on the opposite side. Small superficial bleeders were coagulated. The skin was then reapproximated using 2-0 chromic.

No bleeding or swelling of the testicles was seen. The patient was discharged with instructions on postop care and subsequent birth control procedures.

2. Prostatectomy for Benign Prostatic Hyperplasia

The patient was placed in the dorsal lithotomy position and the perineal area was prepped and draped in the usual manner. The urethra was well lubricated and after a modified meatotomy was dilated to a #32 sound. A #28 resectoscope sheath was advanced with ease into the bladder. Examination of the bladder revealed no abnormalities.

A transurethral resection of approximately 55 g of grossly benign prostatic tissue was carried out without incident. Hemostasis was obtained with electrocoagulation. A #26 Foley catheter with the balloon inflated up to 90 mL was placed and the patient left the Operating Room in good condition.

Estimated blood loss was 350 mL with none replaced.

3. Cone Biopsy for Cervical Dysplasia

J. S. is a 51-year-old female who presented to the Ambulatory Surgical Unit with a history of Pap smear abnormalities. These have ranged from normal in 9/81, to Class I negative for dysplasia, to the most recent of 6/95 showing probable squamous cell carcinoma in situ. During this interval she has had multiple Pap smears, colposcopic-directed biopsies, and endocervical curettages. Every biopsy has been consistent with inflammation and atypia, but has never been confirmatory for cancer. In view of the most recent Pap smear, it was decided to proceed with a cervical cone biopsy to be both diagnostic and therapeutic.

Procedure: The patient was placed into the dorsal lithotomy position. A bivalved speculum was placed into the vagina; the cervix was visualized, and a colposcopic examination was performed with 3% acetic acid. Local anesthesia was administered in a circumferential fashion around the ectocervix. Under colposcopic guidance a hot wire loop was used to scoop out a cone-shaped portion of the cervix. There was a minimal amount of bleeding. Monsel's solution was applied and good hemostasis was achieved. The patient was placed into the supine position and transferred to the recovery room in stable condition.

The pathology report on the cervical cone showed moderate to severe dysplasia (high grade squamous intraepithelial neoplasia) with free surgical margins.

Chapter 14
Case Study Questions

Multiple choice. Select the best answer and write the letter of your choice to the left of each number:

_____ 1. A patient in the dorsal lithotomy position is

- a. lying face down
- b. standing with his arms at his sides
- c. on his left side
- d. on his knees with head and upper chest on the table
- e. on his back with legs flexed and thighs apart

_____ 2. In the first case study, when the ends of the vas were coagulated, they were

- a. probed
- b. dilated
- c. sealed
- d. sutured
- e. clamped

_____ 3. The ectocervix is the

- a. lining of the uterus
- b. lining of the cervix
- c. upper portion of the vagina
- d. hymen
- e. outer portion of the cervix

_____ 4. A curettage is a(n)

- a. scraping
- b. cutting
- c. suturing
- d. examination
- e. incision

_____ 5. A carcinoma in situ is one that

- a. metastasizes rapidly
- b. invades the lungs
- c. remains localized
- d. grows rapidly
- e. spreads to the lymphatic system

Find a term in the case studies that means each of the following:

6. Incision to enlarge the urinary opening _____________________
7. Device used to stop blood flow _____________________
8. Ductus deferens _____________________
9. Pertaining to the area between the thighs _____________________

10. Not malignant ______________________

11. Overgrowth of cells ______________________

12. Within the cervix ______________________

13. Removal of tissue for microscopic examination ______________________

14. Instrument used to dilate and examine a passageway ______________________

Define the following terms:

15. Prostatectomy ____

16. Transurethral ____

17. Resection ____

18. Colposcopic ____

19. Supine ____

REPRODUCTIVE SYSTEM

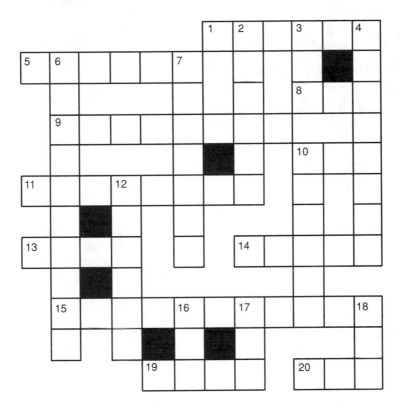

ACROSS

1. appendages, such as those near the uterus
5. the male reproductive glands
8. a contraceptive device (abbr.)
9. the channel through which the testes descend: _____ canal
10. blockage of urine flow at the outlet of the bladder (abbr.)
11. the long, fingerlike extensions of the oviduct that help to capture the released ovum
13. root (with combining vowel): woman
14. the organ above the pituitary
15. introduces semen into the female
19. the inner lining of the uterus: ____ metrium
20. infection of the pelvic cavity (abbr.)

DOWN

2. to widen
3. prefix: upon, over
4. any hormone that produces male characteristics
6. a coiled tube on the surface of the testis that stores sperm
7. cells located between the seminiferous tubules: inter ______ cells
10. mammary gland
12. removal of tissue for microscopic examination
16. root: month, menstruation
17. prefix: new
18. disease spread through sexual activity (abbr.)

Chapter 14 Answer Section

Answers to Chapter Exercises

Exercise 14-1

1. any disease of a testis
2. incision of a testis
3. excision of the epididymis
4. pertaining to the prostate
5. tumor of the scrotum
6. inflammation of the testis and epididymis
7. orchioplasty *(OR-kē-ō-plas-tē)*; also orchidoplasty *(OR-ki-dō-plas-tē)*
8. orchiectomy *(or-kē-EK-tō-mē)*; also orchidectomy *(or-ki-DEK-tō-mē)*
9. orchiopexy *(or-kē-ō-PEK-sē)*; also orchidopexy *(OR-ki-dō-pek-sē)*
10. spermatocyte *(sper-MA-tō-sīt)*
11. spermatolysis *(sper-ma-TOL-i-sis)*
12. spermatogenesis *(sper-ma-tō-JEN-e-sis)*
13. spermatorrhea *(sper-ma-to-RE-a)*
14. spermaturia *(sper-ma-TŪ-rē-a)*
15. hemospermia *(hē-mō-SPER-mē-a)*; also hematospermia *(hem-at-ō-SPER-mē-a)*
16. pyospermia *(pī-ō-SPER-mē-a)*
17. aspermia *(a-SPER-mē-a)*
18. vesiculogram *(ve-SIK-ū-lō-gram)*
19. prostatectomy *(pros-ta-TEK-tō-mē)*
20. vesiculitis *(ve-sik-ū-LĪ-tis)*
21. vasostomy *(vas-OS-tō-mē)*
22. vasorrhaphy *(vas-OR-a-fē)*
23. epididymotomy *(ep-i-did-i-MOT-ō-mē)*
24. oscheoplasty *(OS-kē-ō-plas-tē)*

Exercise 14-2

1. pertaining to an absence of ovulation
2. surgical puncture of the ovary
3. inflammation of the ovary
4. pertaining to the period before menstruation
5. gynecologist *(gī-ne-KOL-ō-jist)*
6. oocyte *(Ō-ō-sīt)*
7. menorrhagia *(men-ō-RĀ-jē-a)*
8. amenorrhea *(a-men-ō-RĒ-a)*
9. dysmenorrhea *(DIS-men-ō-rē-a)*
10. oligomenorrhea *(ol-i-gō-men-ō-RĒ-a)*
11. ovarian *(ō-VAR-ē-an)*
12. ovariocele *(ō-VAR-ē-ō-sēl)*
13. ovariopexy *(ō-var-ē-ō-PEK-sē)*; also oophoropexy *(ō-of-ō-rō-PEK-sē)*
14. oophorotomy *(ō-of-ō-ROT-ō-mē)*
15. oophoroma *(ō-of-ō-RŌ-ma)*

Exercise 14-3

1. excision of an oviduct
2. surgical fixation of the uterus
3. narrowing of the uterus
4. within the uterus
5. plastic repair of the vagina
6. dilatation of the vagina
7. salpingopexy *(sal-PING-gō-pek-sē)*
8. salpingoplasty *(sal-PING-gō-plas-tē)*; also tuboplasty
9. pyosalpinx *(pī-ō-SAL-pinx)*
10. hydrosalpinx *(hī-drō-SAL-pinx)*
11. salpingo-oophorectomy *(sal-ping-gō-ō-of-ō-REK-tō-mē)* also salpingo-ovariectomy *(sal-ping-gō-ō-var-ē-EK-tō-me)*
12. retrouterine *(re-trō-Ū-ter-in)*
13. hysterosalpingogram *(his-ter-ō-sal-PING-gō-gram)*
14. hysterotomy *(his-ter-OT-ō-mē)*
15. metroptosis *(mē-trō-TŌ-sis)*
16. metromalacia *(mē-trō-ma-LĀ-shē-a)*

17. cervicitis *(ser-vi-SĪ-tis)*
18. intracervical *(in-tra-SER-vi-kal)*
19. transvaginal *(trans-VAJ-i-nal)*
20. vaginometer *(vaj-i-NOM-e-ter)*
21. colpocele *(KOL-pō-sēl)*; also vaginocele *(VAJ-in-ō-sēl)*

Exercise 14-4

1. vulvopathy *(vul-VOP-a-thē)*
2. episioplasty *(e-PIZ-ē-ō-plas-tē)*
3. vaginoperineal *(vaj-i-nō-per-i-NĒ-al)*
4. clitoritis *(klit-o-RĪ-tis)*
5. mammogram *(MAM-ō-gram)*
6. mastectomy *(mas-TEK-tō-mē)*; also mammectomy *(ma-MEK-tō-mē)*
7. mastitis *(mas-TĪ-tis)*

Labeling Exercise

Male Genitourinary System

1. kidney
2. ureter
3. peritoneal cavity
4. urinary bladder
5. scrotum
6. testis
7. epididymis
8. vas (ductus) deferens
9. seminal vesicle
10. ejacultory duct
11. prostate
12. bulbourethral (Cowper's) gland
13. urethra
14. penis
15. glans penis
16. prepuce
17. rectum
18. anus

Female Genitourinary System

1. peritoneal cavity
2. ovary
3. oviduct (fallopian tube)
4. uterus
5. round ligament
6. uterosacral ligament
7. cul-de-sac
8. posterior fornix
9. cervix
10. vagina
11. clitoris
12. labium minus
13. labium majus
14. pubis
15. urinary bladder
16. urethra
17. sacrum
18. rectum
19. anus

Chapter Review 14-1

1. e
2. d
3. a
4. b
5. c
6. b
7. e
8. d
9. a
10. c
11. e
12. a
13. b
14. c
15. d
16. b
17. e
18. c
19. a
20. d
21. urethra
22. testis
23. semen
24. testosterone
25. cervix
26. endometrium
27. testis
28. vagina
29. excision of the testis
30. blood in the semen
31. inflammation of the prostate
32. abnormal bleeding from the uterus

33. any disease of the uterus
34. presence of pus in the oviduct
35. vasectomy
36. oscheolith
37. prostatotomy
38. vesiculitis
39. metrorrhexis
40. hysterosalpingectomy
41. oocyte
42. mammography
43. seminal
44. prostatic
45. cervical
46. perineal
47. testes
48. spermatozoa
49. labia
50. fornices

Chapter Review 14-2

1. c
2. e
3. a
4. b
5. d
6. e
7. c
8. a
9. b
10. d
11. a
12. e
13. b
14. c
15. d
16. meiosis
17. ovary
18. scrotum
19. ductus (vas) deferens
20. ovulation
21. uterus
22. breasts (mammary glands)
23. uterus
24. pain in the testis
25. incision of the seminal vesicle
26. instrument for measuring the prostate
27. absence of menstruation
28. below the breast
29. excision of the breast
30. orchiepididymitis
31. vasovesiculitis
32. vasovasostomy
33. oscheoplasty
34. salpingocele
35. transcervical
36. colpoperineoplasty
37. salpingography
38. uterine
39. vaginal
40. labial
41. cervices
42. fimbriae
43. ova
44. benign prostatic hyperplasia
45. gonococcus
46. prostate-specific antigen
47. pelvic inflammatory disease
48. dilation and curettage
49. sexually transmitted disease
50. transurethral resection of the prostate
51. undescended testes
    a. hidden
    b. testis
    c. condition of
52. excessive development of the mammary glands in the male, even to the secretion of milk
    a. woman
    b. breast
    c. condition of
53. Pertaining to the muscular layer of the uterus
    a. muscle
    b. uterus
    c. pertaining to

Answers to Case Study Questions

1. e
2. c
3. e
4. a
5. c
6. meatotomy
7. hemostat
8. vas
9. perineal
10. benign
11. hyperplasia
12. endocervical
13. biopsy
14. speculum
15. surgical removal of the prostate
16. through the urethra
17. partial excision
18. pertaining to examination of the vagina
19. lying face up

Answers to Crossword Puzzle

REPRODUCTIVE SYSTEM

						1 A	2 D	N	3 E	X	4 A
5 T	6 E	S	T	E	7 S		I		P		N
	P				T		L		8 I	U	D
	9 I	N	G	U	I	N	A	L			R
	D				T		T		10 B	N	O
11 F	I	M	12 B	R	I	A	E		R		G
	D		I		A				E		E
13 G	Y	N	O		L		14 B	R	A	I	N
	M		P						S		
	15 I	N	S	E	16 M	I	17 N	A	T	E	18 S
	S		Y		E		E				T
				19 E	N	D	O		20 P	I	D

15 Development

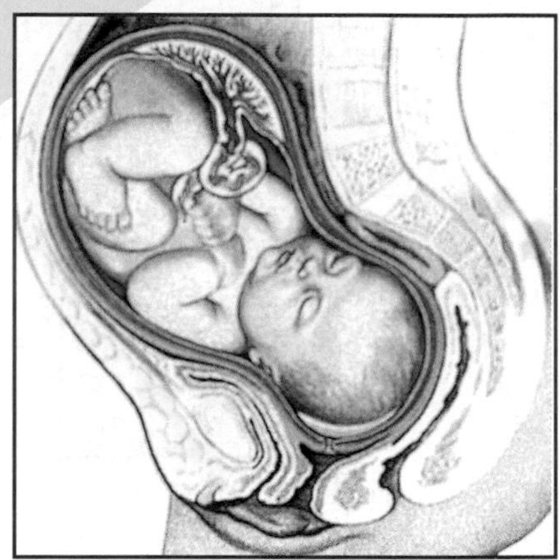

Chapter Contents

Objectives

After study of this chapter you should be able to:

1. Outline the major events that occur in the first 2 months following fertilization
2. Label a diagram of the female reproductive tract that shows fertilization
3. Describe the structure and function of the placenta
4. Describe the three stages of childbirth
5. List the hormonal and nervous controls over lactation
6. Identify and use the roots pertaining to pregnancy and birth
7. Describe the main disorders affecting pregnancy, early development, and birth
8. Compare the terms *congenital* and *hereditary* as applied to birth defects
9. Analyze several case studies concerning pregnancy

Fertilization and Early Development

At the time of **fertilization** (Fig. 15-1) the nuclei of the sperm and egg fuse, restoring the chromosome number of 46 and forming a **zygote**. As the zygote travels through the oviduct toward the uterus, it divides rapidly. Within 6–7 days, the fertilized egg reaches the uterus and implants into the endometrium, and the **embryo** begins to develop.

During the first 8 weeks of growth all of the major body systems are established. Embryonic tissue produces **HCG** (human chorionic gonadotropin), a hormone that keeps the corpus luteum functional in the ovary to maintain the endometrium. (The presence of HCG in urine and blood is the basis for pregnancy tests). After 2 months placental hormones take over this function and the corpus luteum degenerates. At this time the embryo becomes a **fetus**.

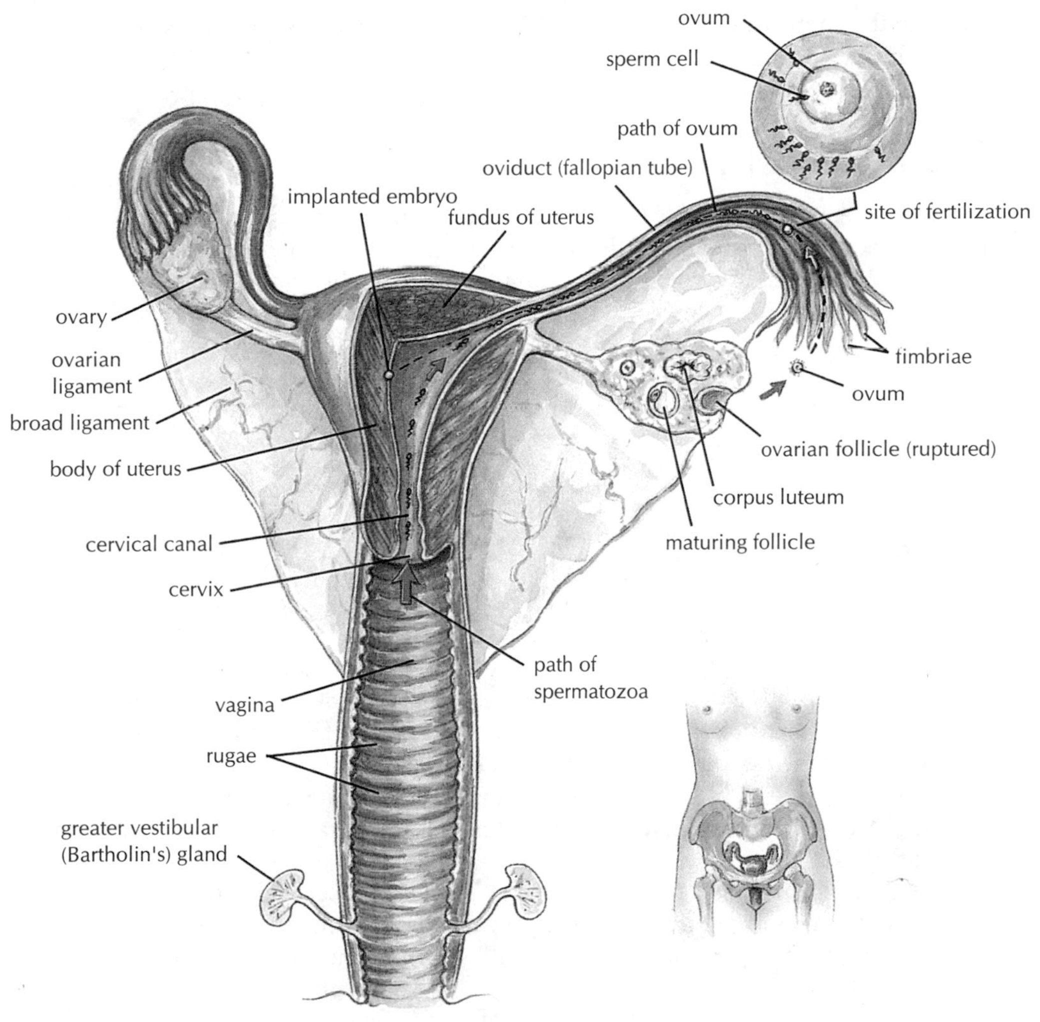

FIGURE 15-1. Female reproductive system showing fertilization.

✳ The Placenta

During development the fetus is nourished by the **placenta**, an organ formed from the outermost layer of the embryo, the **chorion**, and the innermost layer of the uterus, the endometrium (Fig. 15-2). Here, exchanges take place between the bloodstreams of the mother and the fetus through fetal capillaries. The **umbilical cord** contains the blood vessels that link the fetus to the placenta. Fetal blood is carried to the placenta in two umbilical arteries. While traveling through the placenta, the blood picks up nutrients and oxygen and gives up carbon dioxide and metabolic waste. Restored blood is carried from the placenta to the fetus in a single umbilical vein. Although the bloodstreams of the mother and the fetus do not mix, and all exchanges take place through capillaries, some materials do manage to get through the placenta in both directions. For example, some viruses, drugs, and other harmful substances are known to pass from the mother to the fetus; fetal proteins can enter the mother's blood and cause immunologic reactions.

During **gestation** (the period of development), the fetus is cushioned and protected by fluid contained in the **amniotic sac** (amnion; Fig. 15-3), commonly called the bag of waters. This sac ruptures at birth.

✳ Fetal Circulation

The fetus has several adaptations that serve to bypass the lungs, which are not needed to oxygenate the blood. When blood coming from the placenta enters the right atrium, the **foramen ovale**, a small hole in the septum between the atria, allows some of the blood to go directly into the left atrium, thus bypassing the pulmonary artery. Further, blood pumped out of the right ventricle can shunt directly into the aorta through a short vessel, the **ductus arteriosus**, that connects the pulmonary artery with the descending aorta (see Figure 15-2). Both of these passages close off at birth when the pulmonary circuit is established. Their failure to close hampers the work of the heart and may require medical attention.

✳ Childbirth

The length of pregnancy, from fertilization of the ovum to birth, is about 38 weeks or 266 days. In practice, it is calculated as approximately 280 days or 40 weeks from the first day of the last menstrual period (LMP). For study purposes it may be divided into 3-month periods (trimesters) during which defined changes can be observed in the fetus. Childbirth or **parturition** occurs in three stages: 1) onset of regular uterine contractions and dilation of the cervix; 2) expulsion of the fetus; 3) delivery of the placenta and fetal membranes. The third stage is followed by contraction of the uterus and control of bleeding. The factors that start labor are not completely understood, but it is clear that the hormone **oxytocin** from the posterior pituitary gland and other hormones called prostaglandins are involved.

The term **gravida** refers to a pregnant woman. A prefix may be added to show the number of pregnancies, such as primigravida, meaning a woman pregnant for the first time, or a number may be used, such as gravida 1, gravida 2, and so forth. The term **para** refers to a woman who has given birth. This means the production of a viable infant (500 g or more or over 20 weeks' gestation) regardless of whether the infant is alive at birth or whether the birth is single or multiple. Again, prefixes or numerals are used to indicate the number of such pregnancies.

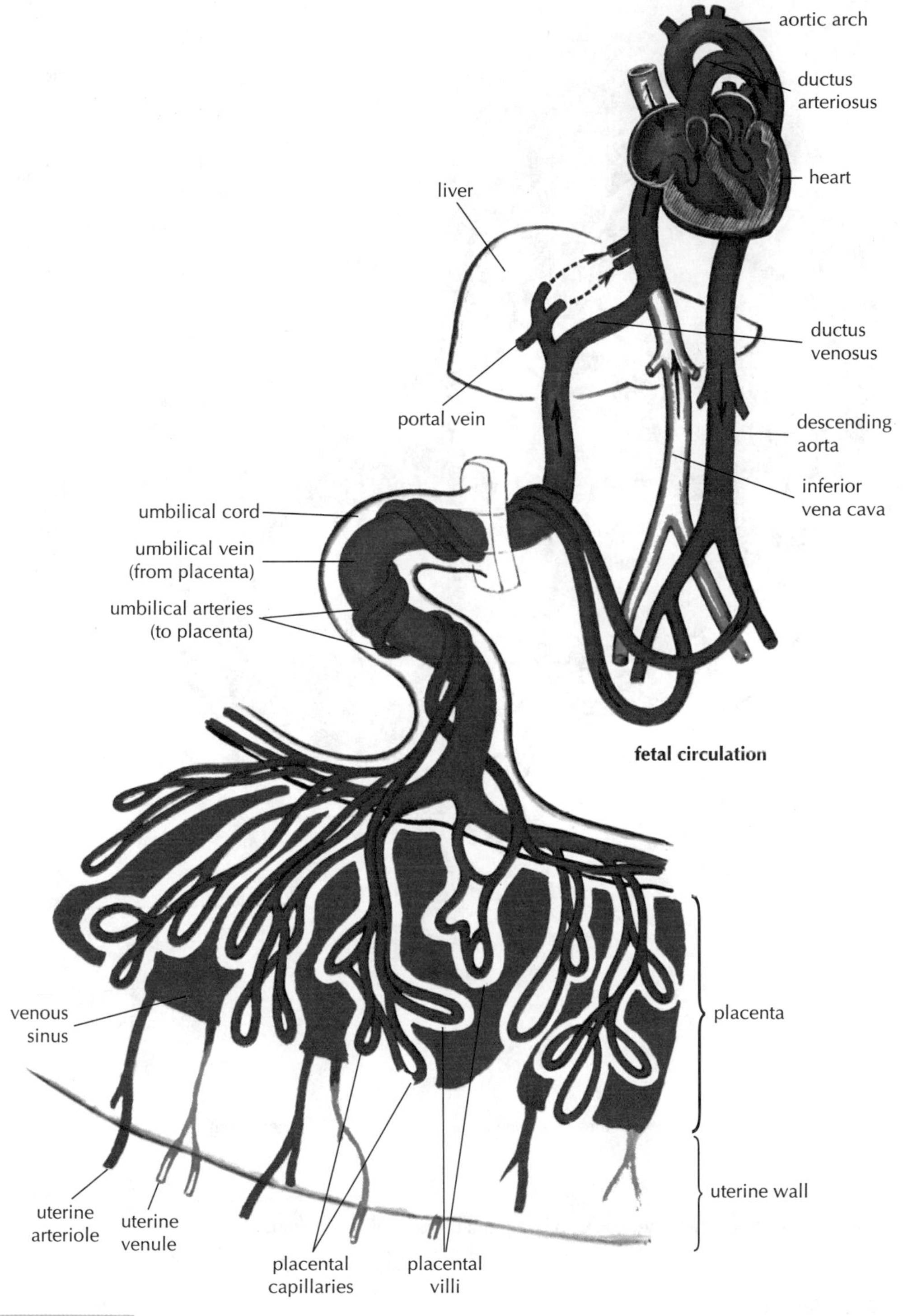

FIGURE 15-2. Fetal circulation and placenta.

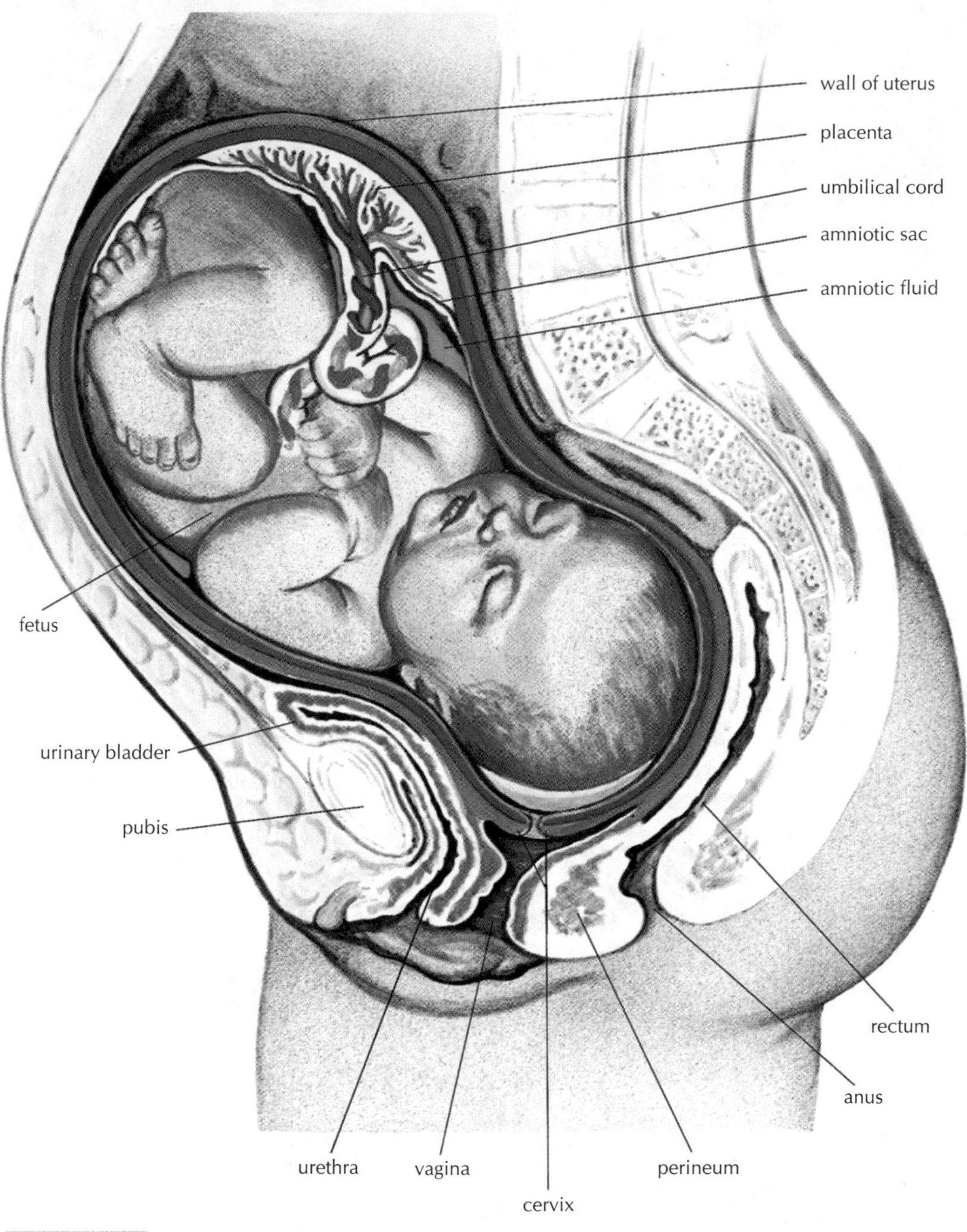

FIGURE 15-3. Midsagittal section of a pregnant uterus with intact fetus.

Lactation

The secretion of milk from the breasts, **lactation**, is started by the hormone prolactin from the anterior pituitary gland, as well as hormones from the placenta. The release of milk is then stimulated by suckling. For the first few days after delivery only **colostrum** is produced. This has a slightly different composition than milk but, like the milk, it has protective antibodies.

KEY TERMS

Normal Structure and Function

Term	Definition
amniotic sac *(am-nē-OT-ik)*	The membranous sac filled with fluid that holds the fetus; also called amnion (root amnio)
chorion *(KOR-ē-on)*	The outermost layer of the embryo that, with the endometrium, forms the placenta (adj. chorionic)
colostrum *(kō-LOS-trum)*	Breast fluid that is secreted in the first few days after birth, before milk is produced
ductus arteriosus *(DUK-tus ar-tēr-ē-Ō-sus)*	A fetal blood vessel that connects the pulmonary artery with the descending aorta, thus allowing blood to bypass the lungs
embryo *(EM-brē-ō)*	The stage in development between the zygote and the fetus, extending from the 2nd to the 8th week of growth in the uterus (adj. embryonic) (root embry/o)
fertilization *(fer-ti-li-ZĀ-shun)*	The union of an ovum and a spermatozoon
fetus *(FĒ-tus)*	The developing child in the uterus from the third month to birth (adj. fetal) (root fet/o)
foramen ovale *(fō-RĀ-men ō-VĀ-lē)*	A small hole in the septum between the atria in the fetal heart that allows blood to pass directly from the right to the left side of the heart
gestation *(jes-TĀ-shun)*	The period of development from conception to birth
gravida *(GRAV-i-da)*	Pregnant woman
lactation *(lak-TĀ-shun)*	The secretion of milk from the mammary glands
neonate *(NĒ-ō-nāt)*	Newborn
oxytocin *(ok-sē-TŌ-sin)*	A pituitary hormone that stimulates contractions of the uterus. It also stimulates release ("letdown") of milk from the breasts.
para	Woman who has produced a viable infant. Multiple births are considered as single pregnancies.
parturition *(par-tū-RI-shun)*	Childbirth; labor (root toc/o, nat/i)
placenta *(pla-SEN-ta)*	The organ, composed of fetal and maternal tissues, that nourishes and maintains the developing fetus
prostaglandins *(PROS-ta-glan-dinz)*	A group of hormones with varied effects, including the stimulation of uterine contractions
umbilical cord *(um-BIL-i-kal)*	The structure that connects the fetus to the placenta. It contains vessels that carry blood between the mother and the fetus.
zygote *(ZĪ-gōt)*	The fertilized ovum

Roots Pertaining to Pregnancy and Birth

Root	Meaning	Example	Definition of Example
amnio	amnion, amniotic sac	diamniotic *di-am-nē-OT-ik*	developing in separate amniotic sacs
embry/o	embryo	embryology *em-brē-OL-ō-jē*	study of the embryo
fet/o	fetus	fetoscope *FĒ-tō-skōp*	endoscope for examining the fetus
toc	labor	eutocia *ū-TŌ-sē-a*	normal labor
nat/i	birth	neonate *NĒ-ō-nāt*	newborn
lact/o	milk	lactation *lak-TĀ-shun*	secretion of milk
galact/o	milk	galactogogue *ga-LAK-ta-gog*	agent that promotes (-agogue) the flow of milk
gravida	pregnant woman	nulligravida *nul-i-GRAV-i-da*	woman who has never (nulli-) been pregnant
para	woman who has given birth	multipara *mul-TIP-a-ra*	woman who has given birth two or more times

Exercise 15-1

Define the following terms:

1. Embryonic
   (em-brē-ON-ik) ____________________
2. Prenatal
   (prē-NĀ-tal) ____________________
3. Neonatalogist
   (nē-ō-nā-TOL-ō-jist) ____________________
4. Monoamniotic
   (mon-ō-am-nē-OT-ik) ____________________
5. Fetoscopy
   (fē-TOS-kō-pē) ____________________
6. Hyperlactation
   (hī-per-lak-TĀ-shun) ____________________
7. Agalactia
   (ā-ga-LAK-shē-a) ____________________

Use the appropriate roots to form words with the following definitions:

8. Rupture of the amniotic sac ____________________
9. Incision of the amnion (to induce labor) ____________________

10. Cell found in amniotic fluid __________
11. Instrument for examination of the embryo __________
12. Measurement of the fetus __________
13. Any disease of an embryo __________
14. After birth __________
15. Woman who is pregnant for the first time (primi-) __________
16. Woman who has been pregnant two or more times __________
17. Woman who has never given birth __________
18. Woman who has given birth to one child __________

Use the suffix *-tocia* meaning "condition of labor" for the following words:

19. Dry labor __________
20. Abnormal or difficult labor __________

Use the root *galact/o* for the following words:

21. Cystic enlargement (-cele) of a milk duct __________
22. Discharge of milk __________

Clinical Aspects of Pregnancy and Development

Preeclampsia, often referred to as toxemia of pregnancy, is a state of hypertension in association with proteinuria and edema. The cause is a hormone imbalance that results in constriction of blood vessels. If untreated, preeclampsia may lead to true **eclampsia** with seizures, coma, and possible death.

Development of a fertilized egg outside its normal position in the uterine cavity is termed an **ectopic pregnancy** (Fig. 15-4). Although it may occur elsewhere in the abdominal cavity, this abnormal development usually takes place in the oviduct, resulting in a **tubal pregnancy**. Salpingitis, endometriosis, and pelvic inflammatory disease (PID) may lead to ectopic pregnancy by blocking passage of the egg into the uterus. Continued growth will rupture the oviduct, causing dangerous hemorrhage. Symptoms of ectopic pregnancy are pain, tenderness, swelling, and shock. A diagnosis is confirmed by laparascopic examination. Prompt surgery is required, sometimes including removal of the tube.

For a variety of reasons, a pregnancy may terminate before the fetus is capable of surviving outside the uterus. An **abortion** is loss of an embryo or fetus before the 20th week of pregnancy or a weight of 500 grams (1.1 lb). When this occurs spontaneously it is commonly referred to as a miscarriage. Most spontaneous abortions occur within the first 3 months of pregnancy. Causes include tumors, hormone imbalance, incompetence (weakness) of the cervix, immune reactions, and most commonly, fetal abnormalities. If all gestational tissues are not eliminated, the abortion is described as incomplete and the remaining tissue must be removed.

An induced abortion is the intentional termination of a pregnancy. A common method is **dilatation and evacuation** (D&E), in which the cervix is dilated and the fetal tissue is removed by suction.

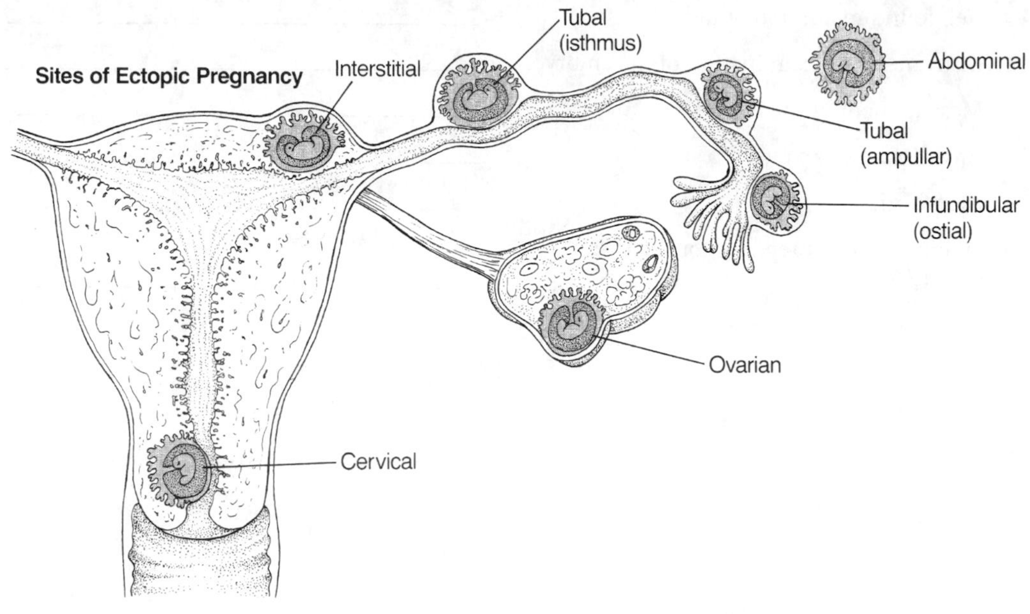

FIGURE 15-4. Possible sites of ectopic pregnancy. (Reeder S, Martin LL, Koniak D: Maternity Nursing, 17th ed, p 777. Philadelphia: JB Lippincott, 1992.)

Placental Abnormalities

If the placenta attaches near or over the cervix instead of in the upper portion of the uterus the condition is termed **placenta previa**. This may cause bleeding in the later stages of pregnancy. **Placental abruption** describes premature separation of the placenta from its point of attachment. If extensive, this may result in fetal death.

Mastitis

Inflammation of the breast, or **mastitis**, may occur at any time but usually occurs in the early weeks of breastfeeding. It is commonly caused by staphylococcus or streptococcus organisms which enter through cracks in the nipple. The breast becomes red, swollen, and tender and the patient may experience chills, fever, and general discomfort.

Congenital Disorders

Congenital disorders are those present at birth (birth defects). They fall into two categories: developmental disorders that occur during growth of the fetus, and hereditary (familial) disorders that can be passed from parents to children through the germ cells. Genetic disorders are any that involve a **mutation** (change) in the genes or chromosomes of the cells. A **carrier** of a genetic disorder is an individual who has a genetic defect that does not appear but can be passed to offspring. Carriers of some genetic disorders can be identified by laboratory tests.

Teratogens are factors that cause malformation of the developing fetus. These include infections, such as **rubella** (German measles), herpes simplex, or syphilis, alcohol, drugs, and radiation. The fetus is most susceptible to teratogenic effects during the first 3 months of pregnancy. Examples

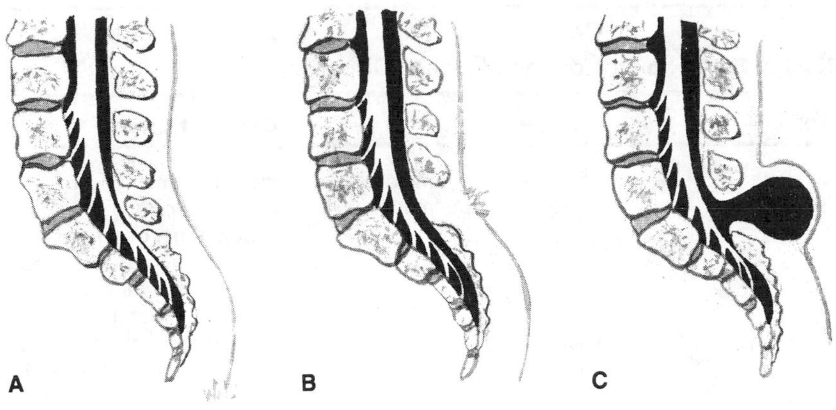

FIGURE 15-5. Spinal defects. **(A)** Normal spine. **(B)** Spina bifida occulta. **(C)** Meningocele. (Pillitteri A: Maternal and Child Health Nursing, p 1169. Philadelphia: JB Lippincott, 1992.)

of developmental disorders are **atresia** (absence or closure of a normal body opening), **anencephalus** (absence of a brain), **cleft lip, cleft palate**, and congenital heart disease. **Spina bifida** is incomplete closure of the spine, through which the spinal cord and its membranes may project (Figs. 15-5, 15-6). This usually occurs in the lumbar region. If there is no herniation of tissue, the condition is spina bifida occulta. Protrusion of the meninges through the opening is a meningocele; in a myelomeningocele, both the spinal cord and membranes herniate through the defect.

Genetic disorders may arise from changes in the number or structure of the chromosomes or changes in single genes. They may also be conditions that involve multiple genes interacting with environmental factors—the diseases that "run in families" such as diabetes mellitus, heart disease, hypertension, and certain forms of cancer. Table 15-1 describes some of the most common genetic disorders.

Many congenital disorders can now be detected before birth. **Ultrasonography** (Fig. 15-7), in addition to being used to monitor pregnancies and determine fetal sex, can also reveal certain fetal abnormalities. In **amniocentesis** (Fig. 15-8), a sample is withdrawn from the amniotic cavity

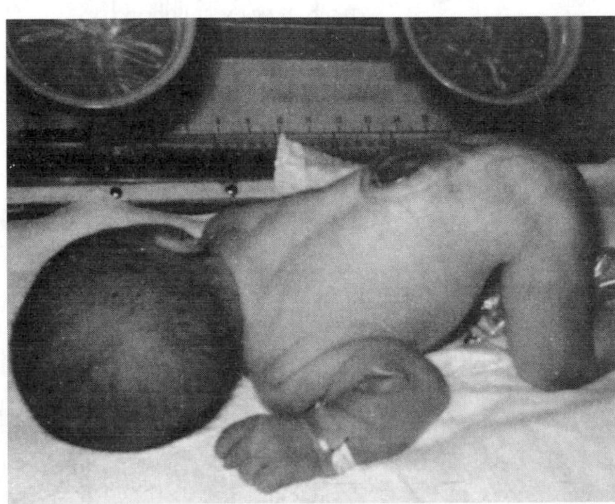

FIGURE 15-6. A myelomeningocele. (Pillitteri A: Maternal and Child Health Nursing, p 1169. Philadelphia: JB Lippincott, 1992.)

TABLE 15-1 Some Common Genetic Disorders*

Disease	Cause	Description
albinism	recessive gene mutation	lack of pigmentation
cystic fibrosis	recessive gene mutation	Affects respiratory system, pancreas, and sweat glands. Most common hereditary disease in white populations (see Chapter 10).
Down syndrome	extra chromosome 21	Slanted eyes, short stature, mental retardation, and others. Incidence increases with increasing maternal age.
hemophilia *(hē-mō-FIL-ē-a)*	recessive gene mutation on the X chromosome	bleeding disease passed from mothers to sons
Huntington's disease	dominant gene mutation	Altered metabolism destroys specific nerve cells. Appears in adulthood and is fatal within about 10 years. Causes motor and mental disorders.
Klinefelter's syndrome	extra sex (X) chromosome	lack of sexual development, lowered intelligence
Marfan's syndrome	dominant gene mutation	disease of connective tissue with weakness of the aorta
neurofibromatosis *(nū-rō-fi-brō-ma-TŌ-sis)*	dominant gene mutation	multiple skin tumors containing nervous tissue
phenylketonuria (PKU) *(fen-il-kē-tō-NŪ-rē-a)*	recessive gene mutation	Lack of enzyme to metabolize an amino acid. Neurologic signs, mental retardation, lack of pigment. Tested for at birth. Special diet can prevent retardation.
sickle cell anemia	recessive gene mutation	Abnormally shaped red cells block blood vessels. Mainly affects black populations.
Tay-Sachs disease	recessive gene mutation	An enzyme deficiency causes lipid to accumulate in nerve cells and other tissues. Causes death in early childhood. Carried in Jewish populations in Eastern Europe.
Turner's syndrome	single sex (X) chromosome	sexual immaturity, short stature, possible lowered intelligence

*A dominant gene is one for a trait that always appears if the gene is present; that is, it will affect the offspring even if inherited from only one parent. A recessive gene is one for a trait that will appear only if the gene is inherited from both parents.

with a needle. The fluid obtained can be analyzed for chemical abnormalities. The cells are grown in the laboratory and tested for biochemical disorders. A **karyotype** is prepared to study the genetic material. In **chorionic villus sampling** (CVS), small amounts of the membrane around the fetus are obtained through the cervix for analysis. This can be done at 8 to 10 weeks of pregnancy in comparison to 14 to 16 weeks for amniocentesis.

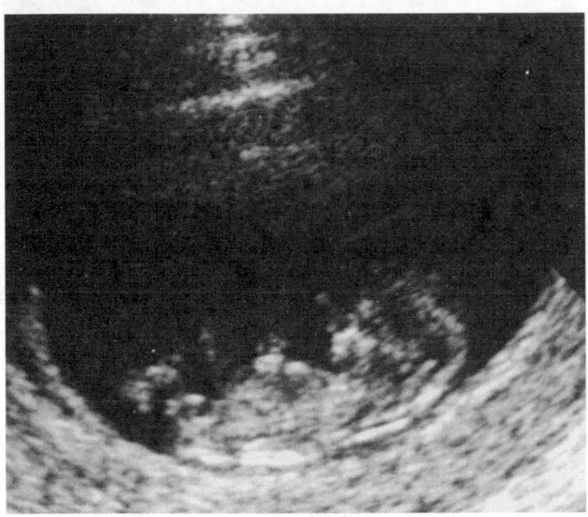

FIGURE 15-7. Sonogram showing fetal profile at 11 weeks. (Benson CB, Jones TB, Lavery MJ et al: Atlas of Obstetrical Ultrasound. Philadelphia: JB Lippincott, 1988.)

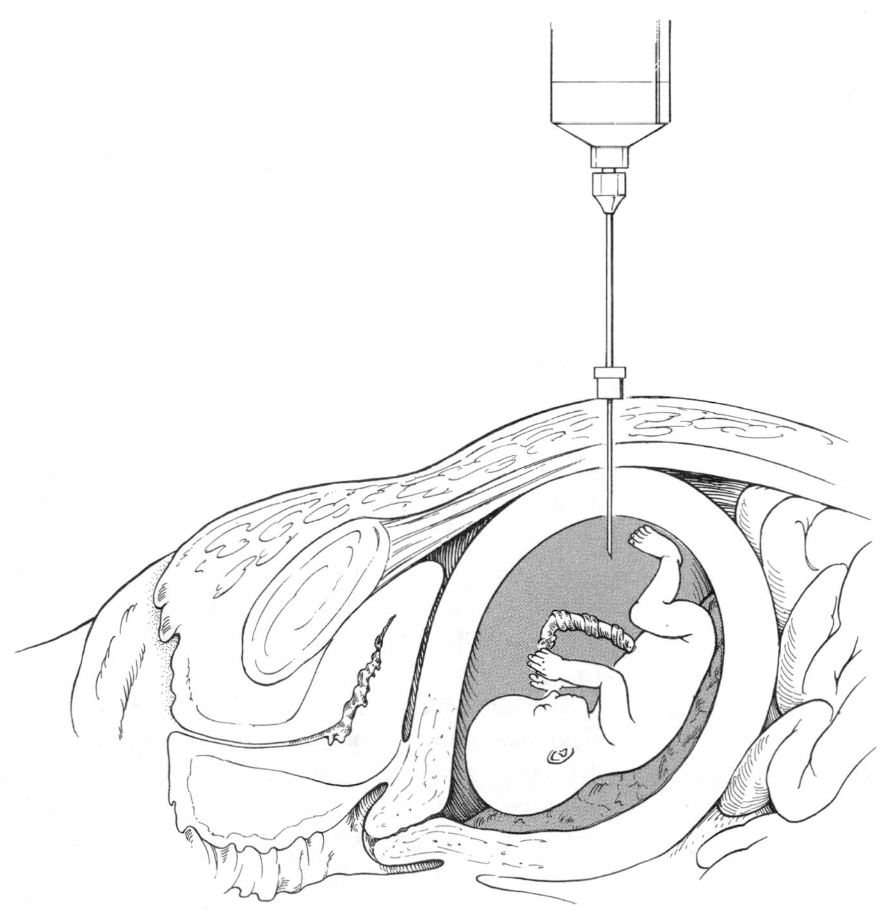

FIGURE 15-8. Amniocentesis. A sample is removed from the amniotic sac. Cells and fluid are tested for fetal abnormalities.

KEY CLINICAL TERMS

Disorders

abortion *(a-BOR-shun)* — Termination of a pregnancy before the fetus is capable of surviving outside the uterus, usually at 20 weeks or 500 grams. May be spontaneous or induced. A spontaneous abortion is commonly called a miscarriage.

anencephalus *(an-en-SEF-a-lus)* — Congenital absence of a brain

atresia *(a-TRĒ-zē-a)* — Congenital absence or closure of a normal body opening

carrier — An individual who has an unexpressed genetic defect that can be passed to his or her children

cleft lip — A congenital separation of the upper lip

cleft palate — A congenital split in the roof of the mouth

congenital disorder — A disorder that is present at birth. May be developmental or hereditary.

eclampsia *(e-KLAMP-sē-a)* — Convulsions and coma occurring during pregnancy or after delivery and associated with the conditions of preeclampsia (see below) (adj. eclamptic)

ectopic pregnancy *(ek-TOP-ik)* — Development of the fertilized ovum outside the body of the uterus. Usually occurs in the oviduct (tubal pregnancy), but may occur in other parts of the reproductive tract or abdominal cavity (see Figure 15-4).

mastitis *(mas-TĪ-tis)* — Inflammation of the breast, usually associated with the early weeks of breastfeeding

mutation *(mū-TĀ-shun)* — A change in the genetic material of the cell. Most mutations are harmful. If the change appears in the sex cells it can be passed to future generations.

placental abruption — Premature separation of the placenta; abruptio placentae

placenta previa *(PRĒ-vē-a)* — A placenta that is attached in the lower portion of the uterus instead of the upper portion, as is normal. May result in hemorrhage late in pregnancy.

preeclampsia *(prē-e-KLAMP-sē-a)* — A toxic condition of late pregnancy associated with hypertension, edema, and proteinuria which, if untreated, may lead to eclampsia. Also called toxemia of pregnancy.

rubella *(rū-BEL-la)* — German measles. The virus can cross the placenta and cause fetal abnormalities, such as eye defects, deafness, heart abnormalities, and mental retardation. The virus is most damaging during the first trimester.

spina bifida *(SPĪ-na BIF-i-da)* — A congenital defect in the closure of the spinal column through which the spinal cord and its membranes may project (see Figures 15-4 and 15-5)

teratogen *(ter-AT-ō-jen)* — A factor that causes developmental abnormalities in the fetus (adj. teratogenic)

Diagnosis and Treatment

amniocentesis *(am-nē-ō-sen-TĒ-sis)* — Transabdominal puncture of the amniotic sac to remove amniotic fluid for testing. Tests on the cells and fluid obtained can reveal congenital abnormalities, blood incompatibility, and sex of the fetus (see Figure 15-8).

chorionic villus sampling (CVS) — Removal of chorionic cells through the cervix for prenatal testing. Can be done earlier in pregnancy than amniocentesis.

dilatation and evacuation (D&E) — Widening of the cervix and removal of the products of conception by suction

karyotype *(KAR-ē-ō-tīp)* — A picture of the chromosomes of a cell arranged in order of decreasing size; can reveal abnormalities in the chromosomes themselves or in their number or arrangement (root *kary/o* means "nucleus")

ultrasonography — The use of high frequency sound waves to produce a photograph of an organ or tissue (see Figure 15-7). Used in obstetrics to diagnose pregnancy, multiple births, and abnormalities as well as to study and measure the fetus. The picture obtained is a sonogram or ultrasonogram.

ADDITIONAL TERMS

Normal Structure and Function

afterbirth — The placenta and membranes delivered after birth of a child

antepartum *(an-tē-PAR-tum)* — Before childbirth, with reference to the mother

fontanel *(fon-tan-EL)* — A membrane-covered space between cranial bones in the fetus that later becomes ossified; a soft spot. Also spelled fontanelle.

intrapartum *(in-tra-PAR-tum)* — Occurring during childbirth

lochia *(LŌ-kē-a)* — The mixture of blood, mucus, and tissue discharged from the uterus after childbirth

meconium *(me-KŌ-nē-um)* — The first feces of the newborn

postpartum — After childbirth, with reference to the mother

premature — Describing an infant born before the organ systems are fully developed; immature

preterm — Occurring before the 37th week of gestation; describing an infant born before the 37th week of gestation

puerperium *(pū-er-PĒR-ē-um)* — The period of 42 days after childbirth, during which the mother's reproductive organs usually return to normal (root *puer* means "child")

(continued)

umbilicus
(um-BIL-i-kus)
The scar in the middle of the abdomen that marks the point of attachment of the umbilical cord to the fetus; the navel

vernix caseosa
(VER-niks kā-sē-Ō-sa)
The cheeselike deposit that covers and protects the fetus (literally "cheesy varnish")

Abnormalities of Pregnancy and Childbirth

cephalopelvic disproportion
(sef-a-lō-PEL-vik)
The condition in which the head of the fetus is larger than the pelvic outlet; also called fetopelvic disproportion

choriocarcinoma
(kor-ē-ō-kar-si-NŌ-ma)
A rare malignant neoplasm composed of placental tissue

hydatidiform mole
(hī-da-TID-i-form)
An overgrowth of placental tissue following fertilization of a damaged ovum. The placenta dilates and resembles grapelike cysts. The tissue may invade the wall of the uterus causing rupture. Also called hydatid mole.

hydramnios
(hī-DRAM-nē-os)
An excess of amniotic fluid; also called polyhydramnios.

oligohydramnios
(ol-i-gō-hī-DRAM-nē-os)
A deficiency of amniotic fluid

patent ductus arteriosus (PDA)
(PĀ-tent)
Persistence of the ductus arteriosus after birth so that blood continues to shunt from the pulmonary artery to the aorta

puerperal infection
(pū-ER-per-al)
Infection of the genital tract after delivery

Diagnosis

alpha-fetoprotein (AFP)
A fetal protein that may be elevated in amniotic fluid and maternal serum in cases of certain fetal disorders

Apgar score
A system of rating an infant's physical condition immediately after birth. Five features are rated as 0, 1, or 2 at 1 minute and 5 minutes after delivery, and sometimes thereafter. Infants with low scores require medical attention.

pelvimetry
(pel-VIM-e-trē)
Measurement of the pelvis by manual examination or x-ray study to determine whether it will be possible to deliver a fetus through the vagina

presentation
Term describing the part of the fetus that can be felt by vaginal or rectal examination. Normally the head presents first (vertex presentation), but sometimes the buttocks (breech presentation), face, or other part presents first.

Treatment

cesarean section
(se-ZAR-ē-an)
Incision of the abdominal wall and uterus for delivery of a fetus

ECMO
Extracorporeal membrane oxygenation. A technique for pulmonary bybass in which deoxygenated blood is removed, passed through a circuit that oxygenates the blood, and then returned. Used for selected newborn and pediatric patients in respiratory failure with an otherwise good prognosis.

obstetrics
(ob-STET-riks)
The branch of medicine that treats women during pregnancy, childbirth, and the puerperium. Usually combined with the practice of gynecology.

pediatrics
(pē-dē-AT-riks)
The branch of medicine that treats children and diseases of children (root *ped/o* means "child")

Pitocin
(pi-TŌ-sin)
Trade name for oxytocin; used to induce and hasten labor

ABBREVIATIONS

AB abortion
AFP alpha-fetoprotein
AGA appropriate for gestational age
C section cesarean section
CVS chorionic villus sampling
D&E dilatation and evacuation
ECMO extracorporeal membrane oxygenation
EDC estimated date of confinement
FHR fetal heart rate
FHT fetal heart tone
FTND full-term normal delivery
FTP full-term pregnancy
GA gestational age
HCG human chorionic gonadotropin
LMP last menstrual period
NB newborn
NICU neonatal intensive care unit
OB obstetrics
PDA patent ductus arteriosus
PIH pregnancy-induced hypertension
PKU phenylketonuria
SVD spontaneous vaginal delivery
UC uterine contractions
UTP uterine term pregnancy
VBAC vaginal birth after cesarean section

Chapter 15
Labeling Exercise

Write the name of each numbered part of the female reproductive system on the corresponding line of the answer sheet.

body of uterus	greater vestibular (Bartholin's) gland	oviduc (fallopian tube)
cervix	implanted embryo	ovum
corpus luteum	maturing follicle	site of fertilization
fimbriae	ovarian follicle (ruptured)	sperm cell
fundus of uterus	ovary	vagina

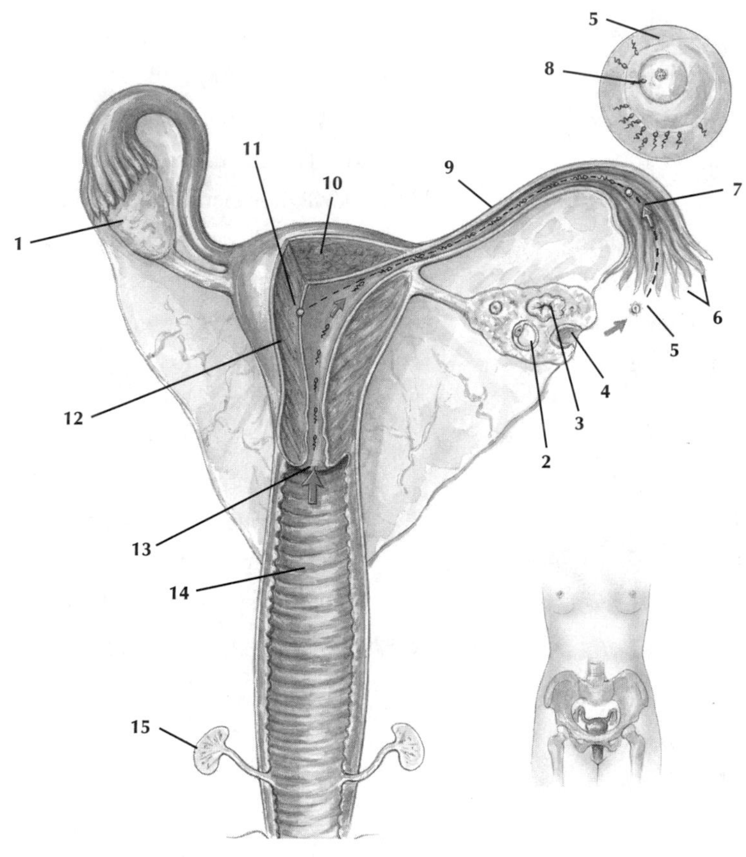

Female reproductive system showing fertilization

1. ______________ 9. ______________

2. ______________ 10. ______________

3. ______________ 11. ______________

4. ______________ 12. ______________

5. ______________ 13. ______________

6. ______________ 14. ______________

7. ______________ 15. ______________

8. ______________

CHAPTER REVIEW 15

Matching. Match the words in each of the sets below with their definitions and write the appropriate letter (a–e) to the left of each number:

_____	1. chorion	a. childbirth
_____	2. gestation	b. outermost layer of the embryo
_____	3. zygote	c. connects the fetus to the placenta
_____	4. umbilical cord	d. period of development in the uterus
_____	5. parturition	e. fertilized egg

_____	6. oxytocin	a. uterine discharge after childbirth
_____	7. HCG	b. embryonic hormone
_____	8. atresia	c. first breast fluid
_____	9. lochia	d. congenital absence of a body opening
_____	10. colostrum	e. hormone that stimulates labor

_____	11. vernix caseosa	a. feces of newborn
_____	12. meconium	b. soft spot in fetal skull
_____	13. fontanel	c. small hole between the fetal atria
_____	14. puerperium	d. material that covers the fetus
_____	15. foramen ovale	e. period after childbirth

_____	16. mutation	a. hereditary disease of protein metabolism
_____	17. hemophilia	b. picture of chromosomes
_____	18. PKU	c. genetic change
_____	19. Klinefelter's syndrome	d. hereditary bleeding disease
_____	20. karyotype	e. congenital abnormality in sex chromosomes

_____	21. prostaglandins	a. congenital absence of a brain
_____	22. eclampsia	b. hormones involved in parturition
_____	23. galactocele	c. cystic enlargement of a milk duct
_____	24. umbilicus	d. condition associated with hypertension during pregnancy
_____	25. anencephalus	e. navel

Fill in the blanks:

26. The stage in development between the zygote and the fetus is the

____.

27. The tissue that nourishes and maintains the developing fetus is the

____.

28. The fluid-filled sac in which the fetus floats is the ______________________.
29. The secretion of milk from the mammary glands is called ______________________.
30. The vessel that carries oxygenated blood from the placenta to the fetus is the ______________________.
31. Loss of an embryo or fetus before 20 weeks or 500 g is termed a(n) ______________________.
32. A physician who specializes in the care of women during pregnancy and childbirth is a(n) ______________________.
33. Hydramnios is an excess of ______________________.
34. A teratogen is an agent that causes ______________________.
35. A woman who has been pregnant two or more times is described as a(n) ______________________.

Definitions. Write the meaning of the following terms:

36. congenital ______________________
37. prenatal ______________________
38. extraembryonic ______________________
39. neonatology ______________________
40. hyperlactation ______________________
41. tripara *(TRIP-a-ra)* ______________________
42. agalactia ______________________

Word building. Write a word for each of the following definitions:

43. Rupture of the amniotic sac ______________________
44. An amniotic cell ______________________
45. Study of the embryo ______________________
46. Direct examination of a fetus ______________________
47. Poisonous (-toxic) to the fetus ______________________
48. Slow labor ______________________

Write one word that means the same as each of the following:

49. neonate ______________________
50. para 1 ______________________
51. gravida 0 ______________________

Write a word that means the opposite of each of the following:

52. postpartum ______________________
53. prenatal ______________________
54. dystocia ______________________

Write the adjective form of each of the following words:

55. fetus ______________________
56. embryo ______________________
57. neonate ______________________
58. placenta ______________________
59. amnion ______________________

Unscrambles. Form a word from each of the following groups of letters and write it in the blank:

60. tscborites ______________________
61. ismuibcul ______________________
62. catlneap ______________________
63. blaleur ______________________
64. ycniotxo ______________________

Word analysis. Define each of the following words and give the meaning of the word parts in each. Use a dictionary if necessary.

65. Amniocentesis ______________________

____

a. amnio ______________________

b. centesis ______________________

66. Ectopic ______________________

____

a. ec- ______________________

b. topos place

c. -ic ______________________

67. Oxytocia ______________________

____

a. oxy sharp, acute

b. toc ______________________

c. -ia ______________________

68. Oligohydramnios ______________________

____

a. oligo- ______________________

b. hydr/o ______________________

c. amnio(s) ______________________

Chapter 15

Case Studies

1. Preeclamptic Pregnancy and Induced Delivery

This 32-year-old female, gravida 2, para 0, was admitted on 21 March at 40.4 weeks gestation for possible induction of labor. This patient had been diagnosed at 36 weeks gestation as having mild preeclampsia evidenced by an increase in blood pressure, headaches, weakness, dizziness, and swelling of the hands and feet. At this time there was an elevation in BUN and uric acid and also traces of protein in 24 hour urine. BP on admission was 145/110. PMH unremarkable except for a tendency toward hypertension.

X-ray pelvimetry on 22 March showed a single fetus in right occiput posterior position. Pelvis of adequate size for induction. Labor induced with Pitocin on 23 March at 9:00 AM. Female infant born 4:10 PM. Weight 6 lb 12 oz. Apgar 9/9. Placenta intact; three vessels. Patient discharged on 27 March in satisfactory condition.

2. Left Ectopic Pregnancy

This is a 29-year-old gravida 1 female with LMP on 15 June. She was seen in the ER on 6 August complaining of left-sided pain following 5 days of heavy menstrual flow. Vaginal ultrasound was negative. HCG was 6600. Pelvic examination showed a normal-size uterus with some tenderness on the left.

On 8 August under general endotracheal anesthesia, the patient had a diagnostic laparoscopy, laparotomy, and resection of a 2 × 2-cm left adnexal mass. The finding was identified as an ectopic pregnancy. The tube was unruptured with proximal endometriosis. The patient did well postop and was discharged on 11 August with an appointment for a follow-up in 2 weeks.

3. Premature Newborn With RDS and Neonatal Jaundice

This preterm neonate was admitted to the Newborn Pediatrics Section on 20 July with respiratory distress syndrome and hyperbilirubinemia of prematurity. Patient J.S. is a male, birth weight 2760 g GA 34 weeks, intrauterine growth AGA, 5-minute Apgar 9. On admission, the infant was endotracheally intubated and placed on a ventilator. Administration of Exosurf was begun. Cardiorespiratory condition was monitored continuously. In view of hypoglycemia and stress gastritis, TPN was initiated on 21 July. This was administered for 1 week, with NPO for the first 5 days.

Outcome was satisfactory. On 23 July, surfactant was discontinued and phototherapy for hyperbilirubinemia was begun. This was continued until resolution on 27 July. The patient was switched to an oxygen hood on 26 July for 3 days. A fourth pulmonary function test on 3 August showed, on 31 breaths, tidal volume 5.0, compliance 0.794, total pulmonary resistance 72.0. A pneumogram on 4 August showed 1.2% periodic breathing, no bradycardia or tachycardia. J.S. was discharged on 6 August with a home apnea monitor, medication: polyvisol 1 mL po qd; nutrition: oral breast milk ad lib on demand. He will be reevaluated at 1 week with pulmonary function tests at 3 months. A sleep study is scheduled for 23 September.

Chapter 15
Case Study Questions

Multiple choice. Select the best answer and write the letter of your choice to the left of each number:

_____ 1. Preeclampsia is also called

a. tubal pregnancy
b. congenital mutation
c. ectopic pregnancy
d. toxemia of pregnancy
e. placenta previa

_____ 2. The occiput of the fetus is the

a. forehead
b. foot
c. back of the head
d. chin
e. shoulder

_____ 3. The term resection means

a. excision
b. x-ray examination
c. biopsy
d. analysis
e. induction

_____ 4. The three vessels mentioned in the first case study refer to

a. two umbilical veins and one pulmonary artery
b. two umbilical arteries and one umbilical vein
c. one umbilical artery and two umbilical veins
d. two pulmonary arteries and one pulmonary vein
e. one pulmonary artery and two coronary veins

_____ 5. Hyperbilirubinemia is associated with

a. edema
b. jaundice
c. malnutrition
d. hypoglycemia
e. gastritis

_____ 6. Pitocin is the trade name for

a. progesterone
b. estrogen
c. chorionic gonadotropin
d. FSH
e. oxytocin

Write a term from the case studies that means each of the following:

7. Measurement of the pelvis _____
8. Within the trachea _____
9. Incision of the abdomen _____
10. Out of the normal position _____
11. Within the uterus _____
12. Treatment with light _____
13. Slow heart rate _____
14. Cessation of breathing _____

Write the meaning of the following abbreviations:

15. PMH _____
16. BUN _____
17. LMP _____
18. HCG _____
19. AGA _____
20. RDS _____
21. TPN _____

DEVELOPMENT

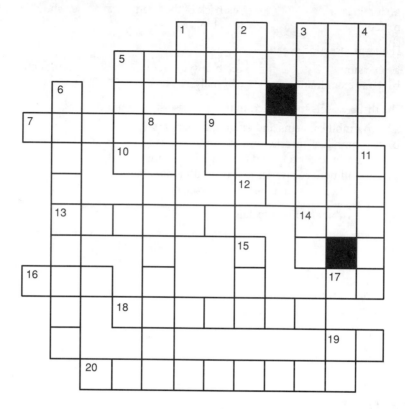

ACROSS

3. prefix: bad, poor
5. newborn
7. childbirth
10. prefix: not
12. prefix: three
13. the membranous sac that holds the fetus
14. prefix: one
16. high blood pressure caused by pregnancy (abbr.)
17. by mouth, orally (abbr.)
18. outside the normal position, such as certain abnormal pregnancies
19. suffix: pertaining to
20. fluid secreted from the breast before milk is produced

DOWN

1. root: ovum
2. root: milk
3. the first feces of the newborn
4. date used to establish the length of a pregnancy (abbr.)
5. root (with combining vowel): birth
6. secretion of milk from the breasts
8. the structure that connects the fetus to the placenta: ________ cord
9. a route for administering drugs into the blood (abbr.)
11. a deficiency of amniotic fluids ______ hydramnios
15. a protein that may be elevated in cases of certain fetal disorders (abbr.)
19. a route for drug administration (abbr.)

Chapter 15
Answer Section

Answers to Chapter Exercises

Exercise 15-1

1. pertaining to the embryo
2. before birth
3. a physician who specializes in care and treatment of the newborn
4. developing in one amniotic sac
5. direct examination of the fetus
6. excess secretion of milk
7. lack of milk production
8. amniorrhexis *(am-nē-ō-REK-sis)*
9. amniotomy *(am-nē-OT-ō-mē)*
10. amniocyte *(AM-nē-ō-sīt)*
11. embryoscope *(EM-brē-ō-skōp)*
12. fetometry *(fē-TOM-e-trē)*
13. embryopathy *(em-brē-OP-a-thē)*
14. postnatal *(post-NĀ-tal)*
15. primigravida *(pri-mi-GRAV-i-da)*
16. multigravida *(mul-ti-GRAV-i-da)*
17. nullipara *(nul-IP-a-ra)*
18. primipara *(pri-MIP-a-ra)*
19. xerotocia *(zē-rō-TŌ-sē-a)*
20. dystocia *(dis-TŌ-sē-a)*
21. galactocele *(ga-LAK-tō-sēl)*; also lactocele *(LAK-tō-sēl)*
22. galactorrhea *(ga-lak-tō-RĒ-a)*; also lactorrhea *(lak-tō-RĒ-a)*

Labeling Exercise

Female Reproductive System Showing Fertilization

1. ovary
2. maturing follicle
3. corpus luteum
4. ovarian follicle (ruptured)
5. ovum
6. fimbriae
7. site of fertilization
8. sperm cell
9. oviduct (fallopian tube)
10. fundus of uterus
11. implanted embryo
12. body of uterus
13. cervix
14. vagina
15. greater vestibular (Bartholin's) glands

Answers to Chapter Review 15

1. b
2. d
3. e
4. c
5. a
6. e
7. b
8. d
9. a
10. c
11. d
12. a
13. b
14. e
15. c
16. c

17. d
18. a
19. e
20. b
21. b
22. d
23. c
24. e
25. a
26. embryo
27. placenta
28. amniotic sac (amnion)
29. lactation
30. umbilical vein
31. abortion
32. obstetrician
33. amniotic fluid
34. fetal malformation
35. multigravida
36. present at birth
37. before birth
38. outside the embryo
39. physician who specializes in care of the newborn
40. excessive secretion of milk
41. a woman who has given birth three times
42. lack of milk production
43. amniorrhexis
44. amniocyte
45. embryology
46. fetoscopy
47. fetotoxic
48. bradytocia
49. newborn
50. primipara
51. nulligravida
52. antepartum
53. postnatal
54. eutocia
55. fetal
56. embryonic
57. neonatal
58. placental
59. amniotic
60. obstetrics
61. umbilicus
62. placenta
63. rubella
64. oxytocin
65. transabdominal puncture of the amnion to remove cells and fluid for testing
    a. amnion
    b. puncture of a cavity
66. Occuring outside of the normal position
    a. out, outside
    b. place
    c. pertaining to
67. extreme rapidity of labor
    a. sharp, acute
    b. labor
    c. condition of
68. A deficiency of amniotic fluid
    a. few, scanty
    b. fluid
    c. amnion

Answers to Case Study Questions

1. d
2. c
3. a
4. b
5. b
6. e
7. pelvimetry
8. endotracheal
9. laparotomy
10. ectopic
11. intrauterine
12. phototherapy
13. bradycardia
14. apnea
15. past medical history
16. blood urea nitrogen
17. last menstrual period
18. human chorionic gonadotropin
19. appropriate for gestational age
20. respiratory distress syndrome
21. total parenteral nutrition

Answers to Crossword Puzzles

DEVELOPMENT

				1 O			2 L		3 M	A	4 L
			5 N	E	O	N	A	T	E		M
	6 L		A				C	■	C		P
7 P	A	R	T	8 U	R	9 I	T	I	O	N	
	C		10 I	M		V			N		11 O
	T			B			12 T	R	I		L
	13 A	M	N	I	O	N			14 U	N	I
	T			L			15 A		M	■	G
16 P	I	H		I			F			17 P	O
	O		18 E	C	T	O	P	I	C		
	N			A						19 I	C
		20 C	O	L	O	S	T	R	U	M	

16 The Endocrine System

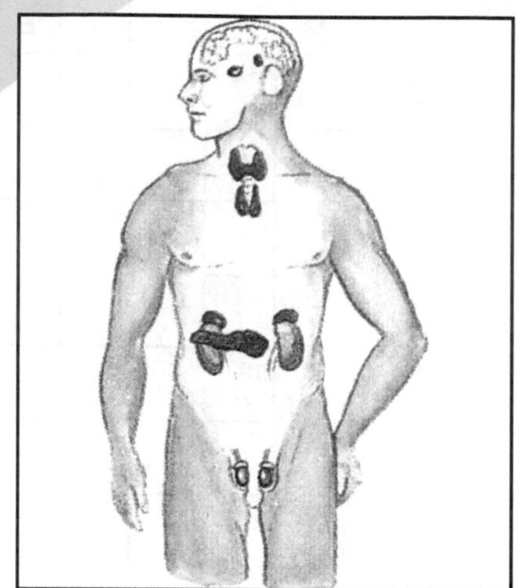

Chapter Contents

Objectives

After study of this chapter you should be able to:

1. Define hormones
2. Compare steroid and amino acid hormones
3. Label a diagram of the endocrine system
4. Name the hormones produced by the endocrine glands and briefly describe the function of each
5. Identify and use roots pertaining to the endocrine system
6. Describe the main disorders of the endocrine system
7. Interpret abbreviations used in endocrinology
8. Analyze several case studies concerning disorders of the endocrine system

The endocrine system consists of a widely distributed group of glands that secretes regulatory substances called **hormones**. Because these substances are released directly into the blood, the endocrine glands are known as the *ductless glands*. Despite the fact that hormones in the blood reach all parts of the body, only certain tissues respond. The tissue that is influenced by a specific hormone is called the **target tissue**. The cells that make up this tissue have specific **receptors** on their membranes to which the hormone attaches, enabling it to act on the cells.

Hormones

Hormones are produced in extremely small amounts and are highly potent. By means of their actions on various target tissues they affect growth, metabolism, reproductive activity, and behavior.

Chemically, they fall into two categories: **steroids**, made from lipids, and hormones made of amino acids, which include proteins and proteinlike compounds. Steroids are produced by the sex glands (gonads) and the outer region (cortex) of the adrenal glands. All the remaining endocrine glands produce amino acid hormones.

The production of hormones is controlled mainly by negative feedback. That is, the hormone itself, or some product of hormone activity, acts as a control over further manufacture of the hormone—a self-regulating system. Hormone production also may be controlled by nervous stimulation or by other hormones.

Endocrine Glands and Hormones

Refer to Figure 16-1 to locate the endocrine glands described below. Table 16-1 lists the main endocrine glands and summarizes the main hormones secreted by each and their functions.

Pituitary

The **pituitary** (hypophysis) is a small gland beneath the brain. It is divided into an anterior lobe (adenohypophysis) and a posterior lobe (neurohypophysis). Both lobes are connected to and controlled by the **hypothalamus**, a part of the brain. The anterior pituitary releases six hormones. One of these is **growth hormone** (somatotropin), which stimulates the growth of bones and acts on other tissues as well. The remainder of the pituitary hormones regulate other glands, including the thyroid, adrenals, gonads, and mammary glands. These hormones are released in response to substances (releasing hormones) that are sent to the anterior pituitary from the hypothalamus. They can be identified by the ending *-tropin*, as in *gonadotropin*. The adjective ending is *-tropic*.

The posterior pituitary releases two hormones that are actually produced in the hypothalamus. These are stored in the posterior pituitary until nervous signals arrive from the hypothalamus to trigger their release. **Antidiuretic hormone** (ADH) acts on the kidneys to conserve water and also promotes constriction of blood vessels. Both these actions serve to raise blood pressure. **Oxytocin** stimulates uterine contractions and promotes milk "letdown" in the breasts during lactation.

Thyroid and Parathyroids

The **thyroid gland** consists of two lobes on either side of the larynx and upper trachea. It secretes a mixture of hormones, mainly **thyroxine** (T_4) and **triiodothyronine** (T_3). Because thyroid hormones contain iodine, their levels can be measured and the activity of the thyroid gland can be studied by following uptake of iodine. Most thyroid hormone in the blood is bound to protein, mainly thyroid binding globulin (TBG).

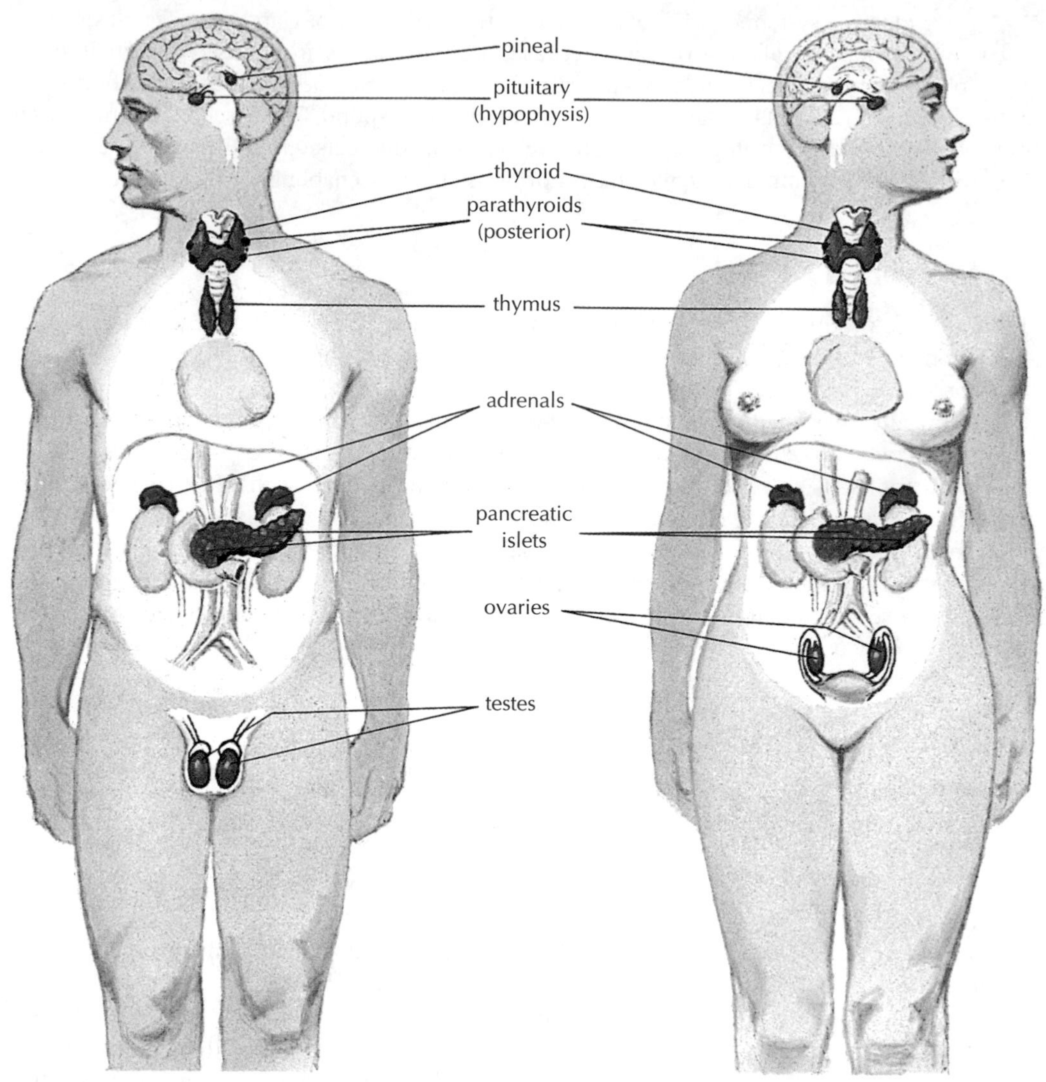

FIGURE 16-1. Glands of the endocrine system

On the posterior surface of the thyroid are four to six tiny **parathyroid glands** that affect calcium metabolism. **Parathyroid hormone** raises the blood level of calcium. It works with the thyroid hormone **thyrocalcitonin**, which lowers blood calcium, to regulate calcium balance.

Adrenals

The **adrenal glands**, located atop each kidney, are divided into two distinct regions: an outer cortex and an inner medulla. The hormones produced by this gland are involved in the body's response to stress. The cortex produces steroid hormones. **Cortisol** (hydrocortisone) mobilizes reserves of fats and carbohydrates to raise the levels of these nutrients in the blood. It also acts to reduce inflammation, and is used clinically for this purpose. **Aldosterone** acts on the kidneys to conserve sodium and water while eliminating potassium. The adrenal cortex also produces small amounts of sex hormones, but their importance is not well understood.

TABLE 16-1 The Endocrine Glands and Their Hormones

Gland	Hormone	Principal Functions
anterior pituitary	GH (growth hormone); also called somatotropin	promotes growth of all body tissues
	TSH (thyroid-stimulating hormone)	stimulates thyroid gland to produce thyroid hormones
	ACTH (adrenocorticotropic hormone)	stimulates adrenal cortex to produce cortical hormones; aids in protecting body in stress situations (injury, pain)
	FSH (follicle-stimulating hormone)	stimulates growth and hormone activity of ovarian follicles; stimulates growth of testes; promotes development of sperm cells
	LH (luteinizing hormone); ICSH (interstitial cell-stimulating hormone) in males	causes development of corpus luteum at site of ruptured ovarian follicle in female; stimulates secretion of testosterone in male
	PRL (prolactin)	stimulates secretion of milk by mammary glands
posterior pituitary	ADH (antidiuretic hormone; vasopressin)	promotes reabsorption of water in kidney tubules; stimulates smooth muscle tissue of blood vessels to constrict
	oxytocin	causes contraction of uterus; causes ejection of milk from mammary glands
thyroid	thyroid hormone: thyroxine (T_4) and triiodothyronine (T_3)	increases metabolic rate, influencing both physical and mental activities; required for normal growth
	calcitonin	decreases calcium level in blood
parathyroids	parathyroid hormone	regulates exchange of calcium between blood and bones; increases calcium level in blood
adrenal medulla	epinephrine and norepinephrine	active in response to stress; increases respiration, blood pressure, and heart rate
adrenal cortex	cortisol (hydrocortisone)	aids in metabolism of carbohydrates, proteins, and fats; active during stress
	aldosterone	aids in regulating electrolytes and water balance
	sex hormones	may influence secondary sexual characteristics
pancreatic islets	insulin	aids transport of glucose into cells; required for cellular metabolism of foods, especially glucose; decreases blood sugar levels
	glucagon	stimulates liver to release glucose, thereby increasing blood sugar levels
testes	testosterone	stimulates growth and development of sexual organs plus development of secondary sexual characteristics; stimulates maturation of sperm cells

(continued)

TABLE 16-1 The Endocrine Glands and Their Hormones *(Continued)*

Gland	Hormone	Principal Functions
ovaries	estrogens	stimulate growth of primary sexual organs and development of secondary sexual characteristics
	progesterone	stimulates development of secretory parts of mammary glands; prepares uterine lining for implantation of fertilized ovum; aids in maintaining pregnancy
thymus	thymosin	important in development of T cells needed for immunity and in early development of lymphoid tissue

The medulla of the adrenal gland produces two similar hormones, **epinephrine** (adrenaline) and **norepinephrine** (noradrenaline). These are released in response to stress and work with the nervous system to help the body meet challenges.

Pancreas

The endocrine portions of the pancreas are the **islets**. They produce two hormones that regulate sugar metabolism. **Insulin** increases cellular use of glucose, thus lowering sugar levels in the blood. **Glucagon** has the opposite effect of raising blood sugar levels.

Other Endocrine Tissues

The **thymus**, described in Chapter 9, is considered an endocrine gland because it secretes a hormone, thymosin. The **gonads** (Chapter 14) are also included because, in addition to producing the sex cells, they secrete hormones.

Other organs, including the stomach, kidney, and small intestine, also produce hormones. However, they have other major functions and are discussed with the systems to which they belong.

Finally, **prostaglandins** are a group of hormones produced by many cells. They have a variety of effects, including stimulation of uterine contractions, promotion of the inflammatory response, and vasomotor activities.

KEY TERMS

TERMS

Normal Structure and Function

adrenal gland
(a-DRĒ-nal)
A gland on the upper surface of the kidney. The outer region (cortex) secretes steroid hormones; the inner region (medulla) secretes epinephrine (adrenaline) and norepinephrine (noradrenaline) (root adren/o)

endocrine
(EN-dō-krin)
Pertaining to a ductless gland that secretes directly into the blood

hormone *(HOR-mōn)*	A secretion of an endocrine gland. A substance that travels in the blood and has a regulatory effect on tissues, organs, or glands.
hypothalamus *(hī-pō-THAL-a-mus)*	A portion of the brain that controls the pituitary gland and is active in maintaining homeostasis
pancreatic islets *(Ī-lets)*	Clusters of endocrine cells in the pancreas that secrete hormones which regulate sugar metabolism. Also called islets of Langerhans or islet cells (root insul/o).
parathyroid gland *(par-a-THĪ-royd)*	A small gland on the back of the thyroid that acts to increase blood calcium levels; there are usually four to six parathyroid glands (root parathyr/o, parathyroid/o)
pituitary gland *(pi-TŪ-i-tar-ē)*	A small endocrine gland at the base of the brain. The anterior lobe secretes growth hormone and hormones that stimulate other glands; the posterior lobe releases ADH and oxytocin manufactured in the hypothalamus. Also called the hypophysis *(hī-POF-i-sis)* (root pituitar, hypophys).
prostaglandins *(pros-ta-GLAN-dinz)*	A group of hormones produced throughout the body that has a variety of effects, including stimulation of uterine contractions and regulation of blood pressure, blood clotting, and inflammation
receptor	A site on the cell membrane to which a substance, such as a hormone, attaches
steroid hormone *(STER-oyd)*	A hormone made from lipids and including the sex hormones and the hormones of the adrenal cortex
target tissue	The specific tissue on which a specific hormone acts. May also be referred to as the target organ.
thyroid gland *(THĪ-royd)*	An endocrine gland on either side of the larynx and upper trachea. It secretes hormones that affect metabolism and growth and a hormone that regulates calcium balance (root thyr/o, thyroid/o).

Roots Pertaining to the Endocrine System

Root	Meaning	Example	Definition of Example
endocrin/o	endocrine glands or system	endocrinology *en-dō-kri-NOL-ō-jē*	study of the endocrine glands
pituitar	pituitary gland, hypophysis	pituitarism *pi-TŪ-i-ta-rizm*	condition caused by any disorder of pituitary function
hypophys	pituitary gland, hypophysis	hypophyseal* *hī-pō-FIZ-ē-al*	pertaining to the pituitary gland

(continued)

Root	Meaning	Example	Definition of Example
thyr/o, thyroid/o	thyroid gland	thyrolytic *thī-rō-LIT-ik*	destructive to thyroid tissue
parathyr/o, parathyroid/o	parathyroid gland	parathyrotropic *par-a-thī-rō-TROP-ik*	acting on the parathyroid gland
adren/o, adrenal/o	adrenal gland, epinephrine	adrenergic *ad-ren-ER-jik*	activated by or related to epinephrine (adrenaline)
adrenocortic/o	adrenal cortex	adrenocortical *ad-rē-nō-KOR-ti-kal*	pertaining to the adrenal cortex
insul/o	pancreatic islets	insulin *IN-sū-lin*	hormone secreted by the islet cells

*Note spelling.

Exercise 16-1

Define the following terms:

1. Hypophysectomy *(hī-pof-i-SEK-tō-mē)* ______
2. Thyropathy *(thī-ROP-a-thē)* ______
3. Adrenomegaly *(a-drē-nō-MEG-a-lē)* ______
4. Insular *(IN-sū-lar)* ______

Words for conditions resulting from endocrine dysfunctions are formed by adding the suffix *-ism* to the name of the gland or its root and adding the prefix *hyper-* or *hypo-* for overactivity or underactivity of the gland. Use the full name of the gland to form words with the following meanings:

5. Condition of underactivity of the thyroid gland ______
6. Condition of overactivity of the parathyroid gland ______
7. Condition of overactivity of the adrenal gland ______

Use the word root for the gland to form the following words:

8. Condition of underactivity of the adrenal cortex ______
9. Condition of overactivity of the pituitary gland (use pituitar) ______

Word building. Write a word for each of the following definitions:

10. Any disease of the endocrine system ______
11. Incision into the thyroid gland ______

12. Surgical removal of the thyroid gland (use thyroid/o) ____________________
13. Any disease of the adrenal gland ____________________
14. Inflammation of the adrenal gland ____________________
15. Inflammation of the pancreatic islets ____________________
16. Tumor (-oma) of the pancreatic islets ____________________

Clinical Aspects of the Endocrine System

Endocrine diseases usually result from the overproduction (hypersecretion) or underproduction (hyposecretion) of hormones. They also may result from secretion at the wrong time or from failure of the target tissue to respond. Some of the common endocrine disorders are described below. Conditions resulting from hypersecretion or hyposecretion of hormones are summarized in Table 16-2.

Pituitary

A pituitary **adenoma** (tumor) usually increases secretion of growth hormone or ACTH. Less commonly it affects the secretion of prolactin. An excess of growth hormone in children causes **gigantism**. In adults it causes **acromegaly**, characterized by enlargement of the hands, feet, jaw, and facial features. Treatment is by surgery to remove the tumor (adenomectomy) or by drugs to reduce the level of growth hormone in the blood. Excess ACTH overstimulates the adrenal cortex, resulting in **Cushing's disease**. Increased prolactin causes milk secretion, or galactorrhea, in both males and females. X-ray studies in cases of pituitary adenoma usually show enlargement of the bony structure in the skull that contains the pituitary.

Hypofunction of the pituitary, as caused by tumor or interruption of blood supply to the gland, may involve a single hormone but usually affects all functions, and is referred to as **panhypopituitarism**. The widespread effects of this condition include dwarfism (from lack of growth hormone), lack of sexual development and sexual function, fatigue, and weakness.

TABLE 16-2 Disorders Associated With Endocrine Dysfunction*

Hormone	Hypersecretion	Hyposecretion
growth hormone	gigantism (children), acromegaly (adults)	dwarfism (children)
antidiuretic hormone	syndrome of inappropriate ADH (SIADH)	diabetes insipidus
aldosterone	aldosteronism	Addison's disease
cortisol	Cushing's syndrome	Addison's disease
thyroid hormone	Graves' disease, thyrotoxicosis	cretinism (children), myxedema (adults)
insulin	hypoglycemia	diabetes mellitus
parathyroid hormone	bone degeneration	tetany (muscle spasms)

*Refer to key terms for pronunciations and descriptions.

A specific lack of ADH from the posterior pituitary results in **diabetes insipidus** in which there is decreased ability of the kidneys to conserve water. Symptoms are polyuria (elimination of large amounts of urine) and polydipsia (intake of large amounts of water).

Thyroid

Because thyroid hormone affects the growth and function of many tissues, a deficiency of this hormone in infancy causes physical and mental retardation as well as other symptoms that together constitute **cretinism**. In the adult, thyroid deficiency causes **myxedema**, in which there is weight gain, lethargy, rough, dry skin, and facial swelling. Both of these conditions are easily treated with thyroid hormone. Most U.S. states now require testing of newborns for hypothyroidism. If not diagnosed at birth, hypothyroidism will lead to mental retardation within 6 months.

The most common form of hyperthyroidism is **Graves' disease**, also called diffuse toxic goiter. This is an autoimmune disorder in which antibodies stimulate an increased production of thyroid hormone. There is weight loss, irritability, hand tremors, and rapid heart rate (tachycardia). A most distinctive sign is a bulging of the eyeballs, termed **exophthalmos**, caused by swelling of the tissues behind the eyes. Treatment for Graves' disease may include antithyroid drugs, surgical removal of all or part of the thyroid, or radiation delivered in the form of radioactive iodine.

A common sign in thyroid disease is an enlarged thyroid, or **goiter**. However, a goiter is not necessarily accompanied by malfunction of the thyroid. A simple or nontoxic goiter is caused by a deficiency of iodine in the diet. With the addition of iodine to salt and other commercial foods, this form of goiter has become a thing of the past.

Thyroid function is commonly tested by measuring radioactive iodine uptake (RIU) in the blood. Thyroid stimulating hormone (TSH) from the pituitary may also be measured. Thyroid scans following the administration of radioactive iodine also are done in studying this gland.

Parathyroids

Overactivity of the parathyroid glands, usually from a tumor, causes a high level of calcium in the blood. Since this calcium is obtained from the bones, there is also degeneration of the skeleton and bone pain. A common side effect is the development of kidney stones from the high levels of circulating calcium.

Damage to the parathyroids or surgical removal, as during thyroid surgery, results in a drop of blood calcium levels. This causes numbness and tingling in the arms and legs and around the mouth (perioral) as well as **tetany** (muscle spasms). Treatment consists of supplying calcium.

Adrenals

Hypofunction of the adrenal cortex, or **Addison's disease**, is usually caused by autoimmune destruction of the gland. The lack of aldosterone results in water loss, low blood pressure, and electrolyte imbalance. There is also weakness, nausea, and increase of brown pigmentation. This last symptom is due to release of a hormone from the pituitary that stimulates the pigment cells (melanocytes) in the skin. Once diagnosed, Addison's disease is treated with replacement cortical hormones.

An excess of adrenal cortical hormones results in **Cushing's syndrome**. Patients have a moon-shaped face, obesity localized in the torso, weakness, excess hair growth (hirsutism), and fluid retention. The most common cause of Cushing's syndrome is the therapeutic administration of steroid hormones. It also may be caused by a tumor. If the disorder is caused by a pituitary tumor that increases production of ACTH, it is referred to as Cushing's *disease*.

Pancreas

The most common endocrine disorder is **diabetes mellitus**, a failure of the body cells to use glucose effectively. The excess glucose accumulates in the blood, causing **hyperglycemia**. Increased urination (polyuria) marks the effort to eliminate the excess glucose in the urine (glycosuria). The result is dehydration and great thirst (polydipsia). There is also weakness, weight loss, and extreme hunger (polyphagia). Unable to use carbohydrates, the body burns more fat. This leads to accumulation of ketone bodies in the blood and a shift toward acidosis, a condition termed **ketoacidosis**. If untreated, diabetes will lead to starvation of the central nervous system and coma. Diabetic patients are prone to circulatory and vision problems, infections, and sometimes renal failure.

There are two types of diabetes mellitus. Heredity seems to be a factor in the appearance of both. Type I, insulin-dependent diabetes mellitus (IDDM), usually appears in children and teenagers. It is caused by a failure of the pancreatic islets to produce insulin, resulting, perhaps, from autoimmune destruction of the cells. Because insulin levels are very low or absent, patients need careful monitoring and injections of this hormone. The insulin is obtained from animals and is now also made by genetic engineering.

The more common Type II, non–insulin-dependent diabetes mellitus (NIDDM), usually appears in adults, most of whom are overweight. These individuals may have normal insulin levels, but their cells do not respond to the hormone. They are often treated successfully with diet, exercise, and oral medications (hypoglycemics) that improve insulin production and increase its effectiveness.

Excess insulin may result from a pancreatic tumor, but more often, it follows administration of too much hormone to a diabetic patient. Hypoglycemia leads to **insulin shock**, which is treated by administration of glucose.

KEY CLINICAL TERMS

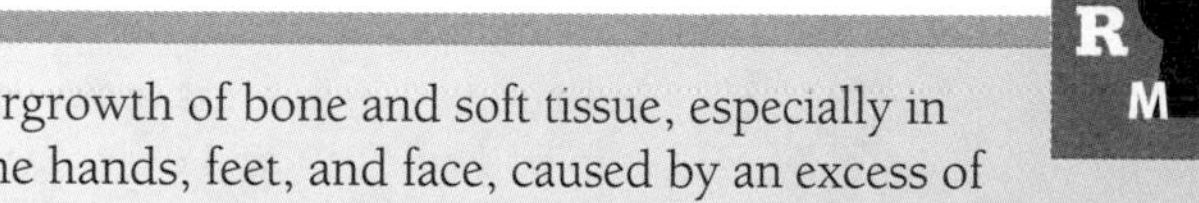

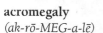

acromegaly *(ak-rō-MEG-a-lē)* — Overgrowth of bone and soft tissue, especially in the hands, feet, and face, caused by an excess of growth hormone in an adult

Addison's disease — A disease resulting from deficiency of adrenocortical hormones. It is marked by darkening of the skin, weakness, and alterations in salt and water balance.

adenoma *(ad-e-NŌ-ma)* — A neoplasm of a gland

cretinism *(KRĒ-tin-izm)* — A condition due to congenital lack of thyroid secretion and marked by arrested physical and mental development

Cushing's disease — Overactivity of the adrenal cortex resulting from excess production of ACTH by the pituitary

Cushing's syndrome — A condition resulting from an excess of hormones from the adrenal cortex. It is associated with obesity, weakness, hyperglycemia, hypertension, and hirsutism (excess hair growth).

diabetes insipidus *(dī-a-BĒ-tēz in-SIP-i-dus)* — A disorder caused by insufficient release of ADH from the posterior pituitary. It results in excessive thirst and production of large amounts of very dilute urine. (The word *diabetes* is from the Greek meaning "siphon," referring to the large urinary output in both forms of diabetes.)

(continued)

diabetes mellitus (*MEL-i-tus*) — A disorder of glucose metabolism caused by deficiency of insulin production or failure of the tissues to respond to insulin. Type I is juvenile or insulin-dependent diabetes mellitus (IDDM); type II is adult-onset or non–insulin-dependent diabetes mellitus (NIDDM).

exophthalmos (*ex-of-THAL-mos*) — Protrusion of the eyeballs as seen in Graves' disease

giantism (*JĪ-an-tizm*) — Overgrowth due to an excess of growth hormone from the pituitary during childhood; also called gigantism

glycosuria — Excess sugar in the urine

goiter (*GOY-ter*) — Enlargement of the thyroid gland. May be toxic or nontoxic. Simple (nontoxic) goiter is caused by iodine deficiency.

Graves' disease — An autoimmune disease resulting in hyperthyroidism. A prominent symptom is exophthalmos (protrusion of the eyeballs). Also called exophthalmic goiter.

hyperglycemia — Excess sugar in the blood

insulin shock — A condition resulting from an overdose of insulin, causing hypoglycemia

ketoacidosis (*kē-tō-as-i-DŌ-sis*) — Acidosis (increased acidity of body fluids) caused by an excess of ketone bodies, as in diabetes mellitus; diabetic acidosis

myxedema (*miks-e-DĒ-ma*) — A condition caused by hypothyroidism in an adult. There is dry, waxy swelling most notable in the face.

panhypopituitarism (*pan-hī-pō-pi-TŪ-i-ta-rism*) — Underactivity of the entire pituitary gland

tetany (*TET-a-nē*) — Irritability and spasms of muscles; may be caused by low blood calcium and other factors

ADDITIONAL TERMS

Normal Structure and Function

pineal gland (*PIN-ē-al*) — A small gland in the brain (see Figure 16-1). Its function in humans is not clear, but it appears to regulate behavior and sexual development in response to environmental light.

sella turcica (*SEL-a TUR-si-ka*) — A saddle-shaped depression in the sphenoid bone that contains the pituitary gland

sphenoid bone (*SFĒ-noyd*) — A bone at the base of the skull that houses the pituitary gland

Symptoms and Conditions

Conn's syndrome — Hyperaldosteronism caused by an adrenal tumor

craniopharyngioma (*krā-nē-ō-far-in-jē-Ō-ma*) — A tumor of the pituitary gland

Hashimoto's disease — A chronic thyroiditis with an autoimmune origin

ketosis *(kē-TŌ-sis)* — Accumulation of ketone bodies, such as acetone, in the body. Usually results from deficiency or faulty metabolism of carbohydrates, as in cases of diabetes mellitus and starvation.

multiple endocrine neoplasia (MEN) — A hereditary disorder that causes tumors in several endocrine glands. Classified according to the combination of glands involved.

pheochromocytoma *(fē-ō-krō-mō-sī-TŌ-ma)* — A usually benign tumor of the adrenal medulla or other structures containing chromaffin cells (cells that stain with chromium salts). It results in increased production of epinephrine and norepinephrine.

pituitary apoplexy *(AP-ō-plek-sē)* — Sudden massive degeneration of the pituitary gland associated with a pituitary tumor

Simmonds' disease — Hypofunction of the anterior pituitary (panhypopituitarism), usually due to an infarction; pituitary cachexia

thyroid storm — A sudden onset of the symptoms of thyrotoxicosis occurring in patients with the disease who are untreated or poorly treated. Also called thyroid crisis.

thyrotoxicosis *(thī-rō-tok-si-KŌ-sis)* — Condition resulting from overactivity of the thyroid gland. The main example is Graves' disease

von Recklinghausen's disease — Degeneration of bone caused by excess production of hormone from the parathyroid glands. Also called Recklinghausen's disease of bone.

Diagnosis and Treatment

fasting blood sugar (FBS) — Measurement of glucose in the blood following a 12-hour fast

free thyroxine index — Calculation based on certain laboratory measurements that indicates the amount of unbound thryoxine in the blood

glucose tolerance test (GTT) — Measurement of glucose levels in blood plasma following administration of a challenge dose of glucose to a fasting patient. Used to measure patient's ability to metabolize glucose.

glycosylated hemoglobin (HbA_{1c}) **test** *(glī-KŌ-si-lā-ted)* — A test that measures the binding of glucose to hemoglobin during the lifespan of a red blood cell. It reflects the average blood glucose level over 2 to 3 months and is useful in evaluating long-term therapy for diabetes mellitus. Also called glycohemoglobin test.

radioactive iodine uptake test (RAIU) — A test that measures thyroid uptake of radioactive iodine as an evaluation of thyroid function

radioimmunoassay (RIA) — A method for measuring very small amounts of a substance, especially hormones, in blood plasma using radioactively labelled hormones and specific antibodies

thyroid scan — Visualization of the thyroid gland following administration of radioactive iodine

(continued)

thyroxine binding globulin (TBG) **test** — Test that measures the main protein that binds T_4 in the blood

transsphenoidal adenomectomy *(trans-sfē-NOY-dal ad-e-nō-MEK-tō-mē)* — Removal of a pituitary tumor through the sphenoid sinus (space in the sphenoid bone)

Also used to diagnose endocrine disorders are imaging techniques, measurements of hormones or their metabolites in plasma and urine, and studies involving hormone stimulation or suppression.

ABBREVIATIONS

ACTH adrenocorticotropic hormone

ADH antidiuretic hormone

DM diabetes mellitus

FBS fasting blood sugar

FTI free thyroxine index

GH growth hormone

GIT glucose tolerance test

HbA_{1c} hemoglobin A_{1c}; glycohemoglobin; glycosylated hemoglobin

^{131}I iodine 131 (radioactive iodine)

IDDM insulin-dependent diabetes mellitus

IGT impaired glucose tolerance

MEN multiple endocrine neoplasia

NIDDM non–insulin-dependent diabetes mellitus

NPH neutral protamine Hagedorn (insulin)

RAIU radioactive iodine uptake

RIA radioimmunoassay

SIADH syndrome of inappropriate antidiuretic hormone (secretion)

T_3 triiodothyronine

T_4 thyroxine

TBG thyroxine-binding globulin

TSH thyroid-stimulating hormone

Chapter 16
Labeling Exercise

Write the name of each numbered gland of the endocrine system on the corresponding line of the answer sheet.

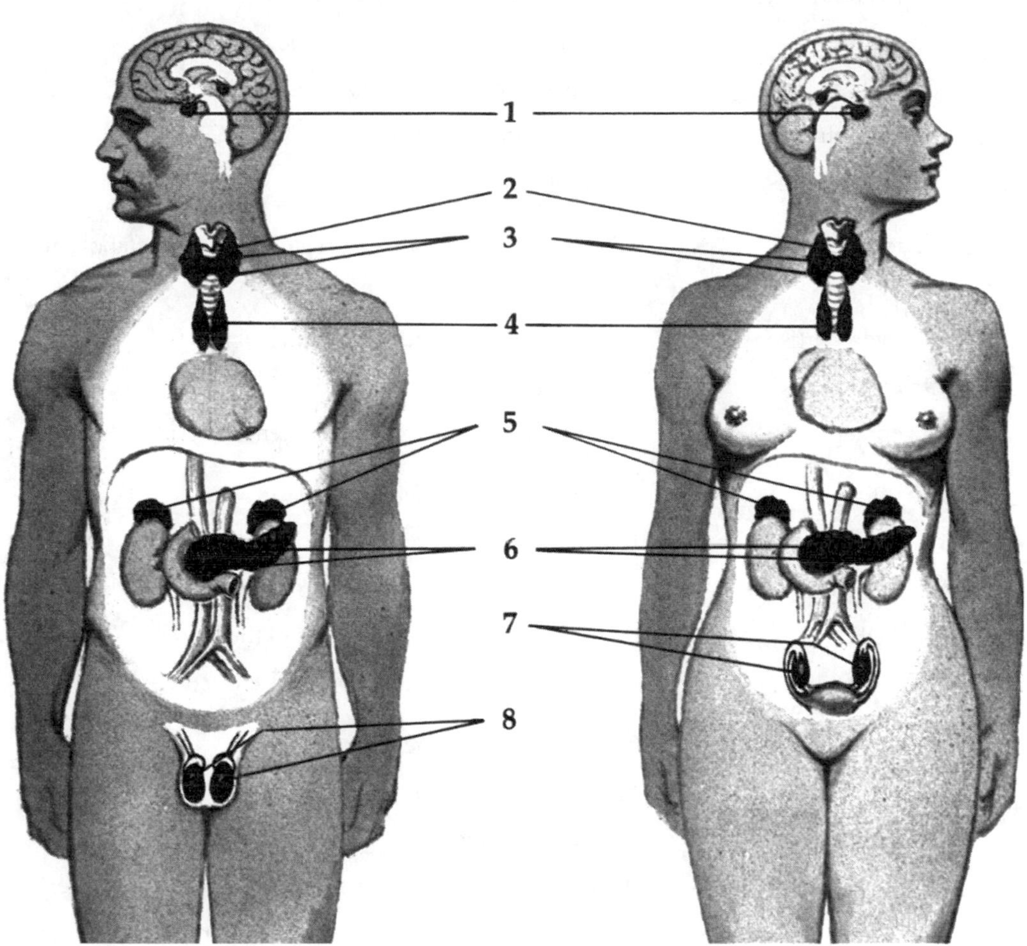

Glands of the endocrine system

adrenals	pituitary (thypophysis)
ovaries	testes
pancreatic islets	thymus
parathyroids	thyroid

1. ______________________ 5. ______________________
2. ______________________ 6. ______________________
3. ______________________ 7. ______________________
4. ______________________ 8. ______________________

CHAPTER REVIEW 16

Matching. Match the terms in each of the sets below with their definitions and write the appropriate letter (a–e) to the left of each number:

_____	1. hypothalamus	a.	inner region of an organ
_____	2. medulla	b.	glands that regulate calcium levels
_____	3. islets	c.	part of the brain that controls the pituitary
_____	4. hypophysis	d.	pancreatic endocrine cells
_____	5. parathyroids	e.	pituitary
_____	6. iodine	a.	pancreatic hormone that regulates sugar metabolism
_____	7. oxytocin	b.	adrenaline
_____	8. hydrocortisone	c.	hormone that produces uterine contractions
_____	9. insulin	d.	ingredient in thyroid hormone
_____	10. epinephrine	e.	hormone produced by the adrenal cortex
_____	11. GTT	a.	form of diabetes mellitus
_____	12. RIA	b.	test of sugar metabolism
_____	13. ACTH	c.	hormone that increases water reabsorption in the kidneys
_____	14. ADH	d.	test for measuring hormones in the blood
_____	15. NIDDM	e.	hormone that stimulates the adrenal cortex
_____	16. Graves' disease	a.	enlargement of the thyroid
_____	17. acromegaly	b.	disorder caused by underactivity of the adrenal cortex
_____	18. Cushing's syndrome	c.	thyrotoxicosis
_____	19. goiter	d.	disorder caused by overactivity of the adrenal cortex
_____	20. Addison's disease	e.	disorder caused by excess growth hormone in adults

Fill in the blanks:

21. The gland in the neck that affects metabolic rate is the ____________________.
22. The endocrine glands located above the kidneys are the ____________________.
23. The most common endocrine disorder is ____________________.
24. A disease caused by hyposecretion of thyroid hormone in adults is ____________________.
25. The gland in the sella turcica of the sphenoid bone is the ____________________.
26. Excess sugar in the blood is called ____________________.

Definitions. Write the meaning of each of the following terms:

27. Hypophyseal *(hī-pō-FIZ-ē-al)* ____________________
28. Hypopituitarism *(hī-pō-pi-TŪ-i-ta-rizm)* ____________________

29. Adrenalectomy *(ad-rē-nal-EK-tō-mē)* ______

30. Hyperthyroidism *(hī-per-THĪ-royd-ism)* ______

31. Endocrinologist *(en-dō-kri-NOL-ō-jist)* ______

32. Adrenocortical *(ad-rē-nō-KOR-ti-kal)* ______

Word building. Write a word for each of the following definitions:

33. Complete (pan-) underactivity of the pituitary gland ______

34. Inflammation of the pancreatic islets ______

35. Any disease of the adrenal gland ______

Use the full name of the gland as the root for the following words:

36. Removal of one half (hemi-) of the thyroid gland ______

37. Condition of normal function of the thyroid gland ______

38. Surgical removal of parathyroid gland ______

39. Condition caused by underactivity of the adrenal gland ______

Use the root *thyr/o* for the following words:

40. Acting on the thyroid gland ______

41. Destructive of (-lytic) thyroid tissue ______

Unscrambles. Form a word from each of the following groups of letters and write it in the blank:

42. stcloior ______

43. tskosie ______

44. hdoyrit ______

45. honreom ______

46. raledan ______

Word analysis. Define each of the following words and give the meaning of the word parts in each. Use a dictionary if necessary.

47. Acromegaly ______

______

a. acro ______

b. megal/o ______

c. -y ______

48. Thyrotoxicosis ______________________________

____

a. thyr/o ______________

b. toxic/o ______________

c. -sis ______________

49. Epinephrine ______________________________

____

a. epi- ______________

b. nephr/o ______________

c. -ine product of

Chapter 16

Case Studies

1. Hyperparathyroidism

The patient is a 58-year-old female with hyperparathyroidism. She has a history of hypertension and, 4 years ago, had a left partial nephrectomy for renal calculi. Three months prior to admission, total calcium increased to 10.8. Her parathyroid hormone level was within normal limits. Physical examination showed a well-developed, well-nourished female in no apparent distress. The remainder of the examination was non-contributory.

Cervical exploration on 8 October showed an enlarged right superior parathyroid gland. The remaining three parathyroid glands appeared normal. The enlarged gland was excised and a biopsy taken of the remaining glands. Pathology reported the abnormal gland to be an adenoma.

On day 1 postop the patient complained of perioral numbness. She showed no other symptoms, but her serum calcium level was subnormal. She was infused with one ampule of calcium gluconate. Her calcium levels improved by 11 October, and the patient was discharged with an appointment for a follow-up in 1 week.

2. Pituitary Adenoma

This patient is a 53-year-old female with a history of pituitary adenoma. One year ago she underwent transsphenoidal hypophysectomy. Since that time she is unaware of rhinorrhea, headache, galacturia, or symptoms of hypothyroidism. She does report urinary frequency and nocturia, but no polyuria, polydipsia, dysuria, or hematuria.

On physical examination the patient appeared mildly obese, but not cushingoid, with signs of acromegaly. She had no hyperpigmentation, no thyromegaly; her breasts were without galactorrhea. Neurologic function was grossly intact on examination.

Assays of T_3 and T_4 were within normal limits. A Metopirone test of pituitary ACTH activity was normal. The patient was discharged without any complication with instructions for a follow-up visit.

3. Pheochromocytoma

This 33-year-old male presented to the urologic service on 14 July for evaluation of a large right renal cyst discovered coincidently following an MRI for an unrelated problem. The patient reported episodes of palpitations with no associated tremors, diaphoresis, or headaches. There was no right flank pain or hematuria and no history of urogenital disorders. BP 158/120; P 96. He had a puffy facies and generalized obesity with no edema. CT scan of the abdomen showed a 10 × 11 × 12-cm septated heterogeneous tumor in the right adrenal gland.

The mass was compressing the kidney and displacing the vena cava. There was no evidence of adenopathy or of other masses in the abdomen or retroperitoneal space. A 24-hour urine sample showed 4–5 times normal urinary catecholamines (neurotransmitters) and top normal urinary cortisol. Diagnosis was a pheochromocytoma and plans were made for surgical excision of the adrenal mass. Alpha and beta blockers were prescribed to stabilize blood pressure, and the patient donated two units of autologous blood in preparation for surgery.

On 28 July, the patient underwent a right radical adrenalectomy. Microscopic examination showed a pheochromocytoma composed of cell aggregates with abundant vasculature. Most of the cells were similar, but some foci showed more hyperchromatism than others. There was no evidence of metastatic spread. Postoperative laboratory reports showed normal levels of epinephrine, norepinephrine, and dopamine. During recovery blood pressure and pulse were within normal limits. The patient was discharged with instructions for periodic evaluations and routine home monitoring of blood pressure.

Chapter 16 Case Study Questions

Multiple choice. Select the best answer and write the letter of your choice to the left of each number:

_____ 1. Renal calculi are

a. kidney stones
b. gallstones
c. stomach ulcers
d. muscle spasms
e. bile obstructions

_____ 2. The word *septated* means

a. homogeneous
b. excised
c. having many blood vessels
d. divided by partitions
e. staining readily

_____ 3. The word *autologous* means

a. pertaining to one's family
b. treated by cold
c. related to one's self
d. precipitated by centrifugation
e. stored

_____ 4. *Hyperchromatism* means

a. excessive color
b. poor staining properties
c. accelerated growth
d. excessive hormone activity
e. abnormality of a gland

Write a word from the case studies that means each of the following:

5. Tumor of a gland ______________________________

6. Pertaining to the neck ______________________________

7. Surgical removal of the pituitary ______
8. Excessive thirst ______
9. Discharge of watery secretions through the nose ______
10. Presence of blood in the urine ______
11. Behind the peritoneum ______
12. Excision of the adrenal gland ______

Write the meaning of the following abbreviations:

13. T_4 ______
14. ACTH ______
15. MRI ______
16. BP ______
17. P ______

Define the following terms:

18. nephrectomy ______
19. perioral ______
20. transsphenoidal ______
21. diaphoresis ______

ENDOCRINE SYSTEM

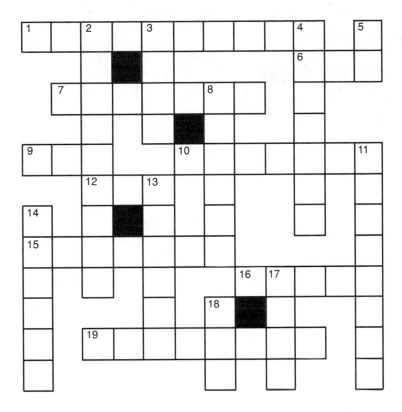

ACROSS

1. alternate name for the pituitary gland
6. hormone that stimulates the thyroid gland (abbr.)
7. a type of hormone made from lipids
9. prefix: three
10. a neoplasm of a gland
12. a blood protein that binds thyroid hormone (abbr.)
15. a regulatory substance secreted by an endocrine gland
16. preix: through, across, beyond
19. the skull bone that houses the pituitary gland

DOWN

2. a small gland beneath the brain that is controlled by the hypothalamus
3. prefix: near, beside
4. a hormone secreted by the testes: testo ______
5. growth hormone (abbr.)
8. the element found in thyroid hormones
11. disorder due to underactivity of the adrenal cortex: ______ disease
13. pituitary hormone that stimulates development of bones and other tissues: ______ hormone
14. a gland in the chest that is active in immunity
17. laboratory test of thyroid function (abbr.)
18. three letter ending for many steroid hormones

Chapter 16 Answer Section

Answers to Chapter Exercises

Exercise 16-1

1. surgical removal of the pituitary gland (hypophysis)
2. any disease of the thyroid gland
3. enlargement of the adrenal gland
4. pertaining to the pancreatic islets
5. hypothyroidism *(hī-pō-THĪ-royd-izm)*
6. hyperparathyroidism *(hī-per-par-a-THĪ-royd-izm)*
7. hyperadrenalism *(hī-per-ad-RĒ-nal-izm)*
8. hypoadrenocorticism *(hī-pō-ad-rē-nō-KOR-ti-sizm)*
9. hyperpituitarism *(hī-per-pi-TŪ-i-ta-rizm)*
10. endocrinopathy *(en-dō-kri-NOP-a-thē)*
11. thyrotomy *(thī-ROT-ō-mē)*; also thyroidotomy *(thī-royd-OT-ō-mē)*
12. thyroidectomy *(thī-royd-EK-tō-mē)*
13. adrenalopathy *(ad-rē-nal-OP-a-thē)*; also adrenopathy *(ad-ren-OP-a-thē)*
14. adrenalitis *(ad-rē-nal-Ī-tis)*; also adrenitis *(ad-re-NĪ-tis)*
15. insulitis *(in-sū-LĪ-tis)*
16. insuloma *(in-sū-LŌ-ma)*

Labeling Exercise

Glands of the Endocrine System

1. pituitary (hypophysis)
2. thyroid
3. parathyroids
4. thymus
5. adrenals
6. pancreatic islets
7. ovaries
8. testes

Answers to Chapter Review 16

1. c
2. a
3. d
4. e
5. b
6. d
7. c
8. e
9. a
10. b
11. b
12. d
13. e
14. c
15. a
16. c
17. e
18. d
19. a
20. b
21. thyroid
22. adrenals
23. diabetes mellitus
24. myxedema
25. pituitary
26. hyperglycemia
27. pertaining to the pituitary gland or hypophysis
28. condition caused by underactivity of the pituitary gland
29. surgical removal of the adrenal gland
30. condition caused by overactivity of the thyroid gland

31. who specializes in study and treatment of endocrine disorders.
32. pertaining to the adrenal cortex
33. panhypopituitarism
34. insulitis
35. adrenalopathy; also adrenopathy
36. hemithyroidectomy
37. euthyroidism
38. parathyroidectomy
39. hypoadrenalism
40. thyrotropic
41. thyrolytic
42. cortisol
43. ketosis
44. thyroid
45. hormone
46. adrenal
47. Disorder caused by excess production of growth hormone in an adult. Characterized by overgrowth of bone and soft tissue, especially in the hands, feet, and face.
    a. extremity
    b. enlargement
    c. condition of
48. A toxic condition caused by hyperactivity of the thyroid gland
    a. thyroid
    b. poisonous
    c. condition of
49. A hormone produced by the adrenal medulla; adrenaline
    a. above
    b. kidney
    c. product of

Answers to Case Study Questions

1. a
2. d
3. c
4. a
5. adenoma
6. cervical
7. hypophysectomy
8. polydipsia
9. rhinorrhea
10. hematuria
11. retroperitoneal
12. adrenalectomy
13. thyroxine
14. adrenocorticotropic hormone
15. magnetic resonance imaging
16. blood pressure
17. pulse
18. surgical removal of the kidney
19. around the mouth
20. through the sphenoid bone
21. profuse sweating

Answers to Crossword Puzzle

ENDOCRINE SYSTEM

1 H	Y	2 P	O	3 P	H	Y	S	I	4 S		5 G
		I		A					6 T	S	H
	7 S	T	E	R	O	8 I	D		E		
		U		A		O			R		
9 T	R	I			10 A	D	E	N	O	M	11 A
		12 T	B	13 G		I			N		D
14 T		A		R		N			E		D
15 H	O	R	M	O	N	E					I
Y		Y		W			16 T	17 R	A	N	S
M				T		18 O		A			O
U		19 S	P	H	E	N	O	I	D		N
S						E		U			S

17 The Nervous System

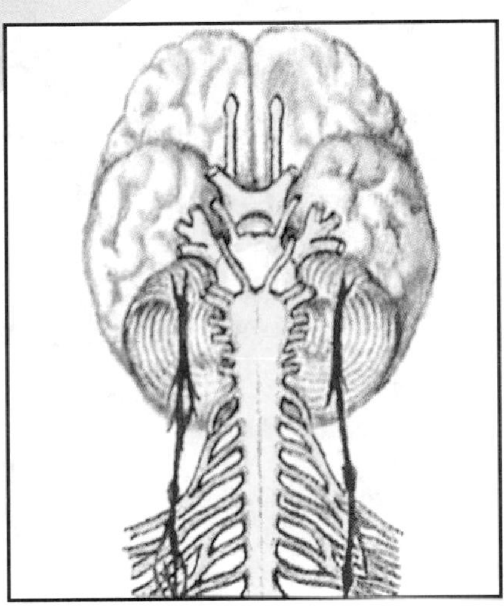

Chapter Contents

Objectives

After study of this chapter you should be able to:

1. Label a diagram showing the structural organization of the nervous system
2. Label a diagram of a neuron
3. Briefly describe the location and functions of the regions of the brain
4. Describe how the central nervous system is protected
5. Label a diagram of the spinal cord in cross section, indicating a reflex pathway
6. Compare the sympathetic and parasympathetic systems
7. Identify and use word parts pertaining to the nervous system
8. Describe the major disorders of the nervous system
9. List some common symptoms of neurologic disorders
10. Define abbreviations used in neurology
11. Interpret case studies involving the nervous system

The nervous system and the endocrine system coordinate and control the body. Together they regulate our responses to the environment and maintain homeostasis. Whereas the endocrine system functions by means of hormones, the nervous system functions by means of electrical impulses. For study purposes, the nervous system may be divided into the **central**

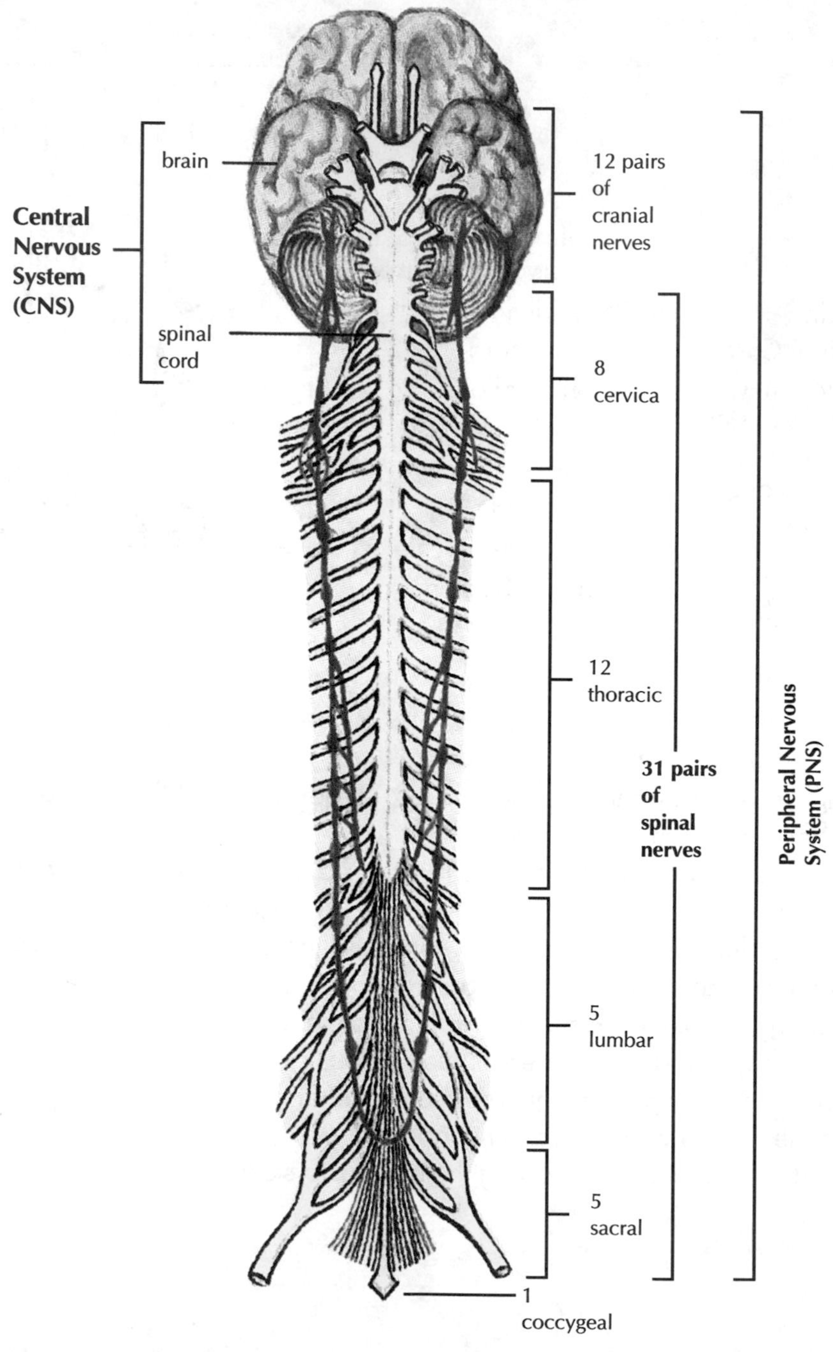

FIGURE 17-1. Anatomic divisions of the nervous system (anterior view).

nervous system (CNS), consisting of the brain and spinal cord, and the **peripheral nervous system** (PNS), consisting of all nervous tissue outside the brain and spinal cord (Fig. 17-1).

Functionally, the nervous system can be divided into the **somatic nervous system**, which controls skeletal muscles, and the visceral or **autonomic nervous system** (ANS), which controls smooth muscle, cardiac muscle, and glands. This system is important in regulating responses to stress and in maintaining homeostasis.

Two types of cells are found in the nervous system:

1. **Neurons**, or nerve cells, that make up the conducting tissue of the nervous system, and
2. **Neuroglia**, the connective tissue cells of the nervous system that support and protect nervous tissue

The Neuron

The neuron is the basic functional unit of the nervous system (Fig. 17-2). Each neuron has two types of fibers extending from the cell body: the **dendrite**, which carries impulses toward the cell body; the **axon**, which carries impulses away from the cell body.

Some axons are covered with **myelin**, a whitish, fatty material that insulates and protects the axon and speeds electrical conduction. Axons so covered are described as *myelinated*, and they make up the **white matter** of the nervous system. Unmyelinated tissue makes up the **gray matter** of the nervous system.

Each neuron is part of a relay system that carries information through the nervous system. A neuron that transmits impulses toward the CNS is a **sensory** neuron; a neuron that transmits impulses away from the CNS is a **motor** neuron. There are also connecting neurons within the CNS. The point of contact between two nerve cells is the **synapse**. At the synapse energy is passed from one cell to another by means of a chemical **neurotransmitter**.

Nerves

Individual neuron fibers are held together in bundles like wires in a cable. If this bundle is part of the PNS, it is called a **nerve**. A collection of cell bodies along the pathway of a nerve is a **ganglion**. A few nerves (sensory nerves) contain only sensory neurons, and a few (motor nerves) contain only motor neurons, but most contain both types of fibers and are described as *mixed nerves*.

The Brain

The **cerebrum** is the largest part of the brain (Fig. 17-3). It is composed largely of white matter with a thin outer layer of gray matter, the **cortex**. It is within the cortex that the higher brain functions of memory, reasoning, and abstract thought occur. The cerebrum is divided into two hemispheres by a deep groove, the longitudinal fissure. Each hemisphere is further divided into lobes with specialized functions.

The **diencephalon** contains the **thalamus**, the **hypothalamus**, and the pituitary gland. The thalamus receives sensory information and directs it to the proper portion of the cortex. The hypothalamus controls the pituitary and forms a link between the endocrine and nervous systems.

The **brain stem** consists of the **midbrain**, the **pons**, and the **medulla oblongata** (see Figure 17-3). The midbrain contains reflex centers for improved vision and hearing. The pons forms a bulge on the anterior surface of the brain stem. It contains fibers which connect different regions of the brain. The medulla connects the brain with the spinal cord. All impulses passing to and from the brain travel through this region. The medulla also has vital centers for control of heart rate, respiration, and blood pressure.

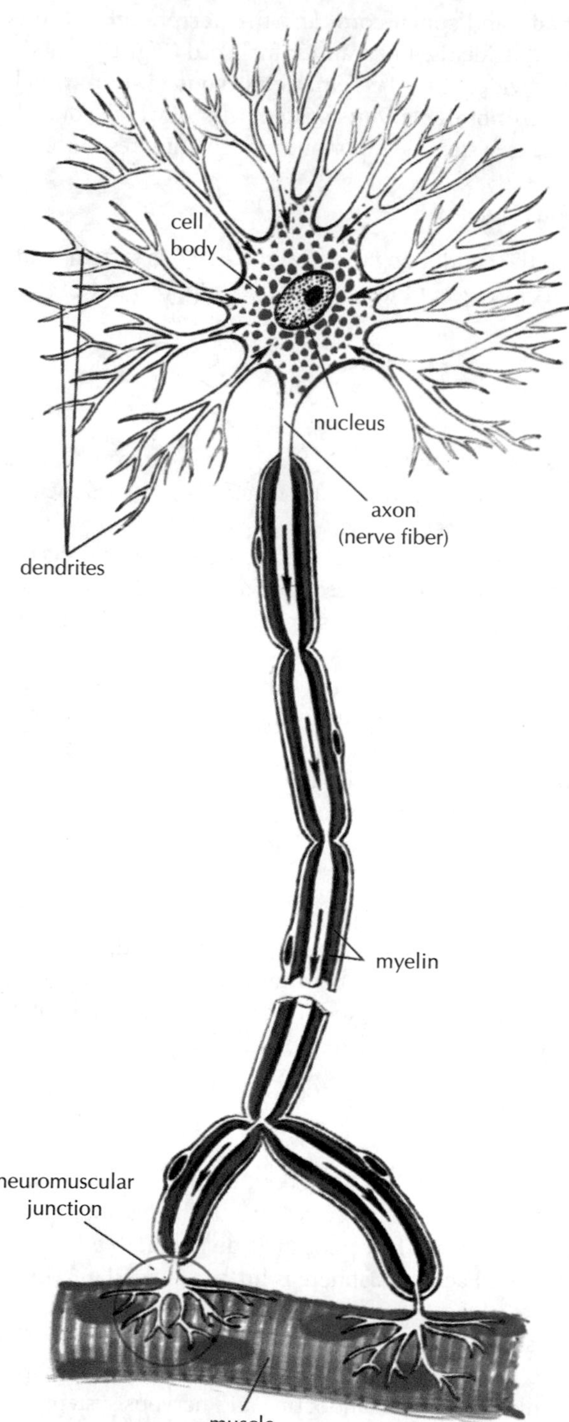

FIGURE 17-2. Motor neuron. The break in the axon denotes length; the arrows show the direction of the nerve impluse.

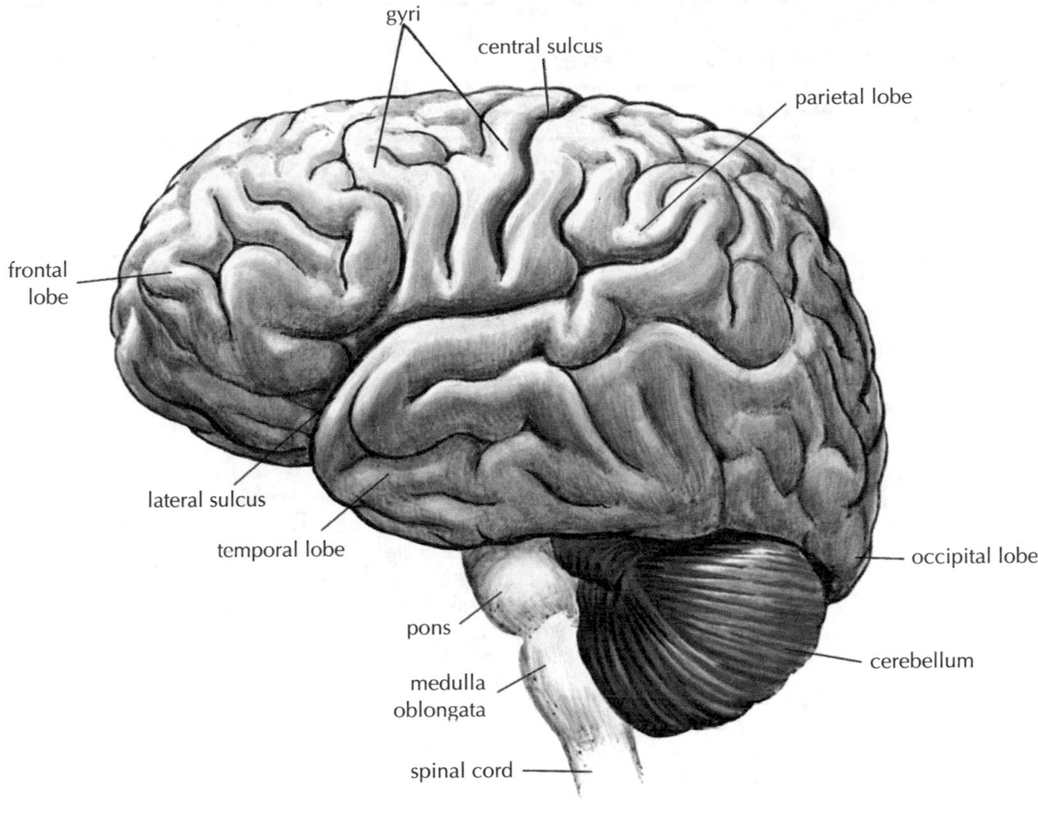

FIGURE 17-3. External surface of the brain showing the main parts and some lobes of the cerebrum.

The **cerebellum** is under the cerebrum and dorsal to the pons and medulla (see Figure 17-3). Like the cerebrum it is divided into two hemispheres. It helps to control voluntary muscle movements and to maintain posture, coordination, and balance.

Within the brain are four **ventricles** (cavities) in which **cerebrospinal fluid** (CSF) is produced. This fluid circulates around the brain and spinal cord acting as a protective cushion for these tissues.

Covering the brain and also the spinal cord are three protective layers, together called the **meninges**. The outermost and toughest of the three is the **dura mater**. The middle layer is the **arachnoid**. The thin, vascular inner layer, attached directly to the tissue of the brain and spinal cord, is the **pia mater**.

Twelve pairs of **cranial nerves** connect with the brain (see Figure 17-1). These are identified by Roman numerals and also by name. See Table 17-1 for a summary chart on the cranial nerves.

The Spinal Cord

The **spinal cord** extends from the medulla oblongata to between the first and second lumbar vertebrae. It has a central area of gray matter surrounded by white matter (Fig. 17-4). The gray matter projects toward the back and the front as the **dorsal** and **ventral horns**. The white mat-

TABLE 17-1 The Cranial Nerves

Number	Name	Function
I	olfactory *ol-FAK-tō-rē*	carries impulses for the sense of smell
II	optic *OP-tik*	carries impulses for the sense of vision
III	oculomotor *ok-ū-lō-MŌ-tor*	controls movement of eye muscles
IV	trochlear *TROK-lē-ar*	controls a muscle of the eyeball
V	trigeminal *trī-JEM-i-nal*	carries sensory impulses from the face; controls chewing muscles
VI	abducens *ab-DŪ-sens*	controls a muscle of the eyeball
VII	facial *FĀ-shal*	controls muscles of facial expression, salivary glands, and tear glands; conducts some impulses for taste
VIII	vestibulocochlear *ves-tib-ū-lō-KOK-lē-ar*	conducts impulses for hearing and equilibrium; also called auditory or acoustic nerve
IX	glossopharyngeal *glos-ō-fa-RIN-jē-al*	conducts sensory impulses from tongue and pharynx; stimulates parotid salivary gland and partly controls swallowing
X	vagus *VĀ-gus*	supplies most organs of thorax and abdomen; controls digestive secretions
XI	spinal accessory *ak-SES-ō-rē*	controls muscles of the neck
XII	hypoglossal *hī-pō-GLOS-al*	controls muscles of the tongue

ter contains the ascending and descending **tracts** (fiber bundles) that carry impulses to and from the brain.

Thirty-one pairs of spinal nerves connect with the spinal cord. Each joins the cord by two **roots**. The dorsal, or posterior, root carries sensory impulses into the cord; the ventral, or anterior, root carries motor impulses away from the cord and out toward a muscle or gland. A simple response that requires few neurons is a **reflex** (see Figure 17-4). In a spinal reflex, impulses travel through the spinal cord only and do not reach the brain. An example is the knee-jerk reflex used in physical examinations. Most neurologic responses, however, involve complex interactions among multiple neurons in the CNS.

✳ The Autonomic Nervous System

The autonomic nervous system (ANS) is the division of the nervous system that controls the involuntary actions of muscles and glands (Fig. 17-5). The ANS itself has two divisions: the **sympathetic nervous system** and the **parasympathetic nervous system**. The sympathetic nervous system motivates our response to stress, the so-called "fight-or-flight" response. It increases heart rate and respiration rate, stimulates the adrenal gland, and delivers more blood to skeletal muscles. The parasympathetic system returns the body to a steady state and stimulates maintenance activities, such as digestion of food. Most organs are controlled by both systems and, in general, the two systems have opposite effects on a given organ.

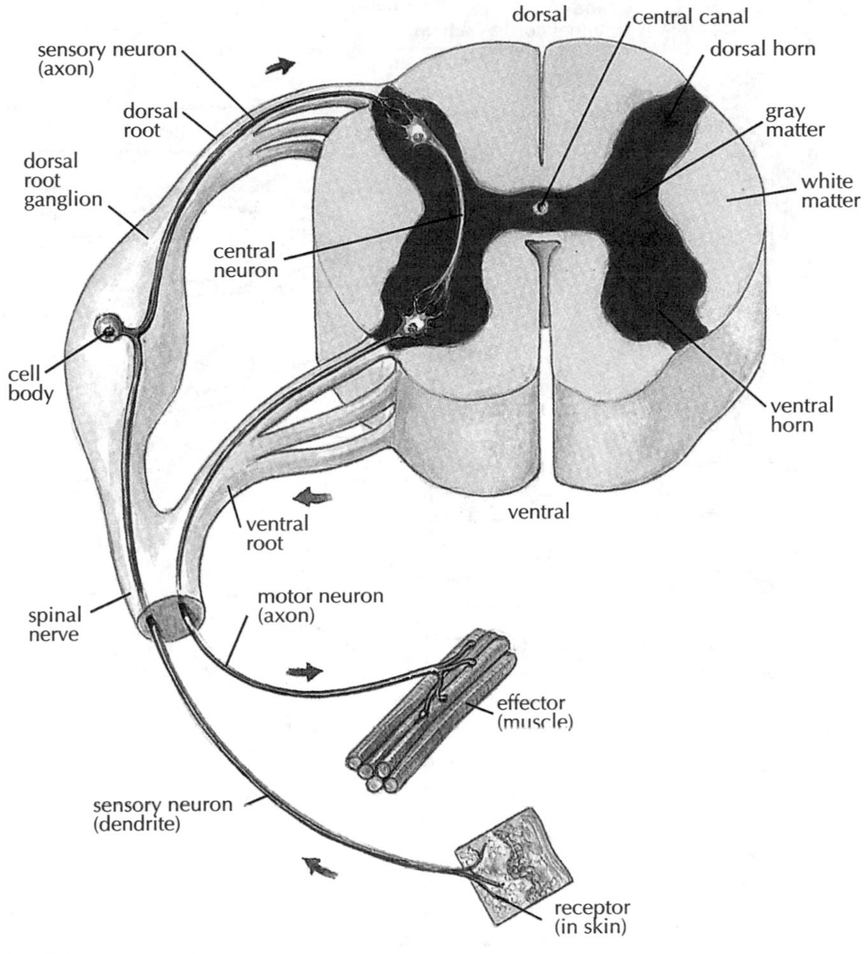

FIGURE 17-4. Cross section of spinal cord showing reflex pathway.

KEY TERMS

Normal Structure and Function

autonomic nervous system (ANS) *(aw-tō-NOM-ik)* — The division of the nervous system that regulates involuntary activities, controlling smooth muscles, cardiac muscle, and glands; the visceral nervous system

axon *(AK-son)* — The fiber of a neuron that conducts impulses away from the cell body

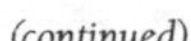

(continued)

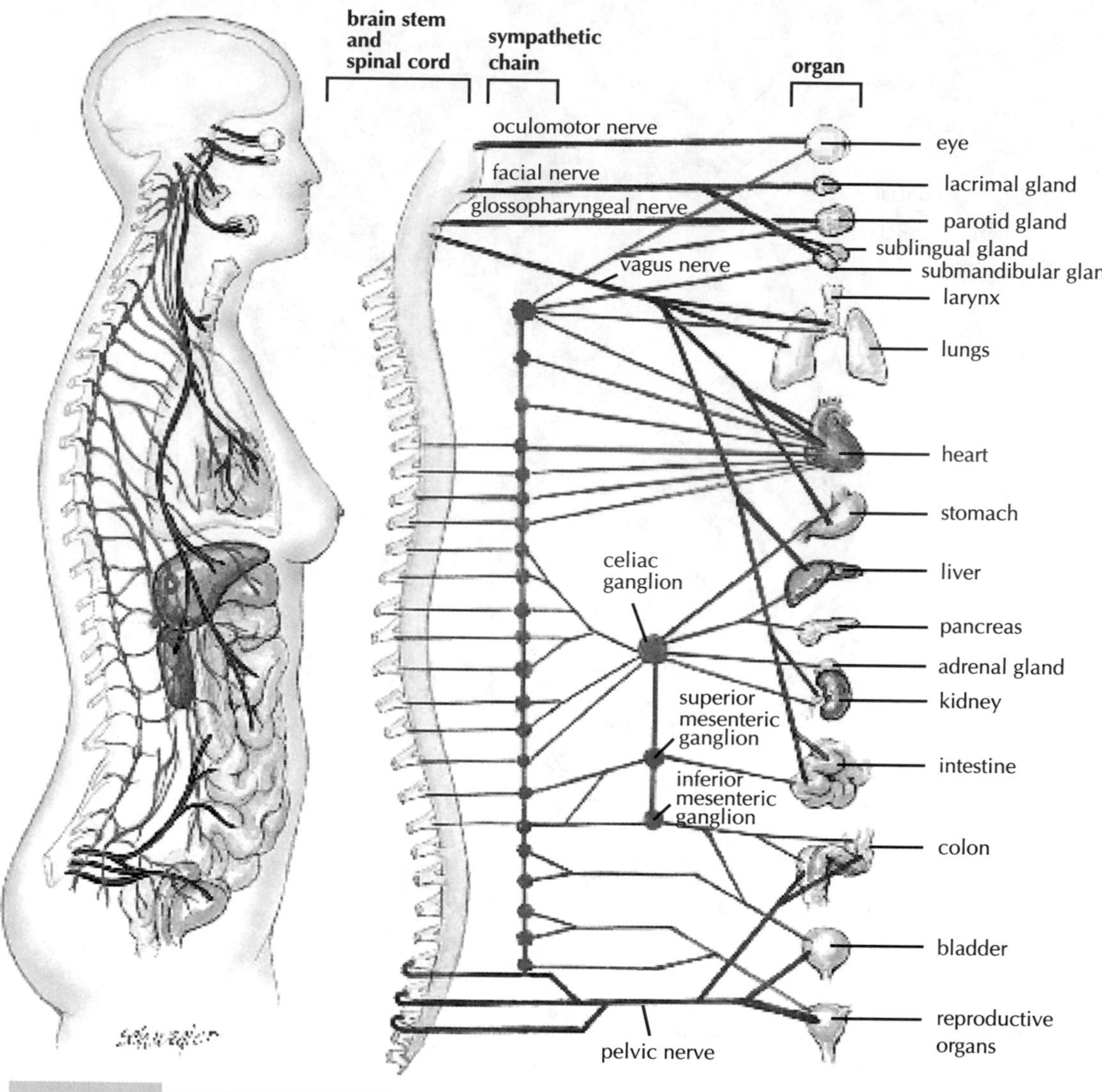

FIGURE 17-5. Autonomic nervous system (only one side is shown). The sympathetic system is shown in green; the parasympathetic system is shown in blue.

brain	The nervous tissue contained within the cranium; consists of the cerebrum, diencephalon, brain stem, and cerebellum (root encephal/o)
brain stem	The part of the brain that consists of the midbrain, pons, and medulla oblongata
central nervous system (CNS)	The brain and spinal cord

cerebellum
(ser-e-BEL-um)
The posterior portion of the brain dorsal to the pons and medulla. It helps to coordinate movement and to maintain balance and posture. (*Cerebellum* means "little brain.") (root cerebell/o)

cerebrum
(SER-e-brum)
The large upper portion of the brain. It is divided into two hemispheres by the longitudinal fissure. (root cerebr/o)

cerebrospinal fluid (CSF)
(ser-e-brō-SPĪ-nal)
The watery fluid that circulates in and around the brain and spinal cord as a protection

cortex
(KOR-teks)
An outer region. The cerebral cortex is the thin surface layer of gray matter of the cerebrum. (root cortic/o)

dendrite
(DEN-drīt)
A fiber of a neuron that conducts impulses toward the cell body

diencephalon
The part of the brain that contains the thalamus, hypothalamus, and pituitary gland. It is located between the cerebrum and the brain stem.

ganglion
(GANG-glē-on)
A collection of nerve cell bodies outside the CNS (pl. ganglia) (root gangli/o, ganglion/o)

gray matter
Unmyelinated tissue of the nervous system

hypothalamus
(hī-pō-THAL-a-mus)
The part of the brain that controls the pituitary gland and maintains homeostasis

medulla oblongata
(me-DUL-la ob-long-GA-ta)
The portion of the brain that connects with the spinal cord. It has vital centers for control of respiration, heart rate, and blood pressure. (root medull/o)

meninges
(men-IN-jēz)
The three membranes that cover the brain and spinal cord: the dura mater, the arachnoid, and the pia mater (s. meninx) (root mening/o, meninge/o)

midbrain
The part of the brain stem between the diencephalon and the pons. It contains centers for coordination of reflexes for vision and hearing.

motor
Producing movement. Describing neurons that carry impulses away from the CNS.

myelin
(MĪ-e-lin)
A whitish, fatty substance that surrounds certain axons of the nervous system

neuroglia
(nū-ROG-lē-a)
The connective tissue cells of the nervous system. Also called glial cells (from *glia* meaning "glue"). (root gli/o)

neuron
(Nū-ron)
A nerve cell

neurotransmitter
A chemical that transmits energy across a synapse

nerve
A bundle of nerve cell fibers outside the CNS (root neur/o)

parasympathetic nervous system
The part of the automatic nervous system that reverses the response to stress and restores homeostasis. It slows heart rate and respiration rate while stimulating activity of the digestive, urinary, and reproductive systems.

(continued)

peripheral nervous system *(per-RIF-er-al)*	The portion of the nervous system outside the CNS
pons *(ponz)*	A rounded area on the ventral surface of the brain stem. It contains fibers that connect regions of the brain. The adjective is pontine *(PON-tēn)*.
reflex *(RĒ-fleks)*	A simple, rapid, and automatic response to a stimulus
Schwann cells *(shvon)*	Cells that produce the myelin sheath around peripheral axons
sensory *(SEN-so-rē)*	Describing neurons that carry impulses toward the CNS
somatic nervous system	The division of the nervous system that controls skeletal (voluntary) muscles
spinal cord	The nervous tissue contained within the spinal column; extends from the medulla oblongata to the second lumbar vertebra (root myel/o)
sympathetic nervous system	The part of the autonomic nervous system that mobilizes a response to stress. It increases heart rate and respiration rate and delivers more blood to skeletal muscles.
synapse *(SIN-aps)*	The junction between two neurons
thalamus *(THAL-a-mus)*	The part of the brain that receives all sensory impulses except those for the sense of smell and directs them to the proper portion of the cerebral cortex (root thalam/o)
tract *(trakt)*	A bundle of nerve cell fibers within the CNS
ventricle *(VEN-trik-l)*	A small cavity, such as one of the cavities in the brain in which CSF is produced (root ventricul/o)
visceral nervous system	The autonomic nervous system
white matter	Myelinated tissue of the nervous system

Word Parts Pertaining to the Nervous System

Roots for the Nervous System and the Spinal Cord

Root	Meaning	Example	Definition of Example
neur/o, neur/i	nervous system, nerve	neurolysis *nū-ROL-i-sis*	destruction of a nerve
gli/o	neuroglia	glioma *gli-Ō-ma*	a neuroglial tumor
gangli/o, ganglion/o	ganglion	ganglionectomy *gang-glē-o-NEK-tō-mē*	surgical removal of a ganglion

(continued)

Roots for the Nervous System and the Spinal Cord (Continued)

Root	Meaning	Example	Definition of Example
mening/o, meninge/o	meninges	meningocele *me-NING-gō-sēl*	hernia of the meninges through the skull or spinal column
myel/o	spinal cord (also bone marrow)	myelogram *MĪ-e-lō-gram*	x-ray of the spinal cord
radicul/o	root of a spinal nerve	radiculopathy *ra-dik-ū-LOP-a-thē*	any disease of a spinal nerve root

Exercise 17-1

Define the following adjectives:

1. neural *(NŪ-ral)* pertaining to a nerve or nerves
2. glial *(GLĪ-al)* ______
3. ganglionic *(gang-glē-ON-ik)* ______
4. meningeal *(me-NIN-jē-al)* ______
5. radicular *(ra-DIK-ū-lar)* ______

Fill in the blanks:

6. Hematomyelia is hemorrhage into the ______ *(hē-ma-tō-mī-Ē-lē-a)*
7. Meningococci are bacteria that infect the ______ *(me-ning-gō-KOK-sī)*
8. Polyradiculitis is inflammation of many ______ *(pol-ē-ra-dik-ū-LĪ-tis)*

Define the following terms:

9. neuralgia *(nū-RAL-jē-a)* ______
10. myeloradiculitis *(mī-e-lō-ra-dik-u-LĪ-tis)* ______
11. meningioma (Note spelling) *(me-nin-jē-Ō-ma)* ______

Write a word for each of the following definitions:

12. Study of the nervous system ______
13. Any disease of the nervous system ______
14. Tumor of a ganglion ______
15. Radiographic study of the spinal cord ______
16. Inflammation of the meninges ______

Roots for the Brain

Root	Meaning	Example	Definition of Example
encephal/o	brain	encephalomalacia *en-sef-a-lō-ma-LĀ-shē-a*	softening of brain tissue
cerebr/o	cerebrum (loosely, brain)	decerebrate *dē-SER-e-brāt*	having no cerebral function
cortic/o	outer portion, cerebral cortex	corticospinal *kor-ti-kō-SPĪ-nal*	pertaining to the cerebral cortex and spinal cord
cerebell/o	cerebellum	intracerebellar *in-tra-ser-e-BEL-ar*	within the cerebellum
thalam/o	thalamus	hypothalamus *hi-pō-THAL-a-mus*	region of brain beneath the thalamus
ventricul/o	cavity, ventricle	supraventricular *sū-pra-ven-TRIK-ū-lar*	above a ventricle
medull/o	medulla oblongata (also spinal cord)	extramedullary *eks-tra-MED-ū-lar-ē*	outside the medulla
psych/o	mind	psychogenic *si-kō-JEN-ik*	originating in the mind
narc/o	stupor, unconsciousness	narcosis *nar-KŌ-sis*	state of stupor induced by drugs
somn/o, somn/i	sleep	somnolent *SOM-nō-lent*	sleepy

Exercise 17-2

Fill in the blanks:

1. An electroencephalogram (EEG) is a record of the electrical activity of the __________
   (ē-lek-trō-en-SEF-a-lō-gram)
2. The term cerebrovascular refers to the blood vessels in the __________
   (ser-ē-brō-VAS-kū-lar)
3. The term *psychosomatic* refers to the body (soma) and the __________
   (sī-kō-sō-MAT-ik)
4. A narcotic is a drug that causes __________
   (nar-KOT-ik)
5. Somnabulism means walking during __________
   (som-NAM-bū-lizm)

Write the adjective for each of the following definitions. Note the endings.

6. Pertaining to the (-al) the cerebrum ______________________
7. Pertaining to (-al) the cerebral cortex ______________________
8. Pertaining to (-ic) the thalamus ______________________
9. Pertaining to (-ar) the cerebellum ______________________
10. Pertaining to (-ar) a ventricle ______________________

Define each of the following terms:

11. encephalitis ______________________
    (en-sef-a-LĪ-tis)
12. medullary ______________________
    (MED-ū-lar-ē
13. psychology ______________________
    (sī-KOL-ō-jē)
14. insomnia ______________________
    (in-SOM-nē-a)

Write a word for each of the following definitions:

15. Any disease of the brain ______________________
16. Within (intra-) the cerebrum ______________________
17. Pertaining to the cerebral cortex and the thalamus ______________________
18. Inflammation of a ventricle ______________________
19. Pertaining to the brain (cerebr/o) and spinal cord ______________________

Suffixes for the Nervous System

Suffix	Meaning	Example	Definition of Example
-phasia	speech	heterophasia *het-er-ō-FĀ-zha*	uttering words that are different from those intended
-lalia	speech, babble	echolalia *ek-ō-LĀ-lē-a*	repetition of words
-lexia	reading	dyslexia *dis-LEK-sē-a*	difficulty in reading
-plegia	paralysis	quadriplegia *kwod-ri-PLĒ-jē-a*	paralysis of all four limbs
-lepsy	seizure	narcolepsy *NAR-kō-lep-sē*	condition marked by sudden episodes of sleep

(continued)

Suffixes for the Nervous System (Continued)

Suffix	Meaning	Example	Definition of Example
Words Pertaining to the Nervous System Used as Suffixes			
-paresis	partial paralysis	myoparesis *mi-ō-pa-RĒ-sis*	partial paralysis of a muscle
-phobia	persistent, irrational fear	claustrophobia *claws-trō-FŌ-bē-a*	fear of being shut in or enclosed (from L. *claudere* "to shut")
-mania	excited state, obsession	megalomania *meg-a-lō-MĀ-nē-a*	exaggerated self-importance; "delusions of grandeur"

Exercise 17-3

Fill in the blanks:

1. A person who is aphasic has a loss or defect in ____________________
   (a-FĀ-sik)
2. Epilepsy is a disease characterized by ____________________
   (EP-i-lep-sē)
3. In one affected with hemiparesis, one side of the body shows ____________________
   (hem-i-pa-RĒ-sis)
4. A person with alexia lacks the ability to ____________________
   (a-LEK-sē-a)

Define the following terms:

5. bradylalia ____________________
   (brad-ē-LĀ-lē-a)
6. pyromania ____________________
   (pī-rō-MĀ-nē-a)
7. gynephobia ____________________
   (jin-e-FŌ-bē-a)

Write a word for each of the following definitions:

8. Slowness in reading ____________________
9. Paralysis of one side (hemi-) of the body ____________________
10. Paralysis of one (mono-) limb ____________________
11. Fear of night and darkness ____________________
12. Fear of (or abnormal sensitivity to) light ____________________

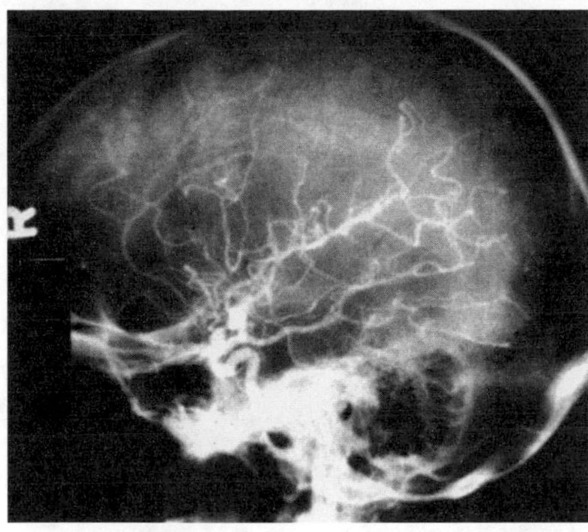

FIGURE 17-6. Cerebral angiogram showing the lateral view of filling of the left carotid and its branches. (Sheldon H: Boyd's Introduction to the Study of Disease, 11th ed, p 522. Philadelphia: Lea & Febiger, 1992. Used with permission.)

Clinical Aspects of the Nervous System

Vascular Disorders

The term **cerebrovascular accident** (CVA), or **stroke**, applies to any occurrence that deprives brain tissue of oxygen. These include blockage (thrombosis or embolism) in a vessel that supplies the brain, a ruptured aneurysm, or some other event that leads to hemorrhage within the brain. Stroke is the third leading cause of death in developed countries, following cancer and heart attack (myocardial infarction). Risk factors for a stroke include hypertension, atherosclerosis (hardening of the arteries), heart disease, diabetes mellitus, and cigarette smoking. Heredity is also a factor.

Thrombosis is the formation of a blood clot in a vessel. Often, in cases of CVA, thrombosis occurs in the carotid artery, the large vessel in the neck that supplies the brain. Sudden blockage by an obstruction traveling from another part of the body is described as an **embolism**. In cases

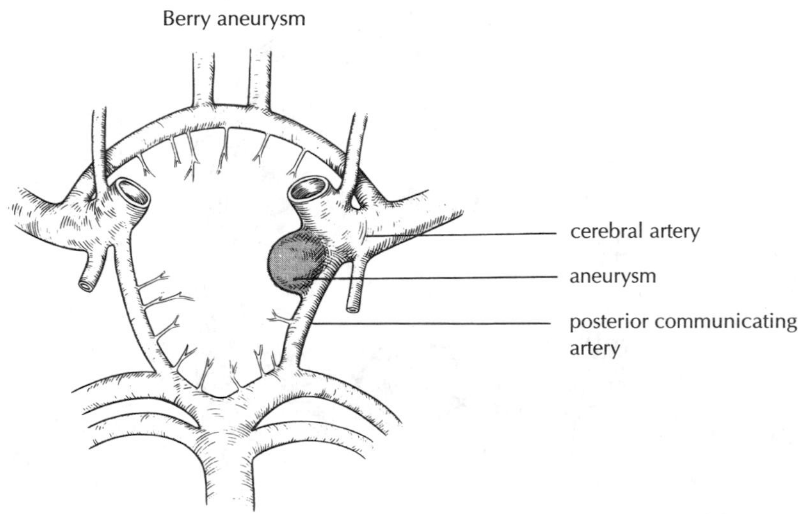

FIGURE 17-7. A cerebral aneurysm in the circle of Willis. (Porth CM: Pathophysiology, 3rd ed, p 275. Philadelphia: JB Lippincott, 1990.)

of stroke, the embolus usually originates in the heart. These obstructions can be diagnosed by **cerebral angiography** (Fig. 17-6) with radiopaque dye, CT scans, and other radiographic techniques. In cases of thrombosis it is sometimes possible to remove the section of a vessel that is blocked and insert a graft. If the carotid artery is involved a **carotid endarterectomy** may be performed to open the vessel, and methods for dissolving such clots are now under study.

An **aneurysm** (Fig. 17-7) is a localized dilation of a vessel that may rupture and cause hemorrhage. An aneurysm may be congenital or may arise from other causes, especially atherosclerosis, which weakens the vessel wall. Hypertension then contributes to its rupture. The effects of cerebral hemorrhage vary from massive loss of function to mild impairment of sensory or motor

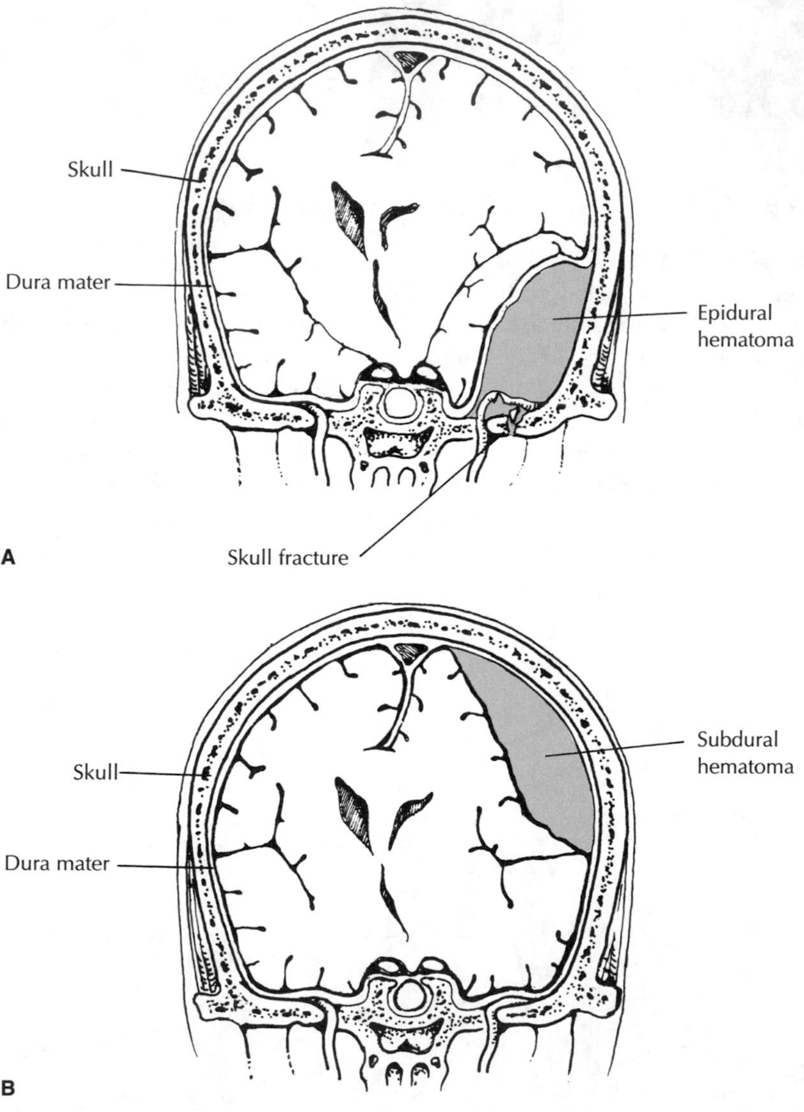

FIGURE 17-8. Hematoma. **(A)** Epidural hematoma. **(B)** Subdural hematoma. (Jones SA, Weigel A, White RD, McSwain NE Jr, Breiter M: Advanced Emergency Care for Paramedic Practice, pp 315–316. Philadelphia: JB Lippincott, 1992.)

activity, depending on the degree of damage. **Aphasia**, loss or impairment of speech communication, is a common aftereffect. **Hemiplegia** (paralysis of one side of the body) on the side opposite the damage is also seen. It has been found in cases of hemorrhage, as in other forms of brain injury, that immediate retraining therapy may help to restore lost function.

Trauma

A blow to the head is the usual cause of bleeding into or around the meninges, forming a hematoma. Damage to an artery from a skull fracture, usually on the side of the head, may be the cause of an **epidural hematoma** (Fig. 17-8A), which appears between the dura mater and the skull bone. The rapidly accumulating blood puts pressure on local vessels and interupts blood flow to the brain. There may be headache, loss of consciousness, or **hemiparesis** (partial paralysis) on the side opposite the blow. Diagnosis is made by CT scan or MRI. If pressure is not relieved within 1 or 2 days, death results.

A **subdural hematoma** (Fig. 17-8B) often results from a blow to the front or back of the head, as when the moving head hits a stationary object. The force of the blow separates the dura from the membrane below, the arachnoid. Blood from a damaged vessel, usually a vein, slowly enters this space. The gradual accumulation of blood puts pressure on the brain causing headache, weakness, and **dementia**. If there is continued bleeding, death results.

A cerebral **concussion** results from a blow to the head or from a fall. It may be followed by headache, dizziness, vomiting, loss of consciousness, and even paralysis, among other symptoms. Damage that occurs on the side of the brain opposite the blow as the brain is thrown against the skull is described as a **contrecoup injury** (from the French, meaning "counterblow").

Other injuries may damage the brain directly. Injury to the base of the brain may involve vital centers in the medulla and interfere with respiration and cardiac function.

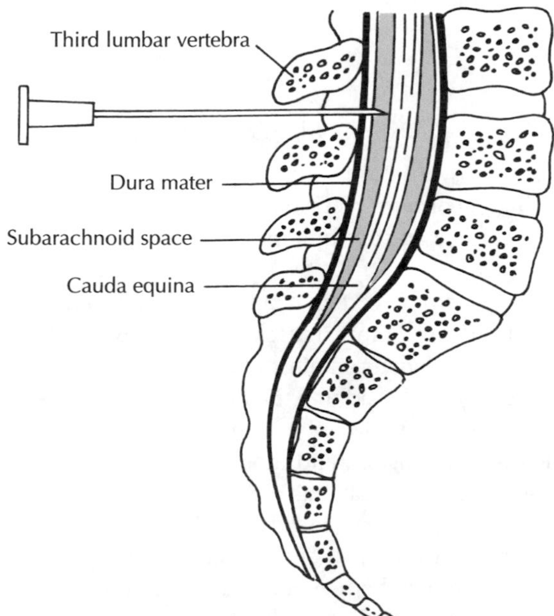

FIGURE 17-9. Lumbar tap. (Taylor C, Lillis CA, LeMone P: Fundamentals of Nursing, 2nd ed, p 543. Philadelphia: JB Lippincott, 1993.)

Infection

Inflammation of the meninges, or **meningitis**, is usually caused by bacteria that enter through the ear, nose, or throat, or are carried by the blood. One organism, the meningococcus, is responsible for epidemics of meningitis among individuals living in close quarters. A stiff neck is a common symptom. The presence of pus or lymphocytes in spinal fluid is also characteristic. Fluid is withdrawn for diagnosis by a **lumbar** (spinal) **puncture** (Fig. 17-9), in which a needle is used to remove cerebrospinal fluid from the meninges in the lumbar region of the spine. This fluid can be examined for white blood cells and bacteria in the case of meningitis, for red blood cells in the case of brain injury, or for tumor cells. Also, the fluid can be analyzed chemically. Normally, it is clear, with glucose and chlorides but no protein and very few cells.

Other conditions that can cause meningitis and **encephalitis** (inflammation of the brain) include viral infections, tuberculosis, and syphilis. Among viral infections, the polio and rabies viruses, herpes virus, HIV (the cause of AIDS), and rarely, common infections such as measles and chickenpox, can involve the central nervous system. Herpes zoster, the chickenpox virus, is also responsible for **shingles**, which spreads along peripheral nerves causing lesions and inflammation.

Neoplasms

Almost all tumors that originate in the nervous system are tumors of nonconducting support cells, the neuroglia. These growths are termed **gliomas** and may be named for the specific type of cell involved, such as astrocytoma, oligodendroglioma, or schwannoma (neurilemoma). Because they tend not to metastasize, these tumors may be described as benign. However, they do harm by compressing brain tissue. The symptoms they cause depend on their size and location. There may be seizures, headache, vomiting, muscle weakness, or interference with a special sense, such as vision or hearing. If present, edema and **hydrocephalus** add to the effects of the tumor.

A **meningioma** is a tumor of the meninges. Because a meningioma does not spread and is localized at the surface, it can usually be removed completely by surgery.

Tumors of neural tissue generally occur in childhood, and may even originate before birth, when nervous tissue is actively multiplying.

Finally, cancer may metastasize to the brain from elsewhere in the body. For unknown reasons, certain forms of cancer, especially melanoma, breast cancer, and lung cancer, tend to spread to the brain.

Degenerative Diseases

Multiple sclerosis (MS) commonly attacks people in their 20s or 30s and progresses at intervals and at varying rates. It involves patchy loss of myelin with hardening (sclerosis) of tissue in the CNS. The symptoms include vision problems, tingling or numbness in the arms and legs, urinary incontinence, tremor, and stiff gait. MS is thought to be an autoimmune disorder, but the exact cause is not known.

Parkinson's disease occurs when, for unknown reason, certain neurons in the midbrain fail to secrete the neurotransmitter dopamine. This leads to tremors, muscle rigidity, flexion at the joints, and emotional problems. Parkinson's is treated with daily adminstration of the drug **L-dopa** (levodopa), a form of dopamine that can be carried by the blood into the brain.

Alzheimer's disease results from unexplained degeneration of neurons and atrophy of the cerebral cortex. This causes loss of recent memory, confusion, and mood changes. Originally called presenile dementia and used only to describe cases in patients about 50 years of age, the term is now applied to these same changes when they occur in the elderly. Alzheimer's is diagnosed by CT or MRI scans and confirmed at autopsy. Histology (tissue) studies show deposits in the tissues of a substance called **amyloid**. The disease may be hereditary. It is also known that people with Down syndrome commonly develop Alzheimer's disease after age 40.

Epilepsy

A prime characteristic of **epilepsy** is recurrent seizures brought on by abnormal electrical activity of the brain. These may vary from brief and mild episodes known as absence (petit mal) seizures to major tonic-clonic (grand mal) seizures with loss of consciousness, **convulsion**, (intervals of violent involuntary muscle contractions), and sensory disuturbances. In other cases (psychomotor seizures) there is a 1- to 2-minute period of disorientation. Epilepsy may be the result of a tumor, injury, or neurologic disease, but in most cases the cause in unknown.

Electroencephalography (EEG) studies reveal abnormalities in brain activity and can be used in diagnosis and treatment. Epilepsy is treated with antiepileptic and anticonvulsive drugs to control seizures, and sometimes surgery is of help. If seizures can not be controlled, the individual with epilepsy may have to avoid certain activities that can lead to harm.

Others

Many hereditary diseases affect the nervous system. Some of these are described in Chapter 15. Hormonal imbalances that involve the nervous system are described in Chapter 16. Finally, drugs, alcohol, toxins, and nutritional deficiencies may act on the nervous system in a variety of ways.

KEY CLINICAL TERMS

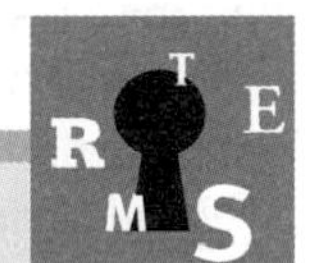

Disorders

Alzheimer's disease *(ALTS-hī-merz)*	A form of dementia caused by atrophy of the cerebral cortex; presenile dementia
amyloid *(AM-i-loyd)*	A starchlike substance of unknown composition that accumulates in the brain in Alzheimer's and other diseases
aneurysm *(AN-ū-rizm)*	A localized abnormal dilation of a blood vessel that results from weakness of the vessel wall (see Figure 17-7). An aneurysm may eventually burst.
aphasia *(a-FĀ-zē-a)*	Specifically, loss or defect in speech communication (from G. *phasis* meaning "speech"). In practice the term is applied more broadly to a range of language disorders, both spoken and written. May affect ability to understand speech (receptive aphasia) or the ability to produce speech (expressive aphasia). Both forms are combined in global aphasia.
astrocytoma *(as-trō-sī-TŌ-ma)*	A neuroglial tumor composed of astrocytes
cerebrovascular accident (CVA)	Sudden damage to the brain resulting from reduction of cerebral blood flow. Possible causes are atherosclerosis, thrombosis, or a ruptured aneurysm. Commonly called *stroke*.
coma *(KŌ-ma)*	A deep stupor caused by illness or injury
concussion *(kon-KUSH-un)*	Injury resulting from a violent blow or shock. A concussion of the brain usually results in loss of consciousness.
contrecoup injury *(kon-tr-KŪ)*	Damage to the brain on the side opposite the point of a blow as a result of the brain's hitting the skull

(continued)

convulsion *(kon-VUL-shun)*	A series of violent, involuntary muscle contractions. A tonic convulsion involves prolonged contraction of the muscles; in a clonic convulsion there is alternation of contraction and relaxation. Both forms appear in grand mal epilepsy.
dementia *(dē-MEN-shē-a)*	A gradual and usually irreversible loss of intellectual function
embolism *(EM-bō-lizm)*	Obstruction of a blood vessel by a blood clot or other material carried in the circulation
encephalitis *(en-sef-a-LĪ-tis)*	Inflammation of the brain
epidural hematoma	Accumulation of blood in the epidural space (between the dura mater and the skull) (see Figure 17-8A)
epilepsy *(EP-i-lep-sē)*	A chronic disease involving periodic sudden bursts of electrical activity from the brain resulting in seizures
glioma *(glī-Ō-ma)*	A tumor of neuroglia cells
hemiparesis *(hem-i-pa-RĒ-sis)*	Partial paralysis or weakness of one side of the body
hemiplegia *(hemi-i-PLĒ-jē-a)*	Paralysis of one side of the body
hydrocephalus *(hī-drō-SEF-a-lus)*	Increased accumulation of CSF in or around the brain as a result of obstruction to flow. May be caused by tumor, inflammation, hemorrhage, or congenital abnormality.
meningioma *(men-nin-jē-Ō-ma)*	Tumor of the meninges
meningitis *(men-in-JĪ-tis)*	Inflammation of the meninges
multiple sclerosis	A chronic, progressive disease involving loss of myelin in the CNS
neurilemoma *(nū-ri-lem-Ō-ma)*	A tumor of the sheath (neurilemma) of a peripheral nerve; Schwannoma
paralysis *(pa-RAL-i-sis)*	Temporary or permanent loss of function. Flaccid paralysis involves loss of muscle tone and reflexes and degeneration of muscles. Spastic paralysis involves excess muscle tone and reflexes but no degeneration.
Parkinson's disease	A disorder originating in the basal ganglia and characterized by slow movements, tremor, rigidity, masklike face. Also called *Parkinsonism*.
seizure *(SĒ-zhur)*	A sudden attack, as seen in epilepsy. The most common forms of seizure are 1) tonic-clonic, or grand mal (gran mal), from French meaning "great illness"; 2) absence seizure, or petit mal (pet-Ē mal), meaning "small illness;" and 3) psychomotor seizure.
shingles	An acute viral infection that follows nerve pathways causing small lesions on the skin. Also called herpes zoster (HER-pēz ZOS-ter), and caused by the same virus that causes chickenpox.

subdural hematoma — Accumulation of blood beneath the dura mater (see Figure 17-8B)

thrombosis *(throm-BŌ-sis)* — Development of a blood clot within a vessel

tremor *(TREM-or)* — A shaking or involuntary movement

Diagnosis and Treatment

carotid endarterectomy *(end-ar-ter-EK-tō-mē)* — Surgical removal of the lining of the carotid artery, the large artery in the neck that suppplies blood to the brain

cerebral angiography — Radiographic study of the blood vessels of the brain following injection of a contrast medium (see Figure 17-6)

electroencephalography *(ē-lek-trō-en-sef-o-LOG-ra-fē)* — Amplification, recording, and interpretation of the electrical activity of the brain

L-dopa *(DŌ-pa)* — A drug used in the treatment of Parkinson's disease; levodopa

lumbar puncture — Puncture of the subarachnoid space in the lumbar region of the spinal cord; spinal puncture. Done to remove spinal fluid for diagnosis or to inject anesthesia (see Figure 17-9).

ADDITIONAL TERMS

Normal Structure and Function

acetylcholine *(as-ē-til-KŌ-lēn)* — A neurotransmitter. Activity involving acetylcholine is described as *cholinergic*.

afferent *(AF-er-ent)* — Carrying toward a central point, such as the sensory neurons and nerves that transmit impulses toward the CNS

basal ganglia — Four masses of gray matter in the cerebrum and upper brain stem that are involved in movement and coordination

blood–brain barrier — A special membrane between circulating blood and the brain that prevents certain damaging substances from reaching brain tissue

Broca's area *(BRŌ-kas)* — An area in the left frontal lobe of the cerebrum that controls speech production

circle of Willis — An interconnection (anastomosis) of several arteries supplying the brain. Located at the base of the cerebrum (see Figure 17-7).

contralateral *(kon-tra-LAT-er-al)* — Affecting the opposite side of the body

(continued)

corpus callosum (*KOR-pus ka-LŌ-sum*) — A large band of connecting fibers between the cerebral hemispheres

dermatome (*DER-ma-tōm*) — The area of the skin supplied by a spinal nerve

efferent (*EF-er-ent*) — Carrying away from a central point, such as the motor neurons and nerves that transmit impulses away from the CNS

epinephrine (*ep-i-NEF-rin*) — A neurotransmitter. Also called *adrenaline*. Activity involving epinephrine is described as *adrenergic*.

gyrus (*JĪ-rus*) — A raised convolution of the surface of the cerebrum (see Figure 17-3) (pl. gyri)

ipsilateral (*ip-si-LAT-er-al*) — On the same side; unilateral

leptomeninges (*lep-to-men-IN-jēz*) — The pia mater and arachnoid together

nucleus (*NŪ-klē-us*) — A collection of nerve cells within the central nervous system

plexus (*PLEKS-us*) — A network, as of nerves or blood vessels

pyramidal tracts (*pi-RAM-i-dal*) — A group of motor tracts involved in fine coordination. Most of the fibers in these tracts cross in the medulla to the opposite side of the spinal cord and affect the opposite side of the body. Fibers not included in the pyramidal tracts are described as *extra-pyramidal*.

reticular activating system (RAS) (*re-TIK-ū-lar*) — A widespread system in the brain that maintains wakefulness

sulcus (*SUL-kus*) — A shallow furrow or groove, as on the surface of the cerebrum (see Figure 17-3) (pl. sulci)

Wernicke's area (*VER-ni-kēz*) — An area in the temporal lobe concerned with speech comprehension

Symptoms and Conditions

amyotrophic lateral sclerosis (ALS) (*a-mī-ō-TROF-ik*) — A disorder marked by muscular weakness, spasticity, and exaggerated reflexes caused by degeneration of motor neurons; Lou Gehrig's disease

amnesia (*am-NĒ-zha*) — Loss of memory

apraxia (*a-PRAK-sē-a*) — Inability to move with purpose or to use objects properly

ataxia (*a-TAK-sē-a*) — Lack of muscle coordination; dyssynergia

athetosis (*ath-e-TŌ-sis*) — Involuntary, slow, twisting movements in the arms, especially the hands and fingers

Bell's palsy (*PAWL-zē*) — Paralysis of the facial nerve

berry aneurysm	A small saclike aneurysm of a cerebral artery (see Figure 17-7)
cerebral palsy	A nonprogressive motor disorder usually caused by a brain defect or injury to the brain at birth
chorea *(KOR-ē-a)*	A nervous condition marked by involuntary twitching of the limbs or facial muscles
delirium *(de-LIR-ē-um)*	A sudden and temporary state of confusion marked by excitement, physical restlessness, and incoherence
dysarthria *(dis-AR-thrē-a)*	Defect in speech articulation due to lack of control over the required muscles
dysmetria *(dis-MĒ-trē-a)*	Disturbance in the path or placement of a limb during active movement. In *hypometria* the limb falls short; in *hypermetria* the limb extends beyond the target.
glioblastoma *(glī-ō-blas-TŌ-ma)*	A malignant astrocytoma
Guillain-Barré syndrome *(gē-YAN-bar-RĀ)*	An acute polyneuritis with progressive muscular weakness that usually occurs after infection. In most cases recovery is complete.
hematomyelia *(hē-ma-tō-mī-Ē-lē-a)*	Hemorrhage of blood into the spinal cord, as from an injury
hemiballism *(hem-ē-BAL-izm)*	Jerking, twitching movements of one side of the body
Huntington's disease	A hereditary disease of the CNS that usually appears between 30 and 50. The patient shows progressive dementia and chorea.
ictus *(IK-tus)*	A blow or sudden attack, such as an epileptic seizure
lethargy *(LETH-ar-jē)*	A state of sluggishness or stupor
neurofibromatosis *(nū-rō-fī-brō-ma-TŌ-sis)*	A condition involving multiple tumors of peripheral nerves
paraplegia *(par-a-PLĒ-jē-a)*	Paralysis of the legs and lower part of the body
Reye's syndrome *(rīz)*	A rare acute encephalopathy occurring in children following viral infections
stupor *(STŪ-por)*	A state of unconsciousness or lethargy with loss of responsiveness
syringomyelia *(sir-in-gō-mī-Ē-lē-a)*	A progressive disease marked by formation of fluid-filled cavities in the spinal cord
tic douloureux *(tik dū-lū-RŪ)*	Episodes of extreme pain in the area supplied by the trigeminal nerve. Also called *trigeminal neuralgia*.
tabes dorsalis *(TĀ-bēz dor-SAL-is)*	Destruction of the dorsal (posterior) portion of the spinal cord with loss of sensation and awareness of body position, as seen in advanced cases of syphilis
transient ischemic attack (TIA)	A sudden, brief, and temporary cerebral dysfunction usually due to interruption of blood flow to the brain

(continued)

Wallerian degeneration *(wahl-LĒ-rē-an)* — Degeneration of a nerve distal to an injury

Additional terms related to neurologic symptoms can be found in the chapters on the senses (18) and the muscular system (20).

Psychiatry

anxiety *(ang-ZĪ-e-tē)* — A feeling of fear, worry, uneasiness, or dread

autism *(AW-tizm)* — A disorder of unknown cause consisting of self-absorption, separateness, oversensitivity, repetitive speech and movements

catatonia *(kat-a-TŌ-nē-a)* — A phase of schizophrenia in which the patient is unresponsive. There is a tendency to remain in a fixed position without moving or talking.

compulsion *(kom-PUL-shun)* — A repetitive, stereotyped act performed to relieve tension

delusion *(dē-LŪ-zhun)* — A false belief inconsistent with knowledge and experience

depression *(dē-PRESH-un)* — An altered mood characterized by loss of interest in pleasurable activities

euphoria *(ū-FOR-ē-a)* — An exaggerated feeling of well-being; elation

hallucination *(ha-lū-si-NĀ-shun)* — A false perception unrelated to reality or external stimuli

hypochondriasis *(hī-pō-kon-DRĪ-a-sis)* — Abnormal anxiety about one's health

neurosis *(nū-RŌ-sis)* — An emotional disorder due to unresolved conflicts with anxiety as a main characteristic

paranoia *(par-a-NOY-a)* — A mental disorder characterized by jealousy and delusions of persecution

psychosis *(sī-KŌ-sis)* — A mental disorder extreme enough to cause personality disintegration and loss of contact with reality

schizophrenia *(skiz-ō-FRĒ-nē-a)* — A poorly understood group of severe mental disorders with features of psychosis, delusions, hallucinations, and withdrawn or bizarre behavior (root *phren* means "mind")

Diagnosis and Treatment

Babinski's reflex — A spreading of the outer toes and extension of the big toe over the others when the sole of the foot is stroked. This response is normal in infants but indicates a lesion of specific motor tracts in adults.

evoked potentials — Record of the electrical activity of the brain following sensory stimulation. Included are visual evoked potentials (VEP), brainstem auditory evoked potentials (BAEP), and somatosensory evoked potentials (SEP), obtained by stimulating the hand or leg. These tests are used to evaluate CNS function.

Romberg's sign — Inability to maintain balance when the eyes are shut and the feet are close together

sympathectomy *(sim-pa-THEK-tō-mē)* — Interruption of transmission by sympathetic nerves either surgically or chemically

trephination *(tref-i-NĀ-shun)* — Cutting a piece of bone out of the skull. The instrument used is a trepan (tre-PAN) or trephine (tre-FĪN).

Also used are EEG, cerebral angiography, CT scan, brain scan (scintiscan), ultrasonography, and MRI.

ABBREVIATIONS

ACh acetylcholine
ALS amyotrophic lateral sclerosis
ANS autonomic nervous system
BAEP brainstem auditory evoked potentials
CBF cerebral blood flow
CNS central nervous system
CSF cerebrospinal fluid
CVA cerebrovascular accident
CVD cerebrovascular disease
DTR deep tendon reflexes
EEG electroencephalogram; electroencephalograph
ICP intracranial pressure
LMN lower motor neuron
LOC level of consciousness
LP lumbar puncture
MS multiple sclerosis
NPH normal-pressure hydrocephalus
NREM non-rapid eye movement (stage of sleep)
PNS peripheral nervous system
RAS reticular activating system
REM rapid eye movement (stage of sleep)
SEP somatosensory evoked potentials
TIA transient ischemic attack
UMN upper motor neuron
VEP visual evoked potentials

Chapter 17
Labeling Exercise

Write the name of each numbered part on the corresponding line of the answer sheet.

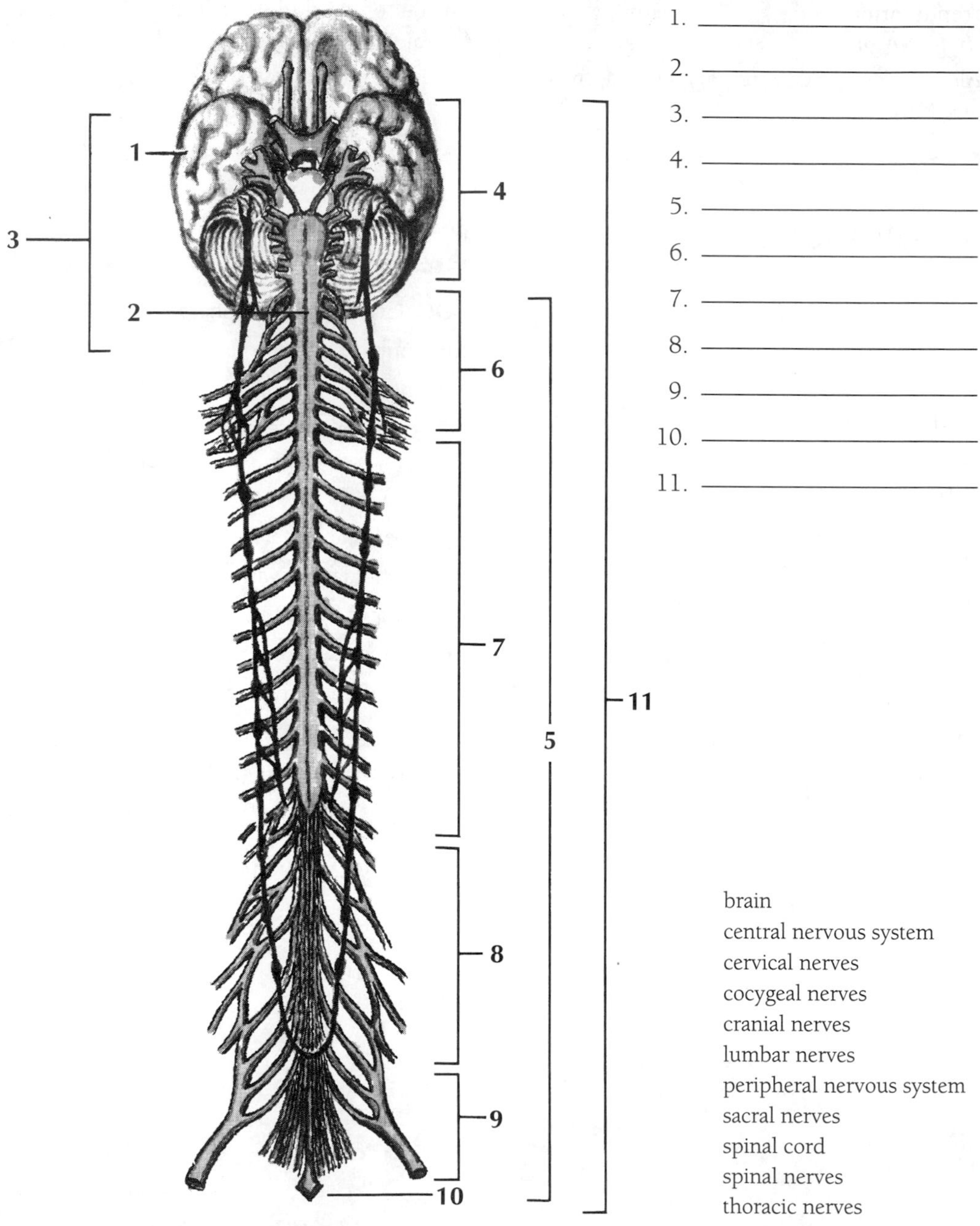

1. ____________
2. ____________
3. ____________
4. ____________
5. ____________
6. ____________
7. ____________
8. ____________
9. ____________
10. ____________
11. ____________

brain
central nervous system
cervical nerves
cocygeal nerves
cranial nerves
lumbar nerves
peripheral nervous system
sacral nerves
spinal cord
spinal nerves
thoracic nerves

Anatomic divisions of the nervous system

Write the name of each numbered part on the corresponding line of the answer sheet.

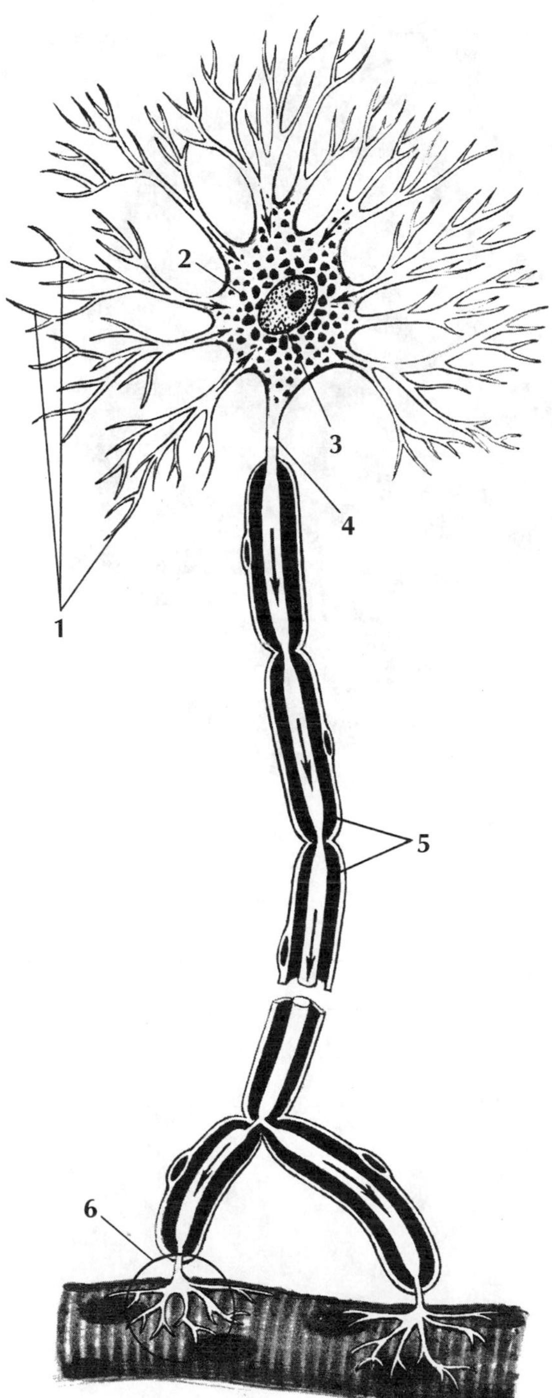

Motor neuron

axon
cell body
dendrites
myelin
neuromuscular junction
nucleus

1. ______________________
2. ______________________
3. ______________________
4. ______________________
5. ______________________
6. ______________________

Write the name of each numbered part on the corresponding line of the answer sheet.

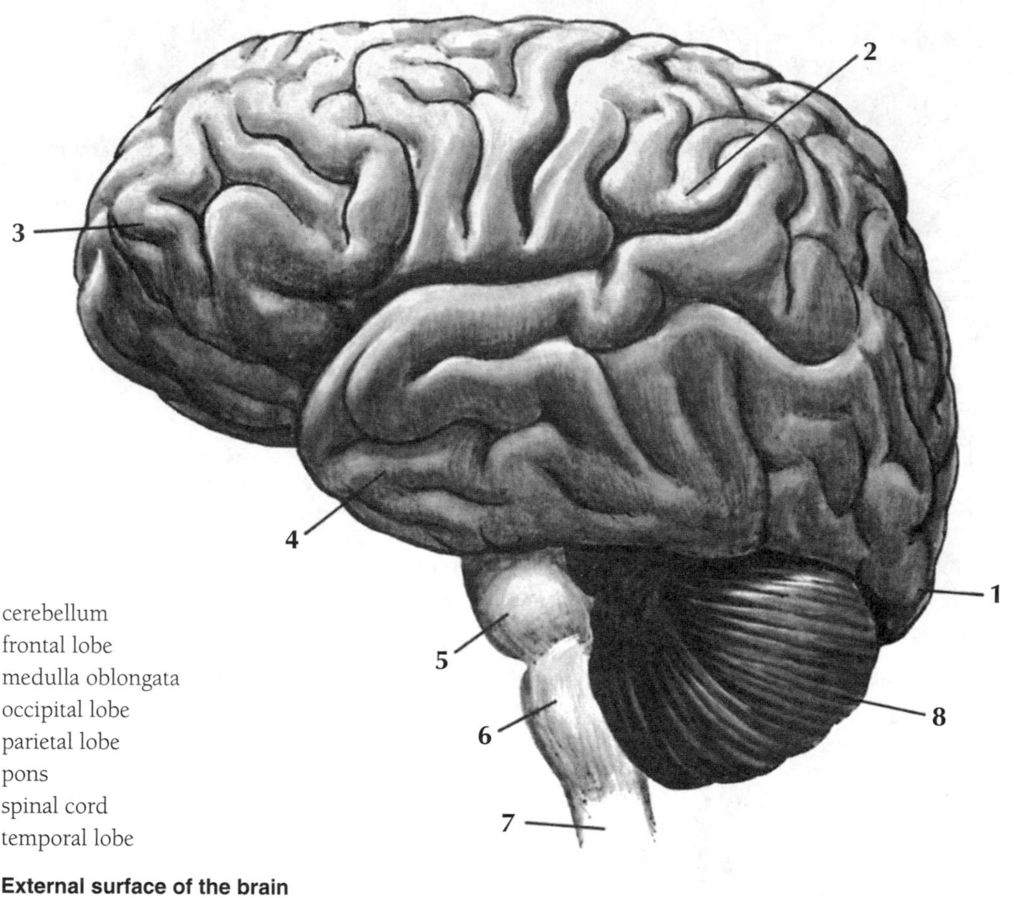

cerebellum
frontal lobe
medulla oblongata
occipital lobe
parietal lobe
pons
spinal cord
temporal lobe

External surface of the brain

1. ______________________
2. ______________________
3. ______________________
4. ______________________
5. ______________________
6. ______________________
7. ______________________
8. ______________________

Write the name of each numbered part of the spinal cord and reflex arc on the corresponding line of the answer sheet.

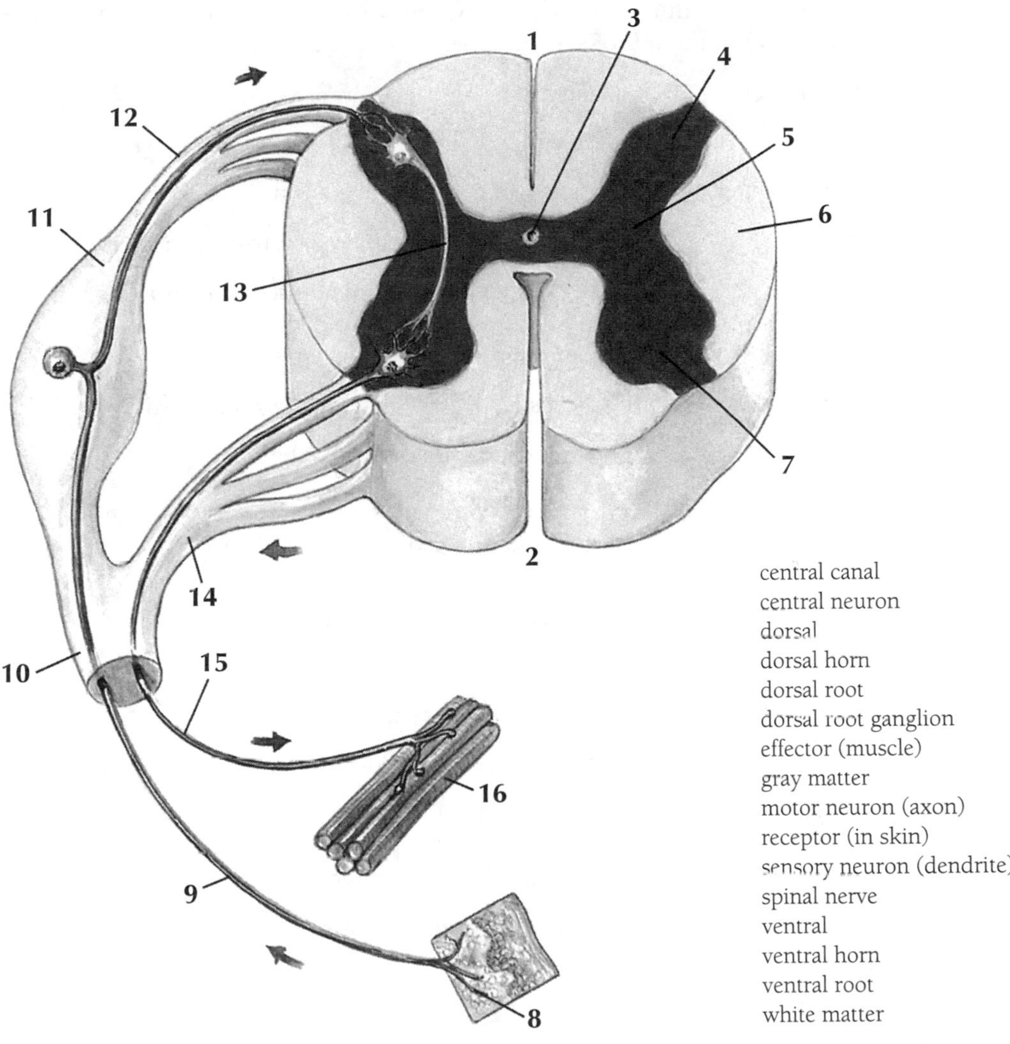

Cross section of spinal cord showing reflex pathway

1. ______________________
2. ______________________
3. ______________________
4. ______________________
5. ______________________
6. ______________________
7. ______________________
8. ______________________
9. ______________________
10. ______________________
11. ______________________
12. ______________________
13. ______________________
14. ______________________
15. ______________________
16. ______________________

CHAPTER REVIEW 17-1

Matching. Match the terms in each of the sets below with their definitions and write the appropriate letter (a–e) to the left of each number:

_____ 1. ganglion	a. fatty material that covers some nerve fibers
_____ 2. tract	b. collection of nerve cell bodies along a nerve
_____ 3. neurotransmitter	c. bundle of nerve cell fibers within the CNS
_____ 4. myelin	d. chemical that carries energy across a synapse
_____ 5. axon	e. nerve fiber that carries impulses away from the cell body

_____ 6. circle of Willis	a. neurotransmitter
_____ 7. Babinski's reflex	b. extension of gray matter in the spinal cord
_____ 8. epinephrine	c. union of arteries leading to the brain
_____ 9. horn	d. diagnostic sign
_____ 10. Broca's area	e. region of the cerebrum that controls speech

_____ 11. euphoria	a. trigeminal neuralgia
_____ 12. odynophobia	b. elation, exaggerated well-being
_____ 13. hydrocephalus	c. abnormal fear of pain
_____ 14. tic douloureux	d. injury caused by a violent blow
_____ 15. concussion	e. excess fluid in the brain

_____ 16. ACh	a. fluid that circulates in the central nervous system
_____ 17. CVA	b. degenerative nerve disease of unknown cause
_____ 18. MS	c. stroke
_____ 19. EEG	d. neurotransmitter
_____ 20. CSF	e. study of brain waves

Fill in the blanks:

21. The brain and spinal cord together make up the _______________.
22. The scientific name for a nerve cell is _______________.
23. The junction between two nerve cells is a(n) _______________.
24. A simple, rapid, automatic response to a stimulus is a(n) _______________.
25. The membranes that cover the brain and spinal cord are the _______________.
26. A psychotropic (*sī-kō-TROP-ik*) drug is one that acts on the _______________.
27. Somnolence (*SOM-nō-lens*) is _______________.

Definitions. Write the meaning of each of the following terms:

28. anencephaly *(an-en-SEF-a-lē)* ______
29. encephalomyelitis *(en-sef-a-lō-mī-e-LĪ-tis)* ______
30. meningocele *(men-IN-gō-sēl)* ______
31. polyneuritis *(pol-ē-nū-RĪ-tis)* ______
32. panplegia *(pan-PLĒ-jē-a)* ______
33. radicular *(ra-DIK-ū-lar)* ______

Word building. Write a word for each of the following definitions:

34. Study of the nervous system ______
35. A tumor of a nerve ______
36. Excision of a ganglion ______
37. Inflammation of a spinal nerve root ______
38. Paralysis of one side of the body ______
39. Within (intra-) the cerebellum ______
40. Difficulty in reading ______

Opposites. Write a word that means the opposite of each of the following:

41. intramedullary ______
42. ipsilateral ______
43. preganglionic ______
44. tachylalia ______
45. sensory ______
46. dorsal ______

Plurals. Write the plural form of each of the following terms:

47. ganglion ______
48. ventricle ______
49. meninx ______
50. sulcus ______

Word analysis. Define each of the following words and give the meaning of the word parts in each. Use a dictionary if necessary.

51. Poliomyelitis *(pō-lē-ō-mī-e-LĪ-tis)* ______

______

a. polio ___gray___
b. myel/o ______
c. -itis ______

52. Dysmetria (*dis-MĒ-trē-a*) ______________________________

____

a. dys- ______________

b. metr/o ______________

c. -ia ______________

53. Polyneuroradiculitis ______________________________

____

a. poly- ______________

b. neur/o ______________

c. radicul/o ______________

d. -itis ______________

CHAPTER REVIEW 17-2

Matching. Match the terms in each of the sets below with their definitions and write the appropriate letter (a–e) to the left of each number:

_____ 1. pons — a. ventral bulge on the brain stem
_____ 2. gyrus — b. connects the brain and spinal cord
_____ 3. cerebrum — c. largest part of the brain
_____ 4. cortex — d. raised area on the surface of the brain
_____ 5. medulla oblongata — e. outer layer of the cerebrum

_____ 6. myelodysplasia — a. inflammation of the pia mater and arachnoid
_____ 7. meningomyelocele — b. development of fluid-filled spaces in the spinal cord
_____ 8. meningorrhagia — c. abnormal development of the spinal cord
_____ 9. leptomeningitis — d. hemorrhage of the meninges
_____ 10. syringomyelia — e. hernia of the meninges and spinal cord

_____ 11. astrocytoma — a. unresponsive state
_____ 12. catatonia — b. partial paralysis of a muscle
_____ 13. myoparesis — c. disorder of the basal ganglia
_____ 14. herpes zoster — d. neuroglial tumor
_____ 15. Parkinson's disease — e. shingles

_____ 16. hypersomnolent — a. paralysis of the bladder
_____ 17. aphasia — b. paralysis that originates in the spinal cord
_____ 18. cystoplegia — c. obsession with a single idea

_____ 19. monomania d. excessively sleepy

_____ 20. myeloplegia e. loss of speech communication

Fill in the blanks:

21. The connective tissue cells of the nervous system are called ____________________.
22. The nerve tissue outside the central nervous system makes up the ____________________.
23. The sympathetic and parasympathetic systems make up the ____________________.
24. The posterior portion of the brain that coordinates muscle movement is the ____________________.
25. The term *epidural* means above the layer of the meninges named the ____________________.
26. Atelencephalia *(a-tel-en-se-FĀ-lē-a)* is incomplete *(atel/o)* development of the ____________________.
27. A neurotoxin *(nū-rō-TOK-sin)* is harmful or poisonous to the ____________________.

Definitions. Write the meaning of each of the following terms:

28. meningoencephalitis *(me-ning-gō-en-sef-a-LĪ-tis)* ____________________
29. corticothalamic *(kor-ti-kō-tha-LAM-ik)* ____________________
30. narcotic *(nar-KOT-ik)* ____________________
31. hemiparesis *(hem-i-pa-RĒ-sis)* ____________________

Word building. Write a word for each of the following definitions:

32. Any disease of the nervous system ____________________
33. A tumor of neuroglial cells ____________________
34. Inflammation of the spinal cord and meninges ____________________
35. Pain in a nerve ____________________
36. Surgical excision of a spinal nerve root ____________________
37. Incision into the brain ____________________
38. Hardening of the brain ____________________
39. Surgical creation of an opening in a brain ventricle ____________________
40. Within (intra-) a ventricle ____________________
41. Total (pan-) paralysis ____________________
42. Fear of water ____________________

Adjectives. Write the adjective form of each of the following words:

43. ganglion ____________________
44. cortex ____________________
45. dura ____________________

46. meninges ______________________

47. psychosis ______________________

Word analysis. Define each of the following words and give the meaning of the word parts in each. Use a dictionary if necessary.

48. Pachymeningitis *(pak-ē-men-in-JĪ-tis)* ______________________

____

a. pachy ______________

b. mening/o ______________

c. -itis ______________

49. Dyssynergia (dis-sin-ER-jē-a) ______________________

____

a. dys- ______________

b. syn- ______________

c. erg ______________

d. -ia ______________

Chapter 17

Case Studies

1. Cerebrovascular Accident (CVA)

This 62-year-old male was admitted with right hemiplegia and aphasia due to a CVA on 21 September. The patient has a history of hypertension, but was in good health and active when he experienced the sudden onset of right-sided weakness. He was awake in the ER but was aphasic with right hemiparesis and BP of 220/120. Subsequent CT scan of the brain showed a left frontotemporal infarct.

The patient was evaluated by Physical Medicine and Rehabilitation for the development of a comprehensive recovery program. He will have speech therapy on an outpatient basis; he will have PT, OT and a home health aide 2× per week for the next 6 weeks. He also has instructions for a home exercise program.

2. Epilepsy

This 70-year-old white male was seen following a generalized seizure during which he felt sleepy, began to shake, turned blue in the lips, and began to foam from the mouth. Postictally, he was disoriented, confused, and tired. A similar incident apparently had occurred 1 year previously.

The patient was a nonsmoker, nondiabetic, normotensive, and nonalcoholic. He suffered a head injury 10 years ago, but showed no seizure activity at that time. Neurologic examination showed the patient to be fully oriented with normal speech but poor memory. He forgot two objects out of three. He could not do serial sevens. He could subtract 7 from 10 correctly. He could obey one and two step commands. He could name objects correctly. He could not spell a five-digit word correctly backwards. Sensory examination showed some hypalgesia in all four limbs and loss of vibratory sensation in the toes. Reflexes are absent in the lower extremities.

The patient is diagnosed as having recurrent generalized tonic-clonic seizures. He has mild dementia and polyneuropathy of unknown etiology. Dilantin is recommended. A loading dose of 1 g and then 350 to 400 mg per day.

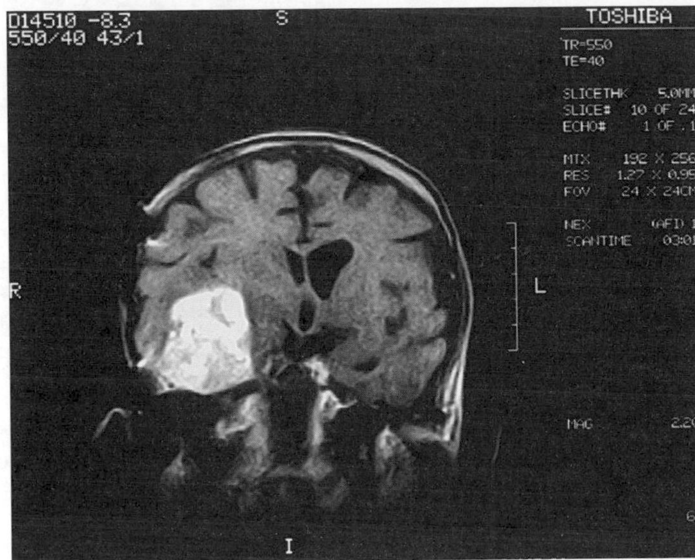

FIGURE 17-10. MRI scan showing tumor in right inferior temporal lobe.

3. Temporal Lobe Glioblastoma with Cyst

This patient was a 42-year-old female seen in October 1997 for symptoms of left hemiparesis, headache, lethargy, confusion, and decreased visual function in the left visual field. MRI scan revealed a large (7 cm × 4 cm) tumor in the right inferior temporal lobe (Fig. 17-10). The tumor enhanced irregularly and there was evidence of a moderately large cyst. This tumor was located at a site where a grade 1–2 glioma measuring 5 cm × 4 cm had been removed 10 years before this consultation. Follow-up studies since that initial surgery had shown no evidence of recurrence.

The patient underwent surgery in which a significant bulk of the tumor was resected and the cyst was partially removed. The tumor had progressed in malignancy and the diagnosis was now grade 4 glioma (also called glioblastoma multiforme). Postoperatively, the cyst reformed and became a chronic problem. A shunt inserted for drainage of the cyst continually became plugged with heavy proteinaceous tumor fluid, requiring further surgery. In November she underwent exploration of the craniotomy site. Tissue was removed from the wall of the capsule and the catheter was realigned. Following this, the cyst had an excellent appearance. The area was well decompressed, the midline shift was relieved, and the patient seemed to be improving with physical therapy.

Symptoms returned in early December. CT scan showed evidence of massive tumor regrowth. It was apparent that the tumor had enlarged substantially and again filled the right temporal lobe. Further treatment was unlikely to be of any lasting benefit. The patient died about 6 weeks later.

Chapter 17
Case Study Questions

Multiple choice. Select the best answer and write the letter of your choice to the left of each number:

_____ 1. The term *postictally* means

a. following a meal
b. before a seizure
c. before a meal
d. following examination
e. following an attack

_____ 2. In case study 3, when the tumor was resected it was

a. drained
b. examined by x-ray
c. compressed
d. surgically removed
e. examined by CT

_____ 3. The term *normotensive* refers to

a. normal muscle tone
b. normal blood pressure
c. chronic illness
d. normal mental state
e. abnormal reflexes

Write the meaning of the following abbreviations:

4. CVA _____
5. CT _____
6. PT _____
7. OT _____
8. MRI _____

Write a word from the case histories that means each of the following:

9. High blood pressure _____
10. Loss of speech communication _____
11. Weakness of one side of the body _____
12. Localized death of tissue caused by lack of blood supply _____
13. Decreased sensitivity to pain _____
14. Loss of intellectual function _____
15. Disorder involving several nerves _____

Define the following words:

16. Hemiplegia _____
17. Glioma _____
18. Cyst _____
19. Craniotomy _____

NERVOUS SYSTEM

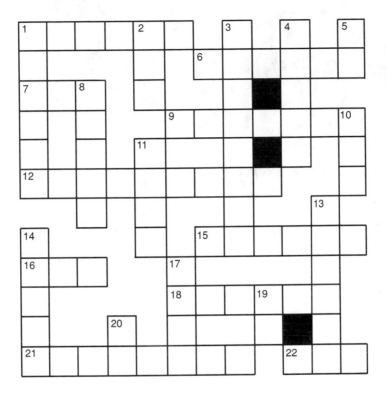

ACROSS

1. root for the membranes that cover the brain and spinal cord
6. a nerve cell
7. study of the electrical activity of the brain (abbr.)
9. root for the part of a spinal nerve that joins the cord
12. the connective tissue cells of the nervous system
15. root for the part of the brain that connects to the spinal cord, also for the cord itself
16. the involuntary nervous system (abbr.)
18. a simple, rapid, and automatic response to a stimulus
21. a localized abnormal dilation of a blood vessel
22. the fluid that circulates in and around the brain and spinal cord (abbr.)

DOWN

1. the whitish, fatty substance that surrounds certain axons
2. term describing hydrocephalus (abbr.)
3. the fiber of a neuron that conducts impulses toward the cell body
4. a bundle of neuron fibers within the central nervous system
5. prefix: not, without, lack of
8. a raised convolution on the surface of the cerebrum
10. describing the location of a motor neuron (abbr.)
11. part of the brain stem
13. a network, as of nerves or blood vessels
14. excited, state, obsession
17. unmyelinated tissue of the nervous system: ______ matter
19. procedure for removing spinal fluid (abbr.)
20. prefix: true, good, easy, normal

Chapter 17
Answer Section

Answers to Chapter Exercises

Exercise 17-1

1. pertaining to a nerve or nerves
2. pertaining to neuroglia
3. pertaining to a ganglion
4. pertaining to the meninges
5. pertaining to a spinal nerve root
6. spinal cord
7. meninges
8. spinal nerve roots
9. pain in a nerve
10. inflammation of the spinal cord and spinal nerve roots
11. tumor of the meninges
12. neurology *(nū-ROL-ō-jē)*
13. neuropathy *(nū-ROP-a-thē)*
14. ganglioma *(gang-glē-Ō-ma)*
15. myelography *(mī-e-LOG-ra-fē)*
16. meningitis *(men-in-JĪ-tis)*

Exercise 17-2

1. brain
2. cerebrum, brain
3. mind
4. stupor, unconsciousness
5. sleep
6. cerebral *(se-RĒ-bral)*
7. cortical *(KOR-ti-kal)*
8. thalamic *(tha-LAM-ik)*
9. cerebellar *(ser-e-BEL-ar)*
10. ventricular *(ven-TRIK-u-lar)*
11. inflammation of the brain
12. pertaining to the medulla
13. study of the mind
14. lack of sleep, inability to sleep
15. encephalopathy *(en-sef-a-LOP-a-thē)*
16. intracerebral *(in-tra-se-RĒ-bral)*
17. corticothalamic *(kor-ti-kō-tha-LAM-ik)*
18. ventriculitis *(ven-trik-ū-LĪ-tis)*
19. cerebrospinal

Exercise 17-3

1. speech communication
2. seizures
3. partial paralysis
4. read
5. slowness of speech
6. obsession with fire
7. fear of women
8. bradylexia *(brad-ē-LEK-sē-a)*
9. hemiplegia *(hem-i-PLĒ-jē-a)*
10. monoplegia *(mon-ō-PLĒ-jē-a)*
11. noctiphobia *(nok-ti-FŌ-bē-a)*; also nyctophobia *(nik-tō-FŌ-bē-a)*
12. photophobia *(fō-tō-FŌ-bē-a)*

Labeling Exercise

Anatomic Divisions of the Nervous System

1. brain
2. spinal cord
3. central nervous system
4. cranial nerves
5. spinal nerves
6. cervical (nerves)
7. thoracic (nerves)
8. lumbar (nerves)
9. sacral (nerves)
10. coccygeal (nerve)
11. peripheral nervous system

Motor Neuron

1. dendrites
2. cell body
3. nucleus
4. axon
5. myelin
6. neuromuscular junction

External Surface of the Brain

1. occipital lobe
2. parietal lobe
3. frontal lobe
4. temporal lobe
5. pons
6. medulla oblongata
7. spinal cord
8. cerebellum

Cross Section of Spinal Cord Showing Reflex Pathway

1. dorsal
2. ventral
3. central canal
4. dorsal horn
5. gray matter
6. white matter
7. ventral horn
8. receptor (in skin)
9. sensory neuron (dendrite)
10. spinal nerve
11. dorsal root ganglion
12. dorsal root
13. central neuron
14. ventral root
15. motor neuron (axon)
16. effector (muscle)

Chapter Review 17-1

1. b
2. c
3. d
4. a
5. e
6. c
7. d
8. a
9. b
10. e
11. b
12. c
13. e
14. a
15. d
16. d
17. c
18. b
19. e
20. a
21. central nervous system
22. neuron
23. synapse
24. reflex
25. meninges
26. mind
27. sleepiness
28. absence of a brain
29. inflammation of the brain and spinal cord
30. hernia of the meninges
31. inflammation of many nerves
32. total paralysis
33. pertaining to a spinal nerve root
34. neurology

35. neuroma
36. ganglionectomy
37. radiculitis
38. hemiplegia
39. intracerebellar
40. dyslexia
41. extramedullary
42. contralateral
43. postganglionic
44. bradylalia
45. motor
46. ventral
47. ganglia
48. ventricles
49. meninges
50. sulci
51. An acute viral disease causing inflammation of the gray matter of the spinal cord
    a. gray
    b. spinal cord
    c. inflammation
52. Disturbance in the path or placement of a limb during active movement
    a. difficult
    b. measure
    c. condition of
53. Inflammation of many nerves, nerve roots, and spinal ganglia
    a. many
    b. nerve
    c. spinal nerve root
    d. inflammation

Chapter Review 17-2

1. a
2. d
3. c
4. e
5. b
6. c
7. e
8. d
9. a
10. b
11. d
12. a
13. b
14. e
15. c
16. d
17. e
18. a
19. c
20. b
21. neurologia
22. peripheral nervous system
23. autonomic nervous system
24. cerebellum
25. dura mater
26. brain
27. nervous system
28. inflammation of the meninges and brain
29. pertaining to the cerebral cortex and the thalamus
30. inducing stupor or unconsciousness
31. partial paralysis of one side of the body
32. neuropathy
33. glioma
34. myelomeningitis
35. neuralgia
36. radiculectomy
37. encephalotomy; cerebrotomy
38. encephalosclerosis
39. ventriculostomy
40. intraventricular
41. panplegia
42. hydrophobia
43. ganglionic
44. cortical
45. dural
46. meningeal
47. psychotic
48. Inflammation of the dura mater
    a. thick, heavy
    b. meninges
    c. inflammation of
49. Disturbance of muscle coordination
    a. abnormal, difficult
    b. together
    c. work
    d. condition of

Answers to Case Study Questions

1. e
2. d
3. b
4. cerebrovascular accident
5. computed tomography
6. physical therapy

7. occupational therapy
8. magnetic resonance imaging
9. hypertension
10. aphasia
11. hemiparesis
12. infarct
13. hypalgesia
14. dementia
15. polyneuropathy
16. paralysis of one side of the body
17. tumor of neuroglial cells
18. filled sac or pouch
19. incision into the cranium

Answers to Crossword Puzzle

NERVOUS SYSTEM

1 M	E	N	I	2 N	G		3 D		4 T		5 A
Y				P		6 N	E	U	R	O	N
7 E	E	8 G		H			N	■	A		
L		Y			9 R	A	D	I	C	U	10 L
I		R		11 P			R	■	T		M
12 N	E	U	R	O	G	L	I	A			N
		S		N			T			13 P	
14 M				S		15 M	E	D	U	L	L
16 A	N	S			17 G					E	
N					18 R	E	F	19 L	E	X	
I			20 E		A			P	■	U	
21 A	N	E	U	R	Y	S	M		22 C	S	F

18 The Senses

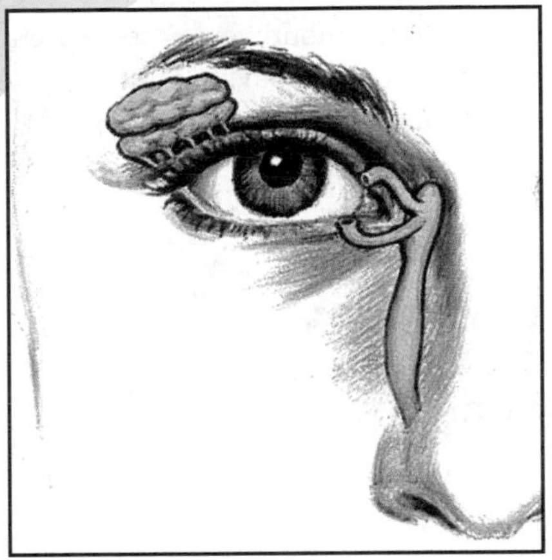

Chapter Contents

Objectives

After study of this chapter you should be able to:

1. Explain the role of the sensory system
2. Label diagrams of the ear and the eye and briefly describe the function of each part
3. Describe the pathway of nerve impulses from the ear to the brain
4. Describe the roles of the retina and the optic nerve in vision
5. Identify and use word parts pertaining to the senses
6. Describe the main disorders pertaining to the ear and the eye
7. Interpret abbreviations used in the study of the ear and the eye
8. Analyze several case studies pertaining to vision or hearing

The sensory system is our network for detecting stimuli from the internal and external environments. It is needed to maintain homeostasis, provide us with pleasure, and protect us from harm. Pain, for example, is an important warning sign of tissue damage. The energy generated in the various **receptors** of the sensory system must be transmitted to the CNS for interpretation.

The general senses are widely distributed throughout the body. These include pain, touch, pressure, temperature, and **proprioception**, the awareness of body position. The special senses are localized within complex sense organs. These include the chemical senses of taste and smell, located in the mouth and nose respectively; the senses of hearing and equilibrium, located in the ear; and the sense of vision in the eye. After a brief introduction, this chapter will concentrate on the ear and the eye.

KEY TERMS

Senses

Term	Definition
gustation *(gus-TĀ-shun)*	The sense of taste
olfaction *(ol-FAK-shun)*	The sense of smell
proprioception *(prō-prē-ō-SEP-shun)*	The awareness of posture, movement, and changes in equilibrium. Receptors are located in muscles, tendons, and joints.
receptor *(rē-SEP-tor)*	A sensory nerve ending or a specialized structure associated with a sensory nerve that responds to a stimulus
tactile *(TAK-til)*	Pertaining to the sense of touch

Suffixes Pertaining to the Senses

Suffix	Meaning	Example	Definition of Example
-esthesia	sensation	cryesthesia *krī-es-THĒ-zē-a*	sensitivity to cold
-algesia	pain	hypalgesia* *hī-pal-JĒ-zē-a*	decreased sensitivity to pain
-osmia	sense of smell	parosmia *par-OS-mē-a*	abnormal (para-) sense of smell
-geusia	sense of taste	pseudogeusia *sū-dō-GŪ-zē-a*	false sense of taste

*prefix hyp/o.

Exercise 18-1

Define the following terms:

1. Hyperesthesia *(hī-per-es-thē-zē-a)* ______________________________

2. Pseudosmia *(sū-DOZ-mē-a)* ______________________________

3. Ageusia *(a-GŪ-zē-a)* ______________________________

Write a word to fit each of the following definitions:

4. Lack (an-) of sensation ______________________________

5. Sensitivity to temperature ______________________________

6. Excess sensitivity to pain ______________________________

7. Abnormal (dys-) sense of taste ______________________________

The Ear

The ear is the receptor for both hearing and equilibrium. For study purposes, it may be divided into three parts: the outer, middle, and inner ear (Fig. 18-1).

The outer ear consists of the projecting **pinna** and the **external auditory canal (meatus)**. This canal ends at the **tympanic membrane** or eardrum, which transmits sound waves to the middle ear.

Spanning the middle ear cavity are three **ossicles** (small bones) each named for its shape: the **malleus** (hammer), **incus** (anvil), and **stapes** (stirrup). Sound waves traveling over the ossicles are transmitted from the footplate of the stapes to the inner ear. The **eustachian tube** connects the middle ear with the nasopharynx and serves to equalize pressure between the outer and middle ear.

The inner ear, because of its complex shape, is described as a *labyrinth*. It consists of an outer bony framework containing a similarly-shaped membranous channel. The entire labyrinth is filled with fluid. The **cochlea**, shaped like the shell of a snail, has the specialized **organ of Corti** concerned with hearing. Cells in this receptor respond to sound waves traveling through the fluid-filled ducts of the cochlea.

The sense of equilibrium is localized in the **vestibular apparatus**. This consists of the chamberlike **vestibule** and three projecting **semicircular canals**. Special cells within these structures respond to movement. (The senses of vision and proprioception are also important in maintaining balance.)

Nerve impulses are transmitted from the ear to the brain by way of the **vestibulocochlear nerve**, the 8th cranial nerve, also called the acoustic or auditory nerve. The cochlear branch of this nerve transmits impulses for hearing from the cochlea; the vestibular branch transmits impulses concerned with equilibrium from the vestibular apparatus.

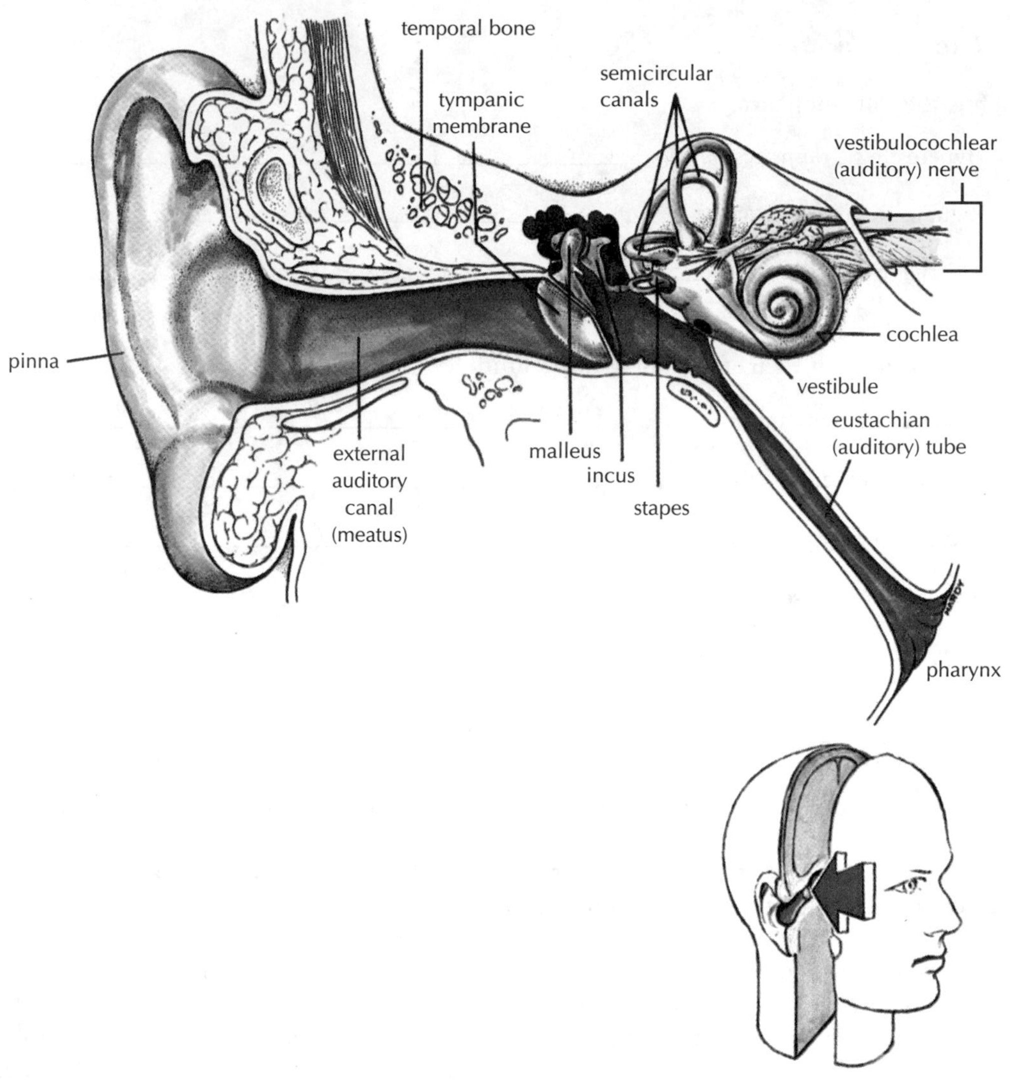

FIGURE 18-1. The ear, showing the outer, middle, and inner subdivisions. (Chaffee EE, Lytle IM: Basic Physiology and Anatomy, 4th ed, p 277. Philadelphia, JB Lippincott, 1980.)

KEY TERMS

Normal Structure and Function

cochlea (*KOK-lē-a*) — The coiled portion of the inner ear that contains the receptors for hearing (root cochle/o)

eustachian tube (*ū-STĀ-shen*) — The tube that connects the middle ear with the nasopharynx and serves to equalize pressure between the outer and middle ear (root salping/o)

ossicles
(OS-i-klz)
The small bones of the middle ear. They are the malleus *(MAL-ē-us)*, incus *(ING-kus)*, and stapes *(STA-pēz)*.

organ of Corti
(KOR-tē)
The hearing receptor located in the cochlea

pinna
(PIN-a)
The projecting part of the outer ear

stapes
(STĀ-pēz)
The ossicle that is in contact with the inner ear (root staped, stapedi/o)

tympanic membrane
(tim-PAN-ik)
The membrane between the external auditory canal and the middle ear (tympanic cavity); the eardrum. It serves to transmit sound waves to the ossicles of the middle ear. (root myring/o, tympan/o)

vestibular apparatus
(ves-TIB-ū-lar)
The portion of the inner ear that is concerned with the sense of equilibrium. It consists of the vestibule and the semicircular canals. (root vestibul/o)

Roots Pertaining to the Ear and Hearing

Root	Meaning	Example	Definition of Example
audi/o	hearing	audition *aw-DISH-un*	act of hearing
acous, acus, cus	sound, hearing	acoustic *a-KŪ-stik*	pertaining to sound or hearing
ot/o	ear	otogenic *ō-tō-JEN-ik*	originating in the ear
myring/o	tympanic membrane	myringotome *mi-RING-gō-tōm*	knife used for surgery on the eardrum
tympan/o	tympanic cavity (middle ear), tympanic membrane	tympanometry *tim-pa-NOM-e-trē*	transmission through the tympanic membrane and middle ear
salping/o	tube, eustachian tube	salpingoscope *sal-PING-gō-skōp*	instrument for examining the eustachian tube
staped/o, stapedi/o	stapes	stapedoplasty *stā-pē-dō-PLAS-tē*	plastic repair of the stapes
labyrinth/o	labyrinth (inner ear)	labyrinthotomy *lab-i-rin-THOT-ō-mē*	incision of the labyrinth
vestibul/o	vestibule, vestibular apparatus	vestibulopathy *ves-tib-ū-LOP-a-thē*	any disease of the vestibule of the inner ear
cochle/o	cochlea of inner ear	retrocochlear *ret-rō-KOK-lē-ar*	behind the cochlea

Exercise 18-2

Fill in the blanks:

1. Hyperacusis (*hī-per-a-KŪ-sis*) is abnormally high sensitivity to ______________.
2. Ototoxic (*ō-tō-TOK-sik*) means poisonous or harmful to the ______________.

Define the following adjectives:

3. Cochlear (*KOK-lē-ar*) ______________
4. Vestibular (*ves-TIB-ū-lar*) ______________
5. Labyrinthine (*lab-i-RIN-thēn*) ______________
6. Stapedial (*stā-PĒ-dē-al*) ______________
7. Auditory (*AW-di-tor-ē*) ______________
8. Otic (*Ō-tik*) ______________

Build words for the following definitions:

9. An instrument for measuring hearing (audi/o-) ______________
10. Pain in the ear ______________
11. Plastic repair of the middle ear ______________
12. Incision of the tympanic membrane ______________
13. Excision of the stapes ______________
14. Pertaining to the vestibular apparatus and cochlea ______________
15. Inflammation of the labyrinth ______________
16. Examination of the eustachian tube ______________

Define the following terms:

17. Audiologist (*aw-dē-OL-ō-jist*) ______________
18. Otitis (*ō-TĪ-tis*) ______________
19. Myringoscope (*mi-RING-gō-skōp*) ______________
20. Salpingopharyngeal (*sal-ping-gō-fa-RIN-jē-al*) ______________
21. Vestibulotomy (*ves-tib-ū-LOT-ō-mē*) ______________

Clinical Aspects of the Ear and Hearing

Hearing Loss

Hearing impairment may result from disease, injury, or developmental problems that affect the ear itself or any nervous pathways concerned with the sense of hearing. **Sensorineural hearing loss** results from damage to the eighth cranial nerve or to central auditory pathways. Heredity, toxins, exposure to loud noises, and the aging process are possible causes for this type of hearing loss. It may range from inability to hear certain frequencies of sound to a complete loss of hearing (deafness). **Conductive hearing loss** results from blockage in sound transmission to the inner ear. Causes include obstruction, severe infection, or fixation of the middle ear ossicles. Often the conditions that cause conductive hearing loss can be treated successfully.

Otitis Media

Otitis is any inflammation of the ear. **Otitis media** refers to an infection that leads to the accumulation of fluid in the middle ear cavity. One cause is malfunction or obstruction of the eustachian tube, such as by allergy, enlarged adenoids, injury, or congenital abnormalities. Another cause is infection that spreads to the middle ear, most commonly from the upper respiratory tract. Continued infection may lead to accumulation of pus and perforation of the eardrum. Otitis media usually affects children under 5 years of age and may result in hearing loss. If untreated, the infection may spread to other regions of the ear and head. Treatment is with antibiotics. A tube also may be placed in the tympanic membrane to ventilate the middle ear cavity, a procedure called a **myringotomy**.

Otosclerosis

In **otosclerosis** the bony structure of the inner ear deteriorates then reforms into spongy bone tissue that may eventually harden. Most commonly, the stapes becomes fixed against the inner ear and is unable to vibrate, resulting in conductive hearing loss. The cause is unknown, but some cases are hereditary. The damaged bone can usually be removed surgically. In a **stapedectomy** the stapes is removed and a prosthetic bone is inserted.

Meniere's Disease

Meniere's disease is a disorder that affects the inner ear. It appears to involve the production and circulation of the fluid that fills the inner ear, but the cause is unknown. The symptoms are **vertigo** (dizziness), hearing loss, pronounced **tinnitus** (ringing in the ears), and feeling of pressure in the ear. The course of the disease is uneven, and symptoms may become less severe with time. Meniere's disease is treated with drugs to control nausea and dizziness, such as those used to treat motion sickness. In severe cases, the inner ear or part of the eighth cranial nerve may be destroyed surgically.

Acoustic Neuroma

An **acoustic neuroma** (also called a schwannoma or neurilemoma) is a tumor that arises from the neurilemma (sheath) of the eighth cranial nerve. As the tumor enlarges, it presses on surrounding nerves and interferes with blood supply. This leads to tinnitus, dizziness, and progressive hearing loss. Other symptoms develop as the tumor presses on the brain stem and other cranial nerves. Usually it is necessary to remove the tumor surgically.

KEY CLINICAL TERMS

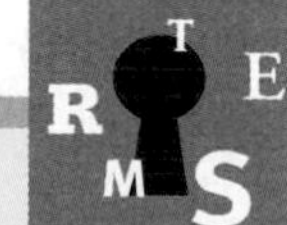

Disorders

acoustic neuroma *(a-KŪ-stik)* — A tumor of the eighth cranial nerve sheath. Although benign, it can press on surrounding tissue and produce symptoms.

conductive hearing loss — Hearing impairment that results from blockage of sound transmission to the inner ear

(continued)

Meniere's disease *(men-ē-ARZ)* — A disease of the inner ear of unknown cause characterized by hearing loss, vertigo, and tinnitus

otitis media *(ō-TĪ-tis MĒ-dē-a)* — Inflammation of the middle ear with accumulation of watery (serous) or mucoid fluid

otosclerosis *(ō-tō-skle-RŌ-sis)* — Formation of abnormal and sometimes hardened bony tissue in the ear. It usually occurs around the oval window and the footplate (base) of the stapes causing immobilization of the stapes and progressive loss of hearing.

sensorineural hearing loss — Hearing impairment that results from damage to the eighth cranial nerve or to auditory pathways in the brain

tinnitus *(tin-Ī-tus)* — A sensation of noises, such as ringing or tinkling, in the ear

vertigo *(VER-ti-gō)* — An illusion of movement, as of the body moving in space or the environment moving about the body. Usually caused by disturbances in the vestibular apparatus. Loosely used to mean dizziness or lightheadedness.

Treatment

myringotomy *(mir-in-GOT-ō-mē)* — Surgical incision of the tympanic membrane. It is done to drain the middle ear cavity or to insert a tube into the tympanic membrane for drainage.

otorhinolaryngology (ORL) *(ō-tō-rī-nō-lar-in-GOL-ō-jē)* — The branch of medicine that deals with diseases of the ear(s), nose, and throat (ENT)

stapedectomy *(stā-pē-DEK-tō-mē)* — Surgical removal of the stapes. It may be done to treat otosclerosis with insertion of a prosthesis.

ADDITIONAL TERMS

Normal Structure and Function

aural *(AW-ral)* — Pertaining to or perceived by the ear

cerumen *(se-RŪ-men)* — The brown, waxlike secretion formed in the external canal of the ear

decibel (dB) *(DES-i-bel)* — A unit for measuring the relative intensity of sound

hertz *(Hz)* — A unit for measuring the frequency of sound

mastoid process — A small projection of the temporal bone behind the external auditory canal. It consists of loosely arranged bony material and small, air-filled cavities.

oval window — An oval opening in the inner ear which is in contact with the footplate of the stapes

stapedius *(stā-PĒ-dē-us)* — A small muscle attached to the stapes. It contracts in the presence of a loud sound, producing the acoustic reflex.

Symptoms and Conditions

cholesteatoma
(kō-lē-stē-a-TŌ-ma)
A cystlike mass containing cholesterol that is most common in the middle ear and mastoid region; a possible complication of chronic middle ear infection

labyrinthitis
(lab-i-rin-THĪ-tis)
Inflammation of the labyrinth of the ear; otitis interna

mastoiditis
(mas-toyd-Ī-tis)
Inflammation of the air cells of the mastoid process

presbyacusis
(prez-bē-a-KŪ-sis)
Loss of hearing due to aging. Also presbyacusia, presbycusis.

Diagnosis and Treatment

electronystagmography (ENG)
(ē-lek-trō-nis-tag-MOG-ra-fē)
A method for recording eye movements by means of electrical responses. Such movements may reflect vestibular dysfunction.

otoscope
(Ō-tō-skōp)
Instrument for examining the ear (see Figure 7-2)

spondee
(spon-dē)
A two-syllable word with equal stress on each syllable; used in hearing tests. Examples are: toothbrush, baseball, cowboy, pancake

ABBREVIATIONS

ABR auditory brain stem response
AC air conduction
AD right ear (L. *auris dexter*)
AS left ear (L. *auris sinistra*)
BAEP brain stem auditory evoked potentials
BC bone conduction
dB decibel
ENG electronystagmography
ENT ear(s), nose, and throat
HL hearing level
Hz Hertz
ORL otorhinolaryngology
ST speech threshold
TM tympanic membrane
TTS temporary threshold shift

The Eye and Vision

The wall of the eye is composed of three layers (Fig. 18-2). The outermost is a tough protective layer, the **sclera**, commonly called the *white of the eye*. This layer extends over the front of the eye as the transparent **cornea**. The middle layer is a vascular layer, the **uvea**, which consists of the **choroid**, the **ciliary body**, and the **iris**. The iris, by which we assign the color of the eye, is a muscular ring that controls the size of the **pupil**, thus regulating the amount of light that enters the eye. The ciliary body contains a muscle that controls the shape of the **lens** to allow for near and far vision, a process known as **accommodation**.

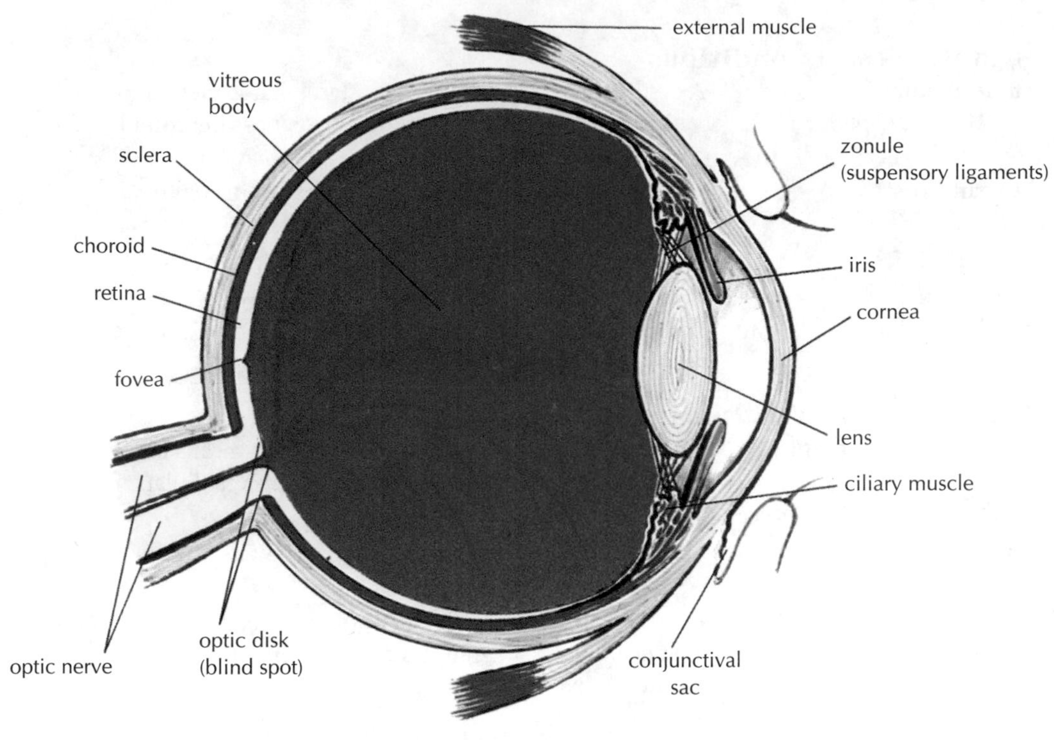

FIGURE 18-2. The eye.

The **retina** is the innermost layer and the actual visual receptor. It consists of specialized cells, **rods** and **cones**, which respond to light. Proper vision requires the **refraction** (bending) of light rays as they pass through the structures of the eye to focus on a specific point on the retina. The energy generated within the rods and cones is transmitted to the brain by way of the optic nerve (2nd cranial nerve). In the retina, near the optic nerve, is the **fovea**, a tiny depression that has a high concentration of cone cells and is the point of greatest **visual acuity** (sharpness). The fovea is surrounded by a yellowish spot called the **macula**.

The eye is protected by its position within a bony socket or **orbit**. It is also protected by the eyelids, eyebrows, eyelashes, and tears. The **lacrimal** (tear) **glands** (Fig. 18-3) constantly bathe the eyes with a lubricating fluid that drains into the nose. There is also the protective **conjunctiva**, a thin membrane that lines the eyelids and covers the anterior portion of the eye.

The eyeball is filled with a jellylike **vitreous body**.

Six muscles attached to the outside of each eye coordinate eye movements.

KEY TERMS

Normal Structure and Function

accommodation *(a-kom-ō-DĀ-shun)* — Adjustment of the curvature of the lens to allow for vision at various distances

conjunctiva *(kon-junk-TĪ-va)* — The mucous membrane that lines the eyelids and covers the anterior portion of the eyeball

choroid *(KOR-oyd)* — The dark, vascular, middle layer of the eye. Part of the uvea (see below) (root chori/o, choroid/o)

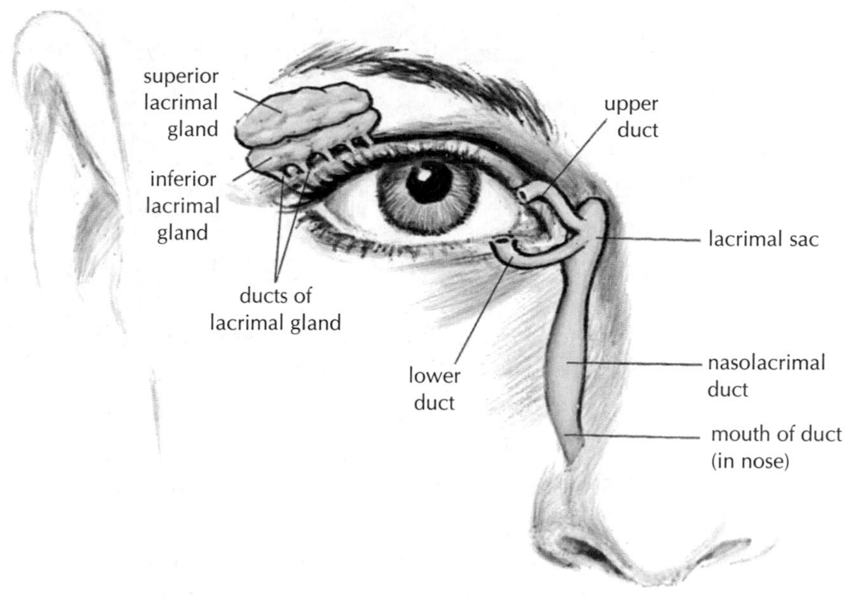

FIGURE 18-3. Lacrimal apparatus.

ciliary body *(SIL-ē-ar-ē)*	The muscular portion of the uvea that surrounds the lens and adjusts its shape for near and far vision (root cycl/o)
cornea *(KOR-nē-a)*	The clear, anterior portion of the sclera (root corne/o, kerat/o)
eye	The organ of vision (root opt/o, ocul/o, ophthalm/o)
eyelid	A protective fold (upper and lower) that closes over the anterior surface of the eye (root palpebr/o, blephar/o)
fovea *(FŌ-vē-a)*	The tiny depression in the retina that is the point of sharpest vision
iris *(Ī-ris)*	The muscular colored ring between the lens and the cornea. It regulates the amount of light that enters the eye by altering the size of the pupil at its center (*pl.* irides) (root ir, irid/o, irit/o)
lacrimal *(LAK-ri-mal)*	Pertaining to tears (root lacrim/o, dacry/o)
lens *(lenz)*	The transparent, biconvex structure in the anterior portion of the eye that refracts light and functions in accommodation (root lent/i, phak/o)
macula *(MAK-ū-la)*	A small spot or colored area. Used alone to mean the yellowish spot in the retina that contains the fovea.
optic disk	The point where the optic nerve joins the retina. At this point there are no rods or cones. Also called the *blind spot* or *optic papilla*.

(continued)

pupil *(PŪ-pil)*	The opening at the center of the iris (pupill/o)
refraction *(rē-FRAK-shun)*	The bending of light rays as they pass through the eye to focus on a specific point on the retina. Also the determination of ocular refractive errors and their correction.
retina *(RET-i-na)*	The innermost, light sensitive layer of the eye. It contains the rods and cones, the specialized receptor cells for vision (root retin/o).
sclera *(SKLĒR-a)*	The tough, white, and fibrous outermost layer of the eye; the white of the eye (root scler/o)
uvea *(Ū-vē-a)*	The middle, vascular layer of the eye. It consists of the choroid, ciliary body, and iris (root uve/o).
visual acuity *(a-KŪ-i-tē)*	Sharpness of vision; commonly measured with the Snellen eye chart
vitreous body *(VIT-rē-us)*	The transparent jellylike mass that fills the main cavity of the eyeball. Also called vitreous humor.

Word Parts Pertaining to the Eye and Vision

Roots for External Eye Structures

Root	Meaning	Example	Definition of Example
palpebr/o	eyelid	palpebral *PAL-pe-bral*	pertaining to an eyelid
blephar/o	eyelid	symblepharon *sim-BLEF-a-ron*	adhesion of the eyelid to the eyeball
lacrim/o	tear, lacrimal apparatus	lacrimation *lak-ri-MĀ-shun*	secretion of tears
dacry/o	tear, lacrimal apparatus	dacryolith *DAK-rē-ō-lith*	stone in the lacrimal apparatus
dacryocyst/o	lacrimal sac	dacryocystocele *dak-rē-ō-SIS-tō-sēl*	hernia of the lacrimal sac

Exercise 18-3

Define the following terms:

1. Interpalpebral *(in-ter-PAL-pe-bral)* ________________
2. Blepharospasm *(BLEF-a-rō-spazm)* ________________
3. Nasolacrimal *(nā-zō-LAK-ri-mal)* ________________
4. Dacryocystectomy *(dak-rē-ō-sis-TEK-tō-mē)* ________________

Build words that fit the following definitions using the roots indicated:

5. Paralysis of the eyelid (blephar/o) ____________________
6. Discharge from the lacrimal apparatus (dacry/o) ____________________
7. Inflammation of a lacrimal sac (dacryocyst/o) ____________________

Roots for the Eye and Vision

Root	Meaning	Example	Definition of Example
opt/o	eye, vision	optometer *op-TOM-e-ter*	instrument for measuring the refractive power of the eye
ocul/o	eye	intraocular *in-tra-OK-ū-lar*	within the eye
ophthalm/o	eye	exophthalmos *eks-of-THAL-mos*	protrusion of the eyeball
scler/o	sclera	subscleral *sub-SKLĒR-al*	below the sclera
corne/o	cornea	circumcorneal *sir-kum-KOR-nē-al*	around the cornea
kerat/o	cornea	keratoplasty *KER-a-tō-plas-tē*	plastic repair of the cornea; corneal transplant
lent/i	lens	lenticular *len-TIK-ū-lar*	pertaining to the lens
phak/o, phac/o	lens	aphakia *a-FĀ-kē-a*	absence of a lens
uve/o	uvea	uveitis *ū-vē-Ī-tis*	inflammation of the uvea
chori/o, choroid/o	choroid	choroidal *kor-OYD-al*	pertaining to the choroid
cycl/o	ciliary body, ciliary muscle	cycloplegia *si-klō-PLĒ-jē-a*	paralysis of the ciliary muscle
ir, irit/o, irid/o	iris	iridoschisis *ir-i-DOS-ki-sis*	separation of the iris into two layers
pupill/o	pupil	iridopupillary *ir-i-dō-PŪ-pi-ler-ē*	pertaining to the iris and the pupil
retin/o	retina	retinitis *ret-i-NĪ-tis*	inflammation of the retina

Exercise 18-4

Fill in the blanks:

1. The science of orthoptics *(or-THOP-tiks)* deals with correcting defects in ____________________.
2. The oculomotor *(ok-ū-lō-MŌ-tor)* nerve controls movements of the ____________________.

3. A keratometer *(ker-a-TOM-e-ter)* is an instrument for measuring the curves of the ____________________.
4. The term *phacolysis (fa-KOL-i-sis)* means destruction of the ____________________.
5. Lenticonus is conical protrusion of the ____________________.

Identify and define the roots pertaining to the eye in the following words:

	Root	Meaning of Root
6. Optometrist *(op-TOM-e-trist)*	________	________
7. Microphthalmus *(mī-krof-THAL-mus)*	________	________
8. Lentiform *(LEN-ti-form)*	________	________
9. Phakotoxic *(fak-ō-TOK-sik)*	________	________
10. Iridodilator *(ir-id-ō-DĪ-lā-tor)*	________	________
11. Interpupillary *(in-ter-PŪ-pi-ler-ē)*	________	________
12. Uveal *(Ū-vē-al)*	________	________
13. Retinoscopy *(ret-in-OS-kō-pē)*	________	________

Write a word that fits each of the following definitions:

14. Inflammation of the uvea and sclera ____________________
15. Softening of the lens (use phac/o) ____________________
16. Inflammation the the ciliary body ____________________
17. Any disease of the retina ____________________

Use *ophthalm/o* for the following words:

18. An instrument used to examine the eye ____________________
19. The medical specialty that deals with the eye and diseases of the eye ____________________

Use *irid/o* for the following words:

20. Surgical removal of (part of) the iris ____________________
21. Paralysis of the iris ____________________

Define the following terms:

22. Optical *(OP-ti-kal)* ____________________
23. Extraocular *(eks-tra-OK-ū-lar)* ____________________
24. Sclerotome *(SKLĒR-ō-tōm)* ____________________
25. Keratitis *(ker-a-TĪ-tis)* ____________________
26. Retrolental *(ret-RŌ-LEN-tal)* ____________________

27. Cyclotomy *(sī-KLOT-ō-mē)* __________
28. Chorioretinal *(kor-ē-ō-RET-i-nal)* __________
29. Iridocyclitis *(ir-i-dō-sī-KLĪ-tis)* __________

*Suffixes for the Eye and Vision**

Suffix	Meaning	Example	Definition of Example
-opsia	vision	heteropsia *het-er-OP-sē-a*	unequal vision in the two eyes
-opia	eye, vision	hemianopia *hem-ē-an-Ō-pē-a*	blindness in half the visual field

*Compounds of *-ops* (eye) + *-ia*

Exercise 18-5

Use *-opsia* for the following words:

1. A visual defect in which objects seem larger (macr/o) than they are __________
2. Lack of (a-) color (chromat/o) vision (complete color blindness) __________

Use *-opia* for the following words:

3. Double vision __________
4. Changes in vision due to old age (use the prefix *presby-* meaning "old") __________

The suffix *-opia* is added to the root *metr/o* (measure) to form words pertaining to the refractive power of the eye. Add a prefix to *-metropia* to form the following words:

5. A lack of perfect refractive power in the eye __________
6. Unequal refractive powers in the two eyes __________

Clinical Aspects of the Eye and Vision

Errors of Refraction

If the eyeball is too long, images will form in front of the retina. In order to focus clearly, an object must be brought closer to the eye. This condition of nearsightedness is technically called **myopia**. The opposite condition is **hyperopia**, or farsightedness, in which the eyeball is too short and images form behind the retina. Objects must be moved away from the eye in order to focus clearly.

The same effect is produced by **presbyopia**, which accompanies aging. The lens loses elasticity and can no longer accommodate for near vision. The person becomes increasingly farsighted. An **astigmatism** is an irregularity in the curve of the cornea or lens that distorts light entering the eye and blurs vision. Most of these impairments can be compensated for with glasses.

Infection

Several microorganisms can cause **conjunctivitis** (inflammation of the conjunctiva). This is a highly infectious disease commonly called "pinkeye."

The bacterium *Chlamydia trachomatis* causes **trachoma**, inflammation of the cornea and conjunctiva that results in scarring. This disease is rare in the United States, but is a common cause of blindness in underdeveloped countries, even though it is easily cured with sulfa drugs and antibiotics.

Gonorrhea is the usual cause of an acute conjuntivitis in newborns called **ophthalmia neonatorum**. An antibiotic ointment is routinely used to prevent such eye infections in newborns.

Disorders of the Retina

Retinal detachment, separation of the retina from the underlying layer of the eye (the choroid), may be caused by a tumor, hemorrhage, or injury to the eye. This interferes with vision and is commonly repaired with laser surgery.

Degeneration of the macula, the point of sharpest vision, is a common cause of visual problems in the elderly. When associated with aging, this deterioration is described as **senile macular degeneration** (SMD). Other causes are drug toxicity and hereditary diseases.

Circulatory problems associated with diabetes mellitus eventually cause changes in the retina referred to as **diabetic retinopathy**. In addition to vascular damage there is a yellowish, waxy exudate high in lipoproteins. With time, new blood vessels form and penetrate the vitreous humor causing hemorrhage, detachment of the retina, and blindness.

Cataract

A **cataract** is an opacity (cloudiness) of the lens. Causes of cataract include disease, injury, chemicals, and exposure to physical forces, especially the ultraviolet radiation in sunlight. The cataracts that frequently appear with age may result from exposure to environmental factors in combination with degeneration due to aging. To prevent blindness, the cloudy lens must be removed surgically. Commonly, the anterior capsule of the lens is removed along with the cataract, leaving the posterior capsule in place (Fig. 18-4). In a newer method, phacoemulsification, the lens is fragmented with high frequency ultrasound and extracted through a small incision. Often, following cataract removal, an artificial intraocular lens (IOL) is implanted to compensate for the missing lens. Alternatively, the person can wear a contact lens or special glasses.

Glaucoma

Glaucoma is an abnormal increase in pressure within the eyeball. It occurs when more aqueous humor is produced than can be drained away from the eye. There is pressure on blood vessels in the eye and on the optic nerve, leading to blindness. There are many causes of glaucoma, and screening for glaucoma should be a part of every routine eye examination. Fetal infection with German measles (rubella) early in pregnancy can cause glaucoma, as well as cataracts and hearing impairment. Glaucoma is usually treated with medication to reduce pressure in the eye, and occasionally is treated with surgery.

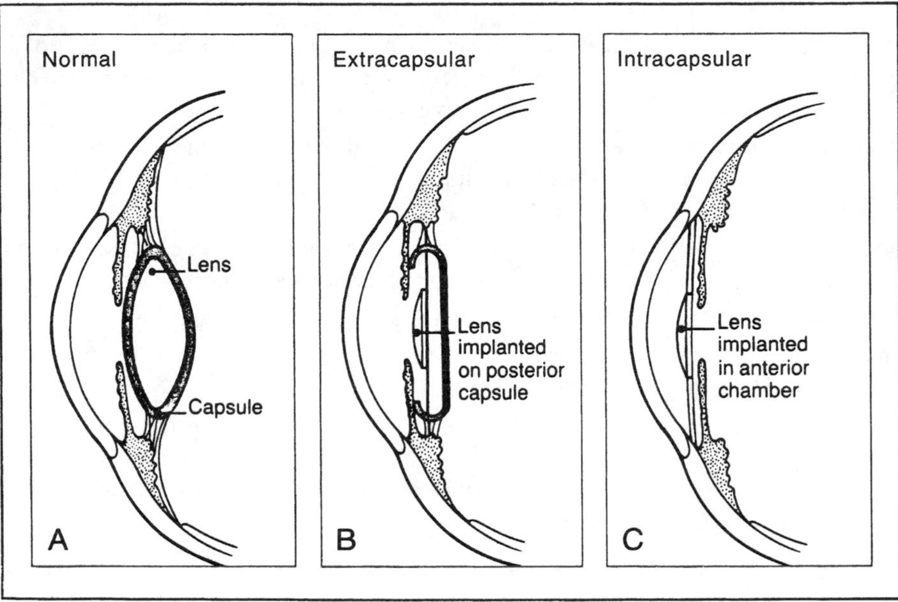

FIGURE 18-4. Cataract extraction surgeries. **(A)** Cross section of normal eye anatomy. **(B)** Extracapsular lens extraction involves removing the lens but leaving the posterior capsule intact to receive a synthetic intraocular lens. **(C)** Intracapsular lens extraction involves removing the lens and lens capsule and implanting a synthetic intraocular lens in the anterior chamber. (Reproduced with permission from Patient Care, Patient Care Communications, Inc., Darien CT. Artist, Paul J. Singh-Roy. All rights reserved.)

KEY CLINICAL TERMS

astigmatism *(a-STIG-ma-tizm)* — An error of refraction due to irregularity in the curvature of the cornea or lens

cataract *(KAT-a-rakt)* — Opacity of the lens of the eye

conjunctivitis *(kon-junk-ti-VĪ-tis)* — Inflammation of the conjunctiva; pinkeye

diabetic retinopathy *(ret-i-NOP-a-thē)* — Degenerative changes in the retina associated with diabetes mellitus

glaucoma *(glaw-KŌ-ma)* — A disease of the eye caused by increased intraocular pressure that damages the optic disk and causes loss of vision. Usually results from faulty drainage of fluids from the anterior portion of the eye.

hyperopia *(hī-per-Ō-pē-a)* — An error of refraction in which light rays focus behind the retina and objects can be seen clearly only when far from the eye; farsightedness. Also called hypermetropia.

(continued)

myopia *(mī-Ō-pē-a)* — An error of refraction in which light rays focus in front of the retina and objects can be seen clearly only when very close to the eye; nearsightedness

ophthalmia neonatorum *(of-THAL-mē-a nē-ō-nā-TOR-um)* — Severe conjunctivitis usually caused by infection with gonococcus during birth

presbyopia *(prez-bē-Ō-pē-a)* — Changes in the eye that occur with age. The lens loses elasticity and the ability to accommodate for near vision.

retinal detachment — Separation of the retina from the underlying layer of the eye

senile macular degeneration (SMD) — Deterioration of the macula associated with aging. Impairs central vision.

trachoma *(tra-KŌ-ma)* — An infection caused by *Chlamydia trachomatis* leading to inflammation and scarring of the cornea and conjunctiva. A common cause of blindness in underdeveloped countries.

ADDITIONAL TERMS

Normal Structure and Function

canthus *(KAN-thus)* — The angle at either end of the slit between the eyelids

convergence *(kon-VER-jens)* — Coordinated movement of the eyes toward fixation on the same point

diopter *(DĪ-op-ter)* — A unit of measurement for the refractive power of a lens

emmetropia *(em-e-TRŌ-pē-a)* — The normal condition of the eye in refraction in which parallel light rays focus exactly on the retina

fundus *(FUN-dus)* — A bottom or base. The fundus of the eye is the back portion of the inside of the eyeball as seen with an ophthalmoscope.

meibomian gland *(mī-BŌ-mē-an)* — A sebaceous gland in the eyelid

tarsus *(TAR-sus)* — The framework of dense connective tissue that gives shape to the eyelid; tarsal plate

zonule *(ZON-ūl)* — A system of fibers that holds the lens in place. Also called suspensory ligaments.

Symptoms and Conditions

amblyopia *(am-blē-Ō-pē-a)* — A condition that occurs when visual acuity is not the same in the two eyes in children. (Prefix *ambly* means "dim.") Disuse of the poorer eye will result in blindness if not corrected. Also called "lazy eye."

blepharoptosis *(blef-a-rop-TŌ-sis)*	Drooping of the eyelid
chalazion *(ka-LĀ-zē-on)*	A small mass on the eyelid resulting from inflammation and blockage of a meibomian gland
hordeolum *(hor-DĒ-ō-lum)*	Inflammation of a sebaceous gland of the eyelid; a sty
keratoconus *(ker-a-tō-KŌ-nus)*	Conical protrusion of the center of the cornea
miosis *(mī-Ō-sis)*	Abnormal contraction of the pupils (from G. meaning "diminution")
mydriasis *(mi-DRĪ-a-sis)*	Pronounced or abnormal dilation of the pupil
nyctalopia *(nik-ta-LŌ-pē-a)*	Inability to see well in dim light or at night; night blindness (root *nyct/o* means "night")
nystagmus *(nis-TAG-mus)*	Rapid, involuntary, rhythmic movements of the eyeball. May occur in neurologic diseases or disorders of the vestibular apparatus of the inner ear.
papilledema *(pap-il-e-DĒ-ma)*	Swelling of the optic disk (papilla); choked disk
phlyctenule *(FLIK-ten-ūl)*	A small blister or nodule on the cornea or conjunctiva
pseudophakia *(sū-dō-FĀ-kē-a)*	A condition in which a cataractous lens has been removed and replaced with a plastic lens implant
retinitis *(ret-in-Ī-tis)*	Inflammation of the retina. Causes include systemic disease, infection, hemorrhage, exposure to light.
retinitis pigmentosa *(ret-in-Ī-tis pig-men-TŌ sa)*	A hereditary chronic degenerative disease of the retina that begins in early childhood. There is atrophy of the optic nerve and clumping of pigment in the retina.
retinoblastoma *(ret-in-ō-blas-TŌ-ma)*	A malignant glioma of the retina. Usually appears in early childhood and is sometimes hereditary. Fatal if untreated, but current cure rates are high.
scotoma *(skō-TŌ-ma)*	An area of diminished vision within the visual field
strabismus *(stra-BIZ-mus)*	A deviation of the eye in which the visual lines of each eye are not directed to the same object at the same time. Also called *squint*. The various forms are referred to as *-tropias*, with the direction of turning indicated by a prefix, such as esotropia (inward), exotropia (outward), hypertropia (upward), and hypotropia (downward). The suffix *-phoria* is also used, as in *esophoria*.
synechia *(sin-EK-ē-a)*	Adhesion of parts, especially adhesion of the iris to the lens and cornea (*pl.* synechiae)
xanthoma *(zan-THŌ-ma)*	A soft, slightly raised, yellowish patch or nodule usually on the eyelids. Occurs in the elderly. Also called *xanthalasma*.

(continued)

Diagnosis and Treatment

canthotomy
(kan-THOT-ō-mē) — Surgical division of a canthus

cystitome
(SIS-ti-tōm) — Instrument for incising the capsule of the lens

electroretinography (ERG)
(ē-lek-trō-ret-i-NOG-ra-fē) — Study of the electrical response of the retina to light stimulation

enucleation
(ē-nū-klē-Ā-shun) — Surgical removal of the eyeball

gonioscopy
(gō-nē-OS-kō-pē) — Examination of the angle between the cornea and the iris (anterior chamber angle) where fluids drain out of the eye (root *goni/o* means "angle")

keratometer
(ker-a-TOM-e-ter) — An instrument for measuring the curvature of the cornea

mydriatic
(mid-rē-AT-ik) — A drug that causes dilation of the pupil

phacoemulsification
(fak-ō-ē-MUL-si-fi-kā-shun) — Removal of a cataract by ultrasonic destruction and extraction of the lens

phorometer
(fo-ROM-e-ter) — An instrument for determining the degree and kind of strabismus

retinoscope
(RET-in-ō-skōp) — An instrument used to determine refractive errors of the eye. Also called a skiascope (SKĪ-a-skōp).

slit lamp biomicroscope — An instrument for examining the eye under magnification

tarsorrhaphy
(tar-SOR-a-fē) — Suturing together of all or part of the upper and lower eyelids

tonometer
(tō-NOM-e-ter) — An instrument used to measure the pressure of fluids in the eye

ABBREVIATIONS

A, Acc accommodation
ARC abnormal retinal correspondence
As, AST astigmatism
cc with correction
Em emmetropia
EOM extraocular movement, muscles
ENT ear(s), nose, and throat
ERG electroretinography
ET esotropia
FC finger counting
HM hand movements
IOL intraocular lens
IOP intraocular pressure
NRC normal retinal correspondence
NV near vision
OD right eye (L. *oculus dexter*)
ORL otorhinolaryngology
OS left eye (L. *oculus sinister*)
OU both eyes (L. *oculi unitas*); also each eye (L. *oculus uterque*)
sc without correction
SMD senile macular degeneration
VA visual acuity
VF visual field
XT exotropia

Chapter 18
Labeling Exercises

Write the name of each numbered part on the corresponding line of the answer sheet.

cochlea
eustachian (auditory) tube
external auditory canal (meatus)
incus
malleus
pinna
semicircular canals
stapes
tympanic membrane
vestibulocochlear (auditory) nerve
vestibule

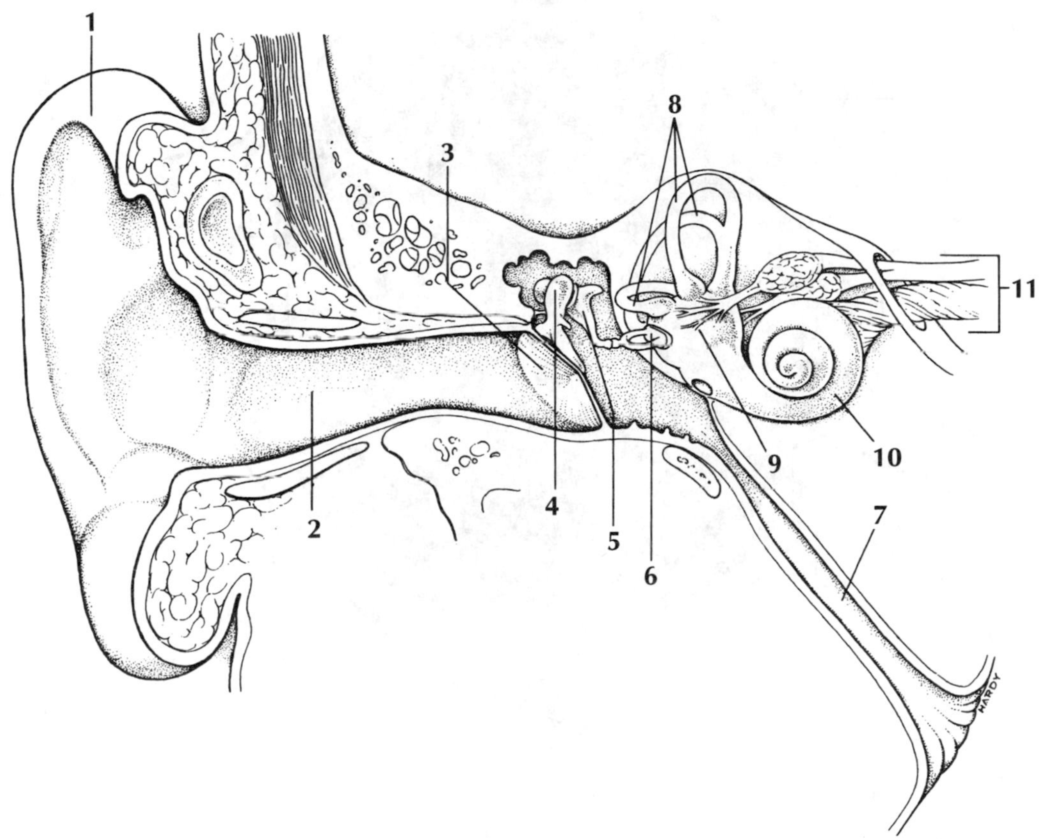

The ear

1. ______________________
2. ______________________
3. ______________________
4. ______________________
5. ______________________
6. ______________________
7. ______________________
8. ______________________
9. ______________________
10. ______________________
11. ______________________

Write the name of each numbered part on the corresponding line of the answer sheet.

choroid
cornea
fovea
iris
lens
optic disk (blind spot)
optic nerve
retina
sclera
vitreous body
zonule (suspensory ligaments)

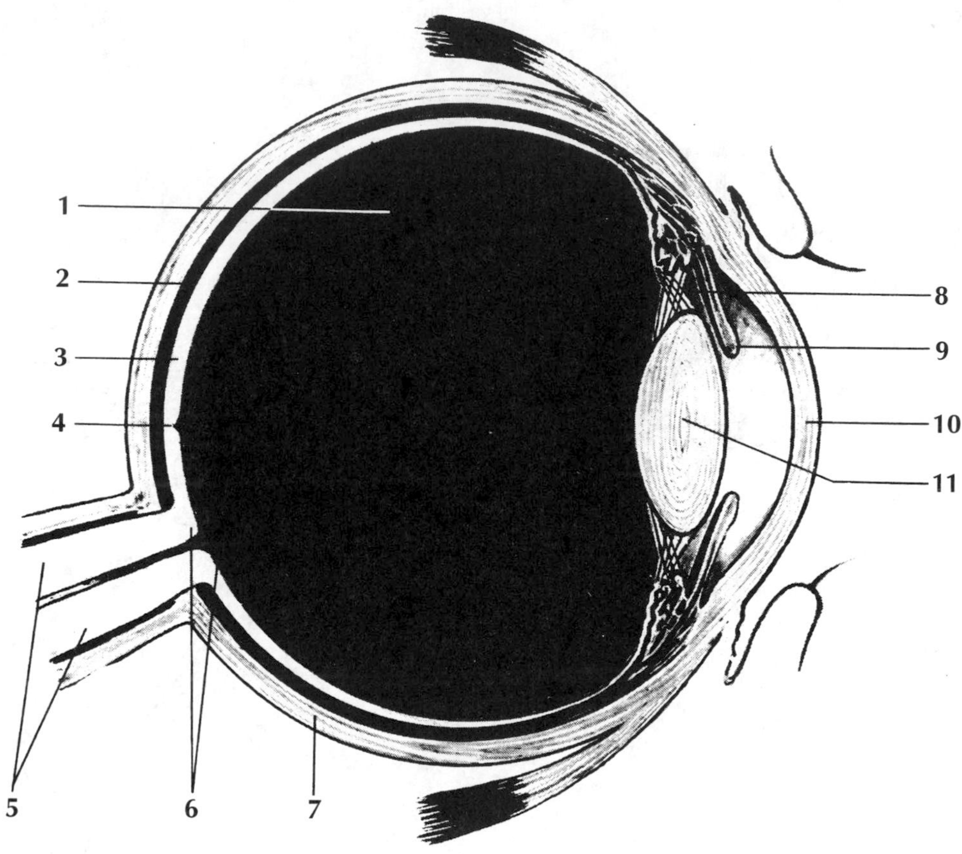

The eye

1. ______________________
2. ______________________
3. ______________________
4. ______________________
5. ______________________
6. ______________________
7. ______________________
8. ______________________
9. ______________________
10. ______________________
11. ______________________

CHAPTER REVIEW 18-1

Matching. Match the terms in each of the sets below with their definitions and write the appropriate letter (a–e) to the left of each number:

_____ 1. proprioception	a. part of the ear concerned with equilibrium
_____ 2. lacrimal gland	b. sense of taste
_____ 3. vestibular apparatus	c. sense of smell
_____ 4. olfaction	d. produces tears
_____ 5. gustation	e. awareness of body position

_____ 6. vitreous body	a. outermost layer of the eye
_____ 7. lens	b. material that fills the eyeball
_____ 8. labyrinth	c. inner ear
_____ 9. sclera	d. passage that connects the middle ear and pharynx
_____ 10. eustachian tube	e. changes in shape for near and far vision

_____ 11. anacusis	a. normal refraction of the eye
_____ 12. fovea	b. complete color blindness
_____ 13. emmetropia	c. instrument used to examine the eye
_____ 14. ophthalmoscope	d. total loss of hearing
_____ 15. achromatopsia	e. point of sharpest vision

_____ 16. strabismus	a. opacity of the lens
_____ 17. tinnitus	b. projection of the temporal bone
_____ 18. cataract	c. nearsightedness
_____ 19. mastoid process	d. sensation of noises in the ear
_____ 20. myopia	e. deviation of the eye

_____ 21. phakosclerosis	a. paralysis of the ciliary muscle
_____ 22. blepharedema	b. corneal transplant
_____ 23. keratoplasty	c. instrument for examining the cornea
_____ 24. cycloplegia	d. hardening of the lens
_____ 25. keratoscope	e. swelling of the eyelid

Fill in the blanks:

26. The coiled portion of the inner ear that contains the receptor for hearing is the _____________________.

27. The ossicle that is in contact with the inner ear is the _____________________.

28. The innermost layer of the eye that contains the receptors for vision is the _____________________.

29. The transparent extension of the sclera that covers the front of the eye is the ____________________.
30. The scientific name for the eardrum is ____________________.
31. The term *dextrocular* (*deks-TROK-u-lar*) refers to the right ____________________.

Definitions. Write the meaning of each of the following terms:

32. Audiologist ____________________
33. Palpebra ____________________
34. Ophthalmectomy ____________________
35. Keratoiritis ____________________
36. Circumlental ____________________
37. Chorioretinal ____________________
38. Myringitis ____________________

Word building. Write a word for each of the following definitions:

39. Absence of pain ____________________
40. Measurement of hearing (audi/o) ____________________
41. Surgical removal of the stapes ____________________
42. Inflammation of the retina ____________________
43. Plastic repair of the ear ____________________
44. Inflammation of the sclera and cornea (use kerat/o-) ____________________
45. Measurement of the pupil ____________________
46. Any disease of the retina ____________________

Adjectives. Write the adjective form of each of the following words:

47. cochlea ____________________
48. uvea ____________________
49. vestibule ____________________
50. sclera ____________________
51. pupil ____________________
52. cornea ____________________

Word analysis. Define each of the following words and give the meaning of the word parts in each. Use a dictionary if necessary.

53. Otorhinolaryngology (*ō-tō-rī-nō-lar-in-GOL-ō-jē*) ____________________

____

   a. ot/o ____________________
   b. rhin/o ____________________

c. laryng/o ____________________

d. -logy ____________________

54. Anisometropia *(an-ī-sō-me-TRŌ-pē-a)* ____

____

a. an- ____________________

b. iso- ____________________

c. metr/o ____________________

d. -opia ____________________

55. Paresthesia *(par-es-THĒ-zē-a)* ____

____

a. par/a ____________________

b. esthesi/o ____________________

c. -ia ____________________

CHAPTER REVIEW 18-2

Matching. Match the terms in each of the sets below with their definitions and write the appropriate letter (a–e) to the left of each number:

_____	1. myesthesia	a.	abnormal smell perception
_____	2. parosmia	b.	night blindness
_____	3. hypergeusia	c.	loss of hearing due to age
_____	4. presbyacusis	d.	muscular sensation
_____	5. nyctalopia	e.	abnormal increase in the sense of taste
_____	6. pinna	a.	receptors for vision
_____	7. accommodation	b.	small bones of the middle ear
_____	8. rods and cones	c.	bending of light rays
_____	9. refraction	d.	projecting portion of the ear
_____	10. ossicles	e.	changes in the eye for vision at various distances
_____	11. hemotympanum	a.	plastic repair of the middle ear
_____	12. blepharoptosis	b.	excessive flow of tears
_____	13. tarsorrhaphy	c.	drooping of the eyelid
_____	14. dacryorrhea	d.	blood in the middle ear
_____	15. tympanoplasty	e.	suturing of the eyelids
_____	16. hyperopia	a.	disease caused by excess pressure in the eye
_____	17. vertigo	b.	farsightedness

_____ 18. scotoma		c. rapid, involuntary movements of the eye
_____ 19. nystagmus		d. an area of decreased vision
_____ 20. glaucoma		e. false sensation of movement

_____ 21. Hz		a. left eye
_____ 22. dB		b. sharpness of vision
_____ 23. sc		c. unit for measuring the intensity of sound
_____ 24. OS		d. unit for measuring frequency of sound
_____ 25. VA		e. without correction

Fill in the blanks:

26. The thin membrane that lines the eyelids and covers the anterior portion of the eye is the_____________________.
27. The middle layer of the eye, consisting of the choroid, ciliary body, and iris is the _____________________.
28. The muscular ring that adjusts the size of the pupil is the _____________________.
29. Mydriasis is abnormal dilation of the _____________________.
30. Otoneurology is study of the nerve supply to the _____________________.
31. An ophthalmometer is an instrument for measuring _____________________.

Definitions. Write the meaning of each of the following terms:

32. Acoustic _____________________
33. Lacrimal _____________________
34. Extraocular _____________________
35. Aphakia _____________________
36. Hyposcleral _____________________

Word building. Write a word for each of the following definitions:

37. Surgical incision of the tympanic membrane _____________________
38. Instrument for examination of the eustachian tube _____________________
39. Pertaining to the vestibular apparatus and cochlea _____________________
40. Discharge from the ear _____________________
41. Inflammation of the uvea and sclera _____________________
42. Excision of (part of) the ciliary body _____________________
43. Inflammation of a lacrimal sac _____________________
44. Incision of the iris (use irid/o) _____________________

Opposites. Write a term that means the opposite of each of the following:

45. miosis ______________________

46. exotropia ______________________

47. cc ______________________

48. OS ______________________

49. hypoesthesia ______________________

Word analysis. Define each of the following words and give the meaning of the word parts in each. Use a dictionary if necessary.

50. Hemianopia *(hem-ē-an-Ō-pē-a)* ______________________

____

a. hemi- ______________________

b. an- ______________________

c. -opia ______________________

51. Hyperchromatopsia *(hī-per-krō-ma-TOP-sē-a)* ______________________

____

a. hyper- ______________________

b. chromat/o ______________________

c. -opsia ______________________

Chapter 18 Case Studies

1. Audiologist's Report

A 55-year-old man was seen with the complaint of decreased hearing sensitivity in the left ear for the past 3 years. In addition to the hearing loss, he was experiencing tinnitus and aural fullness. Pure tone test results revealed normal hearing sensitivity for the right ear and a moderate sensorineural hearing loss for the left ear. Speech thresholds were appropriate for the degree of hearing loss noted. Word recognition was excellent for the right ear and poor for the left ear when the signal was presented at a suprathreshold level: Tympanograms were characterized by normal shape, amplitude, and peak pressure points bilaterally. The contralateral acoustic reflex was normal for the right ear but absent for the left ear at the frequencies tested (500–4000 Hz). The ipsilateral acoustic reflex was present with the probe in the right ear and absent with the probe in the left ear. Brain stem auditory evoked potentials (BAEP) were within the normal range for the right ear. No repeatable response was observed from the left ear. A subsequent MRI showed a 1 cm acoustic neuroma.

2. Temporary Partial Blindness

This 45-year-old female consulted for intermittent episodes of blurred vision over the previous 2 years. The episodes last for approximately 1 hour and are accompanied by headache and malaise but no nausea or vomiting. There is a history of similar attacks in her family. There is no history of hypertension or diabetes.

Neurologic examination shows no disorientation. There is no carotid bruit audible in the neck. The pupils are round and equal and react promptly to light. The optic disks have good color and definition. The retinal vessels appear normal. The visual fields are full. Ocular movements are good in all directions. There is no nystagmus. The corneal reflexes are active and equal. Sensations and movements are normal over the entire face. There is no weakness or ataxia. Reflexes are normal. Pain, touch, position, and vibratory sensations are normal.

Results suggest amaurosis fugax, temporary episodes of partial blindness, associated with stenosis of the carotid artery, resulting in insufficient circulation through the ophthalmic branch. Carotid doppler studies and a CT brain scan are suggested to exclude other abnormalities.

3. Phacoemulsification With Intraocular Lens Implant

The patient and the eye were identified and verbal consent was given. After satisfactory local anesthesia and akinesia were achieved, the patient was prepped and draped. A 5-0 black silk suture was placed under the belly of the superior rectus. A lid speculum was introduced into the lids of the eye. A minimal conjunctival peritotomy was performed and hemostasis was achieved with wetfield cautery. The anterior chamber was entered at the 10:30 o'clock position. A capsulotomy was performed after healon was placed in the anterior chamber. Phacoemulsification was carried out with no difficulty. The remaining cortex was removed by irrigation and aspiration.

An intraocular lens was placed in the posterior chamber. Miochol was injected to achieve pupillary miosis and the wound was closed with one 10-0 suture.

Subconjunctival Celestone and Garamycin were injected. The lid speculum and black silk suture were removed. Following application of Eserine and Bacitracin ointments, the eye was patched and a shield applied. The patient left the operating room in good condition.

Chapter 18
Case Study Questions

Multiple choice. Select the best answer and write the letter of your choice to the left of each number:

_____ 1. Sensorineural hearing loss results from

a. damage to the 8th cranial nerve
b. damage to the 2nd cranial nerve
c. blockage of sound transmission in the ear
d. stapedectomy
e. otitis media

_____ 2. A term that means *on the same side* is

a. contralateral
b. bilateral
c. distal
d. ventral
e. ipsilateral

_____ 3. Another name for an acoustic neuroma is

a. macular degeneration
b. neurilemoma
c. otosclerosis
d. labyrinthitis
e. glaucoma

_____ 4. A carotid bruit is a(n)

a. aneurysm in the carotid artery
b. increased pressure in the carotid vein
c. swelling of the carotid artery
d. obstruction of the carotid vein
e. sound heard in the carotid artery

_____ 5. Another term for optic disk is

a. conjunctiva
b. blind spot
c. fovea
d. macula
e. iris

_____ 6. The term *akinesia* means

a. movement
b. lack of sensation
c. washing
d. lack of movement
e. incision

Find a word in the case studies that means each of the following:

7. Pertaining to or perceived by the ear _______________
8. Record obtained by tympanometry _______________
9. Sensation of ringing or tinkling in the ears _______________
10. Sensation of movement; dizziness or lightheadedness _______________
11. A generalized feeling of discomfort or uneasiness _______________
12. Rapid involuntary movements of the eyes _______________
13. Lack of muscle coordination _______________
14. Destruction of the lens of the eye _______________
15. Removal by suction _______________
16. Abnormal contraction of the pupil _______________

Define the following terms:

17. Suprathreshold _______________
18. Bilaterally _______________
19. Ophthalmic _______________
20. Intraocular _______________
21. Subconjunctival

____

THE SENSES

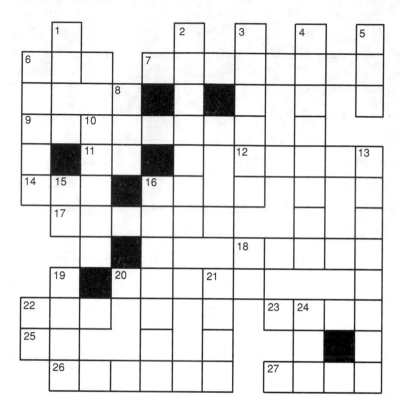

ACROSS

6. a quadrant of the abdomen (abbr.)
7. opacity of the lens of the eye
9. a sensory nerve ending that responds to a stimulus
11. left eye (abbr.)
12. root (with combining vowel) for the iris of the eye
14. organ that contains the tympanic membrane and cochlea
16. under the tongue (abbr.)
17. an ossicle of the ear
18. root that means sound or hearing
20. an ossicle of the ear
22. pressure within the eye (abbr.)
23. root (with combining vowel) that means eye or vision
25. physician (abbr.)
26. the white of the eye
27. a cell in the retina that responds to light

DOWN

1. both eyes; each eye (abbr.)
2. pertaining to the sense of touch
3. root for tear or the structure that produces tears
4. root (with combining vowel) that means tube or eustachian tube
5. root (with combining vowel) for the ear
6. meaning of the prefix mega- or megalo-
8. word part that means "middle"
10. the hearing receptor is named for him
13. instrument for examining the ear
15. left ear (abbr.)
16. a two-syllable word used in hearing tests
18. an error of refraction due to irregularity in the curvature of the cornea or lens (abbr.)
19. specialized cells in the retina that respond to light
21. the middle, vascular layer of the eye
22. prefix: not
24. prefix: before, in front of

Chapter 18
Answer Section

Answers to Chapter Exercises

Exercise 18-1

1. excess sensitivity to stimuli
2. false sense of smell
3. lack of taste sensation
4. anesthesia *(an-es-THĒ-zē-a)*
5. thermesthesia *(ther-mes-THĒ-zē-a)*
6. hyperalgesia *(hī-per-al-JĒ-zē-a)*
7. dysgeusia *(dis-GŪ-zē-a)*

Exercise 18-2

1. sound
2. ear
3. pertaining to the cochlea
4. pertaining to the vestibule or vestibular apparatus
5. pertaining to the labyrinth
6. pertaining to the stapes
7. pertaining to hearing
8. pertaining to the ear
9. audiometer *(aw-dē-OM-e-ter)*
10. otalgia *(ō-TAL-jē-a)*
11. tympanoplasty *(tim-PAN-ō-plas-tē)*
12. myringotomy *(mir-in-GOT-ō-mē)*; also tympanotomy *(tim-pan-OT-ō-mē)*
13. stapedectomy *(stā-pe-DEK-tō-mē)*
14. vestibulocochlear *(ves-tib-ū-lō-KOK-lē-ar)*
15. labyrinthitis *(lab-i-rin-THĪ-tis)*
16. salpingoscopy *(sal-ping-GOS-kō-pē)*
17. a specialist in the diagnosis and treatment of hearing disorders
18. inflammation of the ear
19. instrument used to examine the eardrum
20. pertaining to the eustachian tube and pharynx
21. Surgical incision of the vestibule of the ear

Exercise 18-3

1. between the eyelids
2. spasm of the eyelid
3. pertaining to the nose and lacrimal apparatus
4. excision of a lacrimal sac
5. blepharoplegia *(blef-a-rō-PLĒ-jē-a)*
6. dacryorrhea *(dak-rē-ō-RĒ-a)*
7. dacryocystitis *(dak-rē-ō-sis-TĪ-tis)*

Exercise 18-4

1. vision
2. eye
3. cornea
4. lens of the eye
5. lens
6. opt/o; eye, vision
7. ophthalm/o; eye
8. lent/i; lens
9. phak/o; lens
10. irid/o; iris
11. pupill/o; pupil
12. uve/o; uvea
13. retin/o; retina
14. uveoscleritis *(ū-vē-ō-skle-RĪ-tis)*
15. phacomalacia *(fak-ō-ma-LĀ-shē-a)*
16. cyclitis *(sī-KLĪ-tis)*
17. retinopathy *(ret-i-NOP-a-thē)*
18. ophthalmoscope *(of-THAL-mō-skōp)*
19. ophthalmology *(of-thal-MOL-ō-jē)*
20. iridectomy *(ir-i-DEK-tō-mē)*

21. iridoplegia *(ir-id-ō-PLĒ-jē-a)*
22. pertaining to the eye or vision
23. outside the eye
24. instrument used to incise the sclera
25. inflammation of the cornea
26. behind the lens
27. incision of the ciliary muscle
28. pertaining to the choroid and retina
29. inflammation of the iris and ciliary body

Exercise 18-5

1. macropsia *(mak-ROP-sē-a)*
2. achromatopsia *(a-krō-ma-TOP-sē-a)*
3. diplopia *(dip-LŌ-pē-a)*
4. presbyopia *(pres-bē-Ō-pē-a)*
5. ametropia *(am-e-TRŌ-pē-a)*
6. heterometropia *(het-er-ō-me-TRŌ-pē-a)*

Labeling Exercise

The Ear

1. pinna
2. external auditory canal (meatus)
3. tympanic membrane
4. malleus
5. incus
6. stapes
7. eustachian (auditory) tube
8. semicircular canals
9. vestibule
10. cochlea
11. vestibulocochlear (auditory) nerve

The Eye

1. vitreous body
2. choroid
3. retina
4. fovea
5. optic nerve
6. optic disk (blind spot)
7. sclera
8. zonule (suspensory ligament)
9. iris
10. cornea
11. lens

Chapter Review 18-1

1. e
2. d
3. a
4. c
5. b
6. b
7. e
8. c
9. a
10. d
11. d
12. e
13. a
14. c
15. b
16. e
17. d
18. a
19. b
20. c
21. d
22. e
23. b
24. a
25. c
26. cochlea
27. stapes
28. retina
29. cornea
30. tympanic membrane
31. eye
32. one who studies and treats hearing disorders
33. pertaining to an eyelid
34. surgical excision of the eye
35. inflammation of the cornea and iris
36. around the lens
37. pertaining to the choroid and retina
38. inflammation of the tympanic membrane
39. analgesia *(an-al-JĒ-zē-a)*
40. audiometry
41. stapedectomy
42. retinitis
43. otoplasty
44. sclerokeratitis
45. pupillometry
46. retinopathy
47. cochlear
48. uveal

49. vestibular
50. scleral
51. pupillary
52. corneal
53. The medical specialty that deals with diseases of the ear, nose, and larynx
    a. ear
    b. nose
    c. larynx
    d. study of
54. Unequal refractive powers in the two eyes
    a. not, without
    b. equal
    c. measure
    d. vision
55. Abnormal touch sensation
    a. abnormal
    b. sensation
    c. condition of

Chapter Review 18-2

1. d
2. a
3. e
4. c
5. b
6. d
7. e
8. a
9. c
10. b
11. d
12. c
13. e
14. b
15. a
16. b
17. e
18. d
19. c
20. a
21. d
22. c
23. e
24. a
25. b
26. conjunctiva
27. uvea
28. iris
29. pupil
30. ear
31. the eyes
32. pertaining to sound or hearing
33. pertaining to tears
34. outside the eye
35. absence of a lens
36. beneath the sclera
37. myringotomy; also tympanotomy
38. salpingoscope
39. vestibulocochlear
40. otorrhea
41. uveoscleritis
42. cyclectomy
43. dacryocystitis
44. iridotomy
45. mydriasis
46. esotropia
47. sc
48. OD
49. hyperesthesia
50. blindness in one half the visual field
    a. half
    b. without, lack of
    c. vision
51. Defect of vision in which all objects appear colored
    a. excess
    b. color
    c. vision

Answers to Case Study Questions

1. a
2. e
3. b
4. e
5. b
6. d
7. aural
8. tympanogram
9. tinnitus
10. vertigo
11. malaise
12. nystagmus
13. ataxia
14. phacoemulsification
15. aspiration
16. miosis
17. above threshold level
18. on both sides
19. pertaining to the eye
20. within the eye
21. under or below the conjunctiva

Answers to Crossword Puzzle

THE SENSES

	1 O				2 T		3 L		4 S		5 O
6 L	U	Q		7 C	A	T	A	R	A	C	T
A			8 M	■	C	■	C		L		O
9 R	E	10 C	E	P	T	O	R		P		
G	■	11 O	S	■	I		12 I	R	I	D	13 O
14 E	15 A	R	■	16 S	L		M		N		T
	17 S	T	A	P	E	S			G		O
		I	■	O			18 A	C	O	U	S
	19 R	■	20 I	N	C	21 U	S				C
22 I	O	P		D		V		23 O	24 P	T	O
25 M	D			E		E			R	■	P
	26 S	C	L	E	R	A		27 C	O	N	E

19 *The Skeleton*

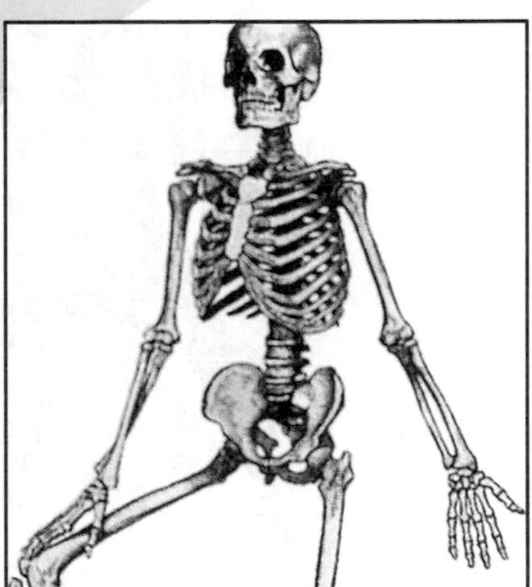

Chapter Contents

Objectives

After study of this chapter you should be able to:

1. Compare the axial skeleton and the appendicular skeleton
2. Compare a suture, a symphysis, and a synovial joint
3. Identify and use roots pertaining to the skeleton
4. Briefly describe formation of bone tissue
5. Describe the main disorders that affect the skeleton and joints
6. Describe the common methods used to diagnose and treat disorders of the skeleton
7. Label diagrams of the skeleton
8. Label a diagram of a long bone
9. Interpret abbreviations used in relation to the skeleton
10. Analyze several case studies pertaining to bones and joints

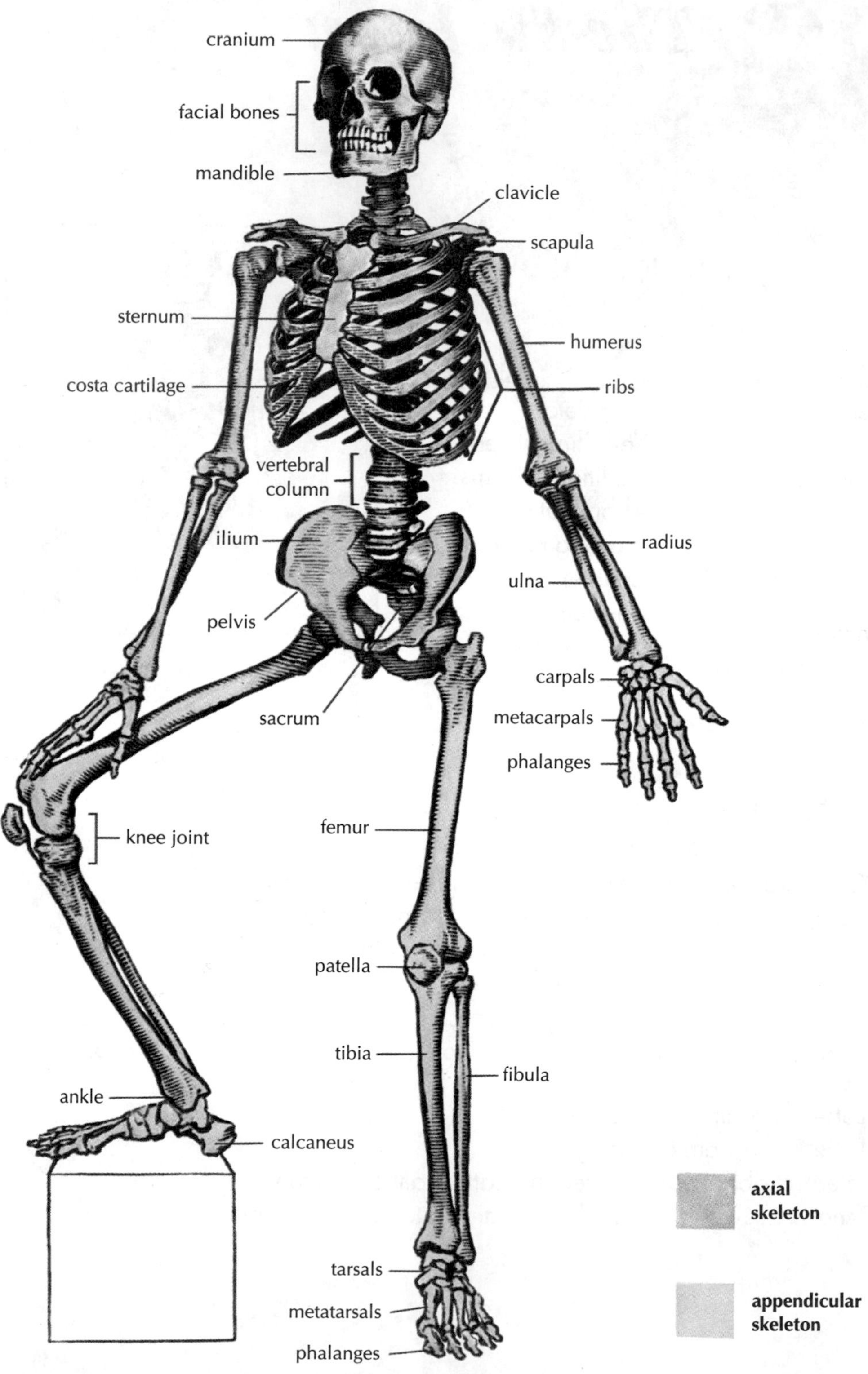

FIGURE 19-1. The skeleton.

Divisions of the Skeleton

The skeleton forms the framework of the body, protects vital organs, and works with the muscular system to produce movement. The human adult skeleton is composed of 206 **bones**. It is divided for study into the axial skeleton and the appendicular skeleton (Fig. 19-1).

The **axial skeleton** consists of the skull (Fig. 19-2), the spinal column, the ribs, and the sternum. As shown in Figure 19-3, the 26 vertebrae of the spinal column are divided into five regions: cervical (7); thoracic (12); lumbar (5); the sacrum (5 fused); and the coccyx (4–5 fused). Between the vertebrae are disks of cartilage that add strength and flexibility to the spine.

The **appendicular skeleton** consists of the bones of the arms and legs, the shoulder girdle, and the pelvis. Each of the two pelvic bones is formed of 3 fused bones (Fig. 19-4). The large, flared, upper bone is the **ilium**.

Bone Formation

Bone is formed by the gradual addition of calcium and phosphorus salts to cartilage or fibrous connective tissue. This process of **ossification** begins before birth and continues to adulthood. Although bone appears to be inert, it is actually living tissue that is constantly being replaced and remodeled throughout life. Three types of bone cells are involved in these changes: **osteoblasts** are the cells that produce bone; **osteocytes** are mature bone cells; and **osteoclasts** are involved in the breakdown of bone tissue to release needed minerals or to allow for reshaping and repair. The process of destroy-

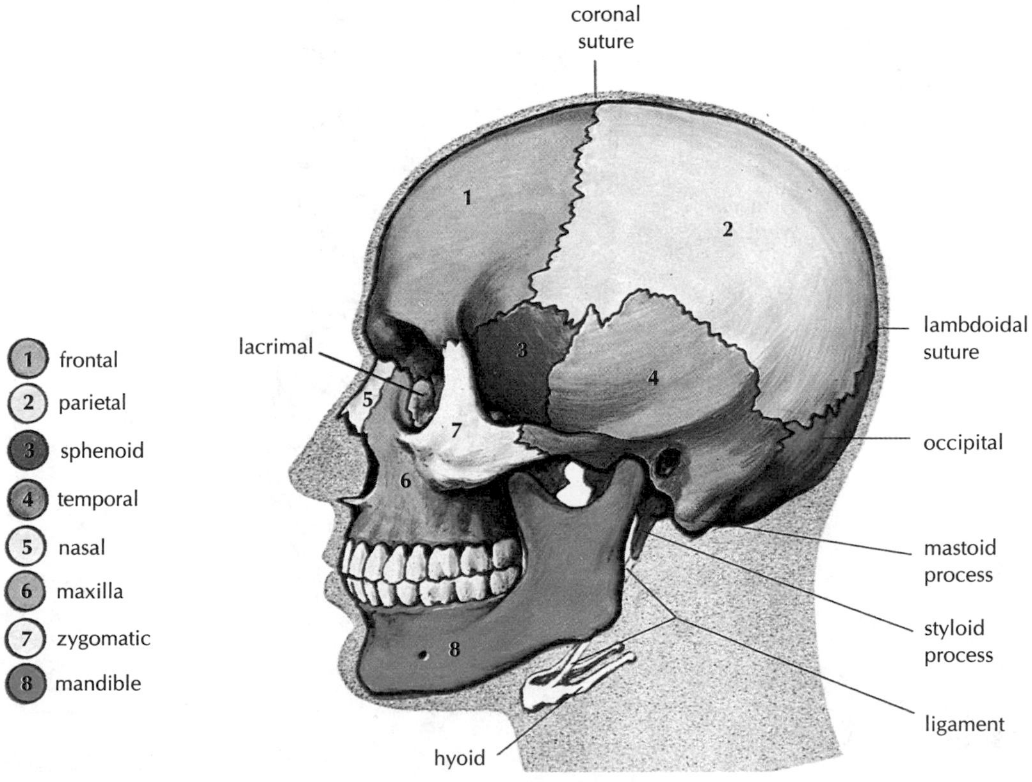

FIGURE 19-2. The skull from the left. An additional cranial bone, the ethmoid, is visible mainly from the interior of the skull.

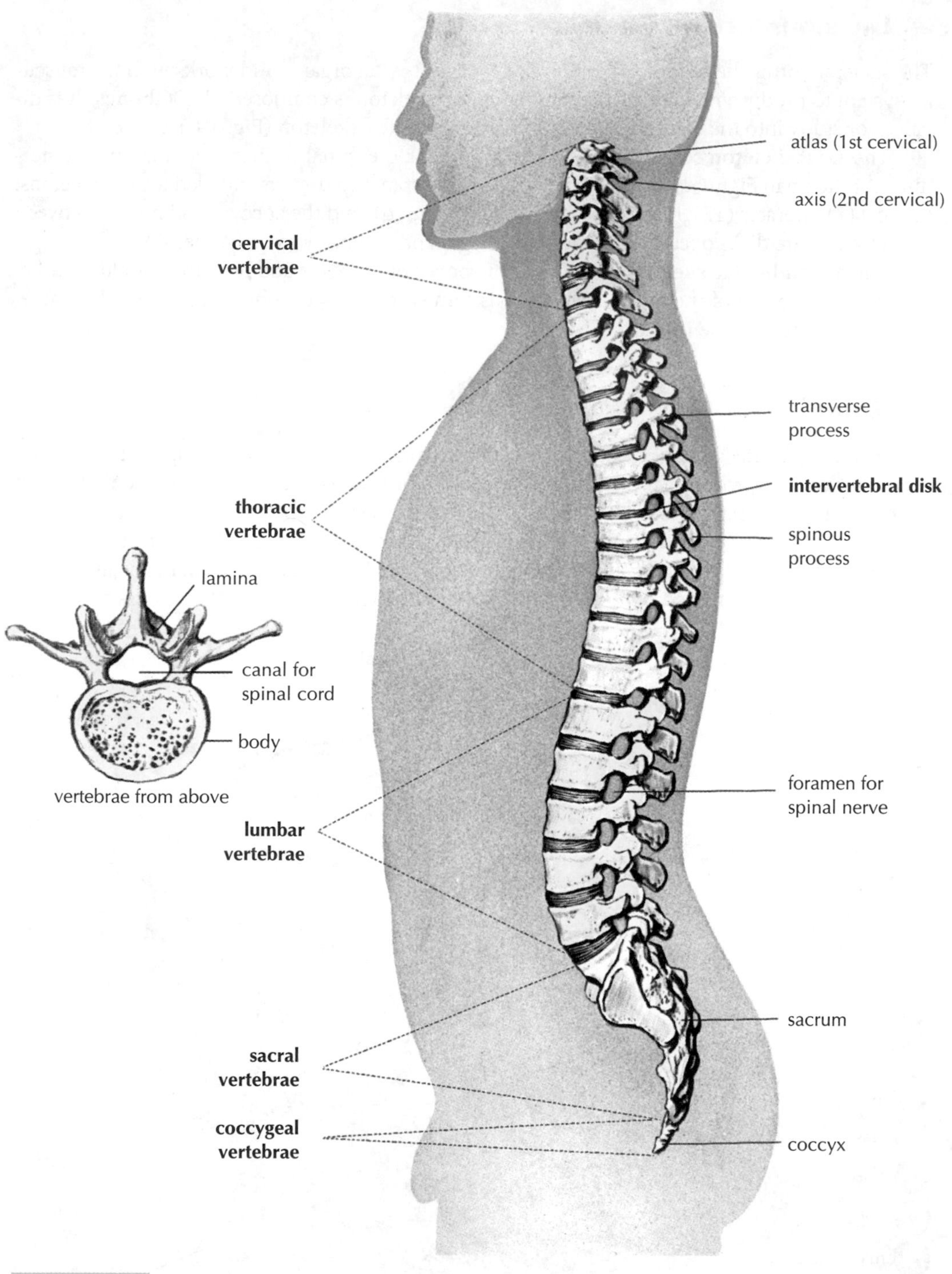

FIGURE 19-3. Vertebral column from the side.

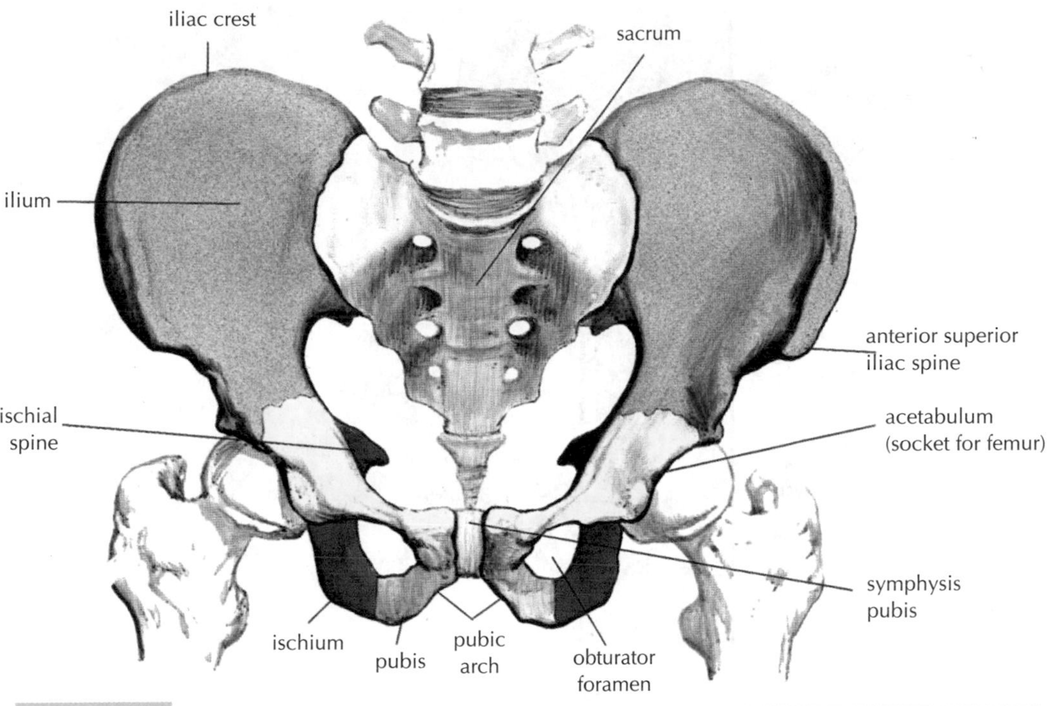

FIGURE 19-4. The pelvis.

ing bone so that its components can be taken into the circulation is called **resorption**. This occurs normally throughout life; in disease states, it may be out of pace with bone production.

Structure of a Long Bone

A typical long bone (Fig. 19-5) has a shaft or **diaphysis** composed of compact bone tissue. Within the shaft is a medullary cavity containing fatty yellow **bone marrow**. The irregular **epiphysis** at either end is made of a less dense, spongy bone tissue containing the blood-forming red bone marrow. A thin layer of cartilage covers the epiphysis and protects the bone surface. Between the diaphysis and the epiphysis at each end of the bone, in a region called the **metaphysis**, is the growth region or **epiphyseal plate**. When the bone stops growing in length, this area becomes fully calcified but remains visible as the epiphyseal line. The thin layer of fibrous tissue that covers the outside of the bone, the **periosteum**, nourishes and protects the bone and also generates new bone cells for growth and repair.

Long bones are found in the arms, legs, hands, and feet. Other types of bones are described as flat (ie, cranial bones), short (ie, wrist and ankle bones), or irregular (ie, facial bones and vertebrae).

Joints

The joints or **articulations** are classified according to the degree of movement they allow. A **suture** is an immovable joint held together by fibrous connective tissue, as is found between the bones of the skull (see Figure 19-2). A **symphysis** is a slightly movable joint connected by cartilage. Examples are the joints between the bodies of the vertebrae (see Figure 19-3) and the joint between the pubic bones (see Figure 19-4). A freely movable joint is called a **synovial joint** or **diarthrosis**.

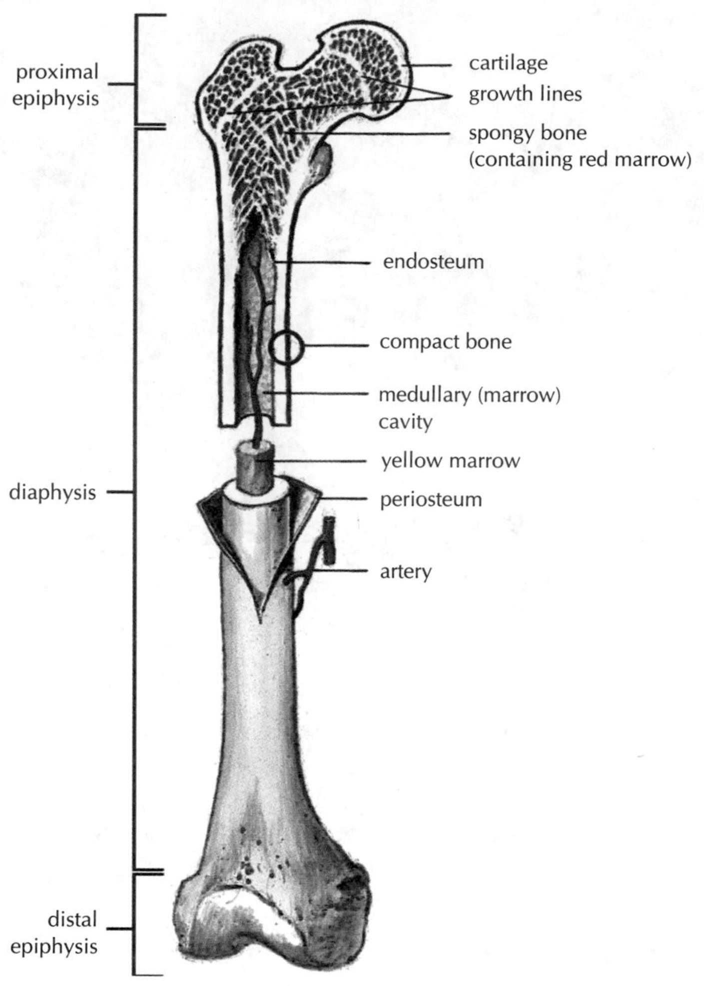

FIGURE 19-5. The structure of a long bone.

Such joints allow for a wide range of movements as described in Chapter 20. The cavity of a diarthrotic joint contains **synovial fluid**, which cushions and lubricates the joint. This fluid is produced by the synovial membrane that lines the joint cavity. Synovial joints are stabilized and strengthened by **ligaments** which connect the articulating bones.

KEY TERMS

Normal Structure and Function

articulation *(ar-tik-ū-LĀ-shun)* — A joint

bone — A calcified form of dense connective tissue; osseous tissue. Also an individual unit of the skeleton made of such tissue (root oste/o).

bone marrow — The soft material that fills the cavities of a bone. Yellow marrow fills the central cavity of the long bones; blood cells are formed in red bone marrow, which is located in spongy bone tissue (root myel/o).

bursa (*BUR-sa*) — A fluid filled sac that reduces friction near a joint (root burs/o)

cartilage (*KAR-ti-lij*) — A type of dense connective tissue that is found in the skeleton, larynx, trachea, and bronchi. It is the precursor to most bone tissue (root chondr/o).

diarthrosis (*di-ar-THRŌ-sis*) — A freely movable joint. Also called a synovial joint (adj. diarthrotic).

diaphysis (*dī-AF-i-sis*) — The shaft of a long bone

epiphysis (*e-PIF-i-sis*) — The irregularly shaped end of a long bone

epiphyseal plate (*ep-i-FIZ-ē-al*) — The growth region of a long bone; located in the metaphysis, between the diaphysis and epiphysis. When bone growth ceases, this area appears as the epiphyseal line.

ilium (*IL-ē-um*) — The large, flared, upper portion of the pelvic bone (adj. iliac; root ili/o)

joint — The junction between two bones; articulation (root arthr/o)

ligament (*LIG-a-ment*) — A strong band of connective tissue that joins one bone to another

metaphysis (*me-TAF-i-sis*) — The region of a long bone between the diaphysis (shaft) and epiphysis (end); during development, the growing region of a long bone

ossification (*os-i-fi-KĀ-shun*) — The formation of bone tissue (from L. *os* meaning "bone")

osteoblast (*OS-tē-ō-blast*) — A cell that produces bone tissue

osteoclast (*OS-tē-ō-clast*) — A cell that destroys bone tissue

osteocyte (*OS-tē-ō-sit*) — A mature bone cell that nourishes and maintains bone tissue

periosteum (*per-ē-OS-tē-um*) — The fibrous membrane that covers the surface of a bone

resorption (*rē-SORP-shun*) — Removal of bone by breakdown and absorption into the circulation

suture (*SŪ-chur*) — An immovable joint

symphysis (*SIM-fi-sis*) — A slightly movable joint

synovial fluid (*sin-O-vē-al*) — The fluid contained in a freely movable (diarthrotic) joint; synovia (root synov/i)

synovial joint — A freely movable joint. It has a joint cavity containing synovial fluid. A diarthrosis.

Roots Pertaining to Skeleton, Bones, and Joints

Roots for Bones and Joints

Root	Meaning	Example	Definition of Example
oste/o	bone	osteopenia *os-tē-ō-PĒ-nē-a*	deficiency of bone tissue
myel/o	bone marrow; also, spinal cord	myeloblast *MĪ-e-lō-blast*	immature bone marrow cell
chondr/o	cartilage	chondrogenesis *kon-drō-JEN-e-sis*	formation of cartilage
arthr/o	joint	arthrosis *ar-THRŌ-sis*	joint; condition affecting a joint
synov/i	synovial fluid, joint, or membrane	asynovia *a-sin-Ō-vē-a*	lack of synovial fluid
burs/o	bursa	bursolith *BUR-sō-lith*	stone in a bursa

Exercise 19-1

Fill in the blanks:

1. The term *osteoid (OS-tē-oyd)* means resembling ______.
2. Arthroplasty *(AR-thrō-plas-tē)* is plastic repair of a(n) ______.
3. A chondrocyte *(KON-drō-sīt)* is a cell found in ______.

Define the following terms:

4. Osteogenesis *(os-tē-ō-JEN-e-sis)* ______
5. Chondromalacia *(kon-drō-ma-LĀ-shē-a)* ______
6. Arthropathy *(ar-THROP-a-thē)* ______
7. Peribursal *(per-i-BER-sal)* ______

Word building. Write a word for each of the following definitions:

8. Inflammation of bone ______
9. Inflammation of bone and bone marrow ______
10. Pertaining to or ressembling (-oid) bone marrow ______
11. Tumor of cartilage ______
12. Instrument for examining the interior of a joint ______

13. Inflammation of a joint ________________
14. Excision of a synovial membrane ________________

The word *ostosis* means "bone growth." Use this as a suffix for the following two words:

15. Excess growth of bone ________________
16. Abnormal growth of bone ________________

Roots for the Skeleton

Root	Meaning	Example	Definition of Example
crani/o	skull, cranium	craniostosis *krā-nē-os-TŌ-sis*	ossification of the cranial sutures
spondyl/o	vertebra	spondylolysis *spon-di-LOL-i-sis*	destruction and separation of a vertebra
vertebr/o	vertebra, spinal column	prevertebral *prē-VER-te-bral*	before or in front of the spinal column
rachi/o	spine	rachischisis *rā-KIS-ki-sis*	fissure of the spine; spina bifida
cost/o	rib	infracostal *in-fra-KOS-tal*	below the ribs
sacr/o	sacrum	craniosacral *krā-nē-ō-SĀ-kral*	pertaining to the skull and sacrum
coccy, coccyg/o	coccyx	coccygeal *kok-SIJ-ē-al*	pertaining to the coccyx
pelvi/o	pelvis	pelvimetry *pel-VIM-e-trē*	measurement of the pelvis
ili/o	ilium	sacroiliac *sak-rō-IL-ē-ak*	pertaining to the sacrum and ilium

Exercise 19-2

Write the adjective that fits each of the following definitions:

1. Pertaining to (-al) the skull ________________
2. Pertaining to (-al) a rib ________________
3. Pertaining to (-ic) the pelvis ________________
4. Pertaining to (-ac) the ilium ________________
5. Pertaining to (-al) the spinal column ________________

Define the following terms:

6. Craniotomy *(krā-nē-OT-ō-mē)* ________________
7. Endocranial *(en-dō-KRĀ-nē-al)* ________________
8. Spondylodynia *(spon-di-lō-DIN-ē-a)* ________________
9. Paravertebral *(par-a-VER-te-bral)* ________________
10. Intrapelvic *(in-tra-PEL-vik)* ________________

Build a word that fits each of the following definitions:

11. Congenital fissure of the skull ________________
12. Inflammation of the vertebrae (use spondyl/o) ________________
13. Surgical puncture of the spine; spinal tap ________________
14. Surgical excision of a rib ________________
15. Pertaining to the ilium and pelvis ________________
16. Near the sacrum ________________
17. Excision of the coccyx ________________
18. Pertaining to the ilium and coccyx ________________

Clinical Aspects of the Skeleton

Disorders of the skeleton often involve surrounding tissues—ligaments, tendons, and muscles—and may be studied together as diseases of the musculoskeletal system. (The muscular system is described in Chapter 20). The medical specialty that concentrates on diseases of the skeletal and muscular systems is **orthopedics**. Physical therapists and occupational therapists must also understand these systems.

Most abnormalities of the bones and joints appear on simple x-rays. (see Figure 19-6 for a normal x-ray of a joint.) Radioactive bone scans, CT, and MRI scans are used as well. Also indicative of disorders are changes in blood levels of calcium and **alkaline phosphatase**, an enzyme needed for calcification of bone.

Infection

Osteomyelitis is an inflammation of bone caused by pus-forming bacteria that enter through a wound or are carried by the blood. Often the blood-rich ends of the long bones are invaded, and the infection then spreads to other regions, such as the bone marrow and even the joints. The use of antibiotics has greatly reduced the threat of osteomyelitis.

Tuberculosis may spread to bone, especially the long bones of the arms and legs and the bones of the wrist and ankle. Tuberculosis of the spine is **Pott's disease**. Infected vertebrae are weakened and may collapse causing pain, deformity, and pressure on the spinal cord. Antibiotics can

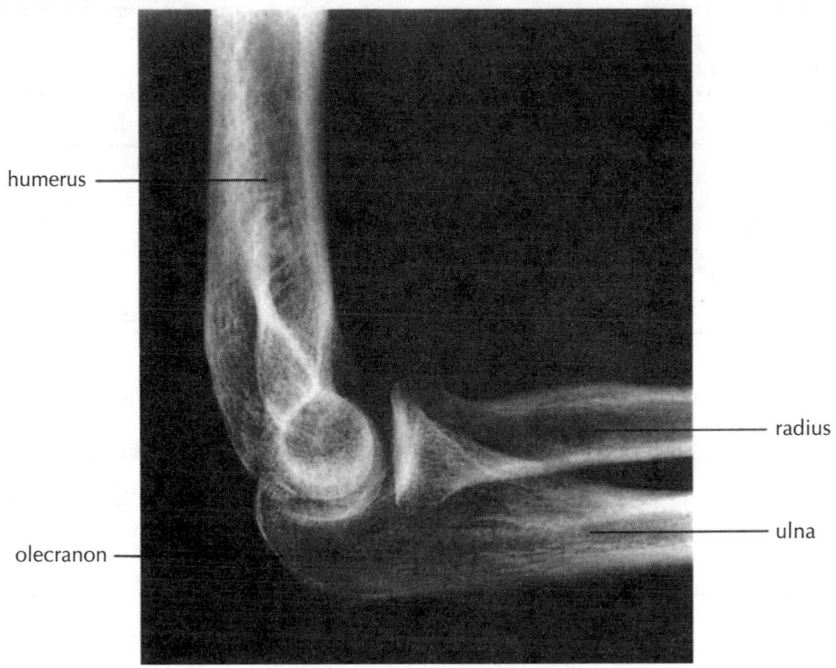

FIGURE 19-6. X-ray of the elbow. Lateral view. (Greenspan A: Orthopedic Radiology, p 319. New York: Gower, 1988.)

be used to control tuberculosis as long as the strains are not resistant to these drugs and the host is not weakened by other diseases.

Fractures

A **fracture** is a break in a bone. The effects of a fracture depend on the location and severity of the break; the amount of associated injury; possible complications, such as infections; and success of healing, which may take months. In a **closed** or **simple fracture**, the skin is not broken. If the fracture is accompanied by a wound in the skin it is described as an **open fracture**. Various types of fractures are listed in Table 19-1 and illustrated in Figure 19-7. **Reduction of a fracture** refers to realignment of the broken bone. If no surgery is required, the reduction is described as closed; an open reduction is one that requires surgery to place the bone in proper position.

Metabolic Bone Diseases

Osteoporosis is a loss of bone mass that results in weakening of the bones. A decline in estrogens after menopause makes women over age 50 most susceptible to this disorder. Efforts to prevent osteoporosis include adequate intake of calcium, engaging in weight-bearing exercise, and estrogen replacement therapy (ERT), also known as hormone replacement therapy (HRT). Osteo-

TABLE 19-1 Types of Fractures

Fracture	Description
closed	a simple fracture with no open wound
Colles' *(KOL-ēz)*	fracture of the distal end of the radius with backward displacement of the hand
comminuted *(COM-i-nū-ted)*	fracture in which the bone is splintered or crushed
compression	fracture due to force from both ends, as to a vertebra
greenstick	one side of the bone is broken and the other side is bent
impacted	one fragment is driven into the other
oblique	break occurs at an angle across the bone; usually one fragment slips by the other
open	fracture is associated with an open wound, or broken bone protrudes through the skin
Pott's	fracture of the distal end of the fibula with injury to the tibial joint
spiral	fracture is in a spiral or S shape; usually caused by twisting injuries
transverse	a break at right angles to the long axis of a bone

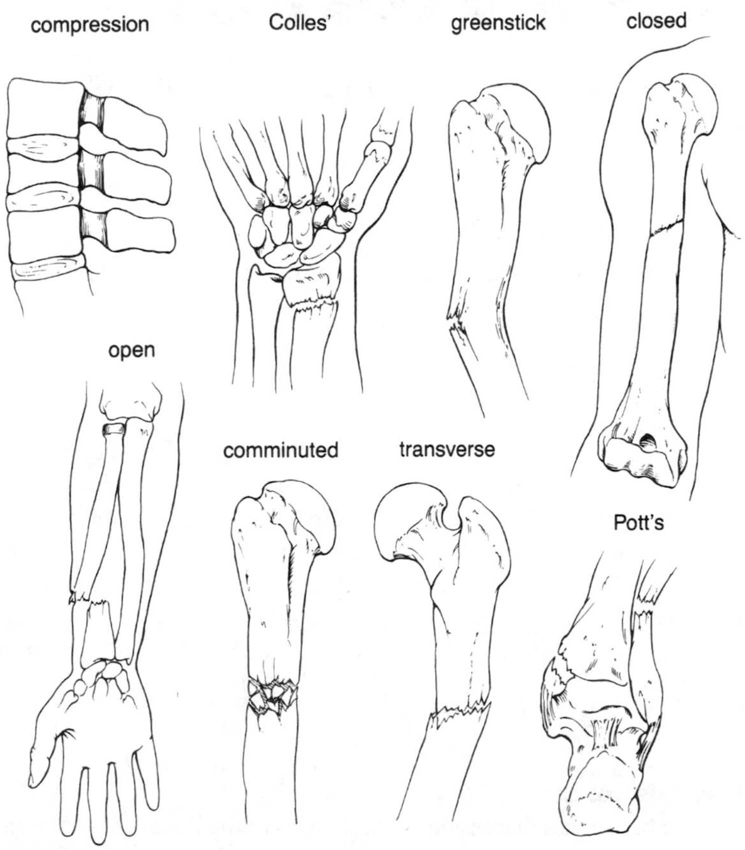

FIGURE 19-7. Types of fractures.

porosis also may be caused by nutritional deficiencies; disuse, as in paralysis or immobilization in a cast; and excess steroids from the adrenal cortex.

In **osteomalacia** there is a softening of bone tissue due to lack of formation of calcium salts. Possible causes include deficiency of vitamin D, needed to absorb calcium and phosphorus from the intestine; renal disorders; liver disease; and certain intestinal disorders. When osteomalacia occurs in children, the disease is called **rickets**. It is usually due to deficiency of vitamin D.

Paget's disease (osteitis deformans) is a disorder of aging in which bones become larger but softer and weaker, resulting in bowing of the long bones. Paget's disease usually involves the bones of the axial skeleton, causing pain, fractures, and hearing loss. With time there may be neurologic signs, heart failure, and predisposition to cancer of the bones.

Neoplasms

Osteogenic sarcoma (osteosarcoma) most commonly occurs in the growing region of a bone, especially around the knee. This is a highly malignant tumor that often requires amputation. It most commonly metastasizes to the lungs.

Chondrosarcoma usually appears in midlife. As the name implies, this tumor arises in cartilage. It may require amputation and most frequently metastasizes to the lungs.

In cases of malignant bone tumors, early surgical removal is important to prevent metastasis. Signs of bone tumors are pain, easy fracture, and increases in serum calcium and alkaline phosphatase. Aside from primary tumors, neoplasms at other sites often metastasize to bone, most commonly to the spine.

Arthritis

In general, **arthritis** means inflammation of a joint. The most common form is **osteoarthritis** or degenerative joint disease (DJD) (Fig. 19-8). This is a gradual degeneration of articular (joint) cartilage due to wear-and-tear. It usually appears at midlife and beyond and involves the weight-bearing joints and joints of the fingers. X-rays show a narrowing of the joint cavity and thickening of the bone. The cartilage may crack and break loose, causing inflammation in the joint and exposing the underlying bone. Osteoarthritis is treated with analgesics to relieve pain, **anti-inflammatory agents**, such as corticosteroids and **nonsteroidal anti-inflammatory drugs** (NSAIDs).

Rheumatoid arthritis is a systemic inflammatory disease of the joints that commonly appears in young adult women. Its exact causes are unknown, but it may involve immunologic reactions. A group of antibodies called **rheumatoid factor** often appears in the blood, but is not always specific for rheumatoid arthritis, as it may occur in other systemic diseases as well. There is an overgrowth of the synovial membrane that lines the joint cavity. As this covers and destroys the joint cartilage, synovial fluid accumulates, causing swelling of the joint. There is degeneration of the underlying bone, eventually causing fusion of the bones, or **ankylosis**. Treatment includes rest, physical therapy, analgesics, and anti-inflammatory drugs.

Gout is caused by an increased level of uric acid in the blood, salts of which are deposited in the joints. It mostly occurs in middle-aged men and almost always involves pain at the base of the great toe. The cause may be a primary metabolic disturbance or a secondary effect of another disease, as of the kidneys. Gout is treated with drugs to suppress formation of uric acid or to increase elimination of uric acid (uricosuric agent).

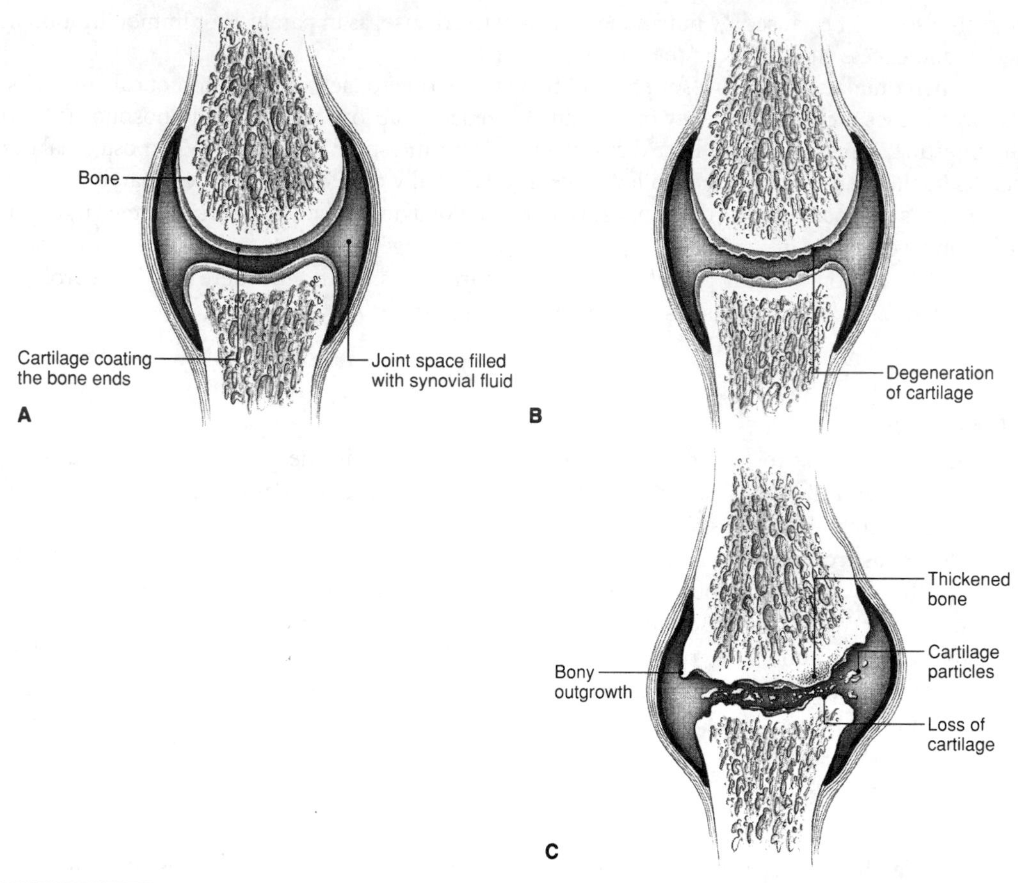

FIGURE 19-8. Osteoarthritis. **(A)** Normal joint. **(B)** Early stage of osteoarthritis. **(C)** Late stage of disease. (Reprinted by permission of Medical Economies Publishing. © Kevin Somerville, artist.)

Disorders of the Spine

Ankylosing spondylitis is a disease of the spine that appears mainly in males. Joint cartilage is destroyed; eventually the disks between the vertebrae calcify and there is fusion of the bones (ankylosis). Changes begin low in the spine and progress upward, limiting mobility.

In cases of a **herniated disk** (Fig. 19-9), the central mass (nucleus pulposus) of the disk between two vertebrae ruptures into the spinal canal. This commonly occurs in the lumbosacral or cervical regions of the spine as a result of injury or heavy lifting. The herniated or "slipped" disk puts pressure on the spinal cord or spinal nerves, often causing pain along the sciatic nerve (sciatica). There may be spasms of the back muscles, leading to disability. Treatment is bed rest; drugs to reduce pain, muscle spasms, and inflammation; followed by an exercise program to strengthen muscles. In severe cases, it may be necessary to remove the disk surgically in a **discectomy**, sometimes followed by fusion of the vertebrae with a bone graft to stabilize the spine. Using techniques of microsurgery, surgery done through a small incision under magnification, it is now possible to remove an exact amount of extruded disk tissue instead of the entire disk.

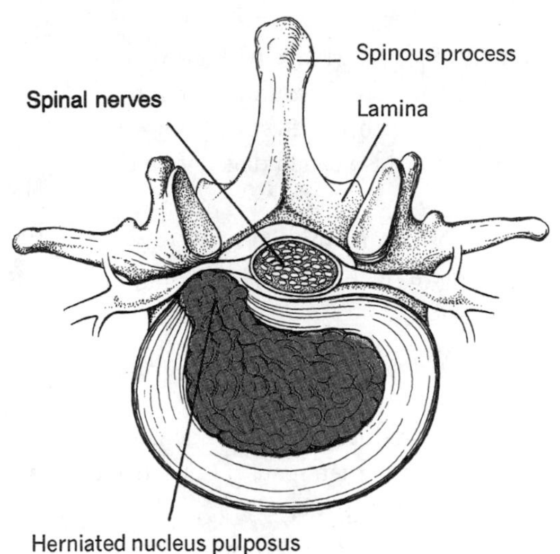

FIGURE 19-9. A ruptured intervertebral disk. The soft central pulp of the disk protrudes into the vertebral canal, putting pressure on the spinal nerve root. (Chaffee EE, Lytle IM: Basic Physiology and Anatomy, 4th ed, p 103. Philadelphia: JB Lippincott, 1980.)

KEY CLINICAL TERMS

Disorders

ankylosing spondylitis *(ang-ki-LŌ-sing spon-di-LĪ-tis)* — A chronic, progressive inflammatory disease involving the joints of the spine and surrounding soft tissue. Most common in young males. Also called rheumatoid spondylitis.

ankylosis *(ang-ki-LŌ-sis)* — Immobility and fixation of a joint

arthritis *(ar-THRĪ-tis)* — Inflammation of a joint

chondrosarcoma *(kon-drō-sar-KŌ-ma)* — A malignant tumor of cartilage

degenerative joint disease (DJD) — Osteoarthritis (see below)

fracture — A break in a bone. In a simple fracture, the broken bone does not penetrate the skin; in an open fracture, there is an accompanying wound in the skin.

gout *(gowt)* — A form of acute arthritis, usually beginning in the knee or foot, caused by deposit of uric acid salts in the joints

herniated disk — Protrusion of the center (nucleus pulposus) of an intervertebral disk into the spinal canal; ruptured or "slipped" disk

nucleus pulposus *(NŪ-klē-us pul-PŌ-sus)* — The central portion of an intervertebral disk

(continued)

osteoarthritis (OA) *(os-tē-ō-ar-THRĪ-tis)*	Progressive deterioration of joint cartilage with growth of new bone and soft tissue in and around the joint. The most common form of arthritis. Results from wear-and-tear, injury, or disease. Also called degenerative joint disease (DJD).
osteogenic sarcoma	A malignant bone tumor; osteosarcoma
osteomalacia *(os-tē-ō-ma-LĀ-shē-a)*	A softening and weakening of the bones due to vitamin D deficiency or other disease
osteomyelitis *(os-tē-ō-mī-e-LĪ-tis)*	Inflammation of bone and bone marrow caused by infection, usually bacterial
osteoporosis *(os-tē-ō-po-RŌ-sis)*	A condition characterized by reduction in bone density. Most common in white women past menopause. Causative factors include, diet, activity, and estrogen levels.
Paget's disease *(PAJ-ets)*	Skeletal disease of the elderly characterized by thickening and softening of bones and bowing of long bones; osteitis deformans
Pott's disease	Inflammation of the vertebrae, usually caused by tuberculosis
rheumatoid arthritis *(RŪ-ma-toyd)*	A chronic autoimmune disease of unknown origin resulting in inflammation of peripheral joints and related structures. More common in women than men.
rheumatoid factor	A group of antibodies found in the blood in cases of rheumatoid arthritis and other systemic diseases
rickets *(RIK-ets)*	Faulty bone formation in children usually due to a deficiency of vitamin D
sciatica *(sī-AT-i-ka)*	Severe pain in the leg along the course of the sciatic nerve

Treatment

alkaline phosphatase *(AL-ka-lin FOS-fa-tās)*	An enzyme needed in the formation of bone. Serum activity of this enzyme is useful in diagnosis.
anti-inflammatory agent	Drug that reduces inflammation
discectomy *(dis-KEK-tō-mē)*	Surgical removal of a herniated intervertebral disk
nonsteroidal anti-inflammatory drug (NSAID)	Drug that reduces inflammation, but is not a steroid. Examples include aspirin and other inhibitors of prostaglandins, naturally produced substances that promote inflammation.
orthopedics *(or-thō-PĒ-diks)*	The study and treatment of disorders of the skeleton, muscles, and associated structures. Literally "straight" (ortho) "child" (ped).
reduction of a fracture	Return of a fractured bone to a normal position. May be closed (not requiring surgery) or open (requiring surgery).

ADDITIONAL TERMS

Normal Structure and Function*

acetabulum
(as-e-TAB-ū-lum)
The bony socket in the hip bone that holds the head of the femur

annulus fibrosus
(AN-ū-lus fi-BRŌ-sus)
The outer ringlike portion of an intervertebral disk

atlas
(AT-las)
The first cervical vertebra (see Figure 19-3); (root *atlant/o*)

axis
The second cervical vertebra (see Figure 19-3)

calvaria
(kal-VAR-ē-a)
The domelike upper portion of the skull

cruciate ligaments
(KRŪ-shē-āt)
Cross-shaped ligaments in the knee

genu
(JE-nu)
The knee

glenoid cavity
(GLEN-oyd)
The bony socket in the scapula that articulates with the head of the humerus

hallux
(HAL-uks)
The great toe

ischium
(IS-kē-um)
The lower portion of the pelvic bone (see Figure 19-4)

malleolus
(ma-LĒ-ō-lus)
The projection of the tibia or fibula on either side of the ankle

meniscus
(me-NIS-kus)
Crescent-shaped cartilage found in certain joints, such as the knee joint

olecranon
(ō-LEK-ra-non)
The process of the ulna that forms the elbow

pubis
(PŪ-bis)
The anterior part of the pelvic bone. The two pubic bones join anteriorly at the pubic symphysis (see Figure 19-4).

symphysis pubis
(SIM-fi-sis)
The anterior joint of the pelvis, formed by the union of the two pubic bones (see Figure 19-4); also called pubic symphysis

Symptoms and Conditions

achondroplasia
(a-kon-drō-PLĀ-zha)
Decreased growth of cartilage in the growth plate of long bones resulting in dwarfism. A genetic disorder.

bursitis
(bur-SĪ-tis)
Inflammation of a bursa, a small fluid-filled sac near a joint. Causes include injury, irritation, and joint disease. The shoulder, hip, elbow, and knee are common sites.

carpal tunnel syndrome
Numbness and weakness of the hand caused by pressure on the median nerve as it passes through a tunnel formed by carpal bones

*See Table 19-2 for a list of bone markings

(continued)

TABLE 19-2 Bone Markings

Marking	Description
condyle *KON-dīl*	smooth, rounded protuberance at a joint
crest	raised, narrow ridge (see iliac crest in Fig. 19-4)
epicondyle *ep-i-KON-dīl*	projection above a condyle
facet *FAS-et*	small, flattened surface
foramen *for-Ā-men*	rounded opening (see foramen for spinal nerve in Fig. 19-3)
fossa *FOS-a*	hollow cavity
meatus *mē-Ā-tus*	long channel within a bone
process	projection (see mastoid process and styloid process in Fig. 19-2)
sinus *SĪ-nus*	air-filled space or channel
spine	sharp projection (see ischial spine in Fig. 19-4)
trochanter *trō-KAN-ter*	large, blunt projection as at the top of the femur
tubercle *TŪ-ber-kl*	small, rounded projection
tuberosity *tū-ber-OS-i-tē*	large, rounded projection

chondroma
(kon-DRŌ-ma)
A benign tumor of cartilage

curvature of the spine
An exaggerated curve of the spine. Includes scoliosis (sideways curve in any region), lordosis (lumbar curve), and kyphosis (thoracic curve).

Ewing's tumor
A bone tumor that usually appears in children 5–15 years of age. It begins in the shaft of a bone and spreads readily to other bones. It may respond to radiation therapy, but then returns. Also called Ewing's sarcoma.

exostosis
(eks-os-TŌ-sis)
A bony outgrowth from the surface of a bone

giant cell tumor
A bone tumor that usually appears in children and young adults. The ends of the bones are destroyed, commonly at the knee, by a large mass that does not metastasize.

Heberden's nodes
(HĒ-ber-denz)
Small, hard nodules formed in the cartilage of the distal joints of the fingers in osteoarthritis

hemarthrosis
(hē-mar-THRŌ-sis)
Bleeding into a joint cavity

kyphosis *(kī-FŌ-sis)*	An exaggerated curve of the spine in the thoracic region; hunchback, humpback
lordosis *(lor-DŌ-sis)*	An exaggerated curve of the spine in the lumbar region; swayback
multiple myeloma	A cancer of blood-forming cells in bone marrow (see Chapter 10)
osteochondroma *(os-tē-ō-kon-DRŌ-ma)*	A benign tumor consisting of cartilage and bone
osteodystrophy *(os-tē-ō-DIS-trō-fē)*	Abnormal bone development
osteogenesis imperfecta	A hereditary disease resulting in the formation of brittle bones that fracture easily. There is faulty synthesis of collagen, the main structural protein in connective tissue.
osteoma *(os-tē-Ō-ma)*	A benign bone tumor that usually remains small and localized
osteopenia *(os-tē-ō-PĒ-nē-a)*	Lack of bone tissue. Decrease of bone density as seen in osteoporosis.
scoliosis *(skō-lē-Ō-sis)*	A sideways curvature of the spine in any region
spondylolisthesis *(spon-di-lō-LIS-the-sis)*	A forward displacement of one vertebra over another (*-listhesis* means "a slipping")
spondylosis *(spon-di-LŌ-sis)*	Degeneration and ankylosis of the vertebrae resulting in pressure on the spinal cord and nerve roots
sprain	Trauma to a joint involving the ligaments
subluxation *(sub-luk-SĀ-shun)*	A partial dislocation
talipes *(TAL-i-pēz)*	A deformity of the foot, especially one occurring congenitally; clubfoot
valgus *(VAL-gus)*	Bent outward
varus *(VAR-us)*	Bent inward
von Recklinghausen's disease	Loss of bone tissue caused by increased parathyroid hormone. Bones become decalcified, deformed, and fracture easily.

Diagnosis and Treatment

arthroclasia *(ar-thrō-KLĀ-zha)*	Surgical breaking of an ankylosed joint to provide movement
arthroscope *(AR-thrō-skōp)*	An endoscope for examining the interior of a joint (Fig. 19-10). May also be used to perform surgery on the joint, for example, to remove damaged cartilage.
arthroscopy *(ar-THROS-kō-pē)*	Use of an arthroscope to examine the interior of a joint or to perform surgery on the joint (see Figure 19-10)

(continued)

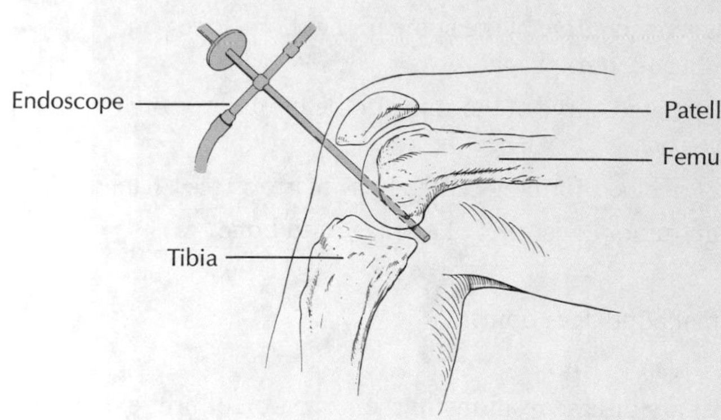

FIGURE 19-10. Arthroscopic examination of the knee. Endoscope is inserted between projections at the end of the femur to view the posterior of the knee.

goniometer *(gō-nē-OM-e-ter)* A device to measure joint angles and movements (root *goni/o* means "angle")

laminectomy *(lam-i-NEK-tō-mē)* Excision of the posterior arch (lamina) of a vertebra (see Figure 19-3)

meniscectomy *(men-i-SEK-tō-mē)* Removal of the cresent-shaped cartilage (meniscus) of the knee joint

myelogram *(MĪ-e-lō-gram)* X-ray of the spinal canal following injection of a radiopaque dye. Used to evaluate a herniated disk.

prosthesis *(PROS-thē-sis)* An artificial organ or part, such as an artificial limb

traction *(TRAK-shun)* The process of drawing or pulling, such as traction of the head in the treatment of injuries to the cervical vertebrae

ABBREVIATIONS

AE above the elbow
AK above the knee
BE below the elbow
BK below the knee.
C cervical vertebra; numbered C1–C7
Co coccyx; coccygeal
DIP distal interphalangeal (joint)
DJD degenerative joint disease
Fx fracture
HNP herniated nucleus pulposus
L lumbar vertebra; numbered L1–L5
MCP metacarpophalangeal (joint)
MTP metatarsophalangeal (joint)
NSAID(s) nonsteroidal anti-inflammatory drug(s)
OA osteoarthritis
ortho, ORTH orthopedics
PIP proximal interphalangeal (joint)
RA rheumatoid arthritis
S sacrum; sacral
T thoracic vertebra; numbered T1–T12
THR total hip replacement
TKR total knee replacement

Chapter 14
Labeling Exercises

Write the name of each numbered part on the corresponding line of the answer sheet.

The skeleton

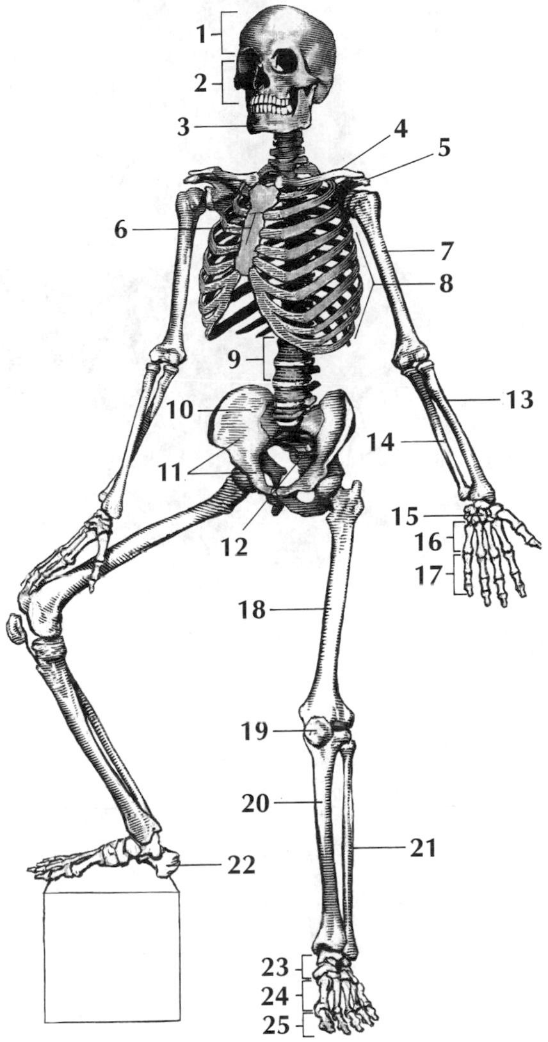

1. ______________________
2. ______________________
3. ______________________
4. ______________________
5. ______________________
6. ______________________
7. ______________________
8. ______________________
9. ______________________
10. ______________________
11. ______________________
12. ______________________
13. ______________________
14. ______________________
15. ______________________
16. ______________________
17. ______________________
18. ______________________
19. ______________________
20. ______________________
21. ______________________
22. ______________________
23. ______________________
24. ______________________
25. ______________________

calcaneus
carpals
clavicle
cranium
facial bones
femur
fibula
humerus
ilium
mandible
metacarpals
metatarsals
patella
pelvis
phalanges
phalanges
radius
ribs
sacrum
scapula
sternum
tarsals
tibia
ulna
vertebral column

Write the name of each numbered part on the corresponding line of the answer sheet.

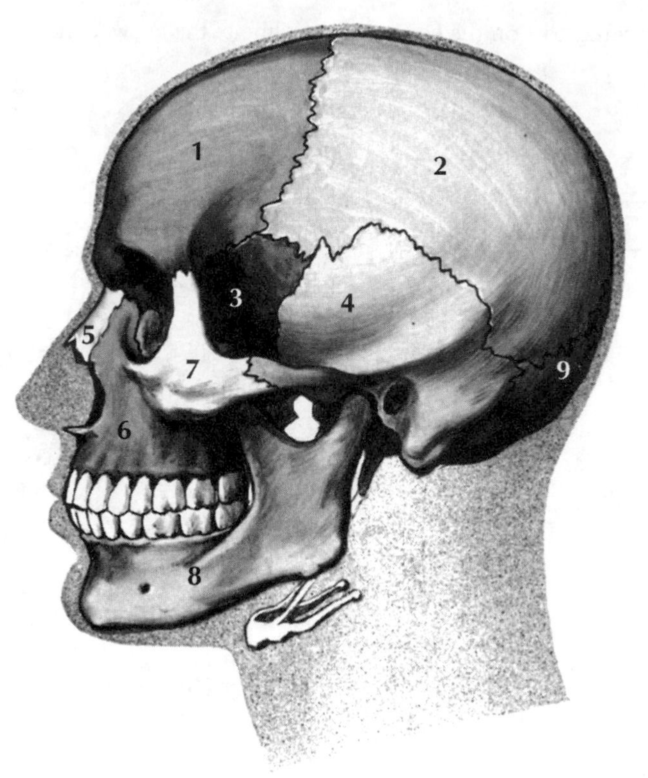

frontal
mandible
maxilla
nasal
occipital
parietal
sphenoid
temporal
zygomatic

1. ______________________
2. ______________________
3. ______________________
4. ______________________
5. ______________________
6. ______________________
7. ______________________
8. ______________________
9. ______________________

Write the name of each numbered part on the corresponding line of the answer sheet.

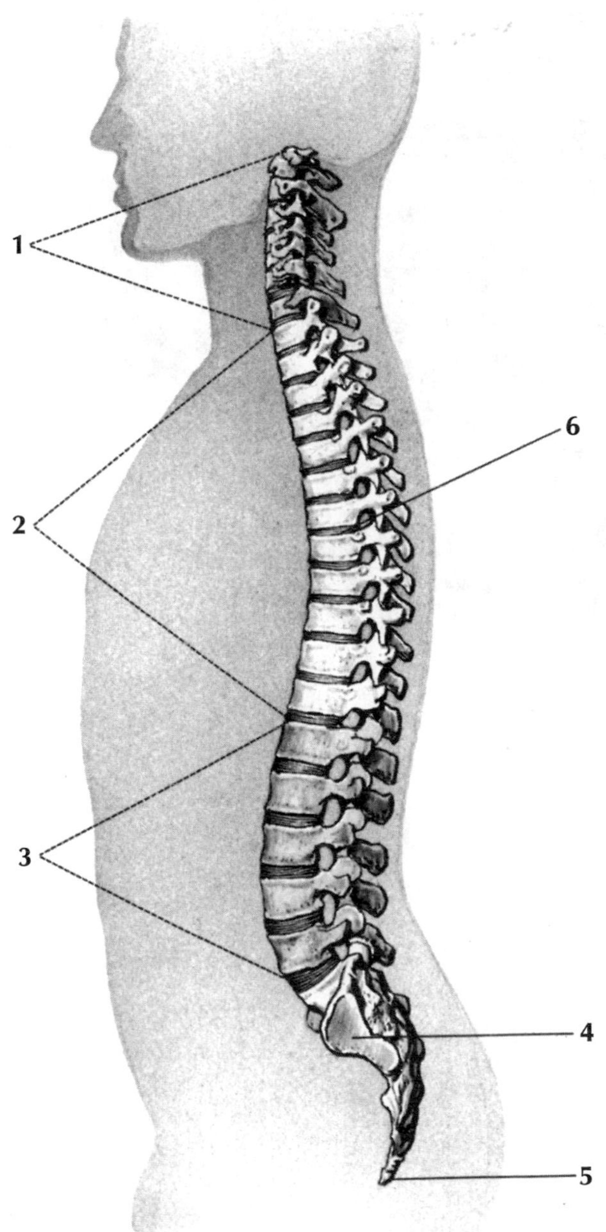

Vertebral column from the side

cervical vertebrae
coccyx
intervertebral disk
lumbar vertebrae
sacrum
thoracic vertebrae

1. ______________________ 4. ______________________

2. ______________________ 5. ______________________

3. ______________________ 6. ______________________

Write the name of each numbered part on the corresponding line of the answer sheet.

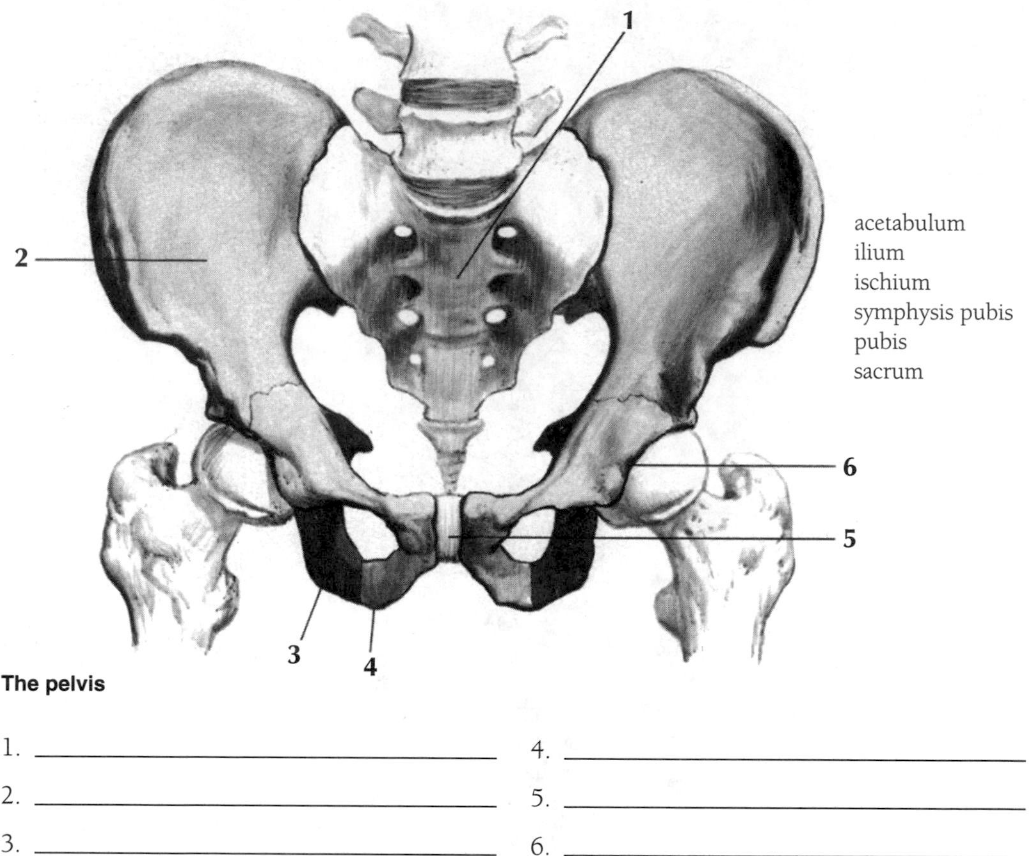

The pelvis

1. ______________________ 4. ______________________

2. ______________________ 5. ______________________

3. ______________________ 6. ______________________

Write the name of each numbered part on the corresponding line of the answer sheet.

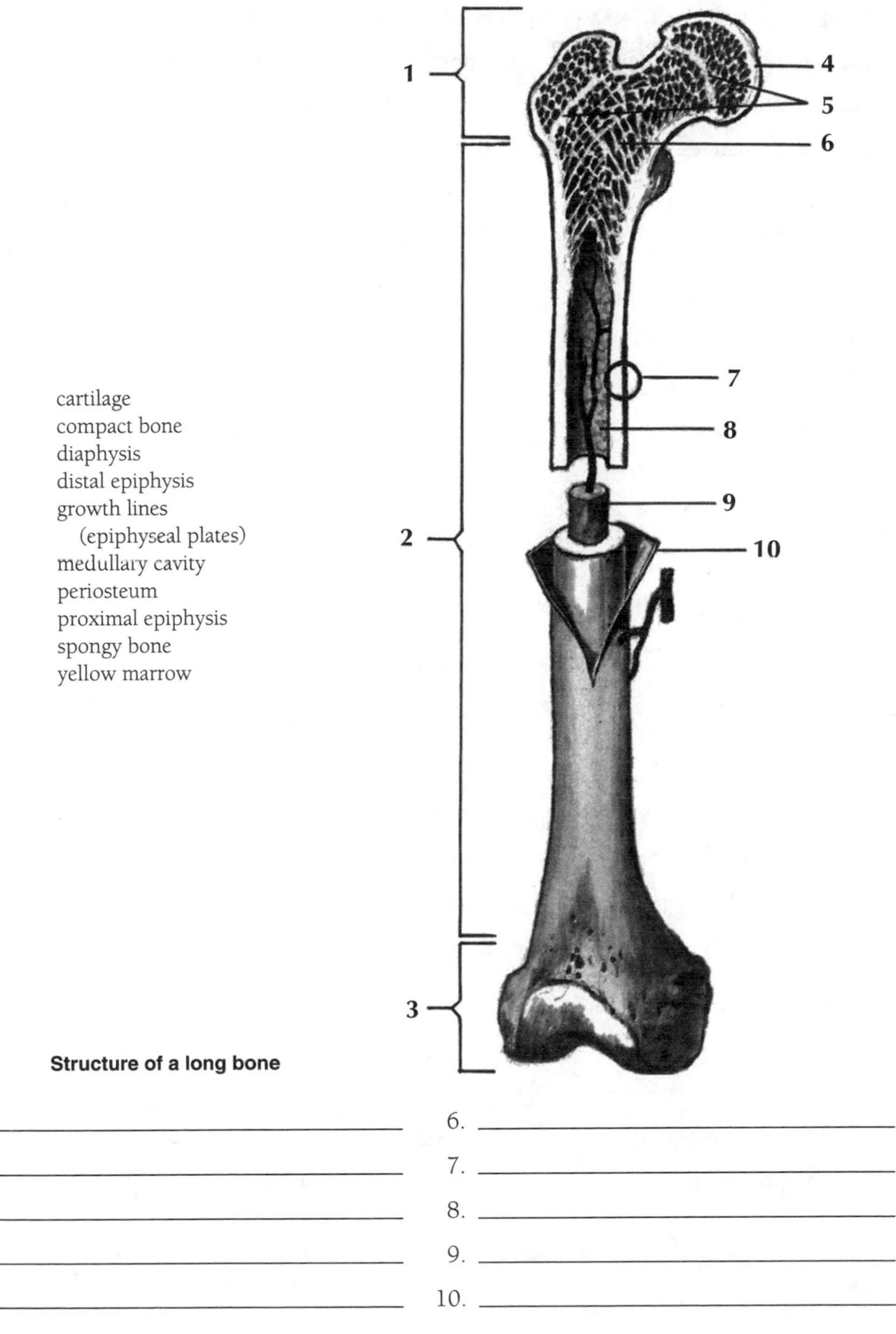

cartilage
compact bone
diaphysis
distal epiphysis
growth lines
(epiphyseal plates)
medullary cavity
periosteum
proximal epiphysis
spongy bone
yellow marrow

Structure of a long bone

1. ______________________
2. ______________________
3. ______________________
4. ______________________
5. ______________________
6. ______________________
7. ______________________
8. ______________________
9. ______________________
10. ______________________

CHAPTER REVIEW 19

Multiple choice. Match the terms in each of the sets below with their definitions and write the appropriate letter (a–e) to the left of each number.

_____ 1. bursa	a. upper portion of the pelvic bone
_____ 2. atlas	b. fluid-filled sac near a joint
_____ 3. phalanges	c. bones of the fingers and toes
_____ 4. ilium	d. a rounded opening, as in a bone
_____ 5. foramen	e. first cervical vertebra
_____ 6. olecranon	a. facial bone
_____ 7. metacarpals	b. kneecap
_____ 8. periosteum	c. bone projection at the elbow
_____ 9. zygomatic	d. membrane that covers a bone
_____ 10. patella	e. bones of the hand
_____ 11. calvaria	a. lower portion of the pelvic bone
_____ 12. metaphysis	b. domelike upper portion of the skull
_____ 13. exostosis	c. growth region of a long bone
_____ 14. malleolus	d. bone projection at the ankle
_____ 15. ischium	e. outgrowth of bone
_____ 16. hemarthrosis	a. immobility of a joint
_____ 17. rachiocentesis	b. formation of bone marrow
_____ 18. spondylolisthesis	c. spinal tap
_____ 19. ankylosis	d. bleeding into a joint cavity
_____ 20. myelopoiesis	e. displacement of a vertebra
_____ 21. meniscectomy	a. artificial organ or part
_____ 22. talipes	b. foot deformity
_____ 23. subluxation	c. partial dislocation
_____ 24. laminectomy	d. removal of knee cartilage
_____ 25. prosthesis	e. removal of part of a vertebra

True-False. Examine each of the following statements. If the statement is true, write T in the first blank. If the statement is false, write F in the first blank and correct the statement by replacing the <u>underlined</u> word in the second blank.

26. The shaft of a long bone is the <u>diaphysis</u>. _____ _______________

27. The carpal bones are found in the <u>ankle</u>. _____ _______________

28. A slightly movable joint is a <u>symphysis</u>. ____ ____________________

29. The humerus is part of the <u>axial</u> skeleton. ____ ____________________

30. The cervical vertebrae are located in the <u>neck</u>. ____ ____________________

31. The bone cells active in bone resorption are the <u>osteoclasts</u>. ____ ____________________

32. Blood cells are formed in <u>yellow</u> bone marrow. ____ ____________________

33. A sideways curvature of the spine is called <u>lordosis</u>. ____ ____________________

34. The term *valgus* means bent <u>outward</u>. ____ ____________________

Fill in the blanks:

35. The term *articulation* is another word for a (n) ____________________.

36. The fluid that fills a freely movable joint is ____________________.

37. A band of connective tissue that connects bone to another bone is a(n) ____________________.

38. The terminal bone of the vertebral column is the ____________________.

39. The thigh bone is the ____________________.

40. The study and treatment of disorders of the, skeleton, muscles, and associated structures is ____________________.

41. The term *costochondral* refers to a rib and its ____________________.

42. Spondylarthritis *(spon-dil-ar-THRĪ-tis)* is arthritis of the ____________________.

43. Sacroiliitis *(sā-krō-il-ē-Ī-tis)* is inflammation of the joint between the sacrum and the ____________________.

Definitions. Write the meaning of each of the following terms:

44. Chondroid *(KON-droyd)* ____________________

45. Osteomalacia *(os-tē-ō-ma-LĀ-shē-a)* ____________________

46. Arthrotome *(AR-thrō-tōm)* ____________________

47. Synovitis *(sin-ō-VĪ-tis)* ____________________

48. Bursotomy *(bur-SOT-ō-mē)* ____________________

49. Craniometry *(krā-nē-OM-e-trē)* ____________________

50. Spondylodynia *(spon-di-lō-DIN-ē-a)* ____________________

51. Subcostal *(sub-KOS-al)* ____________________

52. Iliopelvic *(il-ē-ō-PEL-vic)* ____________________

Word building. Write a word for each of the following definitions:

53. Tumor of bone ______
54. Death (-necrosis) of bone tissue ______
55. Inflammation of bone marrow ______
56. Tumor of bone and cartilage ______
57. Surgical excision of cartilage ______
58. Fusion (-desis) of a joint ______
59. Instrument for examining the inside of a joint ______
60. Inflammation of a synovial membrane ______
61. Stone in a bursa ______
62. Measurement of the pelvis ______
63. Pertaining to a vertebra (use vertebr/o) and a rib ______
64. Surgical excision of the coccyx ______
65. Near the sacrum ______

Adjectives. Write the adjective form of each of the following words:

66. cranium ______
67. ilium ______
68. coccyx ______
69. pelvis ______
70. vertebra ______

Word analysis. Define each of the following words and give the meaning of the word parts in each. Use a dictionary if necessary.

71. Achondroplasia *(a-kon-drō-PLĀ-zha)* ______
    a. a- ______
    b. chondr/o ______
    c. -plasia ______
72. Chondroblastoma *(kon-drō-blas-TŌ-ma)* ______
    a. chondr/o ______
    b. blast ______
    c. -oma ______
73. Spondylosyndesis *(spon-di-lō-SIN-de-sis)* ______
    a. spondyl/o ______
    b. syn- ______
    c. -desis ______

Chapter 19

Case Studies

1. Arthroplasty of the Right TMJ

Patient was a 38-year-old female admitted 3 December 1996. CC: chronic pain in the right temporomandibular joint (TMJ) secondary to an automobile accident 1 year prior to admission. Diagnosis of DJD of the right TMJ was confirmed by CT scan. Prior conservative therapy, including a bite plate and steroid injections had failed. Patient was admitted for arthroplasty of the right TMJ to remove diseased bone on the articulating surface of the right condyle.

On 4 December under general naso-endotracheal anesthesia a vertical incision was made from the superior aspect of the right ear down to the base of the attachment of the right earlobe. After appropriate dissection and retraction, the posterior-superior aspect of the right zygomatic arch was bluntly dissected antero-posteriorly. With a nerve tester, the zygomatic branch of the facial nerve was identified and moved from the surgical field with a plastic loop. The periosteum was then incised along the superior aspect of the arch. An inferior dissection was then made along the capsular ligament which was retracted posteriorly. With a Freer elevator the meniscus was freed and a horizontal incision was made to the condyle. With a Hall drill and saline coolant, a high condylectomy of approximately 3 mm of bone was removed while conserving function of the external pterygoid muscle. The stump of the condyle was filed smooth and irrigated copiously. The lateral capsule, periosteum, subcutaneous tissue, and skin were then closed with sutures. The facial nerve was tested prior to closing and was found to be intact. A pressure pack and Barton bandage were applied. The sponge count, needle count, and instrument count were all correct. Estimated blood loss about 50 mL.

Patient was discharged 6 December with instructions for a soft diet and daily mouth opening exercises. Discharge medications: Keflex, 500 mg po q 6 h; Tylenol #3 po q 4 h prn for pain. She will be followed weekly as an outpatient for 4 weeks.

2. Joint Replacement of the Left Knee

This 68-year-old male had a long history of left knee pain. This had recently worsened and interfered with daily activities, especially on rising from a chair and with ambulation. He had associated general arthritis of the left hip due to an old fracture of the acetabulum and had undergone a total hip arthroplasty with excellent results.

On 11 June a left total knee arthroplasty was done without incident under spinal anesthesia. After recovery, the patient was started on a continuous passive motion machine and began ambulation with weightbearing as tolerated on this knee. On the first postoperative day, his hemoglobin fell to 10.1 and he was transfused with previously donated blood. He was maintained on prophylactic anticoagulant and oral iron.

On 15 June he was transferred to the rehabilitation unit. He will continue with the continuous passive motion machine and with assisted range of motion. He can continue to use a walker as tolerated. He will continue with patellar mobilization and isometric exercises. CBC will be repeated in 3 weeks with follow-up visit after discharge from the rehabilitation center.

3. Bone Scan of Lower Extremities

Triple phase bone scan was carried out using IV injection of 22 mCi 99mTc-MDP.

Phase I—Radionuclide perfusion study over a 1 and ½ minute period from the time of appearance of the tracer in the mid-tibia and fibula demonstrated increased perfusion to the right foot.

Phase II—Post perfusion and blood pool scan demonstrated only slight increased activity in the right lower extremity but moderate increased uptake over the right great toe distally.

Phase III—There is moderate focal increased uptake over the distal right great toe. There is also mild to moderate increased uptake over the distal fourth right digit. There is mild increased uptake over the tarsus bilaterally. There is absence of activity in the distal portions of the 3rd and 4th digits consistent with amputation.

Review of previous radiographs and current findings suggest a low grade focal osteomyelitis involving the distal phalanx of the right great toe.

Chapter 19
Case Study Questions

Multiple choice. Select the best answer and write the letter of your choice to the left of each number:

_____ 1. A condylectomy is
- a. removal of a joint capsule
- b. plastic repair of a vertebra
- c. removal of a rounded bone protuberance
- d. enlargement of a cavity
- e. removal of a tumor

_____ 2. The articulating surface of a bone is located
- a. under the epiphysis
- b. at a joint
- c. around the bone marrow
- d. at a muscle attachment
- e. at a tendon attachment

_____ 3. Ambulation is
- a. walking
- b. sitting erect
- c. undergoing surgery
- d. lifting weights
- e. resting

_____ 4. The acetabulum is
- a. the knee
- b. the distal bone of the finger
- c. a radionuclide
- d. the upper portion of the skull
- e. the bony socket for the femur

_____ 5. Increased perfusion to the right foot means increased
- a. blockage
- b. metabolism
- c. flow of blood
- d. pooling of blood
- e. temperature

_____ 6. The tarsus is the
- a. wrist
- b. ankle
- c. neck
- d. finger
- e. skull

Write a word from the case studies that means each of the following:

7. Pertaining to the cheekbone _____________________________
8. The membrane around a bone _____________________________
9. A crescent-shaped cartilage in a joint _____________________________

10. On both sides ______________________
11. Farthest from the point of attachment, as of a limb ______________________
12. A bone of the fingers or toes ______________________

Define the following terms:

13. Arthritis ______________________
14. Arthroplasty ______________________
15. Prophylactic ______________________
16. Patellar ______________________
17. Osteomyelitis ______________________

Define the following abbreviations:

18. CC ______________________
19. DJD ______________________
20. q 4 h ______________________
21. MRI ______________________
22. R/O ______________________
23. CBC ______________________

THE SKELETON

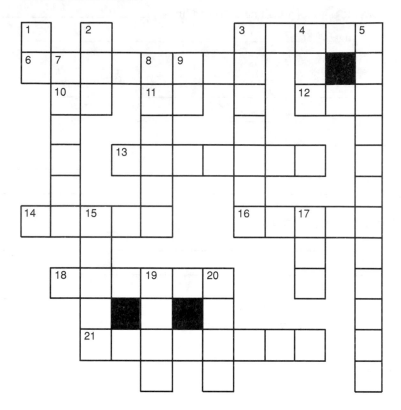

ACROSS

3. root (with combining vowel) that means rib
6. severe pain in the leg along the course of a nerve
10. a form of arthritis (abbr.)
11. suffix: pertaining to
12. meaning of prefixes a-, an-, in-, un-
13. a bone of the pelvis
14. the skull, spinal column, ribs, and sternum make up the ____ skeleton
16. root (with combining vowel) for bone marrow or spinal cord
18. a bone of the leg
21. the bone of the lower jaw

DOWN

1. mouth; body opening
2. the shaft of a long bone ____ physis
3. a mineral needed to form bone
4. prefix: together
5. a loss of bone mass, often developing with age
7. the last portion of the vertebral column
8. pertaining to bones of the ankle
9. suffix: pertaining to
15. the large, flared portion of the pelvic bone
17. the irregular end of a long bone: _____ physis
19. a bone of the forearm
20. the second cervical vertebra

Chapter 19 Answer Section

Answers to Chapter Exercises

Exercise 19-1

1. bone, bone tissue
2. joint
3. cartilage
4. formation of bone
5. softening of cartilage
6. any disease of a joint
7. around a bursa
8. osteitis *(os-tē-Ī-tis)* (note spelling)
9. osteomyelitis *(os-tē-ō-mī-e-LĪ-tis)*
10. myeloid *(MĪ-e-loyd)*
11. chondroma *(kon-DRŌ-ma)*
12. arthroscope *(AR-thrō-skōp)*
13. arthritis *(ar-THRĪ-tis)*
14. synovectomy *(sin-ō-VEK-tō-mē)*
15. hyperostosis *(hī-per-os-TŌ-sis)*
16. dysostosis *(dis-os-TŌ-sis)*

Exercise 19-2

1. cranial
2. costal
3. pelvic
4. iliac
5. vertebral
6. incision of the skull (cranium)
7. within the skull
8. pain in a vertebra
9. near a vertebra or the spinal column
10. within the pelvis
11. cranioschisis *(krā-nē-OS-ki-sis)*
12. spondylitis *(spon-di-LĪ-tis)*
13. rachiocentesis *(rā-kē-ō-sen-TĒ-sis)*; also rachicentesis *(rā-kē-sen-TĒ-sis)*
14. costectomy *(kos-TEK-tō-mē)*
15. iliopelvic *(il-ē-ō-PEL-vik)*
16. parasacral *(par-a-SĀ-kral)*
17. coccygectomy *(kok-si-JEK-tō-mē)*
18. iliococcygeal *(il-ē-ō-kok-SIJ-ē-al)*

Labeling Exercise

The Skeleton

1. cranium
2. facial bones
3. mandible
4. clavicle
5. scapula *(SKAP-ū-la)*
6. sternum
7. humerus *(HŪ-mer-us)*
8. ribs
9. vertebral column
10. ilium
11. pelvis
12. sacrum
13. radius *(RĀ-dē-us)*
14. ulna
15. carpals
16. metacarpals
17. phalanges *(fa-LAN-jēz)*
18. femur *(FĒ-mur)*
19. patella *(pa-TEL-a)*
20. tibia *(TIB-ē-a)*
21. fibula *(FIB-ū-la)*
22. calcaneus *(kal-KĀ-nē-us)*
23. tarsals
24. metatarsals
25. phalanges

Skull From the Left

1. frontal
2. parietal *(pa-RĪ-e-tal)*
3. sphenoid *(SFĒ-noyd)*
4. temporal
5. nasal
6. maxilla
7. zygomatic
8. mandible
9. occipital *(ok-SIP-i-tal)*

Vertebral Column From the Side

1. cervical vertebrae
2. thoracic vertebrae
3. lumbar vertebrae
4. sacrum
5. coccyx
6. intervertebral disk

The Pelvis

1. sacrum
2. ilium
3. ischium *(IS-kē-um)*
4. pubis
5. pubic symphysis
6. acetabulum *(as-e-TAB-ū-lum)*

Structure of a Long Bone

1. proximal epiphysis
2. diaphysis
3. distal epiphysis
4. cartilage
5. growth lines (epiphyseal lines)
6. spongy bone
7. compact bone
8. medullary cavity
9. yellow marrow
10. periosteum

Chapter Review 19

1. b
2. e
3. c
4. a
5. d
6. c
7. e
8. d
9. a
10. b
11. b
12. c
13. e
14. d
15. a
16. d
17. c
18. e
19. a
20. b
21. d
22. b
23. c
24. e
25. a
26. T
27. F wrist
28. T
29. F appendicular
30. T
31. T
32. F red
33. F scoliosis
34. T
35. joint
36. synovial fluid; synovia
37. ligament
38. coccyx
39. femur
40. orthopedics
41. cartilage
42. vertebrae
43. ilium
44. like or ressembling cartilage
45. softening of bone tissue
46. instrument for incising a joint

47. inflammation of the synovial membrane
48. incision into a bursa
49. measurement of the skull (cranium)
50. pain in a vertebra
51. below a rib or the ribs
52. pertaining to the ilium and pelvis
53. osteoma
54. osteonecrosis
55. myelitis
56. osteochondroma
57. chondrectomy
58. arthrodesis
59. arthroscope
60. synovitis
61. bursolith
62. pelvimetry
63. vertebrocostal
64. coccygectomy
65. parasacral
66. cranial
67. iliac
68. coccygeal
69. pelvic
70. vertebral
71. Decreased growth of cartilage in the growth plate of long bones resulting in dwarfism
    a. lack of
    b. cartilage
    c. formation, molding
72. Benign tumor of cartilage-forming cells
    a. cartilage
    b. immature, productive cell
    c. tumor
73. Surgical fusion (ankylosis) between vertebrae
    a. vertebra
    b. together
    c. fusion, binding

Answers to Case Study Questions

1. c
2. b
3. a
4. e
5. c
6. b
7. zygomatic
8. periosteum
9. meniscus
10. bilaterally
11. distal
12. phalanx
13. inflammation of a joint
14. plastic repair of a joint
15. preventive
16. pertaining to the kneecap
17. inflammation of bone and bone marrow
18. chief complaint
19. degenerative joint disease
20. every four hours
21. magnetic resonance imaging
22. rule out
23. complete blood count

Answers to Crossword Puzzle

THE SKELETON

1 O		2 D					3 C	O	4 S	T	5 O
6 S	7 C	I	A	8 T	9 I	C	A		Y	■	S
	10 O	A		11 A	C		L		12 N	O	T
	C			R			C				E
	C		13 I	S	C	H	I	U	M		O
	Y			A			U				P
14 A	X	15 I	A	L			16 M	Y	17 E	L	O
		L							P		R
	18 F	I	B	19 U	L	20 A			I		O
		U	■	L	■	X					S
		21 M	A	N	D	I	B	L	E		I
				A		S					S

20 The Muscular System

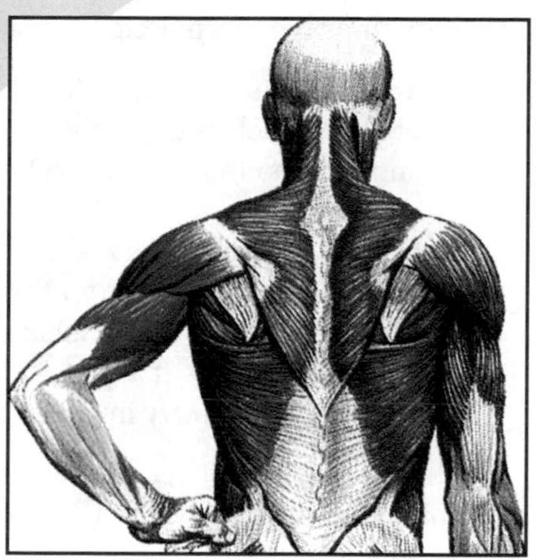

Chapter Contents

Objectives

After study of this chapter you should be able to:

1. Compare the location and function of smooth, cardiac, and skeletal muscle
2. Briefly describe the mechanism of muscle contraction
3. Explain how muscles work together to produce movement
4. List some of the criteria for naming muscles
5. Briefly describe the structure of a muscle
6. Describe the main types of movements produced by muscles
7. Identify and use the roots pertaining to the muscular system
8. Label diagrams of the superficial anterior and posterior muscles
9. Describe the main disorders that affect muscles directly
10. Interpret abbreviations pertaining to muscles
11. Analyze several case studies involving muscles

The main characteristic of muscle tissue is its ability to contract. When stimulated, muscles shorten to produce movement of the skeleton, vessels, or internal organs. Muscles also may remain partially contracted to maintain posture. In addition, the heat generated by muscle contraction is the main source of body heat.

Types of Muscle

There are three types of muscle tissue in the body:

1. **Smooth (visceral) muscle.** This makes up the walls of the hollow organs and the walls of ducts, such as the blood vessels and bronchioles. This muscle operates involuntarily and is responsible for peristalsis, the wavelike movements that propel materials through the systems.
2. **Cardiac muscle**. This makes up the myocardium of the heart wall. It functions involuntarily and is responsible for the pumping of the heart.
3. **Skeletal muscle**. This is attached to the bones of the skeleton and is responsible for voluntary movement. It also maintains posture and generates a large proportion of body heat. All of these voluntary muscles together make up the muscular system.

The discussion which follows describes the characteristics of skeletal muscle, which has been the most extensively studied of the three types of muscle tissue.

Muscle Contraction

Skeletal muscles are stimulated to contract by motor neurons of the nervous system. At the **neuromuscular junction**, the point where a branch of a neuron meets a muscle cell, the neurotransmitter **acetylcholine** is released, prompting contraction of the cell. Two special proteins in the cell, **actin** and **myosin**, interact to produce the contraction. ATP, the cell's energy compound and calcium are needed for this response.

Muscle Action

Muscles work in pairs to produce movement at the joints. (See Table 20–1 for a description of various types of movement.) As one muscle, the **prime mover**, contracts, an opposing muscle, the **antagonist**, must relax. For example, when the biceps brachii on the anterior surface of the upper arm contracts to flex the arm, the triceps brachii on the posterior surface must relax. When the arm is extended, these actions are reversed. In a given movement, the point where the muscle is attached to a stable part of the skeleton is the **origin**; the point where a muscle is attached to a moving part of the skeleton is the **insertion**.

Naming of Muscles

A muscle can be named by its location (near a bone, for example), the direction of its fibers, its size, shape, or number of attachment points (heads), as indicated by the suffix *-ceps*. It may also be named for its action, adding the suffix *-or* to the root for the action. For example, a muscle that produces flexion at a joint is a flexor. Examine the muscle diagrams in Figures 20-1 and 20-2. See how many of these criteria you can find in the names of the muscles. Note that sometimes more than one criterion is used in the name.

TABLE 20-1 Types of Movement Produced by Muscles

Movement	Definition	Example
flexion *FLEK-shun*	closing the angle at a joint	bending at the knee or elbow
extension *eks-TEN-shun*	opening the angle at a joint	straightening at the knee or elbow
abduction *ab-DUK-shun*	movement away from the midline of the body	outward movement of the arms at the shoulders
adduction *a-DUK-shun*	movement toward the midline of the body	return of lifted arms to the body
rotation *rō-TĀ-shun*	turning of a body part on its own axis	turning of the forearm from the elbow
circumduction *ser-kum-DUK-shun*	circular movement from a central point	describing a circle with an outstretched arm
pronation *prō-NĀ-shun*	turning downward	turning the palm of the hand downward
supination *sū-pin-Ā-shun*	turning upward	turning the palm of the hand upward
eversion *ē-VER-zhun*	turning outward	turning the sole of the foot outward
inversion *in-VER-zhun*	turning inward	turning the sole of the foot inward
dorsiflexion *dor-si-FLEK-shun*	bending backward	moving the foot so that the toes point upward, away from the sole of the foot
plantar flexion	bending the sole of the foot	pointing the toes downward

Muscle Structure

Muscles are composed of individual cells, often referred to as *fibers* because they are so long and threadlike. These cells are held together in bundles by connective tissue. Covering each muscle is a sheath of connective tissue or **fascia**. These supporting tissues merge to form the **tendon** that attaches the muscle to a bone.

KEY TERMS

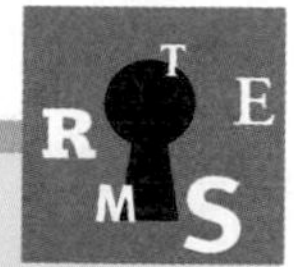

Normal Structure and Function

acetylcholine *(as-e-til-KŌ-lēn)* — A neurotransmitter that stimulates contraction of skeletal muscles

actin *(AK-tin)* — One of the two contractile proteins in muscle cells; the other is myosin

antagonist *(an-TAG-ō-nist)* — The muscle that opposes a prime mover. It must relax when the prime mover contracts.

(continued)

fascia *(FASH-ē-a)*	The fibrous sheath of connective tissue that covers a muscle. Called *deep fascia* to differentiate it from the superficial fascia that underlies the skin. (*pl.* fasciae) (root fasci/o)
insertion	In a given movement, the point where a muscle is attached to a moving part of the skeleton
muscle	An organ which produces movement by contracting; also the tissue that composes such organs (root my/o, muscul/o)
myosin *(MĪ-ō-sin)*	One of the two contractile proteins in muscle cells; the other is actin
neuromuscular junction	The point of contact between a branch of a motor neuron and a muscle cell. Also called the myoneural junction.
origin	In a given movement, the point where a muscle is attached to a stable part of the skeleton.
prime mover	The muscle that carries out a given movement; agonist
tendon *(TEN-dun)*	A fibrous band of connective tissue that attaches a muscle to a bone (root ten/o, tendin/o)
tonus *(TŌ-nus)*	A state of steady, partial contraction of muscle which maintains firmness; muscle tone (root ton/o)

Roots Pertaining to Muscles

Root	Meaning	Example	Definition of Example
my/o	muscle	myositis* *mi-ō-SĪ-tis*	inflammation of muscle
muscul/o	muscle	musculotendinous *mus-kū-lō-TEN-di-nus*	pertaining to muscle and tendon
in/o	fiber	inotropic *in-ō-TROP-ik*	acting on muscle fibers
fasci/o	fascia	fasciodesis *fash-ē-OD-e-sis*	suturing of a fascia to a tendon or other fascia
ten/o, tendin/o	tendon	tenostosis *ten-os-TŌ-sis*	ossification of a tendon
ton/o	tone	cardiotonic *kar-dē-ō-TON-ik*	having a strengthening action on the heart
kine, kinesi/o kinet/o	movement	dyskinesia *dis-ki-NĒ-zē-a*	abnormality of movement

*Note addition of *s* to this root before the suffix *-itis*

text continues on page 497

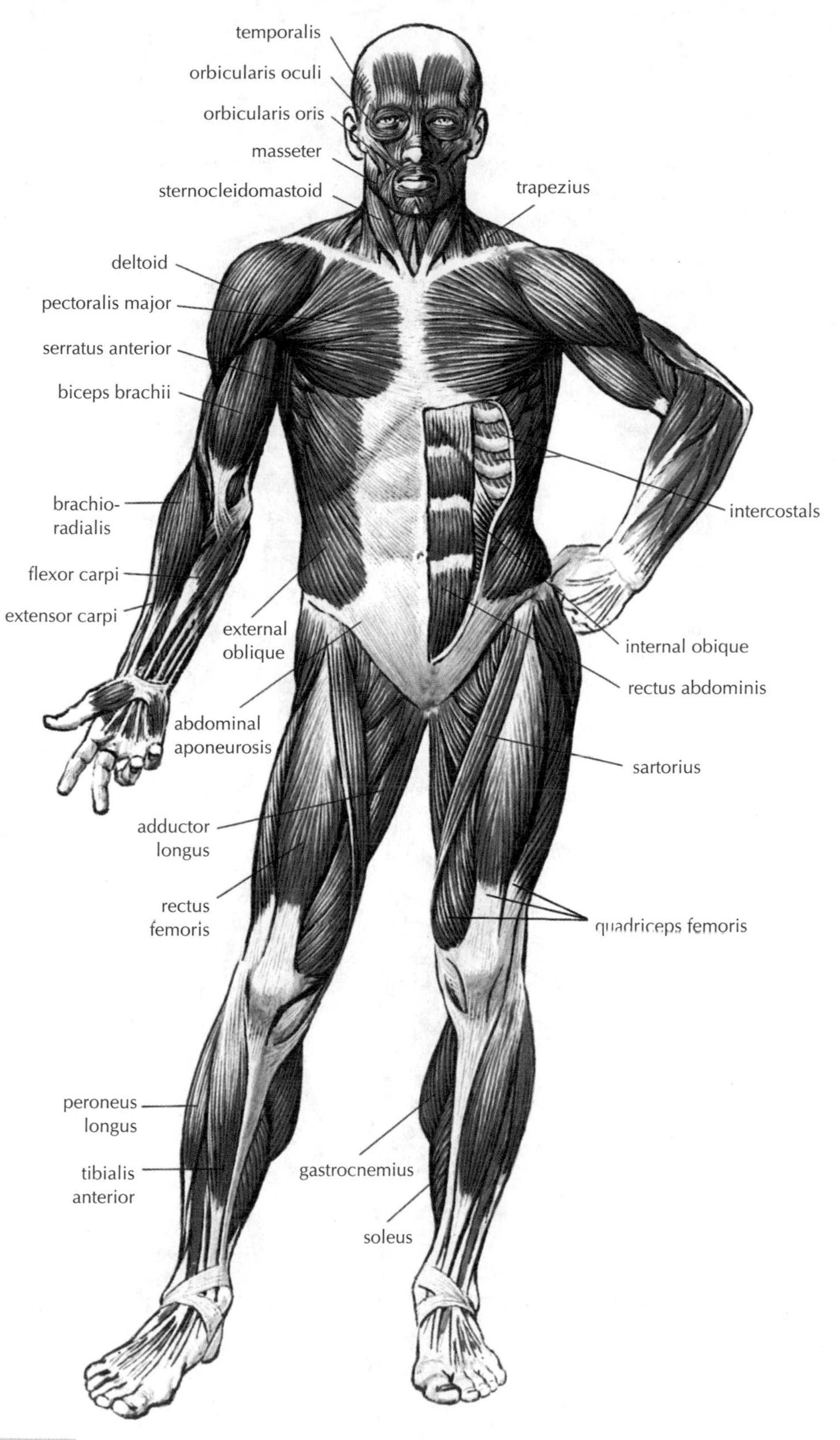

FIGURE 20-1. Superficial muscles (anterior view).

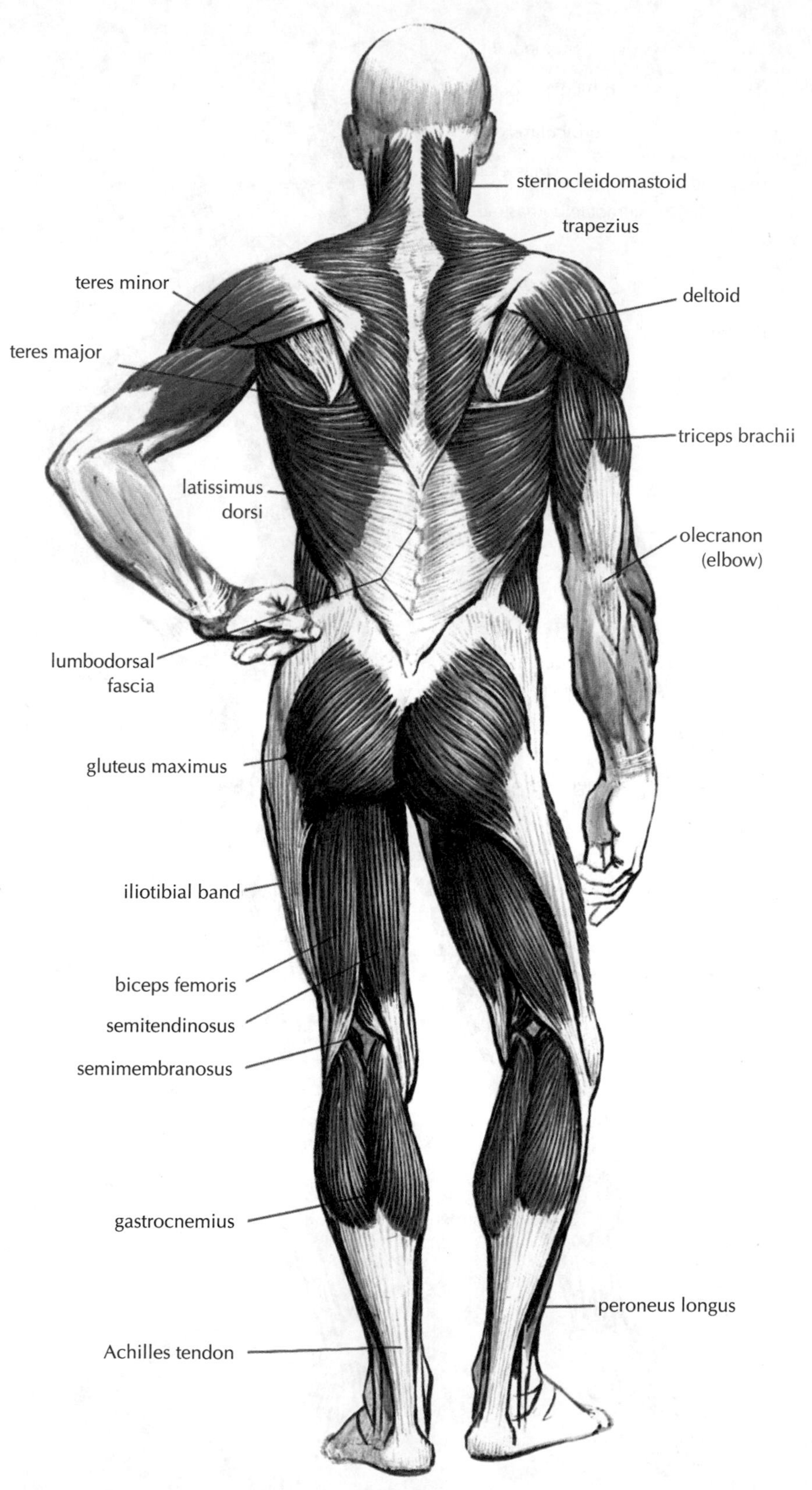

FIGURE 20-2. Superficial muscles (posterior view).

Exercise 20-1

Define the following adjectives:

1. Muscular ______
2. Fascial ______
3. Tendinous ______
4. Kinetic ______

Fill in the blanks:

5. Myoedema *(mī-ō-e-DĒ-ma)* is accumulation of fluid in a(n) ______.
6. Dystonia *(dis-TŌ-nē-a)* is abnormal muscle ______.
7. Kinesitherapy *(ki-nē-se-THER-a-pē)* is treatment by means of ______.
8. Inosclerosis *(in-ō-skle-RŌ-sis)* is hardening of tissue due to increase in ______.
9. Myofibrils *(mī-ō-FĪ-brils)* are small fibers found in ______.

Define the following terms:

10. Atony *(AT-ō-nē)* ______
11. Musculofascial *(mus-kū-lō-FASH-ē-al)* ______
12. Tendinitis *(ten-di-NI-tis)* or tenositis *(ten-ō-SĪ-tis)* (note spelling) ______
13. Hypermyotonia *(hī-per-mī-ō-TŌ-nē-a)* ______
14. Kinesiology *(ki-nē-sē-OL-ō-jē)* ______
15. Fasciorrhaphy *(fash-ē-OR-a-fē)* ______

Word building. Write a word for each of the following definitions:

16. Multiple (poly-) inflammation of muscles ______
17. Any disease of muscle ______
18. Excision of fascia ______
19. Inflammation of a muscle and its tendon (use ten/o) ______
20. Suture of a tendon (use ten/o) ______

Clinical Aspects of the Muscular System

Muscle function may be affected by disorders elsewhere, particularly in the nervous system and connective tissue. The conditions described below affect the muscular system directly. Any disorder of muscles is described as a **myopathy**.

Techniques for diagnosing muscle disorders include electrical studies of muscle in action, **electromyography** (EMG), and serum assay of enzymes released in increased amounts from damaged muscles, mainly **CPK** (creatine phosphokinase).

Muscular Dystrophy

Muscular dystrophy refers to a group of hereditary diseases involving progressive, noninflammatory degeneration of muscles. There is weakness and wasting of muscle tissue with gradual replacement by connective tissue and fat. There also may be cardiomyopathy (disease of cardiac muscle) and mental impairment.

The most common form is **Duchenne muscular dystrophy**, a sex-linked disease passed from mother to son. This appears at age 3 to 4 and patients are incapacitated by age 10 to 15. Death is commonly caused by respiratory failure or infection.

Polymyositis

Polymyositis is inflammation of skeletal muscle leading to weakness, frequently associated with dysphagia (difficulty in swallowing) or cardiac problems. The cause is unknown, and may be related to viral infection or to autoimmunity. Often the disorder is associated with some other systemic disease such as rheumatoid arthritis or lupus erythematosus.

When the skin is involved, the condition is termed **dermatomyositis**. In this case, there is erythema (redness of the skin), dermatitis (inflammation of the skin), and a typical lilac-colored rash, predominantly on the face. In addition to enzyme studies and EMG, muscle biopsy is used in diagnosis.

Myasthenia Gravis

Myasthenia gravis is an acquired autoimmune disease in which antibodies interfere with muscle stimulation at the neuromuscular junction. There is a progressive loss of muscle power, especially in the external eye muscles and other muscles of the face.

KEY CLINICAL TERMS

TERMS

Disorders

Term	Definition
dermatomyositis *(der-ma-tō-mī-ō-SĪ-tis)*	A disease of unknown origin involving inflammation of muscles as well as dermatitis and skin rashes
muscular dystrophy *(DIS-trō-fē)*	A group of hereditary muscular disorders marked by progressive weakness and atrophy of muscles
myasthenia gravis (MG) *(mī-as-THĒ-nē-a GRA-vis)*	A disease characterized by progressive muscular weakness. An autoimmune disease affecting the neuromuscular junction.
polymyositis *(pol-ē-mī-ō-SĪ-tis)*	A disease of unknown cause involving muscle inflammation and weakness

Treatment

Term	Definition
creatine phosphokinase (CK; CPK) *(KRĒ-a-tin fos-fō-KĪ-nās)*	An enzyme found in muscle tissue. The serum level increases in cases of muscle damage.
electromyography (EMG) *(ē-lek-trō-mī-OG-ra-fē)*	Study of the electrical activity of muscles during contraction

ADDITIONAL TERMS

Normal Structure and Function

Achilles tendon *(a-KIL-ēz)* — The strong cordlike tendon that attaches the calf muscles to the heel (see Figure 20-2)

aponeurosis *(ap-ō-nū-RŌ-sis)* — A flat, white, sheetlike tendon that connects a muscle with the part that it moves (see abdominal aponeurosis, Figure 20-1)

creatine *(KRĒ-a-tin)* — A substance in muscle cells that stores energy for contraction

glycogen *(GLĪ-kō-jen)* — A complex sugar that is stored for energy in muscles and in the liver

hamstring muscles — Three muscles of the posterior thigh: the biceps femoris, semitendinosus, and semimembranosus. They flex the leg and adduct and extend the thigh.

isometric *(ī-sō-MET-rik)* — Pertaining to a muscle action in which the muscle tenses but does not shorten

isotonic *(ī-sō-TON-ik)* — Pertaining to a muscle action in which the muscle shortens to accomplish movement

kinesthesia *(kin-es-THĒ-zē-a)* — Awareness of movement; perception of the weight, direction, and degree of movement (*-esthesia* means "sensation")

lactic acid — An acid that accumulates in muscle cells functioning without enough oxygen, as in times of great physical exertion. The lactic acid leads to muscle fatigue after which it is gradually removed from the tissues.

motor unit — A single motor neuron and all of the muscle cells that its branches stimulate

myoglobin *(mī-ō-GLŌ-bin)* — A pigment similar to hemoglobin that stores oxygen in muscle cells

oxygen debt — The period during which muscles are functioning without enough oxygen. Lactic acid accumulates and leads to fatigue.

quadriceps muscle *(KWOD-ri-seps)* — A four-part muscle at the front and sides of the thigh. Includes the rectus femoris, vastus intermedius, vastus lateralis, and vastus medialis. Inserts at the patella and flexes the leg.

rotator cuff — A group of muscles and tendons around the capsule of the shoulder joint that provides mobility and strength to the joint

Symptoms and Conditions

amyotrophic lateral sclerosis (ALS) *(a-mī-ō-TROF-ik)* — A condition caused by degeneration of motor neurons. It is marked by muscular weakness and atrophy with spasticity and hyperreflexia; Lou Gehrig's disease.

asterixis *(as-ter-IK-sis)* — Rapid, jerky movements, especially in the hands, due to intermittent loss of muscle tone

(continued)

asthenia *(as-THĒ-nē-a)*	Weakness. (Prefix *a-* meaning "without" with root *-sthen/o* meaning "strength." The prefix *cali-* in the word calisthenics means "beauty.")
ataxia *(a-TAK-sē-a)*	Lack of muscle coordination (from root *tax/o* meaning "order, arrangement.") (adj. ataxic)
athetosis *(ath-e-TŌ-sis)*	A condition marked by slow, irregular, twisting movements, especially in the hands and fingers. (adj. athetotic)
atrophy *(AT-rō-fē)*	A wasting away; a decrease in the size of a tissue or organ, such as the wasting of muscle from disuse
avulsion *(a-VUL-shun)*	Forcible tearing away of a part
clonus *(KLŌ-nus)*	Alternating spasmodic contraction and relaxation in a muscle (adj. clonic)
contracture *(kon-TRAK-chur)*	Permanent contraction of a muscle
fibromyositis *(fī-brō-mī-ō-SĪ-tis)*	A nonspecific term for pain, tenderness, and stiffness in muscles and joints
fibrositis *(fī-brō-SĪ-tis)*	Inflammation of fibrous connective tissue, especially the muscle fasciae. Marked by pain and stiffness.
rhabdomyolysis *(rab-dō-mī-OL-i-sis)*	An acute disease involving diffuse destruction of skeletal muscle cells. (Root *rhabd/o* means "rod," referring to the long, rodlike muscle cells.)
rhabdomyoma *(rab-dō-mī-Ō-ma)*	A benign tumor of skeletal muscle
rhabdomyosarcoma *(rab-dō-mī-ō-sar-KŌ-ma)*	A highly malignant tumor of skeletal muscle
rheumatism *(rū-ma-tizm)*	A general term for inflammation, soreness, and stiffness of muscles associated with pain in joints (adj. rheumatic, rheumatoid)
spasm	A sudden, involuntary muscle contraction. May be clonic (contraction alternating with relaxation) or tonic (sustained). A strong and painful spasm may be called a cramp. (adj. spastic, spasmodic)
spasticity *(spas-TIS-i-tē)*	Increased tone or contractions of muscles causing stiff and awkward movements
strain	Trauma to a muscle due to overuse or excessive stretch
tendinitis *(ten-di-NĪ-tis)*	Inflammation of a tendon, usually caused by injury or overuse. The shoulder is a common site.
tenosynovitis *(ten-ō-sin-ō-VĪ-tis)*	Inflammation of a tendon sheath
tetanus *(TET-a-nus)*	An acute infectious disease caused by the anaerobic bacillus *Clostridium tetani*. It is marked by persistent painful spasms of voluntary muscles; lockjaw.

tetany
(TET-a-nē)
A condition marked by spasms, cramps, and muscle twitching due to a metabolic imbalance, such as low blood calcium caused by underactivity of the parathyroid glands

torticollis
(tor-ti-KOL-is)
Spasmodic contraction of the neck muscles causing stiffness and twisting of the neck; wryneck

Diagnosis and Treatment

Chvostek's sign
(VOS-teks)
Spasm of facial muscles following a tap over the facial nerve. Evidence of tetany.

rheumatology
(rū-ma-TOL-ō-jē)
The study and treatment of rheumatic diseases

Trousseau's sign
(tru-SŌZ)
Spasmodic contractions caused by pressing the nerve supplying a muscle; seen in tetany

ABBREVIATIONS

Ach acetylcholine
ALS amyotrophic lateral sclerosis
C(P)K creatine phosphokinase; creatine kinase
EMG electromyography, electromyogram
MG myasthenia gravis
MN myoneural (junction)
NM neuromuscular (junction)
OT occupational therapy
PT physical therapy
ROM range of motion

Chapter 20
Labeling Exercises

Write the name of each numbered part on the corresponding line of the answer sheet.

adductor longus
biceps brachii
brachioradialis
deltoid
extensor carpi
external oblique
flexor carpi
gastrocnemius
intercostals
internal oblique
orbicularis oculi
orbicularis oris
pectoralis major
peroneus longus
quadriceps femoris
rectus abdominis
masseter
sartorius
serratus anterior
soleus
sternocleido-mastoid
temporalis
tibialis anterior

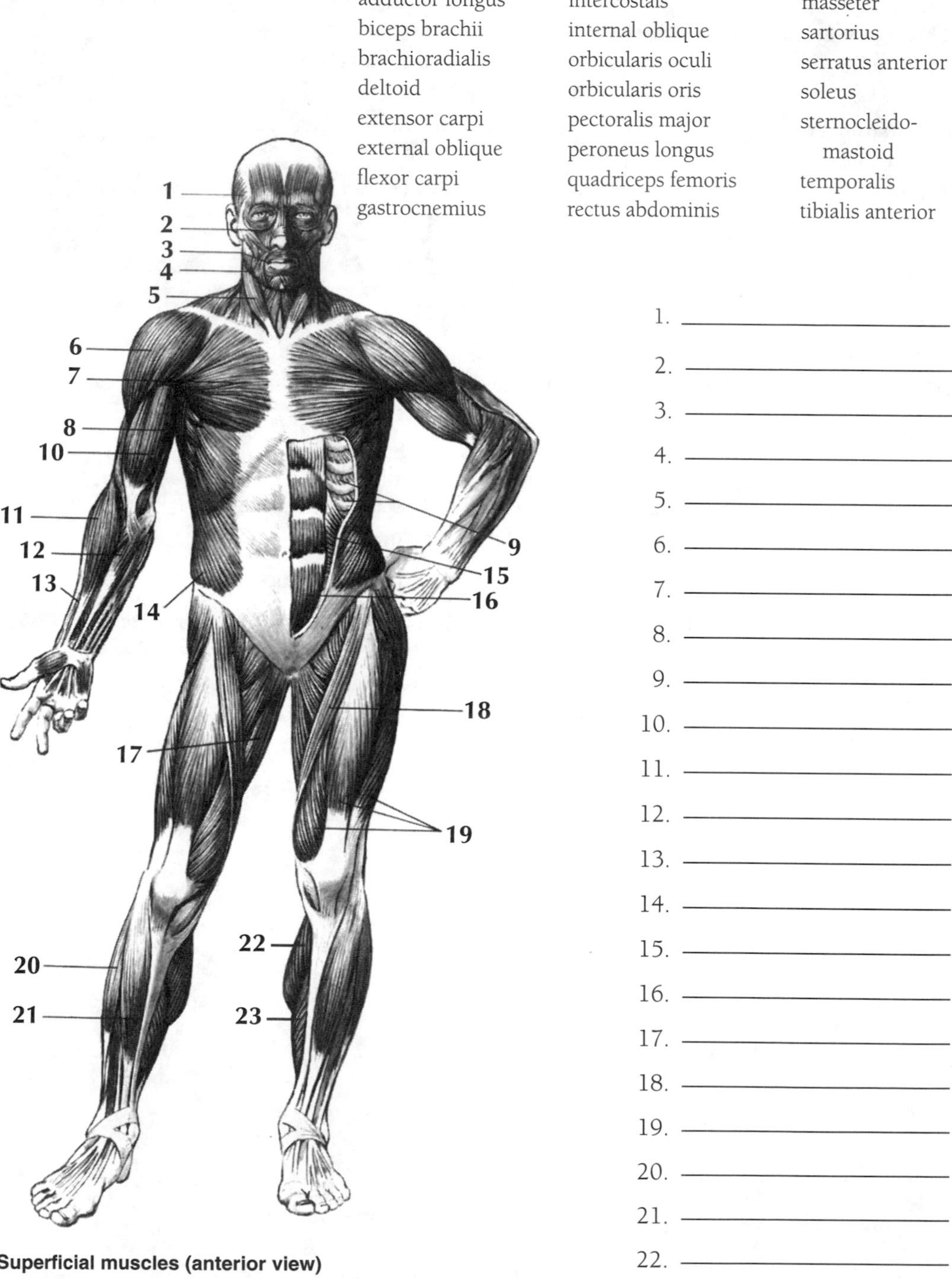

Superficial muscles (anterior view)

1. ____________________
2. ____________________
3. ____________________
4. ____________________
5. ____________________
6. ____________________
7. ____________________
8. ____________________
9. ____________________
10. ____________________
11. ____________________
12. ____________________
13. ____________________
14. ____________________
15. ____________________
16. ____________________
17. ____________________
18. ____________________
19. ____________________
20. ____________________
21. ____________________
22. ____________________
23. ____________________

Write the name of each numbered part on the corresponding line of the answer sheet.

biceps femoris	semitendinosus
gastrocnemius	triceps brachii
gluteus maximus	teres major
latissimus dorsi	teres minor
peroneus longus	trapezius
semimembranosus	

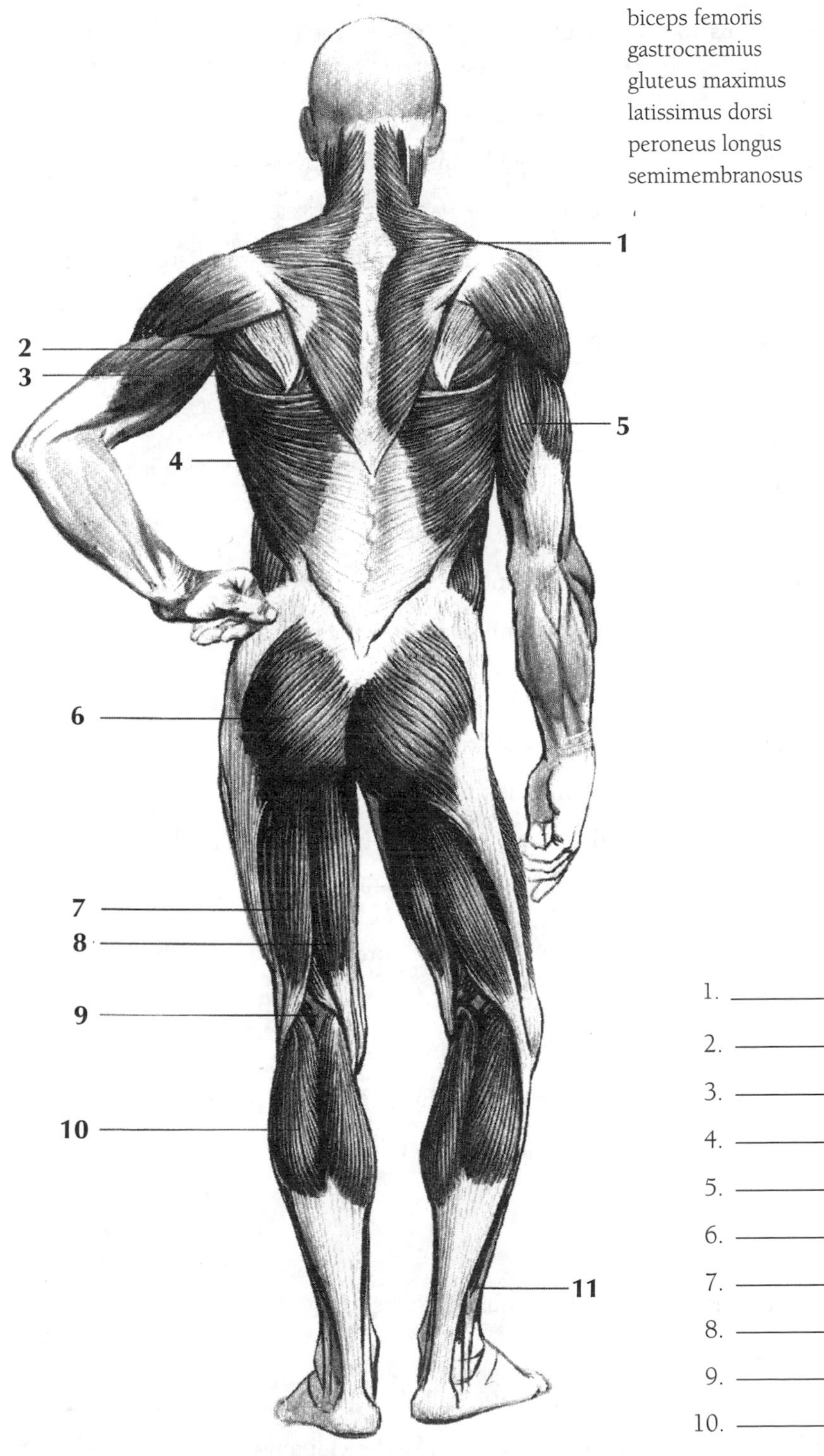

Superficial muscles (posterior view)

1. ____________
2. ____________
3. ____________
4. ____________
5. ____________
6. ____________
7. ____________
8. ____________
9. ____________
10. ____________
11. ____________

CHAPTER REVIEW 20-1

Matching. Match the terms in each of the sets below with their definitions and write the appropriate letter (a–e) to the left of each number (see Figures 20-1 and 20-2 for matches 1–10):

____ 1. semitendinosus	a. main muscle of the calf
____ 2. gastrocnemius	b. triangular muscle that covers the shoulder
____ 3. biceps brachii	c. one of the hamstring muscles
____ 4. deltoid	d. anterior muscle of the upper arm that flexes the forearm
____ 5. quadriceps femoris	e. large muscle group of the anterior thigh
____ 6. intercostal	a. muscle that runs vertically at the center of the anterior trunk
____ 7. rectus abdominis	b. main muscle of the buttocks
____ 8. pectoralis major	c. muscle between the ribs
____ 9. latissimus dorsi	d. large muscle of the upper chest
____ 10. gluteus maximus	e. large muscle across the back below the trapezius
____ 11. tetany	a. abnormal muscle tone
____ 12. bradykinesia	b. oxygen-storing pigment in muscle
____ 13. rhabdomyoma	c. muscle tumor
____ 14. dystonia	d. muscle spasm due to metabolic imbalance
____ 15. myoglobin	e. slowness of movement
____ 16. inosemia	a. lack of muscle coordination
____ 17. aponeurosis	b. wryneck
____ 18. ataxia	c. forcible tearing away of a part
____ 19. torticollis	d. excess fibrin in the blood
____ 20. avulsion	e. flat, sheetlike tendon

Fill in the blanks:

21. The neurotransmitter released at the neuromuscular junction is ____________________.

22. Any muscle that produces extension at a joint is called a(n) ____________________.

23. The number of attachment points (heads) in the triceps brachii muscle is ____________________.

24. The sheath of connective tissue that covers a muscle is called ______________________.
25. A band of connective tissue that attaches a muscle to a bone is a(n) ______________________.
26. The strong, cordlike tendon that attaches the calf muscle to the heel is the______________________.

Definitions. Write the meaning of each of the following terms:

27. Myonecrosis *(mī-ō-ne-KRŌ-sis)* ______________________
28. Inositis *(in-ō-SĪ-tis)* ______________________
29. Tenotomy *(ten-OT-ō-mē)* ______________________
30. Hypotonia *(hī-pō-TŌ-nē-a)* ______________________
31. Hyperkinesia *(hī-per-ki-NĒ-sē-a)* ______________________

Word building. Write a word for each of the following definitions:

32. Study of muscles (use my/o-) ______________________
33. Pain in a muscle (use my/o-) ______________________
34. Pertaining to muscle and fascia ______________________
35. Inflammation of fascia ______________________
36. Suture of fascia ______________________
37. Plastic repair of a tendon (use ten/o-) ______________________

Opposites. Write a word that means the opposite of each of the following terms as they pertain to muscles:

38. prime mover ______________________
39. origin ______________________
40. adduction ______________________
41. pronation ______________________
42. extension ______________________

Adjectives. Write the adjective form of each of the following words:

43. tendon ______________________
44. ataxia ______________________
45. fascia ______________________
46. spasm ______________________
47. clonus ______________________

Word analysis. Define each of the following words and give the meaning of the word parts in each. Use a dictionary if necessary.

48. Isometric ____________________

____

a. iso- ____________

b. metr/o ____________

c. -ic ____________

49. Amyotrophic ____________________

____

a. a- ____________

b. my/o ____________

c. troph/o ____________

d. -ic ____________

50. Myasthenia ____________________

____

a. my/o ____________

b. a- ____________

c. sthen/o ____________

d. -ia ____________

CHAPTER REVIEW 20-2

Naming of Muscles. Below is a list of criteria used in naming muscles. For the following muscles, select the criterion or criteria used to name each and write the appropriate letter or letters in the blank. Be sure to list all of the letters that apply. Refer to Figures 20-1 and 20-2.

a. size

b. shape

c. number of attachment points

d. direction of fibers

e. action

f. location

1. biceps brachii ____________
2. temporalis ____________
3. pectoralis major ____________
4. extensor carpi ____________
5. internal oblique ____________

6. trapezius ____________________
7. brachioradialis ____________________
8. latissimus dorsi ____________________
9. quadriceps femoris ____________________
10. adductor femoris ____________________
11. rectus abdominis ____________________
12. tibialis anterior ____________________
13. deltoid ____________________
14. rectus femoris ____________________

***Chapter* 20**

Case Studies

1. Surgical Repair of Left Rotator Cuff

Patient is a 22-year-old male with a history of recurrent left shoulder dislocations unresponsive to conservative therapy. He is now here for a Bankart repair and surgery as indicated of the left shoulder.

The patient was taken to the Operating Room electively on 25 April 1996 and identified as ____________. The patient was placed in the McConnell beach-chair position and after adequate induction of general endotracheal anesthesia was prepped and draped in the standard fashion. A standard deltopectoral approach was then made to the left shoulder. Hemostasis was achieved by cautery. After retraction of the deltoid and incision of the clavipectoral fascia, the rotator cuff was identified. The subscapularis tendon was incised proximal to its insertion. Following incision of the capsule, inspection showed a large pouch inferiorly in the capsule consistent with laxity (instability). A capsular shift was then performed, repairing the proximal capsule to the labrum (lip) and then tightening the inferior aspect of the capsule. ROM exam showed that external rotation could be performed past neutral and that the shoulder did not dislocate. The wound was copiously irrigated with antibiotic solution and a Jackson-Pratt drain was placed prior to closure. Counts were correct × 2. There were no complications.

2. Cervical and Lumbosacral Strain and Sprain

M.H. is a 28-year-old female suffering from pains in the neck, left arm and shoulder, and lower back following a minor car accident 10 days prior to consultation.

Examination shows the cervical ROM to be restricted in all movements, with pain on rotation of the head to the left and on extension. There is tenderness to palpation over the left lower cervical paravertebral musculature. The lumbar ROM is moderately restricted with pain on flexion and extension. There is tenderness over the lumbosacral paravertebral musculature and over the corresponding interspinous ligaments. There is full abduction and flexion of the left shoulder, but pain over the left upper trapezius muscle, the left rhomboid muscle group, and left levator scapulae muscle.

The diagnosis is acute cervical and lumbosacral strain and sprain with injury to myoligamentous structures. There is also strain and sprain of the left shoulder girdle. The patient will receive NSAID treatment, instructions for self care, and physical therapy to include moist heat, ultrasound, and electrical stimulation to the involved musculature. She will be re-evaluated in 3 weeks.

Chapter 20
Case Study Questions

Multiple choice. Select the best answer and write the letter of your choice to the left of each number.

_____ 1. The insertion of a muscle is

a. the thick middle portion
b. the point of attachment to a moving bone
c. the point of attachment to a stable bone
d. the fibrous sheath
e. the connective tissue

_____ 2. The trapezius is in the

a. arm
b. back
c. abdomen
d. hand
e. hip

_____ 3. The levator scapulae muscle acts to

a. lower the scapula
b. turn the scapula
c. raise the scapula
d. adduct the scapula
e. pronate the scapula

Write a word from the case studies that means each of the following:

4. Within the trachea _____
5. Stoppage of blood flow _____
6. The fibrous sheath around a muscle _____
7. Near the point of attachment, as of a limb _____
8. Turning a body part on its own axis _____
9. Closing the angle at a joint _____
10. Movement away from the midline _____
11. Pertaining to the lower back _____
12. Between vertebrae _____
13. Trauma to a muscle due to overuse _____

Define the following terms:

14. Deltopectoral _____
15. Palpation _____
16. Cervical _____
17. Paravertebral _____
18. Myoligamentous _____

Define the following abbreviations:

19. ROM _____
20. NSAID _____

MUSCULAR SYSTEM

ACROSS

1. a muscle around the mouth: obicularis ______
6. the end of a muscle that remains fixed in a given movement
8. a metric abbreviation
9. a muscle with two attachment points (heads) as in _____ brachii or femoris
10. prefix: out, outside
12. suffix: condition of
13. a nursing degree (abbr.)
14. a muscle of the inner thigh
17. prefix: absence, removal, separation
19. a measurement used in hearing tests (abbr.)
20. rapid, jerky movements, especially of the hands, due to intermittent loss of muscle tone
22. the muscle that contracts to produce a given motion: prime ______
23. the record produced in an electrical study such as the EMG, EEG, or EKG
26. the root (with combining vowel) that means pressure
29. a drug mixture in oil or other liquid intended for external application
30. prefix: down, without, removal, loss

DOWN

2. a muscle of the forearm: brachio______
3. a muscle of the leg
4. root (with combining vowel) meaning movement
5. describing the junction between a nerve and a muscle (abbr.)
7. the end of a muscle attached to a moving part
8. alternating spasmodic contraction and relaxation in a muscle
9. prefix: two, twice
11. prefix: three
15. to dissolve and take back into the circulation, as of bone
16. a muscle of the neck: _____ cleidomastoid
17. root meaning finger or toe
18. trauma to a muscle due to overuse or excessive stretch
21. prefix; not
24. suffix: condition of
25. word part meaning origin, formation
27. movement toward the midline of the body: ____ duction
28. prefix: again, back

Chapter 20
Answer Section

Answers to Chapter Exercises

Exercise 20-1

1. pertaining to muscle
2. pertaining to fascia
3. pertaining to a tendon
4. pertaining to movement
5. muscle
6. tone
7. movement
8. fibers
9. muscle
10. lack of muscle tone
11. pertaining to muscle and fascia
12. inflammation of a tendon
13. excess muscle tone
14. study of movement
15. suture of fascia
16. polymyositis *(pol-ē-mī-ō-SĪ-tis)*
17. myopathy *(mī-OP-a-thē)*
18. fasciectomy *(fash-ē-EK-tō-mē)*
19. myotenositis *(mī-ō-ten-ō-SĪ-tis)*
20. tenorrhaphy *(te-NOR-a-fē)*

Labeling Exercise

Superficial Muscles (anterior view)

1. temporalis *(tem-pō-RĀ-lis)*
2. orbicularis oculi *(or-bik-ū-LĀ-ris OK-ū-li)*
3. orbicularis oris *(OR-is)*
4. masseter *(MAS-e-ter)*
5. sternocleidomastoid *(ster-nō-klī-dō-MAS-toyd)*
6. deltoid *(DEL-toyd)*
7. pectoralis *(pek-tō-RĀ-lis)* major
8. serratus *(ser-Ā-tus)* anterior
9. intercostals
10. biceps brachii *(BĪ-seps BRĀ-kē-ī)*
11. brachioradialis *(brā-kē-ō-rā-dē-AL-is)*
12. flexor carpi
13. extensor carpi
14. external oblique
15. internal oblique
16. rectus abdominis
17. adductor longus
18. sartorius *(sar-TŌ-rē-us)*
19. quadriceps femoris *(KWOD-ri-seps FEM-or-is)*
20. peroneus longus *(per-ō-NĒ-us LONG-us)*
21. tibialis *(tib-ē-Ā-lis)* anterior
22. gastrocnemius *(gas-trok-NĒ-mē-us)*
23. soleus *(SŌ-lē-us)*

Superficial Muscles (posterior view)

1. trapezius *(tra-PĒ-zē-us)*
2. teres *(TĒ-rez)* minor
3. teres major
4. latissimus dorsi *(la-TIS-i-mus DOR-sī)*
5. triceps brachii
6. gluteus *(GLŪ-tē-us)* maximus
7. biceps femoris
8. semitendinosus *(sem-ē-ten-di-NŌ-sus)*
9. semimembranosus *(sem-ē-mem-bra-NŌ-sus)*
10. gastrocnemius
11. peroneus longus

Answers to Chapter Review

Chapter Review 20-1

1. c
2. a
3. d
4. b
5. e
6. c
7. a
8. d
9. e
10. b
11. d
12. e
13. c
14. a
15. b
16. d
17. e
18. a
19. b
20. c
21. acetylcholine
22. extensor
23. three
24. fascia
25. tendon
26. Achilles tendon
27. death of muscle tissue
28. inflammation of fibers (fibrous tissue)
29. incision of a tendon
30. decreased muscle tone
31. abnormally increased movement
32. myology
33. myalgia
34. musculofascial; also myofascial
35. fascitis; also fasciitis
36. fasciorrhaphy
37. tenoplasty
38. antagonist
39. insertion
40. abduction
41. supination
42. flexion
43. tendinous
44. ataxic
45. fascial
46. spastic, spasmodic
47. clonic
48. Pertaining to muscle action in which the muscle tenses but does not shorten
    a. the same, equal
    b. measure
    c. pertaining to
49. Pertaining to muscle wasting, atrophy
    a. lack of
    b. muscle
    c. nourishment
    d. pertaining to
50. Muscular weakness
    a. muscle
    b. lack of
    c. strength
    d. condition of

Chapter Review 20-2

1. c, f
2. f
3. f, a
4. e, f
5. f, d
6. b
7. f
8. f
9. c, f
10. e, f
11. d, f
12. f
13. b
14. d, f

Answers to Case Study Questions

1. b
2. b
3. c
4. endotracheal
5. hemostasis
6. fascia
7. proximal
8. rotation
9. flexion
10. abduction

11. lumbar
12. interspinous
13. strain
14. pertaining to the deltoid and pectoral muscles
15. examination by touching the surface of the body
16. pertaining to the neck
17. near the vertebrae
18. pertaining to muscle and ligament
19. range of motion
20. nonsteroidal anti-inflammatory

Answers to Crossword Puzzle

MUSCULAR SYSTEM

1 O	2 R	I	3 S				4 K				5 N
	A		6 O	R	7 I	G	I	N		8 C	M
	D		L	■	N		N			L	
9 B	I	C	E	P	S		10 E	C	11 T	O	
12 I	A		U	■	E		T	■	13 R	N	
	L		14 S	A	R	T	O	15 R	I	U	16 S
17 D	I	18 S			T			E		19 S	T
20 A	S	T	E	R	I	X	21 I	S			E
C	■	R			O	■	22 M	O	V	E	R
23 T	R	A	C	24 I	N	25 G		R			N
Y	■	I	■	S	■	E		26 B	27 A	28 R	O
29 L	I	N	I	M	E	N	T		30 D	E	

21 *The Skin*

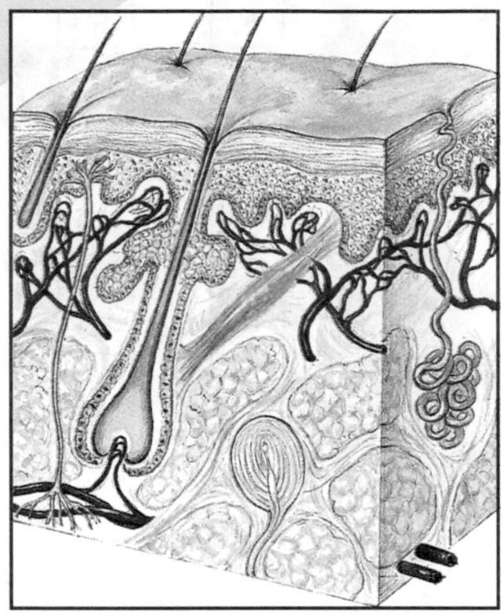

Chapter Contents

Objectives

After study of this chapter you should be able to:

1. Compare the epidermis, dermis, and subcutaneous tissue
2. Describe the roles of keratin and melanin in the skin
3. Name and describe the glands in the skin
4. Describe the structure of hair and of nails
5. Identify and use roots pertaining to the skin
6. Describe the main disorders that affect the skin
7. Label a diagram of the skin
8. Analyze several case studies involving the skin

Like the eyes, the skin is a readily visible reflection of one's health. Its color, texture, and resilience reveal much, as does the condition of the hair and nails. The skin and its associated structures make up the **integumentary system.** This body-covering system protects against infection, dehydration, and injury. Extensive damage to the skin, as by burns, can result in a host of dangerous complications. The skin also serves in temperature regulation and sensory perception.

Anatomy of the Skin

The outermost portion of the skin is the **epidermis**, consisting of 4–5 layers (strata) of epithelial cells (Fig. 21-1). The deepest, basal layer produces new cells. As these cells gradually rise toward the surface they die and become filled with **keratin**, a protein that thickens and toughens the skin. The outermost (horny) layer of the epidermis is composed of flat, dead, protective cells that are constantly being shed and replaced. Some of the cells in the epidermis produce **melanin**, a pigment that gives color to the skin and protects against sunlight.

The **dermis** is beneath the epidermis. It is composed of connective tissue, nerves, blood vessels, and lymphatics. This layer supplies support and nourishment for the skin.

The **subcutaneous tissue** beneath the dermis is composed mainly of connective tissue and fat.

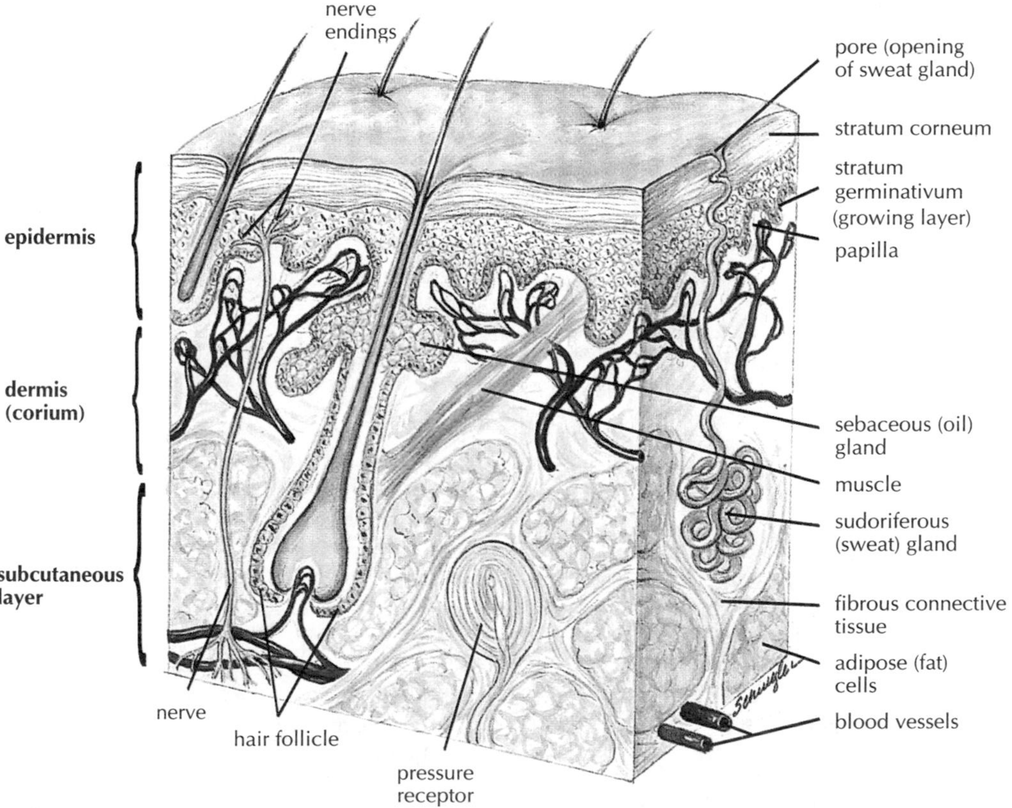

FIGURE 21-1. Cross section of the skin.

Associated Skin Structures

The **sudoriferous** (sweat) **glands** act mainly in temperature regulation by releasing a watery fluid that evaporates to cool the body.

The **sebaceous glands** release an oily fluid, **sebum**, that lubricates the hair and skin and prevents drying.

Hair is widely distributed over the body. Each hair develops within a sheath or **follicle** and grows from its base within the deep layers of the skin. Both hair and nails function in protection. Each nail develops from a growing region at its proximal end. Hair and nails are composed of nonliving material consisting mainly of keratin.

KEY TERMS

Normal Structure and Function

Term	Definition
dermis *(DER-mis)*	The layer of the skin between the epidermis and the subcutaneous tissue. The true skin or corium.
epidermis *(ep-i-DER-mis)*	The outermost layer of the skin
hair	A threadlike keratinized outgrowth from the skin (root trich/o)
hair follicle	The sheath in which a hair develops
integumentary system *(in-teg-ū-MEN-ta-rē)*	The skin and its associated glands, hair, and nails
keratin *(KER-a-tin)*	A protein that thickens and toughens the skin and makes up hair and nails (root kerat/o)
melanin *(MEL-a-nin)*	A dark pigment that gives color to the hair and skin and protects the skin against the sun's radiation (root melan/o)
nail	A platelike keratinized outgrowth of the skin that covers the dorsal surface of the terminal phalanges (root onych/o)
sebaceous gland *(se-BĀ-shus)*	A gland that produces sebum. Usually associated with a hair follicle. (root seb/o)
sebum *(SĒ-bum)*	A fatty secretion of the sebaceous glands that lubricates the hair and skin (root seb/o)
skin	The tissue that covers the body; the integument (root derm/o, dermat/o)
subcutaneous tissue *(sub-kū-TĀ-nē-us)*	The layer of tissue beneath the skin (from L. *cutis* meaning "skin"); also called the hypodermis
sudoriferous gland *(sū-dor-IF-er-us)*	A sweat gland (root hidr/o, idr/o)

Roots Pertaining to the Skin

Root	Meaning	Example	Definition of Example
derm/o, dermato/o	skin	hypodermic *hī-pō-DER-mik*	administered under the skin
kerat/o	keratin, horny layer of the skin	keratosis *ker-a-TŌ-sis*	horny growth of the skin
melan/o	dark, black, melanin	hypomelanosis *hī-pō-mel-a-NŌ-sis*	deficiency of melanin in the skin
hidr/o, idr/o	sweat, perspiration	hydradenitis *hī-drad-i-NĪ-tis*	inflammation of a sweat gland
seb/o	sebum, sebaceous gland	seborrhea *seb-or-Ē-a*	excess flow of sebum
trich/o	hair	trichomycosis *trik-ō-mī-KŌ-si*	fungal infection of the hair
onych/o	nail	onychia *ō-NIK-ē-a*	inflammation of the nail and nail bed (not an *-itis* ending)

Exercise 21-1

Identify the roots in the following words and give the meaning of each:

	Root	Meaning of Root
1. epidermis *(ep-i-DER-mis)*	________	________
2. anidrosis *(an-ī-DRŌ-sis)*	________	________
3. keratogenous *(ker-a-TOJ-e-nus)*	________	________
4. seborrheic *(seb-ō-RĒ-ik)*	________	________
5. hypertrichosis *(hī-per-tri-KŌ-sis)*	________	________
6. hyponychium *(hī-pō-NIK-ē-um)*	________	________

Fill in the blanks.

7. Dyskeratosis *(dis-ker-a-TŌ-sis)* is an abnormality in the skin's formation of ________________.
8. A melanosome *(MEL-a-nō-sōm)* is a small body in a cell that produces ________________.
9. Hypohidrosis *(hī-pō-hī-DRŌ-sis)* is abnormally low production of ________________.
10. Trichoid *(TRIK-oyd)* means resembling a(n) ________________.
11. Onychomycosis *(on-i-kō-mī-KŌ-sis)* is a fungus infection of a(n) ________________.

Word building. Write a word that fits each of the following definitions:

12. A tumor containing melanin ____________
13. Study of the hair ____________
14. Formation (-genesis) of keratin ____________
15. Softening of a nail ____________
16. Cell that produces melanin ____________
17. Study of the skin and skin diseases ____________
18. Excess production of sweat ____________
19. Inflammation of the skin ____________
20. Instrument for cutting the skin ____________

Use the suffix *-derma* meaning "condition of the skin" in the next two words:

21. Hardening of the skin ____________
22. Presence of pus in the skin ____________

Clinical Aspects of the Skin

Many diseases are manifested by changes in the quality of the skin or by specific lesions. Some types of skin lesions are described in Table 21-1 and illustrated in Figure 21-2. The study of the skin and diseases of the skin is **dermatology**, but careful observation of the skin, hair, and nails should be part of every physical examination.

TABLE 21-1 Types of Skin Lesions

Lesion	Description
bulla *BUL-a*	A raised, fluid-filled lesion larger than a vesicle (pl. bullae)
fissure *FISH-ur*	A crack or break in the skin
macule *MAK-ūl*	A flat, colored spot
nodule *NOD-ūl*	A solid, raised lesion larger than a papule. Often indicative of systemic disease.
papule *PAP-ūl*	A small, circular, raised lesion at the surface of the skin
plaque *plak*	A patch
pustule *PUS-tūl*	A raised lesion containing pus. Often in a hair follicle or sweat pore.
vesicle *VES-i-kl*	A small, fluid-filled, raised lesion. A blister or bleb.
wheal *wēl*	A smooth, rounded, slightly raised area often associated with itching. Seen in urticaria (hives) such as resulting from allergy.

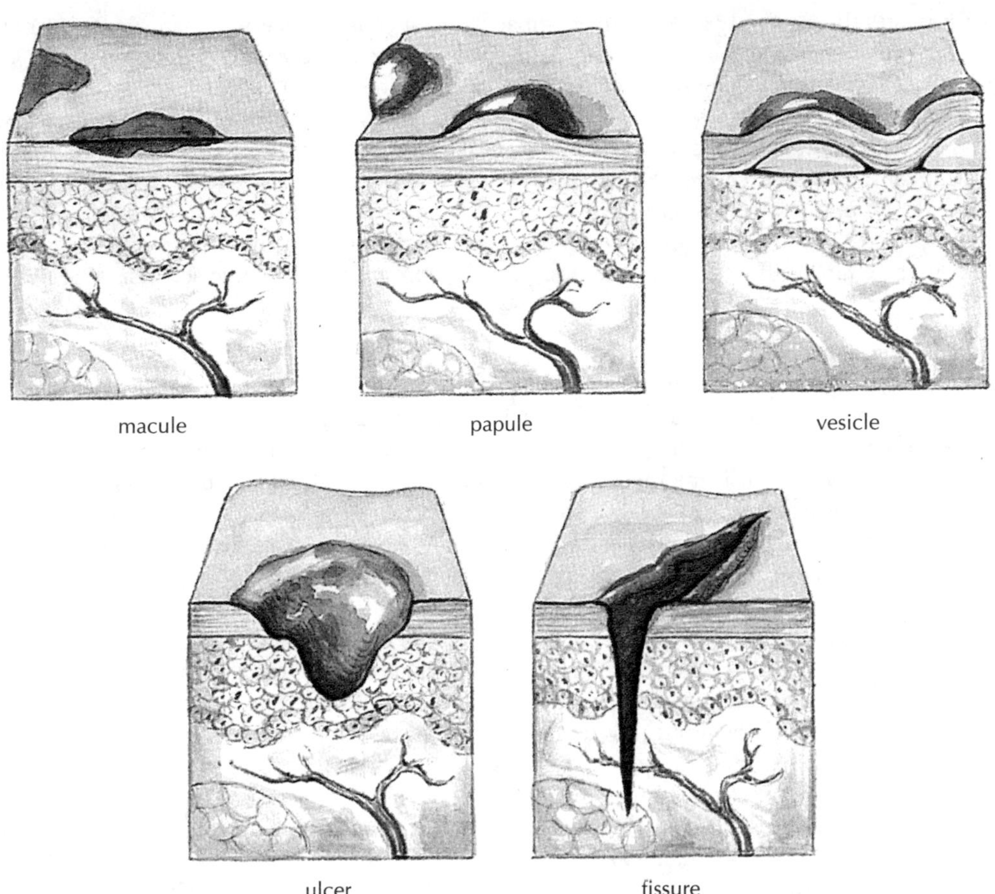

FIGURE 21-2. Some common skin lesions.

Psoriasis

Psoriasis is a chronic overgrowth (hyperplasia) of the epidermis producing large, erythematous (red) plaques with silvery scales. The cause is unknown, but there is sometimes a hereditary pattern. Psoriasis is treated with topical corticosteroids and with exposure to ultraviolet (UV) light. Severe cases have been treated with a combination of a drug, psoralen (P), to increase sensitivity to light, followed by exposure to a form of UV light (UV-A).

Autoimmune Disorders

The diseases discussed below are caused, at least in part, by autoimmune reactions. They are diagnosed by biopsy of lesions and by antibody studies.

Pemphigus is characterized by the formation of blisters (bullae) in the skin and mucous membranes caused by a separation of epidermal cells from underlying layers. Rupture of these lesions leaves deeper areas of the skin unprotected from infection and fluid loss, much as in cases of burns. The cause is an autoimmune reaction to epithelial cells. Pemphigus is fatal unless treated by methods to suppress the immune system.

Systemic lupus erythematosus (SLE) generally involves the skin, and produces a typical butterfly-shaped rash across the nose and cheeks. The disease may also appear in a chronic form that involves the skin only and is termed subacute cutaneous lupus erythematosus (SCLE). It is seen as rough, raised, violet-tinted papules, usually limited to the face and scalp. These skin lesions are worsened by exposure to ultraviolet radiation in sunlight.

Scleroderma is a disease of unknown cause that involves thickening and tightening of the skin. There is gradual fibrosis of the dermis due to overproduction of collagen. Sweat glands and hair follicles are also involved. A very early sign of scleroderma is Raynaud's disease, in which blood vessels in the fingers and toes constrict in the cold, causing numbness, pain, coldness, and tingling. Skin symptoms first appear on the forearms and around the mouth. Internal organs become involved in a diffuse form of scleroderma called progressive systemic sclerosis (PSS).

Skin Cancer

Skin cancer is the most common type of human cancer. Its rate has been increasing in recent years, mainly due to increased exposure to the ultraviolet rays in sunlight.

Malignant melanoma results from an overgrowth of melanocytes, the pigment-producing cells in the epidermis. It is the most dangerous form of skin cancer because of its tendency to metastasize. This cancer appears as a lesion that is variable in color with an irregular border. It may spread superficially for up to 1 or 2 years before it begins to invade the deeper tissues of the skin and to metastasize through blood and lymph. The prognosis for cure is good if the lesion is recognized and removed surgically before it enters this invasive stage.

Squamous cell carcinoma and **basal cell carcinoma** are both cancers of epithelial cells. Both appear in areas exposed to sunlight, such as the face. Squamous cell carcinoma appears as a painless, firm, red nodule or plaque that may develop surface scales, ulceration, or crusting. This cancer may invade underlying tissue, but tends not to metastasize. It is treated by surgical removal, and sometimes with x-irradiation or chemotherapy.

Basal cell carcinoma constitutes more than 75% of all skin cancers. It usually appears as a smooth, pearly papule. Because these cancers are easily seen and do not metastasize, the cure rate following excision is greater than 95%.

Kaposi's sarcoma, once considered rare, is now seen frequently in association with AIDS. It usually appears as distinct brownish areas on the legs. These plaques become raised and firm as the tumor progresses. In those with weakened immune systems, such as AIDS patients, the cancer can metastasize.

KEY CLINICAL TERMS

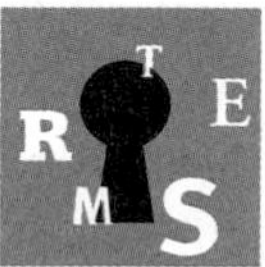

basal cell carcinoma	An epithelial tumor that rarely metastasizes and has a high cure rate with surgical removal
dermatology *(der-ma-TOL-ō-jē)*	Study of the skin and diseases of the skin
Kaposi's sarcoma *(KAP-ō-sēz)*	Cancerous lesion of the skin and other tissues seen most often in patients with AIDS
malignant melanoma	A metastasizing pigmented tumor of the skin
pemphigus *(PEM-fi-gus)*	An autoimmune disease of the skin characterized by sudden, intermittent formation of bullae (blisters). May be fatal if untreated.
psoriasis *(so-RĪ-a-sis)*	A chronic hereditary dermatitis with red lesions covered by silvery scales

scleroderma (*sklēr-ō-DER-ma*) — A chronic disease that is characterized by thickening and tightening of the skin and that often involves internal organs in a form called progressive systemic sclerosis (PSS)

squamous cell carcinoma — An epidermal cancer that may invade deeper tissues but tends not to metastasize

systemic lupus erythematosus (SLE) — A chronic disease of connective tissue that often involves the skin

ADDITIONAL TERMS

Symptoms and Conditions

acne (*AK-nē*) — An inflammatory disease of the sebaceous glands and hair follicles usually associated with excess secretion of sebum

actinic (*ak-TIN-ik*) — Pertaining to the effects of radiant energy, such as sunlight, ultraviolet light, and x-rays

albinism (*AL-bin-izm*) — A hereditary lack of pigment in the skin, hair, and eyes

alopecia (*al-ō-PĒ-shē-a*) — Absence or loss of hair; baldness

Beau's lines (*bōz*) — White lines across the fingernails; usually a sign of systemic disease or injury

bromhidrosis (*brō-mi-DRŌ-sis*) — Sweat which has a foul odor due to bacterial decomposition; also called bromidrosis

carbuncle (*CAR-bung-kl*) — A localized infection of the skin and subcutaneous tissue, usually caused by staphylococcus, and associated with pain and discharge of pus

cicatrix (*SIK-a-triks*) — A scar. Scar formation is called *cicatrization*.

comedo (*KOM-e-dō*) — A plug of sebum, often containing bacteria, in a hair follicle; a blackhead (pl. comedones)

decubitus ulcer (*dē-KŪ-bi-tus*) — An ulcer caused by pressure to an area of the body from a bed or a chair; a bedsore

dermatitis (*der-ma-TĪ-tis*) — Inflammation of the skin, often associated with redness and itching. May be caused by allergy, irritants (contact dermatitis), or a variety of diseases.

dermatophytosis (*der-ma-tō-fi-TŌ-sis*) — Fungal infection of the skin, especially between the toes; athlete's foot (root *phyt/o* means "plant")

diaphoresis (*dī-a-fō-RĒ-sis*) — Profuse sweating

dyskeratosis (*dis-ker-a-TŌ-sis*) — Any abnormality in keratin formation in epithelial cells

(continued)

ecchymosis
(ek-i-MŌ-sis)
A collection of blood under the skin caused by leakage from small vessels

eczema
(EK-zē-ma)
A general term for an inflammation of the skin with redness, lesions, and itching. Also called atopic dermatitis.

erysipelas
(er-i-SIP-e-las)
An acute infectious disease of the skin with localized redness and swelling and systemic symptoms

erythema
(er-i-THĒ-ma)
Diffuse redness of the skin

erythema nodosum
(nō-DŌ-sum)
Inflammation of subcutaneous tissues resulting in tender, erythematous nodules. May be an abnormal immune response to a systemic disease, an infection, or a drug.

exanthem
(eks-AN-them)
Any eruption of the skin which accompanies a disease, such as measles; a rash

furuncle
(FŪ-rung-kl)
A painful skin nodule caused by staphylococci which enter through a hair follicle; a boil

hemangioma
(hē-man-jē-Ō-ma)
A benign tumor of blood vessels. In the skin they are called birthmarks or port wine stains.

herpes simplex
(HER-pēz SIM-pleks)
A group of acute infections caused by herpes simplex virus. Type I herpes simplex virus produces fluid-filled vesicles, usually on the lips, following fever, exposure to the sun, injury, or stress; cold sore, fever blister. Type II infections usually involve the genital organs.

hirsutism
(HIR-sū-tizm)
Excessive growth of hair

ichthyosis
(ik-thē-Ō-sis)
A dry, scaly condition of the skin (from the root *ichthy/o* meaning "fish")

impetigo
(im-pe-TĪ-gō)
A bacterial skin infection with pustules that rupture and form crusts; most commonly seen in children, usually on the face

keloid
(KĒ-loyd)
A raised, thickened scar caused by overgrowth of tissue during scar formation

keratosis
(ker-a-TŌ-sis)
Any skin condition marked by thickened or horny growth. Seborrheic keratosis is a benign tumor, yellow or light brown in color, that appears in the elderly. Actinic keratosis is caused by exposure to sunlight and may lead to squamous cell carcinoma.

mycosis fungoides
(mī-KŌ-sis fun-GOY-dēz)
A rare malignant disease that originates in the skin and involves the internal organs and lymph nodes. There are large, painful, ulcerating tumors.

nevus
(NĒ-vus)
A defined discoloration of the skin. A congenital vascular tumor of the skin. A mole, birthmark.

paronychia
(par-ō-NIK-ē-a)
Infection around a nail

pediculosis
(pe-dik-ū-LŌ-sis)
Infestation with lice

petechiae
(pē-TĒ-kē-ē)
Flat, pinpoint, purplish-red spots caused by bleeding within the skin or mucous membrane (sing. petechia)

pruritus *(prū-RĪ-tus)* — Severe itching

purpura *(PUR-pū-ra)* — A condition characterized by hemorrhages into the skin and other tissues

rosacea *(rō-ZĀ-sē-a)* — A condition of unknown cause involving redness of the skin, pustules, and overactivity of sebaceous glands, mainly on the face

scabies *(SKĀ-bēz)* — A highly contagious skin disease caused by a mite

senile lentigines *(len-TIJ-i-nēz)* — Brown macules that appear on sun-exposed skin in adults; liver spots

shingles — An acute eruption of vesicles along the path of a nerve; herpes zoster *(HER-pēz ZOS-ter)*. Caused by the same virus that causes chicken pox.

tinea *(TIN-ē-a)* — A fungal infection of the skin; ringworm

urticaria *(ur-ti-KĀ-rē-a)* — A skin reaction marked by temporary, smooth, raised areas (wheals) associated with itching; hives

verruca *(ver-RŪ-ka)* — An epidermal tumor; a wart

vitiligo *(vit-i-LĪ-gō)* — Patchy disappearance of pigment in the skin; leukoderma

xeroderma pigmentosum *(zē-rō-DER-ma pig-men-TŌ-sum)* — A fatal hereditary disease that begins in childhood with discolorations and ulcers of the skin and muscle atrophy. There is increased sensitivity to the sun and increased susceptibility to cancer.

Diagnosis and Treatment

cautery *(KAW-ter-ē)* — Destruction of tissue by physical or chemical means; cauterization. Also the instrument or chemical used for this purpose.

debridement *(da-brē-DMON)* — Removal of dead or damaged tissue, as from a wound

dermabrasion *(DERM-a-brā-zhun)* — A plastic surgical procedure for removing scars or birthmarks by chemical or mechanical destruction of epidermal tissue

dermatoplasty *(DER-ma-tō-plas-tē)* — Transplantation of human skin; skin grafting

diascopy *(dī-AS-kō-pē)* — Examination of skin lesions by pressing a glass plate against the skin

escharotomy *(es-kar-OT-ō-mē)* — Removal of scab tissue (eschar) resulting from burns or other skin injuries

fulguration *(ful-gū-RĀ-shun)* — Destruction of tissue by high frequency electric sparks

Wood's lamp — An ultraviolet light used to diagnose fungal infections

ABBREVIATIONS

PSS progressive systemic sclerosis
PUVA psoralen UV-A
SCLE subacute cutaneous lupus erythematosus
SLE systemic lupus erythematosus
UV ultraviolet

CHAPTER REVIEW 21

Multiple choice. Match the terms in each of the sets below with their definitions and write the appropriate letter (a–e) to the left of each number:

_____ 1. macule	a. birthmark or mole
_____ 2. alopecia	b. bedsore
_____ 3. decubitus ulcer	c. baldness
_____ 4. cicatrix	d. flat, colored spot
_____ 5. nevus	e. scar
_____ 6. vesicle	a. removal of scab tissue
_____ 7. erythema	b. profuse sweating
_____ 8. escharotomy	c. blister
_____ 9. diaphoresis	d. thickened scar
_____ 10. keloid	e. redness of the skin
_____ 11. eczema	a. excess growth of hair
_____ 12. shingles	b. infestation with lice
_____ 13. tinea	c. skin disease caused by a herpes virus
_____ 14. hirsutism	d. inflammation of the skin with redness, lesions, and itching
_____ 15. pediculosis	e. fungal infection
_____ 16. petechiae	a. hives
_____ 17. debridement	b. pinpoint spots on the skin
_____ 18. pruritus	c. removal of dead tissue
_____ 19. diascopy	d. method for examining the skin
_____ 20. urticaria	e. severe itching

Chapter 21
Labeling Exercise

Write the name of each numbered part on the corresponding line of the answer sheet.

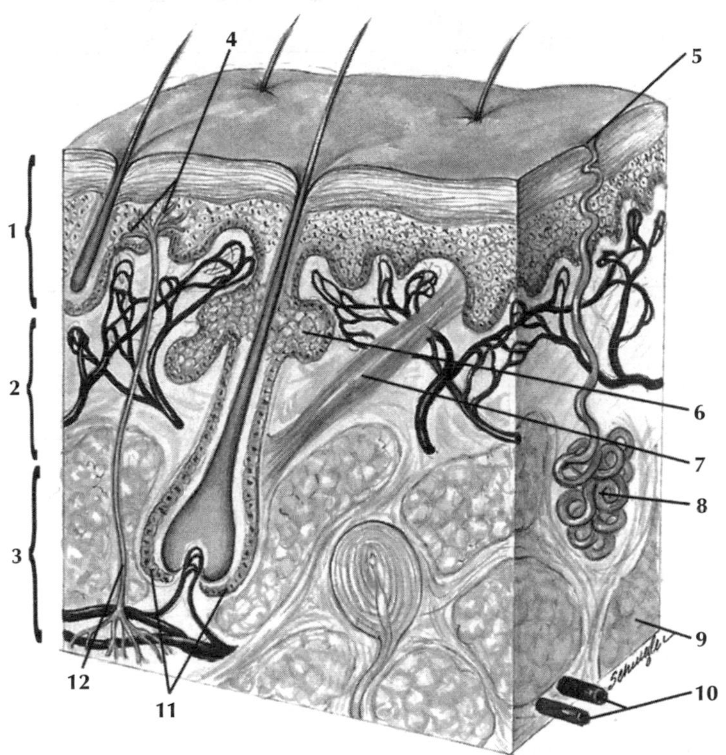

acipose (fat) cells
blood vessels
dermis (corium)
epidermis
hair follicle
muscle
nerve endings
nerve
pore (opening of sweat gland)
sebaceous (oil) gland
subcutaneous layer
sudoriferous (sweat) gland

Cross section of the skin

1. ______________________
2. ______________________
3. ______________________
4. ______________________
5. ______________________
6. ______________________
7. ______________________
8. ______________________
9. ______________________
10. ______________________
11. ______________________
12. ______________________

Fill in the blanks:

21. The skin and its associated structures make up the ______________ system.
22. The main pigment in skin is ______________.
23. The protein that thickens the skin and makes up hair and nails is ______________.
24. The layer of the skin above the dermis is the ______________.
25. A sudoriferous gland produces ______________.
26. The oil-producing glands of the skin are the ______________.

Definitions. Write the meaning of each of the following terms:

27. Xeroderma (*zē-rō-DER-ma*) ______________
28. Pachyderma (*pak-ē-DER-ma*) ______________
29. Keratogenesis (*ker-a-tō-JEN-e-sis*) ______________
30. Hypermelanosis (*hī-per-mel-a-NŌ-sis*) ______________
31. Trichomycosis (*trik-ō-mī-KŌ-sis*) ______________
32. Onychia (*ō-NIK-ē-a*) ______________

Word building. Write a word for each of the following definitions:

33. Pertaining to (-al) the skin ______________
34. Any skin disease ______________
35. Cell that produces melanin ______________
36. Hardening of the skin ______________
37. Discharge of sebum ______________
38. Loosening or separation (-lysis) of a nail ______________

Use the word *hidrosis* (sweating) as an ending for the following words.

The ending *-idrosis* is also used.

39. Absence (an-) of sweating ______________
40. Excess sweating ______________
41. Excretion of colored (chrom/o) sweat ______________

Unscrambles. Form a word from each of the following groups of letters and write it in the blank:

42. lehaw ______________
43. docmoe ______________

44. udolne ______________________________

45. ektniar ______________________________

46. llocifel ______________________________

Word analysis. Define each of the following words and give the meaning of the word parts in each. Use a dictionary if necessary.

47. Onychocryptosis *(on-i-kō-krip-TŌ-sis)* ______________________________

____

   a. onych/o ______________

   b. crypt/o ______________

   c. -sis ______________

48. Achromotrichia *(a-krō-mō-TRIK-ē-a)* ______________________________

____

   a. a- ______________

   b. chrom/o ______________

   c. trich/o ______________

   d. -ia ______________

49. Hidradenoma *(hī-drad-e-NŌ-ma)* ______________________________

____

   a. hidr/o ______________

   b. aden/o ______________

   c. -oma ______________

Chapter 21 Case Studies

1. Cutaneous Lymphoma

The patient is a 52-year-old female with a history of cutaneous T cell lymphoma since 1987. Initial systemic chemotherapy with methotrexate was discontinued due to stomatitis. Since then she has been treated with topical chemotherapeutic agents with some improvement. Past medical history includes hidradenitis.

Physical examination showed diffuse erythroderma with scaling and hyperkeratosis; positive alopecia; leukoplakia and ulcerations of the mouth and tongue.

Two courses of topical chemotherapy were given during hospitalization. The patient was referred to Dental Medicine for treatment of the oral lesions and was discharged in stable condition with an appointment for a follow-up in 4 weeks. Discharge medications included hydrocortisone 1% ointment to body q hs, Keralyt gel bid for hyperkeratosis, Dyclone and Benadryl to mouth prn.

2. Basal Cell Carcinoma (BCC)

This 63-year-old female stated that she noticed a "tiny hard lump" at the base of her left nostril when cleansing her face. The lesion has been present for the past several months. On examination she was noted to have a small pearly white nodule at the lower portion of the left ala. There were no other obvious lesions on her face or neck.

The lesion was excised. Gross findings showed a 8 × 6 × 4-cm fragment of skin and subcutaneous tissue. The specimen was bisected and submitted in toto. The pathology report identified the lesion to be a basal cell carcinoma that was completely excised. Patient will be seen in follow-up in 6 months.

3. Sepsis in a Patient With Severe Burns

Patient is a 43-year-old male admitted 12 November with 20% full thickness burns to the right and left legs. Pulmonary status, evaluated by bronchoscopy, showed the patient to have suffered severe inhalation injury. Patient was taken to surgery for fasciotomies and escharotomies of both legs. The right leg was amputated and the left leg was debrided at that time. On 16 November patient returned to OR for further debridement. He was placed on amphotericin, piperacillin, and Silvadene Cream.

On 26 November patient developed sepsis. Temperature was 103.8. Cultures revealed resistant *staphylococcus, pseudomonas*, and *candida*. Bactrim cleared all but the pseudomonas, and the patient was placed on Amikin. He will be observed for nephrotoxicity, neurotoxicity, and other possible side effects while under treatment for respiratory and cardiac problems.

Chapter 21
Case Study Questions

Multiple choice. Select the best answer and write the letter of your choice to the left of each number:

_____ 1. Hydradenitis is inflammation of a

a. sweat gland
b. salivary gland
c. sebaceous gland
d. ceruminous gland
e. meibomian gland

_____ 2. Leukoplakia is

a. baldness
b. ulceration
c. formation of white patches in the mouth
d. formation of yellow patches on the skin
e. formation of scales on the skin

_____ 3. Hydrocortisone is a(n)

a. vitamin
b. steroid
c. analgesic
d. lubricant
e. diuretic

_____ 4. The term *in toto* means

a. immediately
b. contained in a vial
c. frozen
d. partially
e. entirely

_____ 5. Basal cell carcinoma involves

a. subcutaneous tissue
b. epithelial cells
c. connective tissue
d. adipose tissue
e. hair folicles

_____ 6. Escharotomies were done in case study #3 in order to

a. graft tissue
b. examine the injury
c. set a bone
d. remove scab tissue
e. amputate a limb

Write a word from the case studies that means each of the following:

7. Increased production of keratin in the skin ____________________
8. Redness of the skin ____________________
9. Removal of dead or damaged tissue ____________________
10. Condition of having microorganisms in blood or tissues ____________________

Define the following terms:

11. Lymphoma ____________________
12. Stomatitis ____________________
13. Nephrotoxicity ____________________

THE SKIN

ACROSS

5. the true skin or corium
6. accumulation of fluid in the tissues
9. pertaining to a sweat gland
12. prefix; against
14. fat is stored in adipose _____
17. severe itching
18. prefix: through
19. ichthyosis is a scaly condition of the skin. The name comes from the root ichthy/o meaning _____
20. the main portion of the integumentary system
22. a small mass of lymphoid tissue is a lymph ______

DOWN

1. a fatty secretion that lubricates the hair and skin
2. root (with combining vowel) that means sweat
3. prefix: down, without, removal, loss
4. prefix: again, back
7. inflammation of the skin
8. a degenerative muscle disease (Lou Gehrig's disease) (abbr.)
10. the type of organism that causes mycosis, such as tinea
11. a highly contagious skin disease caused by a mite
13. root (with combining vowel) meaning hair
15. a chronic disease of connective tissue that often involves the skin: systemic ______ erythematosus
16. trauma to a joint involving the ligaments
21. a negative word

Chapter 21
Answer Section

Answers to Chapter Exercises

Exercise 21-1

1. derm/o; skin
2. idr/o; sweat
3. kerat/o; keratin, horny layer of the skin
4. seb/o; sebum
5. trich/o; hair
6. onych/o; nail
7. keratin
8. melanin
9. sweat, perspiration
10. hair
11. nail
12. melanoma *(mel-a-NŌ-ma)*
13. trichology *(trik-OL-ō-jē)*
14. keratogenesis *(ker-a-tō-JEN-e-sis)*
15. onychomalacia *(on-i-kō-ma-LĀ-shē-a)*
16. melanocyte *(MEL-an-ō-sīt)*
17. dermatology *(der-ma-TOL-ō-jē)*
18. hyperhydrosis *(hī-per-hī-DRŌ-sis)*
19. dermatitis *(der-ma-TĪ-tis)*
20. dermatome *(DER-ma-tōm)*
21. scleroderma *(sklēr-ō-DER-ma)*
22. pyoderma *(pī-ō-DER-ma)*

Labeling Exercise

Cross Section of the Skin

1. epidermis
2. dermis (corium)
3. subcutaneous tissue
4. nerve endings
5. pore (opening of sweat gland)
6. sebaceous (oil) gland
7. muscle
8. sudoriferous (sweat) gland
9. adipose (fat) cells
10. blood vessels
11. hair follicle
12. nerve

Answers to Chapter Review 21

1. d
2. c
3. b
4. e
5. a
6. c
7. e
8. a
9. b
10. d
11. d
12. c
13. e
14. a
15. b
16. b
17. c
18. e
19. d
20. a
21. integumentary
22. melanin
23. keratin
24. epidermis

25. sweat
26. sebaceous glands
27. dryness of the skin
28. thickening of the skin
29. formation of keratin
30. excess melanin in the skin
31. fungal infection of the hair
32. inflammation of the nail and nail bed
33. dermal
34. dermatopathy, dermopathy
35. melanocyte
36. scleroderma
37. seborrhea
38. onycholysis
39. anhidrosis, anidrosis
40. hyperhidrosis, hyperidrosis
41. chromhidrosis, chromidrosis
42. wheal
43. comedo
44. nodule
45. keratin
46. follicle
47. Ingrown toenail
    a. nail
    b. hidden
    c. condition of
48. Lack of color or graying of the hair
    a. lack of
    b. color
    c. hair
    d. condition of
49. Benign tumor of a sweat gland
    a. sweat
    b. gland
    c. tumor

Answers to Case Study Questions

1. a
2. c
3. b
4. e
5. b
6. d
7. hyperkeratosis
8. erythroderma
9. debridement
10. sepsis
11. tumor of the lymphatic system
12. inflammation of the mouth
13. harmfulness or toxicity to the kidney

Answers to Crossword Puzzle

THE SKIN

	1 S			2 H			3 D		4 R		
5 D	E	R	M	I	S		6 E	7 D	E	M	8 A
	B			D				E			L
9 S	U	D	O	R	I	10 F	E	R	O	U	S
	M			O		U		M			
11 S						N		12 A	N	13 T	I
14 C	E	15 L	L	16 S		G		T	■	R	
A		U	■	17 P	R	U	R	I	T	I	S
B		18 P	E	R		S	■	T	■	C	
I		U	■	A			19 F	I	S	H	
E		20 S	K	I	21 N			S		O	
S				22 N	O	D	E				

Abbreviations

Abbreviation	Meaning	Chapter
$\bar{a}$	before	7
A, Acc	accommodation	18
$\overline{aa}$	of each	7
Ab	antibody	10
AB	abortion	15
ABC	aspiration biopsy cytology	7
ABG(s)	arterial blood gas(es)	11
ABR	auditory brainstem response	
ac	before meals	18
AC	air conduction	18
ACE	angiotensin converting enzyme	9
ACh	acetylcholine	17, 20
ACTH	adrenocorticotropic hormone	16
AD	right ear	18
ad lib	as desired	7
ADH	antidiuretic hormone	13
AE	above the elbow	19
AF	atrial fibrillation	9
AFB	acid fast bacillus	11
AFP	alpha-fetoprotein	7, 15
Ag	antigen	9
AGA	appropriate for gestational age	15
AIDS	acquired immunodeficiency syndrome	10
AK	above the knee	19
ALL	acute lymphocytic leukemia	10
ALS	amyotrophic lateral sclerosis	17, 20
AMA	against medical advice	7
AMB	ambulatory	7
AMI	acute myocardial infarction	9
AML	acute myelogenous leukemia	9
ANS	autonomic nervous system	16
AP	anteroposterior	7
APAP	acetaminophen	8
APC	atrial premature complex	9
APPT	activated partial thromboplastin time	10
aq	water, aqueous	7
AR	aortic regurgitation	9
ARC	abnormal retinal correspondence	18
ARDS	adult (acute) respiratory distress syndrome	11
ARF	acute respiratory failure	11
ARF	acute renal failure	13
ASA	acetylsalicylic acid (aspirin)	8
As, Ast	astigmatism	18
AS	atrial stenosis; arteriosclerosis	9
AS	left ear	18
ASCVD	arteriosclerotic cardiovascular disease	9
ASD	atrial septal defect	9
ASHD	arteriosclerotic heart disease	9
AST	aspartate aminotransferase (SGOT)	9
AT	atrial tachycardia	9
ATN	acute tubular necrosis	13
AV	atrioventricular	9
BAEP	brainstem auditory evoked potentials	17
BBB	bundle branch block	9
BC	bone conduction	17
BE	barium enema	12
BE	below the elbow	19
bid	twice a day	7
BK	below the knee	19
BM	bowel movement	12
BNO	bladder neck obstruction	14
BP	blood pressure	7
BPH	benign prostatic hyperplasia	14
BRP	bathroom privileges	7
BSE	breast self-examination	14
BT	bleeding time	10
BUN	blood urea nitrogen	13
bx	biopsy	7
$\bar{c}$	with	7
c	Celsius (centigrade)	7
C	compliance	11
C	cervical vertebra	19
C section	cesarean section	15

Abbreviation	Meaning	Chapter
CA	cancer	6
CABG	coronary artery bypass graft	9
CAD	coronary artery disease	9
cap	capsule	7, 8
CAPD	continuous ambulatory peritoneal dialysis	13
CBC	complete blood count	10
CBD	common bile duct	12
CBF	cerebral blood flow	17
CBR	complete bed rest	7
cc	with correction	18
CC	chief complaint	7
CCPD	continuous cyclic peritoneal dialysis	13
CCU	coronary care unit	9
CHD	coronary heart disease	9
CHF	congestive heart failure	9
Ci	Curie	7
CIN	cervical intraepithelial neoplasia	13
CIS	carcinoma in situ	6
CLL	chronic lymphocytic leukemia	10
cm	centimeter	appendix
CML	chronic myelogenous leukemia	10
CNS	central nervous system	16
c/o	complains of	7
Co	coccyx; coccygeal	19
CO_2	carbon dioxide	11
COLD	chronic obstructive lung disease	11
COPD	chronic obstructive pulmonary disease	11
CPAP	continuous positive airway pressure	11
C(P)K	creatine (phospho)kinase	9, 20
CPR	cardiopulmonary resuscitation	9
CRF	chronic renal failure	13
crit	hematocrit	10
C&S	culture and sensitivity	7
CSF	cerebrospinal fluid	17
CT	computed tomography	7
CVA	cerebrovascular accident	17
CVD	cerebrovascular disease	17
CVP	central venous pressure	9
CVS	chorionic villus sampling	15
CXR	chest x-ray	11
D&C	dilatation and curettage	14
dB	decibel	18
dc	discontinue	7
D&E	dilatation and evacuation	14
DES	diethylstilbestrol	14
DIC	disseminated intravascular coagulation	10
DIFF	differential count	10
DIP	distal interphalangeal	19
DJD	degenerative joint disease	19
dL	deciliter	appendix
DM	diabetes mellitus	16
DOE	dyspnea on exertion	9
DTR	deep tendon reflex(es)	17
DUB	dysfunctional uterine bleeding	14
DVT	deep vein thrombosis	7
Dx	diagnosis	7
EBV	Epstein-Barr virus	10
EDC	estimated date of confinement	15
EEG	electroencephalogram; electroencephalograph	16
EKG (ECG)	electrocardiogram	9
ELISA	enzyme-linked immunoabsorbent assay	10
elix	elixir	8
EM	emmetropia	18
EMG	electromyography, electromyogram	20
ENG	electronystagmography	18
ENT	ear(s), nose, and throat	18
EOM	extraocular movement, muscles	18
EOMI	extraocular muscles intact	7
EPO	erythropoietin	13
ERCP	endoscopic retrograde cholangiopancreatography	12
ERT	estrogen replacement therapy	19
ERV	expiratory reserve volume	11
ESR	erythrocyte sedimentation rate	10
ESRD	end-stage renal disease	13
ESWL	extracorporeal shock wave lithotripsy	13
ET	esotropia	18
F	Fahrenheit	7
FAP	familial adenomatous polyposis	12
FBS	fasting blood sugar	16
FC	finger counting	18
FDA	Food and Drug Administration	8
FEV	forced expiratory volume	11
FHR	fetal heart rate	15
FHT	fetal heart tone	15
FRC	functional residual capacity	11
FSH	follicle-stimulating hormone	14
FTI	free thyroxine index	16
FTND	full term normal delivery	15
FTP	full term pregnancy	15

Abbreviation	Meaning	Chapter
FUO	fever of unknown origin	6
FVC	forced vital capacity	11
Fx	fracture	19
g	gram	appendix
GA	gestational age	15
GC	gonococcus	14
GFR	glomerular filtration rate	13
GH	growth hormone	16
GI	gastrointestinal	12
GTT	glucose tolerance test	16
gt(t)	drop(s)	7
GU	genitourinary	13
GYN	gynecology	14
H&P	history and physical	7
HAV	hepatitis A virus	12
Hb, Hgb	hemoglobin	10
HBA_{1c}	hemoglobin A_{1c}; glycohemoglobin; glycosylated hemoglobin	16
HBV	hepatitis B virus	12
HCG	human chorionic gonadotropin	15
HCl	hydrochloric acid	12
Hct, Ht	hematocrit	10
HCV	hepatitis C virus	12
HDL	high-density lipoprotein	9
HEENT	head, eyes, ears, nose, and throat	7
HIV	human immunodeficiency virus	10
HL	hearing level	18
HM	hand movements	18
HNP	herniated nucleus pulposus	19
h/o	history of	7
HPI	history of present illness	7
HPV	human papilloma virus	14
HRT	hormone replacement therapy	14
hs	at bedtime	7
HTN	hypertension	9
Hx	history	7
Hz	Hertz	18
^{131}I	iodine 131	16
I&D	incision and drainage	7
I&O	intake and output	7
IBD	inflammatory bowel disease	12
IBS	inflammatory bowel syndrome	12
IC	inspiratory capacity	11
ICP	intracranial pressure	17
ICSH	interstitial cell-stimulating hormone	14
ICU	intensive care unit	7
ID	intradermal	8
IDDM	insulin-dependent diabetes mellitus	16
IF	intrinsic factor	10
Ig	immunoglobulin	10
IGT	impaired glucose tolerance	16
IM	intramuscular(ly)	7
INH	isoniazid	8, 11
IOL	intraocular lens	18
IOP	intraocular pressure	18
IPPA	inspection, palpation, percussion, auscultation	7
IPPB	intermittent positive pressure breathing	11
IPPV	intermittent positive pressure ventilation	11
IRV	inspiratory reserve volume	11
ITP	idiopathic thrombocytopenic purpura	10
IU	international unit	7
IUD	intrauterine device	14
IV	intravenous(ly)	7, 8
IVC	intravenous cholangiogram	12
IVCD	intraventricular conduction delay	9
IVP	intravenous pyelography	13
IVPB	intravenous piggyback	7
IVU	intravenous urography	13
JVP	jugular venous pulse	9
K	potassium	13
kg	kilogram	appendix
km	kilometer	appendix
KUB	kidney-ureter-bladder	13
KVO	keep vein open	7
L	lumbar vertebra	19
L	liter	appendix
LAD	left anterior descending (coronary artery)	9
LAHB	left anterior hemiblock	9
LDH	lactic dehydrogenase	9
LDL	low-density lipoprotein	9
LH	luteinizing hormone	14
LL	left lateral	7
LLL	left lower lobe (of lung)	11
LLQ	left lower quadrant	5
LMN	lower motor neuron	17
LMP	last menstrual period	15
LOC	level of consciousness	17
LP	lumbar puncture	17
LUL	left upper lobe (of lung)	11
LUQ	left upper quadrant	5
LV	left ventricle	9
LVAD	left ventricular assist device	9
LVEDP	left ventricular end-diastolic pressure	9
lytes	electrolytes	10

Abbreviation	Meaning	Chapter
μg, mcg	microgram	appendix
μL	microliter	appendix
μm	micrometer	appendix
m	meter	appendix
mcg	microgram	appendix
MCH	mean corpuscular hemoglobin	10
MCHC	mean corpuscular hemoglobin concentration	10
MCP	metacarpophalangeal	19
MCV	mean corpuscular volume	9
MED(s)	medicine(s), medication(s)	8
MEFR	maximal expiratory flow rate	11
MEN	multiple endocrine neoplasia	16
mEq	milliequivalent	10
MET	metastasis	7
mg	milligram	appendix
MG	myasthenia gravis	20
MI	myocardial infarction	9
mL	milliliter	appendix
mm	millimeter	appendix
MMFR	maximum midexpiratory flow rate	11
mm Hg	millimeters mercury	9
MN	myoneural	20
MR	mitral regurgitation, reflux	9
MRI	magnetic resonance imaging	7
MS	mitral stenosis	9
MS	multiple sclerosis	17
MTP	metatarsophalangeal	19
MUGA	multigated acquisition (scan)	9
MVP	mitral valve prolapse	9
Na	sodium	13
NAD	no apparent distress	7
n&v	nausea and vomiting	12
NB	newborn	15
NG	nasogastric	12
NGU	nongonococcal urethritis	14
NICU	neonatal intensive care unit	15
NIDDM	non–insulin-dependent diabetes mellitus	16
NM	neuromuscular	20
NPH	neutral protamine Hagedorn (insulin)	16
NPH	normal pressure hydrocephalus	17
NPO	nothing by mouth	7
NRC	normal retinal correspondence	18
NREM	non-rapid eye movement	17
NS	normal saline	7
NSAID(s)	nonsteroidal anti-inflammatory drug(s)	8, 19
NSR	normal sinus rhythm	9
NV	near vision	18
O_2	oxygen	11
OA	osteoarthritis	19
OB	obstetrics	15
OD	right eye	18
OOB	out of bed	7
ORL	otorhinolaryngology	18
ortho, ORTH	orthopedics	19
OS	left eye	18
OT	occupational therapy	20
OTC	over-the-counter	8
OU	both eyes; each eye	18
$\bar{p}$	after, post	7
P	pulse	7
PA	posteroanterior; physician assistant	7
$PACo_2$	arterial partial pressure of carbon dioxide	11
PAO_2	arterial partial pressure of oxygen	11
PAP	pulmonary arterial pressure	9
pc	after meals	7
PCA	patient controlled analgesia	7
PCP	*Pneumocystis carinii* pneumonia; pneumocystic pneumonia	10
PCV	packed cell volume	10
PDA	patent ductus arteriosus	15
PDR	Physicians' Desk Reference	8
PE	physical examination	7
PEP	protein electrophoresis	13
PE(R)RLA	pupils equal, (regular) react to light and accommodation	7
PEEP	positive end-expiratory pressure	11
PEFR	peak expiratory flow rate	11
PET	positron emission tomography	7
PFT	pulmonary function test(s)	11
pH	scale for measuring hydrogen ion concentration (acidity)	10
Ph	Philadelphia chromosome	10
PID	pelvic inflammatory disease	14
PIH	pregnancy induced hypertension	15
PIP	peak inspiratory pressure	11

Abbreviation	Meaning	Chapter
PIP	proximal interphalangeal	19
PKU	phenylketonuria	15
PMH	past medical history	7
PMI	point of maximal impulse	9
PMN	polymorphonuclear (neutrophil)	10
PMS	premenstrual syndrome	14
poly, polymorph	neutrophil	10
PNS	peripheral nervous system	17
po	by mouth, orally	7, 8
post op	postoperative	7
pp	postprandial (following a meal)	7
PPD	purified protein derivative (tuberculin)	11
pre op	preoperative	7
prn	as needed	7
PSA	prostate specific antigen	14
PSS	progressive systemic sclerosis	21
PSVT	paroxysmal supraventricular tachycardia	9
pt	patient	7
PT	physical therapy	20
PT, ProTime	prothrombin time	10
PTCA	percutaneous transluminal coronary angioplasty	9
PTT	partial thromboplastin time	10
PUVA	psoralen UV-A	21
PVC	premature ventricular contraction	9
PVD	peripheral vascular disease	9
PWP	pulmonary (artery) wedge pressure	9
PYP	pyrophosphate	9
qd	every day	7
qh	every hour	7
q__h	every __ hours	7
qid	four times a day	7
qm	every morning	7
qn	every night	7
QNS	quantity not sufficient	7
qod	every other day	7
QS	quantity sufficient	7
R	respiration	7
RA	rheumatoid arthritis	19
RAIU	radioactive iodine uptake	16
RAS	reticular activating system	17
RATx	radiation therapy	7
RBC	red blood cell; red blood (cell) count	10
RDS	respiratory distress syndrome	11
REM	rapid eye movement	17
RIA	radioimmunoassay	16
RL	right lateral	7
RLL	right lower lobe (of lung)	11
RLQ	right lower quadrant	5
RML	right middle lobe (of lung)	11
R/O	rule out	7
ROM	range of motion	20
ROS	review of systems	7
RUL	right upper lobe (of lung)	11
RUQ	right upper quadrant	5
RV	residual volume	11
Rx	drug, prescription, therapy	7, 8
$\bar{s}$	without	7
S	sacrum; sacral	19
S_1	the first heart sound	9
S_2	the second heart sound	9
SA	sinoatrial	9
SaO_2	oxygen percent saturation (arterial)	11
SBE	subacute bacterial endocarditis	9
sc	without correction	18
SC, subcu.	subcutaneous(ly)	7, 8
SCLE	subacute cutaneous lupus erythematosus	21
seg	neutrophil	10
SEP	somatosensory evoked potentials	17
SG	specific gravity	13
SGOT	serum glutamic oxaloacetic transaminase (AST)	9
SIADH	syndrome of inappropriate antidiuretic hormone	16
SIDS	sudden infant death syndrome	11
SK	streptokinase	9
SL	sublingual	8
SLE	systemic lupus erythematosus	10, 21 10, 21
SMD	senile macular degeneration	18
SPECT	single photon emission computed tomography	7
$\overline{ss}$	half	7
ST	speech threshold	18
staph	staphylococcus	6
STAT	immediately	7
STD	sexually transmitted disease	14
strep	streptococcus	6
supp	suppository	7, 8
susp	suspension	7, 8

Abbreviation	Meaning	Chapter
SVD	spontaneous vaginal delivery	15
SVT	supraventricular tachycardia	9
T	thoracic vertebra	19
T	temperature	7
T_3	triiodothyronine	16
T_4	thyroxine	16
T&A	tonsils and adenoids; tonsillectomy and adenoidectomy	11
tab	tablet	8
TB	tuberculosis	11
TBG	thyroxine binding globulin	16
^{99m}Tc	technetium-99m	9
TGV	thoracic gas volume	11
THR	total hip replacement	19
TIA	transient ischemic attack	17
tid	three times a day	7
tinct	tincture	7, 8
TKO	to keep open	7
TKR	total knee replacement	19
TLC	total lung capacity	11
Tm	maximal transport capacity	13
TM	tympanic membrane	18
TNM	(primary) tumor, (regional lymph) nodes, (distant) metastases	7
tPA	tissue plasminogen activator	9
TPN	total parenteral nutrition	12
TPR	temperature, pulse, respiration	7
TPUR	transperineal urethral resection	14
TSE	testicular self-examination	14
TSH	thyroid-stimulating hormone	16
TSS	toxic shock syndrome	14
TT	thrombin time	10
TTP	thrombotic thrombocytopenic purpura	10
TTS	temporary threshold shift	18
TURP	transurethral resection of prostate	14
TV	tidal volume	11
U	units	7
UA	urinalysis	13
UC	uterine contractions	15
UGI	upper gastrointestinal	12
UMN	upper motor neuron	17
ung	ointment	7, 8
URI	upper respiratory infection	11
USP	United States Pharmacopeia	8
UTP	uterine term pregnancy	15
UV	ultraviolet	7, 21
VA	visual acuity	18
VBAC	vaginal birth after cesarean section	15
VC	vital capacity	11
VD	venereal disease	14
VDRL	Venereal Disease Research Laboratory	14
VEP	visual evoked potentials	17
VF	ventricular fibrillation, visual field	18
VPC	ventricular premature complex	9
VS	vital signs	7
VSD	ventricular septal defect	9
VT	ventricular tachycardia	9
VTG	thoracic gas volume	11
vWF	von Willebrand's factor	10
WBC	white blood cell; white blood (cell) count	10
WD	well developed	7
WNL	within normal limits	7
WPW	Wolff-Parkinson-White syndrome	9
×	times	7
XT	exotropia	18

Appendix

Metric Measurements

Unit	Abbreviation	Metric Equivalent	U.S. Equivalent
Units of Length			
kilometer	km	1000 meters	0.62 miles; 1.6 km/mile
meter*	m	100 cm; 1000 mm	39.4 inches; 1.1 yards
centimeter	cm	1/100 m; 0.01 m	0.39 inches; 2.5 cm/inch
millimeter	mm	1/1000 m; 0.001 m	0.039 inches; 25 mm/inch
micrometer	µm	1/1000 mm; 0.001 mm	
Units of Weight			
kilogram	kg	1000 g	2.2 lb
gram*	g	1000 mg	0.035 oz; 28.5 g/oz
milligram	mg	1/1000 g; 0.001 g	
microgram	µg, mcg	1/1000 mg; 0.001 mg	
Units of Volume			
liter*	L	1000 mL	1.06 qt
deciliter	dL	1/10 L; 0.1 L	
milliliter	mL	1/1000 L; 0.001 L	0.034 oz; 29.4 mL/oz
microliter	µL	1/1000 mL; 0.001 mL	

*Basic unit

Glossary

Word Parts and Their Meanings

Word Part	Meaning	Reference
a-	not, without, lack of, absence	21
ab-	away from	22
abdomin/o	abdomen	49
-ac	pertaining to heart	11
acous, acus	sound, hearing	425
acro-	extremity, end	52
ad-	toward, near	22
aden/o	gland	34
adip/o	fat	37
adren/o, adrenal/o	adrenal gland, epinephrine	362, 362
adrenocortic/o	adrenal cortex	362
aer/o	air, gas	86
-al	pertaining to	11
algi/o, algesi/o	pain	108
-algesia	pain	68, 422
-algia	pain	68
ambly-	dim	438
amnio	amnion	336
amyl/o	starch	37
an-	not, without, lack of	21
andr/o	male	292
angi/o	vessel	130
an/o	anus	231
ante-	before	24
anti-	against	21, 108
aort/o	aorta	131
-ar	pertaining to	11
arter/o, arteri/o	artery	130
arteriol/o	arteriole	130
arthr/o	joint	462
-ary	pertaining to	11
-ase	enzyme	36
atel/o	incomplete	201
atri/o	atrium	129
audi/o	hearing	425
auto-	self	173
azot/o	nitrogen compounds	168
bacill/i, bacill/o	bacillus	72
bacteri/o	bacterium	72
bar/o	pressure	86
bi-	two, twice	19
bili	bile	233
blast/o	immature cell, productive cell, embryonic cell	34
blephar/o	eyelid	432
brachi/o	arm	49
brady-	slow	67
bronch/i, bronch/o	bronchus	197
bronchiol	bronchiole	197
bucc/o	cheek	229
burs/o	bursa	462
calc/i	calcium	168
cali, calic	calyx	265
-capnia	carbon dioxide (level of)	196
carcin/o	cancer, carcinoma	66
cardi/o	heart	129
cec/o	cecum	230
-cele	hernia, localized dilation	68
celi/o	abdomen	49
centesis	puncture, tap	88
cephal/o	head	49
cerebell/o	cerebellum	387, 390
cerebr/o	cerebrum	387, 390
cervic/o	neck, cervix	49, 306
cheil/o	lip	229
cheir/o, chir/o	hand	49
chem/o	chemical	108
cholangi/o	bile duct	233
chol/e, chol/o	bile, gall	233
cholecyst/o	gallbladder	233
choledoch/o	common bile duct	233
chondr/o	cartilage	462
chori/o, choroid/o	choroid	433
chrom/o, chromat/o	color, stain	86
chron/o	time	86
circum-	around	54
clasis, -clasia	breaking	69
clitor/o, clitorid/o	clitoris	308
coccy, coccyg/o	coccyx	463
cochle/o	cochlea (of inner ear)	425
col/o, colon/o	colon	231

Word Part	Meaning	Reference
colp/o	vagina	306
contra-	against	21, 108
corne/o	cornea	433
cortic/o	outer portion, cerebral cortex	390
cost/o	rib	463
crani/o	skull, cranium	463
cry/o	cold	86
crypt/o	hidden	295
cus	sound, hearing	425
cyan/o-	blue	20
cycl/o	ciliary body, ciliary muscle (of eye)	433
cyst/o, cyst/i	filled sac or pouch, cyst, bladder, urinary bladder	66, 266
-cyte, cyt/o	cell	34
dacry/o	tear, lacrimal apparatus	432
dacryocyst/o	lacrimal sac	432
dactyl/o	finger, toe	52
de-	down, without, removal, loss	21
dent/o, dent/i	tooth, teeth	229
derm/o, dermat/o	skin	517
-desis	binding, fusion	88
dextr/o-	right	25
di-	two, twice	19
dia-	through	21
dilation, dilatation	expansion, widening	70
dipl/o-	double	19
dis-	absence, removal, separation	21
duoden/o	duodenum	230
dys-	abnormal, painful, difficult	68
ec-	out, outside	25
ectasia, ectasis	dilation, dilatation	70
ecto-	out, outside	25
-ectomy	excision, surgical removal	88
edema	accumulation of fluid, swelling	70
electr/o	electricity	86
embryo/o	embryo	336
emesis	vomiting	239
-emia	condition of blood	166
encephal/o	brain	390
end/o-	in, within	25
endocrin/o	endocrine	361
enter/o	intestine	230
epi-	upon, over	54
epididym/o	epididymis	293
episi/o	vulva	308
erg/o	work	86
erythr/o-	red, red blood cell	20, 167
erythrocyt/o	red blood cell	167

Word Part	Meaning	Reference
esophag/o	esophagus	230
-esthesia, -esthesi/o	sensation	422
eu-	true, good, easy, normal	23
ex/o	away from, outside	25
extra-	outside	54
fasci/o	fascia	494
ferr/i, ferr/o	iron	168
fet/o	fetus	336
fibr/o	fiber	34
-form	like, resembling	11
galact/o	milk	336
gangli/o, ganglion/o	ganglion	388
gastr/o	stomach	230
gen, genesis	origin, formation	35
-geusia	sense of taste	422
gingiv/o	gums	229
gli/o	neuroglia	388
glomerul/o	glomerulus	265
gloss/o	tongue	229
gluc/o	glucose	37
glyc/o	sugar, glucose	37
gnath/o	jaw	229
-gram	record of data	87
-graph	instrument for recording data	87
-graphy	act of recording data	87
gravida	pregnant wowan	336
gyn/o, gynec/o	woman	305
hem/o, hemat/o	blood	167
hemi-	half, one side	19
-hemia	condition of blood	166
hepat/o	liver	233
hetero-	other, different, unequal	23
hidr/o	sweat, perspiration	517
hist/o, histi/o	tissue	34
homo-, homeo-	same, unchanging	23
hydr/o	water, fluid	36
hyper-	over, excess, increased, abnormally high	22
hypn/o	sleep	108
hypo-	under, below, decreased, abnormally low	22
hypophys	pituitary, hypophysis	361
hyster/o	uterus	306
-ia	condition of	10
-ian	specialist	12
-ia/sis	condition of	12
-iatrics	medical specialty	12
-iatry	medical specialty	12
-ic	pertaining to	11
-ical	pertaining to	11
idr/o	sweat, perspiration	517

Word Part	Meaning	Reference
-ile	pertaining to	11
ile/o	ileum	230
ili/o	ilium	463
im-	not	21
immun/o	immunity, immune system	167
in-	not	21
infra-	below	54
in/o	fiber, muscle fiber	494
insul/o	pancreatic islets	362
inter-	between	54
intra-	in, within	54
ir-, irit/o, irid/o	iris	433
-ism	condition of	12
iso-	equal, same	23
-ist	specialist	12
-itis	inflammation	69
jejun/o	jejunum	230
juxta-	near, beside	54
kali	potassium	169
kary/o	nucleus	34
kerat/o	cornea, keratin, horny layer of skin	433, 517
kine, kinesi/o, kinet/o	movement	494
labi/o	lip	229
labyrinth/o	labyrinth (inner ear)	425
lacrim/o	tear, lacrimal apparatus	432
lact/o	milk	336
-lalia	speech, babble	391
lapar/o	abdominal wall	49
laryng/o	larynx	197
lent/i	lens	433
-lepsy	seizure	391
leuk/o-	white, colorless, white blood cell	20, 167
leukocyt/o	white blood cell	167
-lexia	reading	391
lingu/o	tongue	229
lip/o	fat, lipid	37
lith	calculus, stone	66
-logy	study of	12
lumb/o	lumbar region, lower back	49
lymphaden/o	lymph node	132
lymphangi/o	lymphatic vessel	132
lymph/o	lymph, lymphatic system, lymphocyte	132, 167
lymphocyt/o	lymphocyte	167
lysis	separation, loosening, dissolving, destruction	70
-lytic	lysing, destroying	108
macro-	large, abnormally large	23
mal-	bad, poor	68
malacia	softening	70
mamm/o	breast, mammary gland	308
mania	excited state, obsession	392
mast/o	breast, mammary gland	308
medull/o	inner part, medulla oblongata	390
mega-, megalo-	large, abnormally large	23
-megaly	enlargement	69
melan/o-	black, dark,melanin	20, 517
mening/o, meninge/o	meninges	389
men/o, mens	month, menstruation	305
mes/o	middle	25
-meter	instrument for measuring	87
metr/o	measure	435
metr/o, metr/i	uterus	306
-metry	measurement of	87
micro-	small, one millionth	23
-mimetic	mimicking, simulating	108
mon/o	one	19
morph/o	form, structure	34
muc/o	mucus, mucous membrane	34
multi-	many	19
muscul/o	muscle	494
myc/o	fungus, mold	71
myel/o	bone marrow, spinal cord	167, 389 462
my/o	muscle	494
myring/o	tympanic membrane	425
myx/o	mucus	34
narc/o	stupor, unconsciousness	108, 390
nas/o	nose	197
nat/i	birth	336
natri	sodium	169
necrosis	death of tissue	70
neo-	new	23
nephr/o	kidney	265
neur/o, neur/i	nervous system, nerve	388
noct/i	night	90
normo-	normal	23
nucle/o	nucleus	34
nyct/o	night, darkness	90
ocul/o	eye	433
odont/o	tooth, teeth	229
-odynia	pain	69
-oid	like, resembling	11
olig/o-	few, scanty, deficiency of	22
-oma	tumor	69
onc/o	tumor	67

Word Part	Meaning	Reference
onych/o	nail	517
oo	ovum	305
oophor/o	ovary	305
ophthalm/o	eye	433
-opia	eye, vision	435
-opsia	vision	435
opt/o	eye, vision	433
orchid/o, orchi/o	testis	293
or/o	mouth	229
ortho-	straight, correct, upright	23
osche/o	scrotum	293
-ose	sugar	36
-o/sis	condition of	10
-osmia	sense of smell	422
oste/o	bone	462
ot/o	ear	425
-ous	pertaining to	11
ovari/o	ovary	305
ov/o	ovum	305
-oxia	oxygen (level of)	196
ox/y	oxygen, sharp, acute	169
pachy	thick	68
palat/o	palate	229
palpebr/o	eyelid	432
pan-	all	22
pancreat/o	pancreas	233
papill/o	nipple	34
para-	near, beside	54
para	woman who has given birth	336
parathyr/o, parathyroid/o	parathyroid	362
paresis	partial paralysis	392
path/o, -pathy	disease	67, 69
ped/o	foot, child	52, 345
pelvi/o	pelvis	463
-penia	decrease in, deficiency of	166
per-	through	22
peri-	around	54
perine/o	perineum	308
periton, peritone/o	peritoneum	49
-pexy	surgical fixation	88
phac/o, phak/o	lens	433
phag/o	eat, ingest	34
pharmac/o	drug	109
pharyng/o	pharynx	197
-phasia	speech	391
phil, -philic	attracting, absorbing	35
phleb/o	vein	131
phobia	fear	392
phon/o	sound, voice	86
-phonia	voice	196

Word Part	Meaning	Reference
phot/o	light	86
phren/o	diaphragm	198
phrenic/o	phrenic nerve	198
pituitar	pituitary hypophysis	361
plas, -plasia	formation, molding, development	35
-plasty	plastic repair, plastic surgery, reconstruction	88
-plegia	paralysis	391
pleur/o	pleura	198
-pnea	breathing	196
pneum/o, pneumat/o	air, gas, lung respiration	198
pneumon/o	lung	198
pod/o	foot	52
-poiesis	formation, production	166
poikilo-	varied, irregular	23
poly-	many, much	19
post-	after, behind	24
pre-	before, in front of	24
presby-	old	438
prim/i-	first	19
pro-	before, in front of	24
proct/o	rectum	231
prostat/o	prostate	293
prote/o	protein	37
pseudo-	false	23
psych/o	mind	390
ptosis	dropping, downward displacement, prolapse	70
ptysis	spitting	201
pulm/o, pulmon/o	lung	198
pupill/o	pupil	433
pyel/o	renal pelvis	265
pylor/o	pylorus	230
py/o	pus	67
pyr/o, pyret/o	fever, fire	67, 108
quadr/i-	four	19
rachi/o	spine	389, 463
radicul/o	root of spinal nerve	389
radi/o	radiation, x-ray	86
re-	again, back	23
rect/o	rectum	231
ren/o	kidney	265
reticul/o	network	34
retin/o	retina	433
retro-	behind, backward	54
-rhage, -rhagia	bursting forth, profuse flow, hemorrhage	69
-rhaphy	surgical repair, suture	88
-rhea	flow, discharge	69
-rhexis	rupture	69

Word Part	Meaning	Reference
rhin/o	nose	197
sacr/o	sacrum	463
salping/o	tube, oviduct, eustachian (auditory) tube	306, 425
-schisis	fissure, splitting	69
scler/o	hard, sclera (of eye)	67, 433
sclerosis	hardening	67
-scope	instrument for viewing or examining	87
-scopy	examination of	87
seb/o	sebum, sebaceous gland	517
semi-	half, partial	19
semin	semen	293
sial/o	saliva, salivary gland, salivary duct	229
sider/o	iron	169
sigmoid/o	sigmoid colon	231
sinistr/o	left	25
-sis	condition of	10
somat/o	body	34
some	small body	35
somn/i, somn/o	sleep	390
son/o	sound, ultrasound	86
spasm	sudden contraction, cramp	70
sperm/i,	semen,	293
spermat/o	spermatozoa	293
spir/o	breathing	198
splen/o	spleen	132
spondyl/o	vertebra	463
staped/o, stapedi/o	stapes	425
staphyl/o	grapelike cluster, staphylococcus	71
stasis	suppression, stoppage	70
steat/o	fatty	37
stenosis	narrowing, constriction	70
steth/o	chest	86
stoma, stomat/o	mouth	229
-stomy	surgical creation of an opening	88
strept/o-	twisted chain, streptococcus	71
sub-	below, under	54
super-	above, excess	22
supra-	above	54
syn-, sym-	together	25
synov/i	synovial joint, synovial membrane	462
tachy-	rapid	68
tel/e-, tel/o-	end	25
ten/o, tendin/o	tendon	494
terat/o	malformed fetus	336
test/o	testis	293
tetra-	four	19
thalam/o	thalamus	390
therm/o	heat, temperature	86
thorac/o	chest, thorax	49
thromb/o	blood clot	167
thrombocyt/o	platelet, thrombocyte	167
thym/o	thymus gland	132
thyr/o, thyroid/o	thyroid	362
toc/o	labor	336
-tome	instrument for incising (cutting)	88
-tomy	incision of, cutting	88
ton/o	tone	494
tonsill/o	tonsil	132
tox/o, toxic/o	poison, toxin	67, 108
trache/o	trachea	197
trans-	through, across, beyond	22
tri-	three	19
trich/o	hair	517
-tripsy	crushing	88
trop,- tropic	act(ing) on, affect(ing)	35, 108
troph/o, -trophy, -trophia	feeding, growth, nourishment	35
tympan/o	tympanic cavity (middle ear), tympanic membrane	425
un-	not	21
uni-	one	19
ureter/o	ureter	266
urethr/o	urethra	266
-uria	urine, urination	267
ur/o	urine, urinary tract	266
urin/o	urine	266
uter/o	uterus	306
uve/o	uvea (of eye)	433
vagin/o	sheath, vagina	306
valv/o, valvul/o	valve	129
varic/o	twisted and swollen vein	137
vascul/o	vessel	130
vas/o	vessel, duct, vas deferens	108, 130 293
ven/o, ven/i	vein	131
ventricul/o	cavity, ventricle	129, 390
vertebr/o	vertebra, spinal column	463
vesic/o	urinary bladder	266
vesicul/o	seminal vesicle	293
vestibul/o	vestibule, vestibular apparatus (of ear)	425
vir/o	virus	72
vulv/o	vulva	308
xanth/o-	yellow	20
xero-	dry	68
-y	condition of	10

Meanings and Their Corresponding Word Parts

Meaning	Word Part(s)	Reference
abdomen	abdomin/o, celi/o	49
abdominal wall	lapar/o	49
abnormal	dys-	68
abnormally high	hyper-	22
abnormally large	macro-, mega-, megalo-	23
abnormally low	hypo-	22
above	super-, supra-	22, 54
absence	a-, an-, dis-	21
absorb(ing)	phil, -philic	35
accumulation of fluid	edema	70
across	trans-	22
act of recording data	-graphy	87
act(ing) on	trop, -tropic	35, 108
acute	ox/y	169
adrenal gland	adren/o, adrenal/o	362
adrenaline	adren/o	362
adrenal	adren/o	362
adrenal cortex	adrenocortic/o	362
affect(ing)	trop, -tropic	35, 108
after	post-	24
again	re-	23
against	anti-, contra-	21, 108
air	aer/o, pneumat/o	86
all	pan-	22
amnion	amnio	336
anus	an/o	231
aorta	aort/o	131
arm	brachi/o	49
around	circum-, peri-	54
arteriole	arteriol/o	130
artery	arter/o, arteri/o	130
atrium	atri/o	129
attract(ing)	phil, -philic	35
away from	ab-, ex/o-	22, 25
babble	-lalia	391
bacillus	bacill/i, bacill/o	72
back	re-	23
backward	retro-	54
bacterium	bacteri/o	72
bad	mal-	68
before	ante-, pre-, pro-	24
behind	post-, retro-	24, 54
below	hypo-, infra-, sub-	22, 54
beside	para-, juxta-	54
between	inter-	54
beyond	trans-	22
bile	bili, chol/e, chol/o	233
bile duct	cholangi/o	233
binding	-desis	88
birth	nat/i	336
black	melan/o-	20
bladder	cyst/o, cyst/i	66, 266
bladder (urinary)	cyst/o, vesic/o	66, 266
blood	hem/o, hemat/o	167
blood (condition of)	-emià, -hemia	166
blood clot	thromb/o	167
blue	cyan/o-	20
body	somat/o	34
body (small)	some	35
bone	oste/o	462
bone marrow	myel/o	167
brain	encephal/o	390
breaking	clasis, clasia	69
breast	mamm/o, mast/o	308
breathing	-pnea, spir/o	196, 198
bronchiole	bronchiol	197
bronchus	bronch/i, bronch/o	197
bursa	burs/o	461
bursting forth	-rhage, -rhagia	69
calcium	calc/i	168
calculus	lith	66
calyx	cali, calic	265
cancer	carcin/o	66
carbon dioxide	-capnia	196
carcinoma	carcin/o	66
cartilage	chondr/o	462
cavity	ventricul/o	129
cecum	cec/o	230
cell	-cyte, cyt/o	34
cerebellum	cerebell/o	387, 390
cerebral cortex	cortic/o	387, 390
cerebrum	cerebr/o	387, 390
cervix	cervic/o	49, 306
chain (twisted)	strept/o	71
cheek	bucc/o	229
chemical	chem/o	108
chest	thorac/o, steth/o	49
child	ped/o	345
choroid	chori/o, choroid/o	433
ciliary body	cycl/o	433
ciliary muscle	cycl/o	433
clitoris	clitor/o, clitorid/o	308
clot	thromb/o	167
coccyx	coccy, coccyg/o	463
cochlea	cochle/o	425
cold	cry/o	86
colon	col/o, colon/o	231
color	chrom/o, chromat/o	86
colorless	leuk/o-	20, 167
common bile duct	choledoch/o	233
condition of	-ia, -ia/sis, -ism, -o/sis, -sis, -y	10
condition of blood	-emià, -hemia	166
constriction	stenosis	70
contraction (sudden)	spasm	70
cornea	corne/o, kerat/o	433
correct	ortho-	23

Meaning	Word Part(s)	Reference
cramp	spasm	70
cranium	crani/o	463
crushing	-tripsy	88
cutting	-tomy	88
cutting instrument	-tome	88
cyst	cyst/o, cyst/i	66, 266
dark	melan/o-	20, 517
darkness	nyct/o	90
data	-gram	87
death of tissue	necrosis	70
decreased, decrease in	hypo-, -penia	22, 166
deficiency of	oligo-, -penia	22, 166
destruction	lysis	70
destroying	-lytic	108
development	plas, -plasia	35
diaphragm	phren/o	198
different	hetero-	23
difficult	dys-	68
dilatation, dilation	ectasia, ectasis	70
dim	ambly-	438
discharge	-rhea	69
disease	path/o, -pathy	67, 69
dissolving	lysis	70
double	dipl/o-	19
down	de-	21
dropping, downward displacement	ptosis	70
drug	pharmac/o	109
dry	xero-	68
duct	vas/o	108, 130, 293
duodenum	duoden/o	230
ear	ot/o	425
easy	eu-	23
eat	phag/o	34
egg	oo, ov/o	305
electricity	electr/o	86
embryo	embry/o	336
embryonic cell	-blast, blast/o	34
end	tel/e, tel/o, acro	25
endocrine	endocrin/o	361
enlargement	-megaly	69
enzyme	-ase	36
epididymis	epididym/o	293
epinephrine	adren/o	362
equal	iso-	23
esophagus	esophag/o	230
eustachian (auditory) tube	salping/o	306, 425
examination of	-scopy	87
excess	hyper-, super-	22
excision	-ectomy	88
excited state	mania	392

Meaning	Word Part(s)	Reference
expansion	dilation, dilatation, ectasia, ectasis	70
extremity	acro	52
eye	ocul/o, ophthalm/o, opt/o, -opia	433
eyelid	blephar/o, palpebr/o	432
false	pseudo-	23
fascia	fasci/o	494
fat	adip/o, lip/o	37
fatty	steat/o	37
fear	phobia	392
feeding	troph/o, -trophy, -trophia	35
fetus	fet/o	336
fetus (malformed)	terat/o	336
fever	pyr/o, pyret/o	67, 108
few	oligo-	22
fiber	fibr/o, in/o	34
filled sac or pouch	cyst/o, cyst/i	66, 266
finger	dactyl/o	52
fire	pyr/o, pyret/o	67, 102
first	prim/i-	19
fissure	-schisis	69
fixation (surgical)	-pexy	88
flow	-rhea	69
fluid	hydr/o	36
foot	ped/o, pod/o	52
form	morph/o	34
formation	gen, genesis, plas, -plasia, -poiesis	35
four	quadr/i, tetra-	19
fungus	myc/o	71
fusion	-desis	88
gall	chol/e, chol/o	233
gallbladder	cholecyst/o	233
ganglion	gangli/o, ganglion/o	388
gas	aer/o, pneum/o, pneumon/o, pneumat/o	86, 198
gland	aden/o	34
glomerulus	glomerul/o	265
glucose	gluc/o, glyc/o	37
good	eu-	23
grapelike cluster	staphyl/o	71
growth	troph/o, -trophy, -trophia	35
gums	gingiv/o	229
hair	trich/o	517
half	hemi-, semi-	19
hand	cheir/o, chir/o	49
hard	scler/o	67, 433
hardening	sclerosis	67
head	cephal/o	49
hearing	acous, acus, audi/o, cus	425

Meaning	Word Part(s)	Reference
heart	cardi/o	129
heat	therm/o	86
hemorrhage	-rhage, -rhagia	69
hernia	-cele	68
hidden	crypt/o	295
horny layer of skin	kerat/o	433, 517
hypophysis	hypophys, pituitar	361
islets (pancreatic)	insul/o	362
ileum	ile/o	230
ilium	ili/o	463
immature cell	blast	34
immunity	immun/o	167
in	end/o-, intra-	25
in front of	pre-, pro-	24
incision of	-tomy	88
incomplete	atel/o-	201
increased	hyper-	22
inflammation	-itis	69
ingest	phag/o	34
instrument for incising (cutting)	-tome	88
instrument for measuring	-meter	87
instrument for recording data	-graph	87
instrument for viewing or examining	-scope	87
intestine	enter/o	230
iris	ir, irid/o, irit/o	433
iron	ferr/i, ferr/o, sider/o	168
irregular	poikilo-	23
jaw	gnath/o	229
jejunum	jejun/o	230
joint	arthr/o	462
keratin	kerat/o	433, 517
kidney	nephr/o, ren/o	265
labor	toc/o	336
labyrinth	labyrinth/o	425
lack of	a-, an-	21
lacrimal apparatus	dacry/o, lacrim/o	432
lacrimal sac	dacryocyst/o	432
large	macro-, mega-, megalo-	23
larynx	laryng/o	197
left	sinistr/o-	25
lens	lent/i, phac/o, phak/o	433
leukocyte	leuk/o, leukocyt/o	20, 167
level of carbon dioxide	-capnia	196
level of oxygen	-oxia	196
light	phot/o	86
like	-form, -oid	11
lip	cheil/o, labi/o	229
lipid	lip/o	37
liver	hepat/o	233
localized dilation	-cele	68
loosening	lysis	70
loss	de-	21
lumbar region, lower back	lumb/o	49
lung, lungs	pneum/o, pneumat/o, pneumon/o, pulm/o, pulmon/o	198
lymph, lymphatic system	lymph/o	132, 167
lymphocyte	lymph/o, lymphocyt/o	167
lymph node	lymphaden/o	132
lymphatic vessel	lymphangi/o	132
lysing	-lytic	103
male	andr/o	292
malformed fetus	terat/o	336
mammary gland	mamm/o, mast/o	308
many	multi-, poly-	19
marrow	myel/o	167, 389
measure	metr/o	435
measuring instrument	-meter	87
measurement of	metry	87
medical specialty	-iatrics, iatry	12
medulla oblongata	medull/o	390
melanin	melan/o	20, 517
meninges	mening/o, meninge/o	389
menstruation	men/o, mens	305
middle	meso-	25
milk	galact/o, lact/o	336
mimicking	-mimetic	108
mind	psych/o	390
mold	myc/o	71
molding	plas, -plasia	35
month	men/o, mens	305
mouth	or/o, stoma, stomat/o	229
movement	kine, kinesi/o, kinet/o	494
much	poly-	19
mucus	muc/o, myx/o	34
mucous membrane	muc/o	34
muscle	my/o, muscul/o	494
muscle fiber	in/o	494
nail	onych/o	517
narrowing	stenosis	70
near	ad-, juxta-, para-	22
neck	cervic/o	49, 306

Meaning	Word Part(s)	Reference
nerve, nervous system	neur/o, neur/i	388
network	reticul/o	34
neuroglia	gli/o	388
new	neo-	23
night	noct/i, nyct/o	90
nipple	papill/o	34
nitrogen compound	azot/o	168
normal	eu-, normo-	23
nose	nas/o, rhin/o	197
not	a-, an-, in-, im-, un-	21
nourishment	troph/o, -trophy, -trophia	35
nucleus	kary/o	34
obsession	mania	392
old	presby-	438
one	mon/o-, uni-	19
one side	hemi-	19
opening (created surgically)	-stomy	88
origin	gen, genesis	35
other	hetero-	23
out, outside	ec-, ecto-, ex/o, extra-	25
outer portion	cortic/o	390
ovary	ovari/o, oophor/o	305
over	hyper-, epi-	22
oviduct	salping/o	306, 425
ovum	oo, ov/o	305
oxygen	ox/y, -oxia	169
pain	-algia, -odynia	68
pain	-algesia, algi/o, algesi/o	108
painful	dys-	68
palate	palat/o	229
pancreas	pancreat/o	233
pancreatic islets	insul/o	362
paralysis	-plegia	391
paralysis (partial)	paresis	392
parathyroid	parathyr/o, parathyroid/o	362
partial	semi-	19
partial paralysis	paresis	392
pelvis	pelvi/o	463
perineum	perine/o	308
peritoneum	periton, peritone/o	49
perspiration	hidr/o, idr/o	517
pertaining to	-ac, -al, -ar, -ary, -ial, -ic, -ical, -ile, -ous	11
pharynx	pharyng/o	197
pituitary	pituitar, hypophys	361
plastic repair, plastic surgery	-plasty	88
platelet	thrombocyt/o	167
pleura	pleur/o	198
poison	tox/o, toxic/o	67, 108

Meaning	Word Part(s)	Reference
poor	mal-	68
potassium	kali	169
pouch (filled)	cyst/o, cyst/i	66, 266
pregnant woman	gravida	336
pressure	bar/o	86
production	-poiesis	166
productive cell	blast	34
profuse flow	-rhage, -rhagia	69
prolapse	ptosis	70
prostate	prostat/o	293
protein	prote/o	37
puncture	centesis	88
pupil	pupill/o	433
pus	py/o	67
pylorus	pylor/o	230
radiation	radi/o	86
rapid	tachy-	68
reading	-lexia	391
reconstruction	-plasty	88
record of data	-gram	87
recording data (act of)	-graphy	87
rectum	rect/o, proct/o	231
red	erythr/o-	20
red blood cell	erythr/o, erythrocyt/o	20, 161
removal	de-, dis-	21
removal (surgical)	-ectomy	88
renal pelvis	pyel/o	265
repair (plastic)	-plasty	88
repair (surgical)	-rhaphy	88
respiration	pneum/o, pneumon/o, pneumat/o	198
resembling	-form, -oid	11
retina	retin/o	433
rib	cost/o	463
right	dextr/o-	25
root of spinal nerve	radicul/o	389
rupture	-rhexis	69
sac (filled)	cyst/o, cyst/i	66
sacrum	sacr/o	463
saliva, salivary gland, salivary duct	sial/o	229
same	homo-, homeo-, iso-	23
sclera (of eye)	scler/o	67, 433
scanty	oligo-	22
scrotum	osche/o	293
sebum, sebaceous gland	seb/o	517
seizure	-lepsy	391
self	auto-	173
semen	semin, sperm/i, spermat/o	293

Meaning	Word Part(s)	Reference
seminal vesicle	vesicul/o	293
sensation	-esthesia, esthesi/o	422
sense of smell	-osmia	422
sense of taste	-geusia	422
separation	dis-, -lysis	21
sharp	ox/y	169
sheath	vagin/o	306
sigmoid colon	sigmoid/o	231
simulating	-mimetic	108
skin	derm/o, dermat/o	516
skull	crani/o	463
sleep	somn/o, somn/i, hypn/o	390
slow	brady-	67
small	micro-	23
small body	some	35
smell (sense of)	-osmia	422
sodium	natri	169
softening	malacia	70
sound	phon/o, son/o, acous, acus, cus	425
specialist	-ian, -ist, -logist	12
specialty	-iatrics, -iatry	12
speech	-phasia, -lalia	391
sperm, spermatozoa	sperm/i, spermat/o	293
spinal column	vertebr/o	463
spinal cord	myel/o	389, 462
spine	rachi/o	389, 463
spitting	ptysis	201
spleen	splen/o	132
splitting	-schisis	69
stain	chrom/o, chromat/o	86
stapes	staped/o, stapedi/o	425
staphylococcus	staphyl/o	71
starch	amyl/o	21
stomach	gastr/o	230
stone	lith	66
stoppage	stasis	70
straight	ortho-	23
streptococcus	strept/o	71
structure	morph/o	34
study of	-logy	12
stupor	narc/o	108
sugar	glyc/o, -ose	37
sudden contraction	spasm	70
suppression	stasis	70
surgery (plastic)	-plasty	88
surgical creation of an opening	-stomy	88
surgical fixation	-pexy	88
surgical removal	-ectomy	88
surgical repair	-rhaphy	88
suture	-rhaphy	88
sweat	hidr/o, idr/o	88
swelling	edema	70

Meaning	Word Part(s)	Reference
synovial joint, synovial membrane	synov/i	462
tap	centesis	88
taste (sense of)	-geusia	422
tear	dacry/o, lacrim/o	432
teeth	dent/o, denti, odont/o	229
temperature	therm/o	86
tendon	ten/o, tendin/o	494
testis	test/o, orchid/o, orchi/o	293
thalamus	thalam/o	390
thick	pachy-	68
thorax	thorac/o	49
three	tri-	19
thrombocyte	thrombocyt/o	167
through	dia-, per-, trans-	21
thymus gland	thym/o	132
thyroid	thyr/o, thyroid/o	362
time	chron/o	86
tissue	hist/o, histi/o	34
tissue death	necrosis	70
toe	dactyl/o	52
together	syn-, sym-	25
tone	ton/o	494
tongue	gloss/o, lingu/o	229
tonsil	tonsill/o	132
tooth	dent/o, dent/i, odont/o	229
toward	ad-	22
toxin	tox/o, toxic/o	67, 108
trachea	trache/o	197
true	eu-	23
tube	salping/o	306, 425
tumor	onc/o, -oma	67
twice	bi-, di-	19
twisted and swollen vein	varic/o	137
two	bi-, di-, dipl/o-	19
tympanic cavity	tympan/o	425
tympanic membrane	myring/o, tympan/o	425
ultrasound	son/o	86
unchanging	homo-, homeo-	23
unconsciousness	narc/o	108, 390
under	hypo-, sub-	22
unequal	hetero-	23
upon	epi-	54
upright	ortho-	23
ureter	ureter/o	306
urethra	urethr/o	266
urinary bladder	cyst/o, vesic/o	66, 266
urine, urinary tract, urination	ur/o, -uria	266
uterus	hyster/o, metr/o, metr/i, uter/o	306

Meaning	Word Part(s)	Reference
uvea	uve/o	433
vagina	colp/o, vagin/o	306
valve	valv/o, valvul/o	129
varied	poikilo-	23
vas deferens	vas/o	293
vein	ven/o, ven/i, phleb/o	131
vein (twisted, swollen)	varic/o	137
ventricle	ventricul/o	129, 390
vertebra	spondyl/o, vertebr/o	463
vessel	angi/o, vas/o, vascul/o	130
vestibular apparatus, vestibule	vestibul/o	425
virus	vir/o	72
vision	opt/o, -opia, -opsia	433
voice	phon/o, -phonia	86
vomiting	emesis	239
vulva	episi/o, vulv/o	308
water	hydr/o	36
white	leuk/o-	20
white blood cell	leuk/o, leukocyt/o	20, 167
widening	ectasia, ectasis, dilation, dilatation	70
within	end/o-, intra-	25
without	a-, an-, de-	21
woman	gyn/o, gynec/o	305
woman who has given birth	para	336
work	erg/o	86
x-ray	radi/o	86
yellow	xanth/o-	20

Suggested Readings

Books

Andreoli TE (ed): Cecil Essentials of Medicine, 4th ed. San Diego, CA, Harcourt Brace, 1997

Biblis M (ed): Dorland's Medical Abbreviations, Philadelphia, WB Saunders, 1992

Burton GG, Hodgkin JE (eds): Respiratory Care: A Guide to Clinical Practice, 4th ed. Philadelphia, Lippincott-Raven, 1997

Burton GR, Engelkirk PG: Microbiology for the Health Sciences, 5th ed. Philadelphia, Lippincott-Raven, 1996

Cormack DH: Essential Histology, Philadelphia, Lippincott-Raven, 1993

Crouch JE: Functional Human Anatomy, 4th ed. Baltimore, Williams and Wilkins, 1985

Deglin JH, Vallerand, AH (eds): Davis's Drug Guide for Nurses, 3rd ed. Philadelphia, FA Davis, 1996

DeSousa LR et al: Medical Abbreviations, Albany, NY, Delmar, 1995

Dorland's Illustrated Medical Dictionary, 28th ed. Philadelphia, WB Saunders, 1994

Fischbach F: A Manual of Laboratory and Diagnostic Tests, 5th ed. Philadelphia, Lippincott-Raven, 1996

Guyton AC: Textbook of Medical Physiology, 9th ed. Philadelphia, WB Saunders, 1995

Isselbacher KJ et al (eds): Harrison's Principles of Internal Medicine, 13th ed. New York, McGraw Hill, 1994

Magalini SI: Dictionary of Medical Syndromes, 3rd ed. Philadelphia, JB Lippincott, 1990

Martini F: Fundamentals of Anatomy and Physiology, 3rd ed. Englewood Cliffs, NJ, Prentice-Hall, 1995

McDonough JT (ed): Stedman's Concise Medical Dictionary, 2nd ed. Baltimore, Williams and Wilkins, 1994

Memmler RL, Cohen BJ, Wood DL: The Human Body in Health and Disease, 8th ed. Philadelphia, Lippincott-Raven, 1996

Physicians' Desk Reference (PDR). Oradell NJ, Medical Economics Books, Published yearly

Porth CM: Pathophysiology, 4th ed. Philadelphia, Lippincott-Raven, 1994

Rakel RE (ed): Conn's Current Therapy. Philadelphia, WB Saunders, 1998

Rubin E, Farber JL: Essential Pathology, 2nd ed. Philadelphia, Lippincott-Raven, 1995

Scherer JC, Roach SS: Introductory Clinical Pharmacology, 5th ed. Philadelphia, Lippincott-Raven, 1995

Sheldon H: Boyd's Introduction to the Study of Disease, 11th ed. Baltimore, Williams and Wilkins, 1992

Sloane SB: Medical Abbreviations and Eponyms, 2nd ed. Philadelphia, WB Saunders, 1996

Taylor C, Lillis C, LeMone C: Fundamentals of Nursing, 3rd ed. Philadelphia, Lippincott-Raven, 1997

Thomas CL (ed): Taber's Cyclopedic Medical Dictionary, 17th ed. Philadelphia, FA Davis, 1993

Tortora GJ, Grabowski SR: Principles of Anatomy and Physiology, 8th ed. New York, Harper Collins, 1996

VanDeGraaf KM, Fox SI: Concepts of Human Anatomy and Physiology, 4th ed. Dubuque, Wm C Brown, 1995

Volk WA et al: Essentials of Medical Microbiology, 5th ed. Philadelphia, Lippincott-Raven, 1995

Periodicals

American Journal of Nursing. New York, American Journal of Nursing Co.

JAMA. Chicago, American Medical Association

Medical World News. New York, Medical Tribune Inc.

New England Journal of Medicine. Boston, Massachusetts Medical Society

Nursing. Springhouse, PA, Springhouse Corp.

Patient Care. Montvale, NJ, Medical Economics Publishing

The Professional Medical Assistant, Chicago, American Association of Medical Assistants

Respiratory Care. Daedalus Enterprises, Dallas

Respiratory Management. Santa Monica, Macmillan Professional Journals

RN. Montvale, NJ, Medical Economics Publishing

The Surgical Technologist. Englewood, CO, Association of Surgical Technologists

Index

Note: Page numbers followed by f indicate figures; those followed by t indicate tables.

Flashcards

An excellent way to learn this new vocabulary is by means of flashcards. These have proved so successful that a section of flashcards has been included. They are presented in chapter order so that they can be removed in sequence as you progress through the book. Of course, these cards represent only a portion of the necessary vocabulary, and you should add to the collection with cards of your own. Blank cards are included for this purpose. Note also that the flashcards are exactly the size of one half of a 3″ × 5″ index card. You can make additional cards by cutting index cards in half.

word part

-ia, -ia/sis, -ism, -o/sis, -sis, -y

word part

-ac, -al, -ary, -ic, -ile, -ous

word part

a-, an-

word part

ante-, pre-, pro-

word part

anti-, contra-

word part

dia-, per-, trans-

word part

ecto-, ex/o-, extra-

word part

endo-, intra-

meaning **pertaining to**	*meaning* **condition of**
meaning **before**	*meaning* **not, without, lack of**
meaning **through**	*meaning* **against**
meaning **in, within**	*meaning* **out, outside**

word part

erythr/o

word part

hyper-

word part

hypo-

word part

leuk/o

word part

macro-, mega-, megal/o-, -megaly

word part

post-

word part

blast/o

word part

-cyte, cyt/o

meaning

over, excess, increased, abnormally high

meaning

red, red blood cell

meaning

white, colorless, white blood cell

meaning

under, below, decreased, abnormally low

meaning

after, behind

meaning

large, abnormally large, enlargement

meaning

cell

meaning

immature cell, productive cell

word part

gen, genesis

word part

hist/o, histi/o

word part

brachi/o

word part

cephal/o

word part

cervic/o

word part

circum-, peri-

word part

juxta-, para-

word part

lapar/o

meaning

tissue

meaning

origin, formation

meaning

head

meaning

arm

meaning

around

meaning

neck, cervix

meaning

abdominal wall

meaning

near, beside

word part

thorac/o

word part

-algia, -algesia, -odynia, algi/o, algesi/o

word part

brady-

word part

-cele

word part

dys-

word part

ectasia, ectasis

word part

-itis

word part

lysis

meaning

pain

meaning

chest

meaning

hernia, localized dilation

meaning

slow

meaning

dilation, widening

meaning

abnormal, painful, difficult

meaning

separation, loosening, dissolving, destruction

meaning

inflammation

word part

lith

word part

mal-

word part

malacia

word part

-oma, onc/o

word part

path/o, -pathy

word part

ptosis

word part

-rhage, -rhagia

word part

-rhea

meaning

bad, poor

meaning

calculus, stone

meaning

tumor

meaning

softening

meaning

dropping, downward displacement

meaning

disease

meaning

flow, discharge

meaning

bursting forth

word part

-rhexis

word part

scler/o

word part

tachy-

word part

chrom/o, chromat/o

word part

-ectomy

word part

-gram

word part

-graph

word part

-graphy

meaning

hard, sclera of eye

meaning

rupture

meaning

color, stain

meaning

rapid

meaning

record of data

meaning

excision, surgical removal

meaning

act of recording data

meaning

instrument for recording data

word part

-pexy

word part

-plasty

word part

-rhaphy

word part

-stomy

word part

-tomy

word part

angi/o, vas/o, vascul/o

word part

cardi/o

word part

phleb/o, ven/i, ven/o

meaning

plastic repair

meaning

surgical fixation

meaning

surgical creation of an opening

meaning

surgical repair, suture

meaning

vessel, duct

meaning

incision, cutting

meaning

vein

meaning

heart

word part

-emia, -hemia, hem/o, hemat/o

word part

myel/o

word part

-penia

word part

pneum/o, pneumon/o, pulm/o, pulmon/o

word part

chol/e, chol/o

word part

gastr/o

word part

hepat/o

word part

cyst/o, vesic/o

meaning

bone marrow, spinal cord

meaning

blood

meaning

lung, lungs

meaning

decrease in, deficiency of

meaning

stomach

meaning

bile, gall

meaning

urinary bladder

meaning

liver

word part

nephr/o, ren/o

word part

gyn/o, gynec/o

word part

hyster/o, metr/o

word part

cortic/o

word part

medull/o

word part

neur/o

word part

ocul/o, ophthalm/o, -opt/o, -opia, -opsia

word part

arthr/o

meaning

woman

meaning

kidney

meaning

outer portion, cortex

meaning

uterus

meaning

nerve, nervous system

meaning

inner part, medulla oblongata

meaning

joint

meaning

eye, vision

word part

chondr/o

word part

cost/o

word part

crani/o

word part

oste/o

word part

kine, kinesi/o, kinet/o

word part

my/o

word part

derm/o, dermat/o

word part

hidr/o, idr/o

meaning **rib**	*meaning* **cartilage**
meaning **bone**	*meaning* **skull**
meaning **muscle**	*meaning* **movement**
meaning **sweat, perspiration**	*meaning* **skin**